Fluid and Electrolyte Balance

NURSING CONSIDERATIONS

Fluid and Electrolyte Balance

NURSING CONSIDERATIONS

FOURTH EDITION

Norma M. Metheny, PhD, RN, FAAN
Professor and Dorothy A. Votsmier Endowed Chair in Nursing
St. Louis University School of Nursing
St. Louis, Missouri

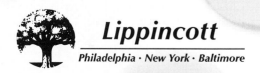

Lippincott
Philadelphia · New York · Baltimore

Acquisitions Editor: Lisa Stead
Assistant Editor: Claudia Vaughn
Senior Project Editor: Sandra Cherrey Scheinin
Senior Production Manager: Helen Ewan
Production Coordinator: Patricia McCloskey
Design Coordinator: Art Director: Carolyn O'Brien
Cover Designer: Jen Marmarinos
Indexer: Lynne Mahan

4th Edition

9 8 7 6 5 4 3 2 1

Library of Congress Cataloging-in-Publication Data
Fluid and electrolyte balance : nursing considerations / [edited by] Norma M. Metheny.—
4th ed.
        p. cm.
     Includes bibliographical references and index.
     ISBN 0-7817-2072-9 (alk. paper)
       1. Body fluid disorders. 2. Body fluid disorders—Nursing. 3. Water-electrolyte
imbalances. 4. Water-electrolyte imbalances—Nursing.   I. Metheny, Norma Milligan.
       [DNLM: 1. Water-Electrolyte Balance—Nurses' Instruction. 2. Water-Electrolyte
Imbalance—Nurses' Instruction. WD 220 F646 2000]
     RC630 .F556 2000
     616.3'992—dc21   99-042877

Care has been taken to confirm the accuracy of the information presented and to describe generally accepted practices. However, the authors, editors, and publisher are not responsible for errors or omissions or for any consequences from application of the information in this book and make no warranty, express or implied, with respect to the contents of the publication.

The authors, editors and publisher have exerted every effort to ensure that drug selection and dosage set forth in this text are in accordance with current recommendations and practice at the time of publication. However, in view of ongoing research, changes in government regulations, and the constant flow of information relating to drug therapy and drug reactions, the reader is urged to check the package insert for each drug for any change in indications and dosage and for added warnings and precautions. This is particularly important when the recommended agent is a new or infrequently employed drug.

Some drugs and medical devices presented in this publication have Food and Drug Administration (FDA) clearance for limited use in restricted research settings. It is the responsibility of the health care provider to ascertain the FDA status of each drug or device planned for use in their clinical practice.

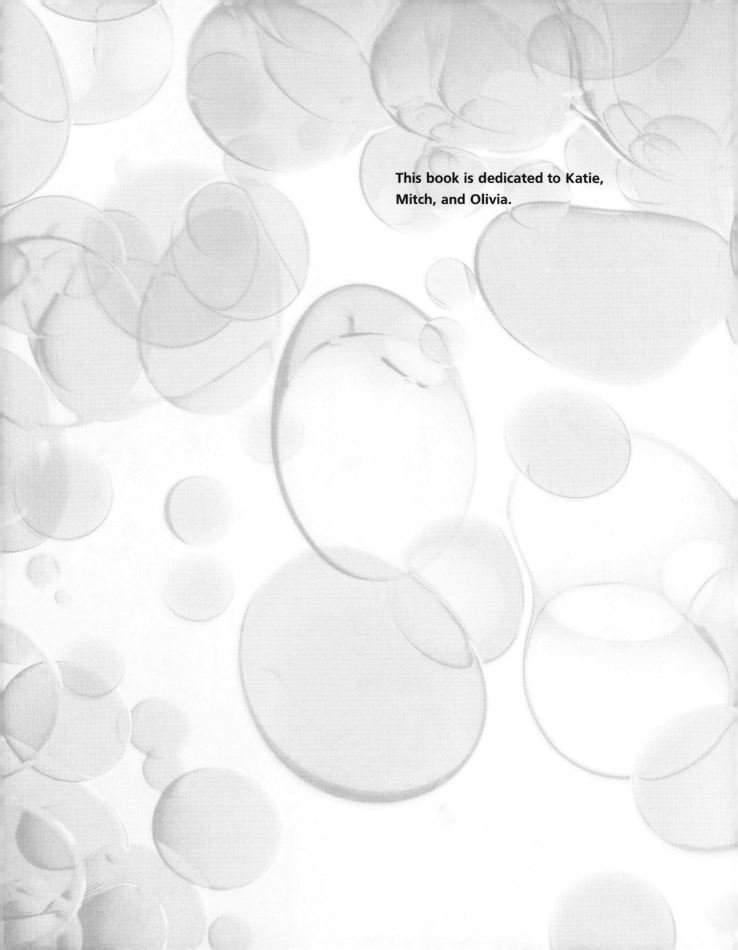

This book is dedicated to Katie, Mitch, and Olivia.

Contributors

Joan Clark, RN, MSN(R), CS, ANP
Clinical Instructor
St. Louis University School of Nursing
Nurse Practitioner
St. Louis Hematology/Oncology Specialists
St. Louis, Missouri

Mary Ellen Grohar-Murray, RN, PhD
Associate Professor of Nursing
St. Louis University
St. Louis, Missouri

J. Keith Hampton, RN, CS, MSN,
Epogen Account Executive
Amgen Incorporated
Warrenton, Missouri

Dorothy C. James, RN, PhD
Assistant Professor
Perinatal Nursing
St. Louis University School of Nursing
St. Louis, Missouri

Mary Kay Macheca, RN, MSN(R), ANP, CDE
Certified Adult Nurse Practitioner/
Certified Diabetes Educator
The Bortz Diabetes Control Center
Richmond Heights, Missouri

Sherry Beth Robinson, RNCS, PhD
Assistant Professor
Division of Geriatrics
Southern Illinois University School of Medicine
Springfield, Illinois

Patsy L. Ruchala, RN, DNSc
Director, Master's Programs in Nursing
Coordinator, Perinatal Master's Specialty
St. Louis University School of Nursing
St. Louis, Missouri

Marilyn Schallom, RN, MSN, CCRN, CS
Surgical Critical Care Certified Nurse Specialist
Barnes-Jewish Hospital
St. Louis, Missouri

Diedre M. Schweiss, MSN, RN, CPNP
Assistant Professor of Nursing
St Louis University
St. Louis, Missouri

Recognition of Former Contributors

Charold L. Baer, PhD, RN, FCCM, CCRN
Professor
Oregon Health Sciences University
School of Nursing
Portland, Oregon

Donna C. Casperson, RN, MSN, OCN
Oncology Clinical Nurse Specialist
St. Louis, Missouri

Susan Cole, RN, MSN, CCRN
Clinical Nurse Specialist
St. Francis Hospital
Cape Girardeau, Missouri

Marilyn Hackenthal, RN, MSN
Former Professor of Nursing
Lewis and Clark Community College
Alton, Illinois

Kathryn Neunaber, RN, BSN, CCRN, CEN
Surgical/Trauma Intensive Care Unit
St. Louis University Health Sciences Center
St. Louis, Missouri

Catherine C. Powers, MSN(R), RN, CCRN
Former Cardiovascular Clinical Nurse Specialist
Barnes Hospital at Washington University
St. Louis, Missouri

Lisa Reed, RN, MSN(R)
Former Research Associate
St. Louis University Health Sciences Center
St. Louis, Missouri

Irene I. Riddle, PhD, RN
Professor and Director of Doctoral Program
  in Nursing
Saint Louis University School of Nursing
St. Louis, Missouri

Reviewers

Ruth LeBlanc, RN, CCRN
Professor, Critical Care Nursing Diploma Program
Continuing Education Department
St. Lawrence College
Kingston, Ohio

Jane V. McCloskey, RN, MSN
Faculty
School of Nursing
Carolinas College of Health Science
Charlotte, North Carolina

Mary B. Neiheisel, BSN, MSN, EdD, CSN, FNP-C
Lafayette General Medical Center LEQSF
  Regents' Professor
Professor of Nursing
Department of Graduate Nursing
College of Nursing
The University of Southwestern Louisiana
Lafayette, Louisiana

Preface

The fourth edition of *Fluid and Electrolyte Balance: Nursing Considerations* carries on in the tradition established by the prior editions of this textbook. It provides current and comprehensive information related to the nursing care of patients with fluid, electrolyte, and acid-base imbalances in a readable and user-friendly manner. Because concepts of fluid and electrolyte balance apply to a broad spectrum of patient problems, the book's scope is wide. While written simply, to promote ease of understanding for students, it contains enough information to stimulate the interests of advanced practitioners. The most current research findings related to conditions affecting fluid and electrolyte balance are integrated throughout the text. All chapters have been completely revised and updated with an increased emphasis on providing care to patients in long-term and ambulatory care settings.

ORGANIZATION

The basic organization remains unchanged. As in prior editions, the first three units present concepts fundamental to understanding the clinical chapters that follow. Unit I—Basic Concepts—includes a chapter on fundamental concepts and definitions, and a completely revised nursing assessment chapter. Unit II—An Overview of Fluid and Electrolyte Problems: Nursing Considerations—provides chapters on fluid volume imbalances, sodium imbalances, potassium imbalances, calcium imbalances, magnesium imbalances, phosphorus imbalances, and acid-base disturbances. Case studies are included to enhance understanding of specific imbalances. Unit III—Parenteral and Enteral Nutrition—has been completely revised and updated to reflect the latest developments in parenteral fluid administration as well as in parenteral and enteral nutrition. Unit IV—Clinical Situations Associated with Fluid and Electrolyte Problems—contains the bulk of the clinical chapters. Included are chapters on gastrointestinal problems, fluid balance in surgical

patients, hypovolemic shock in trauma and postoperative patients, heart failure, renal failure, diabetic ketoacidosis and hyperosmolar syndrome, fluid balance in the brain-injured patient, acute pancreatitis, cirrhosis with ascites, oncologic conditions, and pregnancy. The final unit (Unit V)—Special Considerations in Children and the Elderly—offers a concise explanation of special fluid and electrolyte problems in the very young and the very old.

The book retains its strong nursing focus to help facilitate integration of the information into nursing practice. In all chapters, pathophysiology is discussed to promote an understanding of rationales for nursing interventions. Assessment of fluid and electrolyte balance, based on an understanding of pathophysiology, is integrated throughout the textbook. Because monitoring for the occurrence or worsening of imbalances is an integral part of the nurse's role, patients at risk for specific imbalances are identified throughout the text, as are the common indicators of these problems. Examples of nursing diagnoses related to fluid and electrolyte problems are presented when appropriate, followed by a description of nursing interventions. By their nature, these interventions often involve manipulation of fluid and nutrient intake; therefore, the electrolyte content of common beverages and foods is included as appropriate.

NEW TO THIS EDITION

Each chapter has been completely reviewed, revised, and updated to reflect the latest developments in the study of fluid and electrolyte balance. Extensive reference lists are provided to allow the reader to pursue particular areas of interest. These references include the most recent nursing and medical research related to fluid and electrolyte balance, as well as classic work that provides the foundation for current practice.

The book is formatted to promote easy access to material. Clinical tips are highlighted for easy identification when information is needed in a hurry. Numerous case studies have been added with an eye toward supporting critical concepts with immediate clinical relevance.

Information to help nurses provide care for home patients with fluid and electrolyte problems has been integrated throughout the text. For example, sick day rules for diabetic patients have been updated, and information related to the safe use of laxatives and enemas has been included to allow nurses to prevent fluid and electrolyte imbalances through education of home patients and their families.

I wish to acknowledge the skilled master clinicians who have thoroughly revised their chapters to reflect current practice, and also the contributors to prior editions. Because of these individuals' high level of expertise, the information presented in their clinical chapters is pragmatic and ready for application to practice.

Fluid and Electrolyte Balance: Nursing Considerations, fourth edition, was written with the intent of fostering critical thinking in those providing care to patients with potential or actual fluid and electrolyte disturbances. Designed for students and practicing nurses, it provides the necessary information to deliver safe, effective, scientifically based nursing care.

Norma M. Metheny, PhD, RN, FAAN

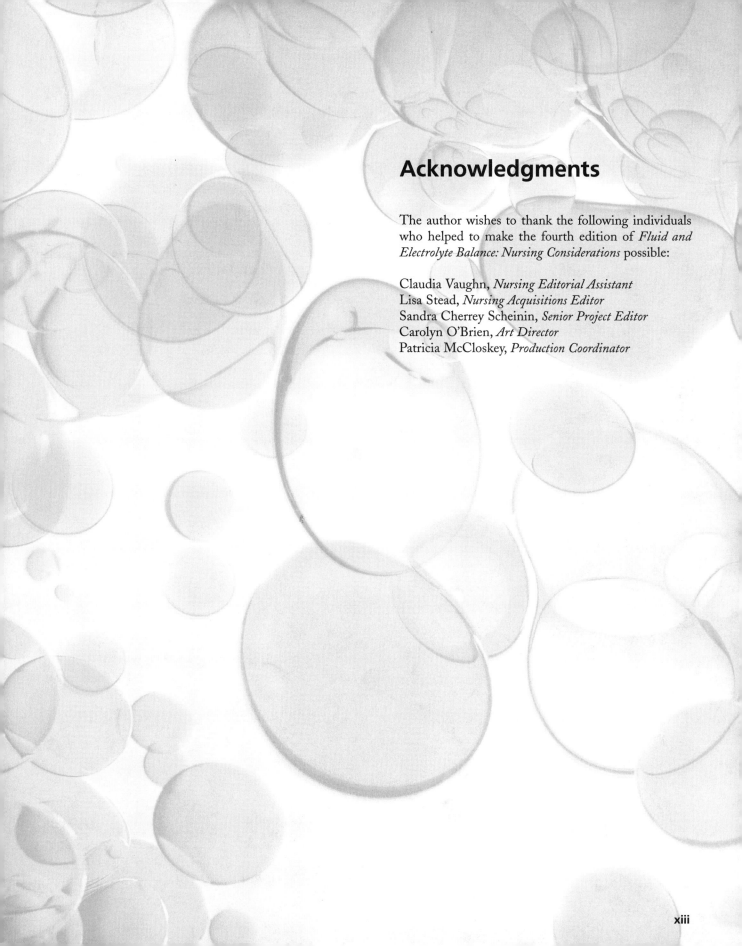

Acknowledgments

The author wishes to thank the following individuals who helped to make the fourth edition of *Fluid and Electrolyte Balance: Nursing Considerations* possible:

Claudia Vaughn, *Nursing Editorial Assistant*
Lisa Stead, *Nursing Acquisitions Editor*
Sandra Cherrey Scheinin, *Senior Project Editor*
Carolyn O'Brien, *Art Director*
Patricia McCloskey, *Production Coordinator*

Contents

Basic Concepts

CHAPTER 1

Fundamental Concepts and Definitions

DISTRIBUTION OF BODY FLUIDS AND ELECTROLYTES

In the typical adult man, about 60% of body weight consists of *fluid* (water and electrolytes); in the typical adult woman, the percentage is lower (about 50% of body weight).[1] This fluid is either *intracellular* (within the cells) or *extracellular* (outside the cells). Extracellular fluid (ECF) is further subdivided into *intravascular fluid* (plasma) and *interstitial fluid* (fluid lying between the cells, or tissue fluid) (Fig. 1-1). Also part of the ECF are transcellular fluids, primarily representing secretions from epithelial cells and having ionic compositions different from the plasma and interstitial fluids. Examples of transcellular fluid include secretions in the salivary glands, pancreas, liver, and biliary tract, as well as fluid in the gastrointestinal (GI) and respiratory tracts, sweat gland ducts, cavities of the eyes, cerebrospinal fluid, and kidneys.[2] In adults, two-thirds of the body fluid exists in the intracellular space (primarily in the skeletal muscle mass). The remaining one-third is primarily found between the cells and in the plasma space. Microscopically, one might visualize the body fluids as in Figure 1-2. A normal man weighing 154 lb (70 kg) has about 30 liters of intracellular fluid, and 15 liters of extracellular fluid.[3]

Total body water content varies with body fat content, sex, and age. Fat cells contain little water, whereas lean tissue is rich in water. Thus, women have less body fluid than men because they have proportionately more body fat. The elderly have less body fluid than their younger counterparts for the same reason. Obese individuals, in general, have considerably less fluid than those of lean build (Fig. 1-3).

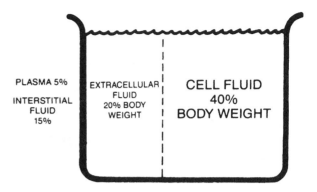

FIGURE 1-1.   Total body fluid, 60% body weight.

Infants have a high body fluid content (about 70% of their body weight). In addition to having proportionately more body fluid than adults, infants have relatively more ECF. Indeed, more than half of the newborn's body fluid is extracellular, whereas in the adult only a third or less is extracellular. Because ECF is more readily lost from the body than is cellular fluid, infants are more vulnerable to fluid volume deficit. As infants become older, their total body fluid percentage decreases; the change is most rapid during the first 6 months of life. By the end of the second year, the total body fluid approaches the adult percentage of about 60% (36% cellular and 24% extracellular). At puberty, the adult body composition is attained (40% cellular and 20% extracellular). For the first time there is a sex differentiation in fluid content (Table 1-1).

After 40 years of age, mean values for total body fluid in percentage of body weight decrease for both men and women; however, the sex differentiation remains. After 60 years of age, the percentage may decrease to about 52% in men and 46% in women (even

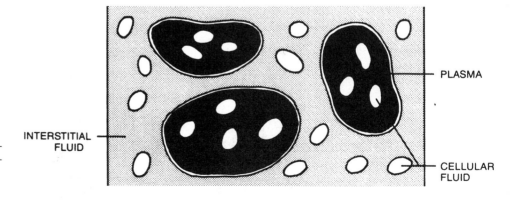

FIGURE 1-2.   Microscopic visualization of body fluid distribution.

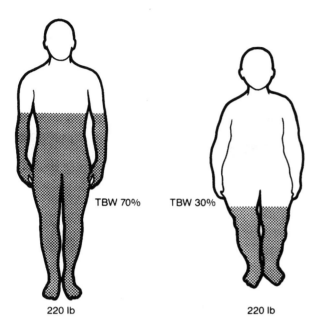

FIGURE 1-3. Body composition of a lean and an obese individual. TBW, total body weight (Adapted from Statland H. *Fluid & Electrolytes in Practice*, 3rd ed. Philadelphia: JB Lippincott; 1963; with permission.)

less in obese persons). Again, the reduction in body fluid is explained by the fact that with aging there is a decrease in lean body mass in favor of fat. Variations in total body fluid with age are listed in Table 1-1.

Body fluid is composed primarily of water and electrolytes. An *electrolyte* is defined as a substance that develops an electrical charge when dissolved in water. Examples of electrolytes are sodium, potassium, calcium, chloride, and bicarbonate. Those that develop a positive charge in water are called *cations*, for example, sodium (Na^+, potassium (K^+), calcium (Ca^{++}), and magnesium (Mg^{++}). Electrolytes that develop negative charges when dissolved in water are called *anions*, for example, chloride (Cl^-) and bicarbonate (HCO_3^-). In all body fluids, anions and cations are always present in equal amounts because positive and negative charges must be equal. In fact, *all* solutions (whether biological or nonbiological) are electrically neutral; this condition of electroneutrality is sometimes called the law of electroneutrality.[4]

The bulk of body fluid is located within the body's intracellular fluid (ICF); this fluid is contained within the body's more than 100 trillion cells.[5] The electrolyte content of ICF differs significantly from that of ECF. Table 1-2 lists the electrolytes in plasma (ECF) and Table 1-3 lists those in ICF. Because special techniques are required to measure the concentration of electrolytes in the ICF, it is customary to measure the electrolytes in the ECF, namely plasma. Plasma electrolyte concentrations are used in assessing and managing patients with electrolyte imbalances. Some tests are performed on serum (the portion of plasma left after clotting); for practical purposes, the terms *serum electrolytes* and *plasma electrolytes* are used interchangeably.

● TABLE 1-1. Approximate Values of Total Body Fluid as a Percentage of Body Weight in Relation to Age and Sex

Age	Total Body Fluid (% Body Weight)
Full-term newborn	70–80%
1 year	64%
Puberty to 39 years	Men: 60%
	Women: 52%
40–60 years	Men: 55%
	Women: 47%
> 60 years	Men: 52%
	Women: 46%

● TABLE 1-2. Plasma Electrolytes

Electrolytes	mEq/L
Cations	
Sodium (Na^+)	142
Potassium (K^+)	5
Calcium (Ca^{++})	5
Magnesium (Mg^{++})	2
Total cations	154
Anions	
Chloride (Cl^-)	103
Bicarbonate (HCO_3^-)	26
Phosphate (HPO_4^{--})	2
Sulfate (SO_4^{--})	1
Organic acids	5
Proteinate	17
Total anions	154

TABLE 1-3. Approximation of Major Electrolyte Content in Intracellular Fluid

Electrolytes	mEq/L
Cations	
Potassium (K^+)	150
Magnesium (Mg^{++})	40
Sodium (Na^+)	10
Total cations	200
Anions	
Phosphates ⎫	
Sulfates ⎬	150
Bicarbonate (HCO_3^-)	10
Proteinate	40
Total anions	200

The major electrolytes in the ECF are sodium (Na^+) and chloride (Cl^-), with a great preponderance of sodium ions (142 mEq/L) compared with other cations. About 90% of the ECF osmolality (concentration) is determined by the sodium concentration. Sodium ions are restricted primarily to the ECF and are of primary importance in regulating body fluid volume.[6] Retention of sodium is associated with fluid retention; in contrast, whenever excessive quantities of sodium are lost, body fluid volume tends to decrease.

The electrolyte content of interstitial fluid is not measured in clinical situations; however, it is essentially the same as that of plasma, except that it contains less proteinate. Recall that plasma protein is necessary to maintain oncotic pressure and keep the intravascular fluid inside the blood vessels; the protein of plasma that is the principal determinant of colloid osmotic pressure is albumin.

The major electrolytes in the ICF are potassium and phosphate. Because the ECF can tolerate only small potassium concentrations (about 5 mEq/L), release of large stores of intracellular potassium through cellular trauma can be extremely dangerous.

The body expends a great deal of energy maintaining the extracellular preponderance of sodium and the intracellular preponderance of potassium. It does so by means of cell membrane pumps, which exchange sodium and potassium ions.

UNITS OF MEASURE FOR ELECTROLYTES

Concentrations of solutes can be expressed in several ways, for example, milligrams per deciliter (mg/dL), milliequivalents per liter (mEq/L), or millimoles per liter (mmol/L). Because all of these units may be used in clinical settings, a brief review of their meanings is appropriate. *Milligrams per 100 mL (deciliter)* expresses the weight of the solute per unit volume. In contrast, a milliequivalent is a measure of chemical activity. By definition, a *milliequivalent of an ion* is its atomic weight expressed in milligrams divided by the valence. This measure is most favored in the United States for expressing the small concentrations of electrolytes in body fluids because it emphasizes the principle that ions combine milliequivalent for milliequivalent, not millimole for millimole or milligram for milligram. Also, the important concept of *electroneutrality* is clarified when using milliequivalents because milliequivalents of cations and anions exist in equal numbers in the body fluids (Fig. 1-4). This obligatory relationship is not evident if the ionic concentrations are measured in millimoles per liter or in milligrams per deciliter. Because electrolytes in body fluids are active chemicals (anions and cations) that unite in varying combinations, it is considered more logical to express their concentration as a measure of chemical activity rather than as a measure of weight.

Countries using the Système Internationale (SI) units express electrolyte content in body fluids in millimoles. To understand millimoles, it is necessary to review the definition of a mole. One *mole* (mol) of a substance is defined as the molecular (or atomic) weight of that substance in grams. For example, a mole of sodium is equivalent to 23 g (the atomic weight of sodium is 23). A *millimole* is one-thousandth of a mole,

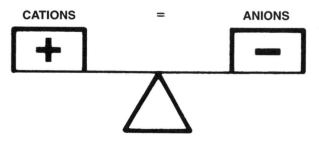

FIGURE 1-4. Number of cations equals number of anions.

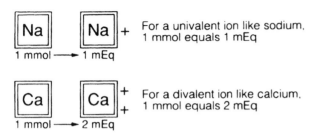

FIGURE 1-5. Millimoles versus milliequivalents for univalent and divalent ions.

or the molecular or atomic weight expressed in milligrams. Thus, a millimole of sodium is equivalent to 23 mg. Univalent elements, such as sodium (Na^+), chloride (Cl^-), and potassium (K^+), have identical numbers for milliequivalents and millimoles; that is, 140 mEq of Na^+ = 140 mmol of Na^+ and 5 mEq of K^+ = 5 mmol of K^+. However, different numbers are required for electrolytes that are not univalent. To convert from units of millimoles per liter to milliequivalents per liter, use the following formula:

$$mEq/L = mmol/L \times valence$$

For example, because the valence of calcium is 2, 1 mmol of calcium = 2 mEq of calcium.[7] (Fig. 1-5). Although the milliequivalent is not an SI unit, it is so widely used and conceptually useful that it is likely to be used for some time.

● FUNCTIONS OF BODY FLUIDS

Body fluids are in constant motion, maintaining healthy living conditions for body cells. The ECF interfaces with the outside world and is modified by it, but the ICF remains stable. Nutrients are transported by the ECF to the cells, and wastes are carried away from the cells by means of the capillary bed. About 10 billion capillaries with a total surface area close to the size of a football field provide this function for the entire body.[8]

Normal movement of fluids through the capillary wall into the tissues depends on two forces: *hydrostatic pressure* (exerted by pumping of the heart) and *oncotic pressure* (exerted by nondiffusible plasma proteins, primarily albumin). At the arterial end of the capillary, fluids are filtered through its wall by a hydrostatic pressure that exceeds the oncotic pressure exerted by plasma proteins. In contrast, because oncotic pressure is greater than hydrostatic pressure in the venous end of the capillary, fluids re-enter the capillary here (Fig. 1-6).

● REGULATION OF BODY FLUID COMPARTMENTS

OSMOSIS

When two different solutions are separated by a membrane impermeable to the dissolved substances, a shift of water occurs through the membrane from the region of low solute concentration to the region of high solute concentration until the solutions are of equal concentration (Fig. 1-7). The magnitude of this force depends on the number of particles dissolved in the solutions and not on their weights.

The number of dissolved particles in a unit of water determines the solution's concentration and can be expressed as either osmolality or osmolarity. *Osmolality*

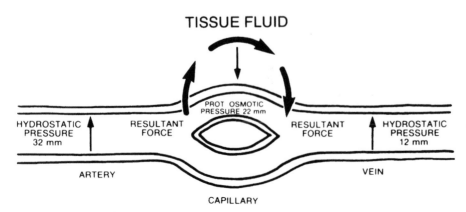

FIGURE 1-6. Fluid movement at capillary bed.

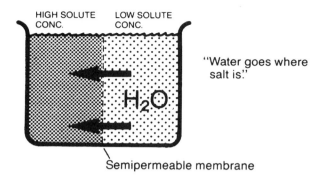

FIGURE 1-7. Osmosis.

refers to the number of osmoles per kilogram of water; thus, the total volume will be 1 liter of water plus the relatively small volume occupied by the solute.[9] *Osmolarity* refers to the number of osmoles per liter of solution. In this instance, the volume of water is less than 1 liter by an amount equal to the solute volume. Because of the very low solute concentration in body fluids, the difference between osmolality and osmolarity is negligible. Nonetheless, osmolality is the correct term to use when referring to body fluids because osmotic activity in the body depends on the concentration of active particles per kilogram of water.[10] The term *tonicity* is sometimes used instead of osmolality. Solutions may be termed isotonic, hypotonic, or hypertonic. Isotonic solutions have the same effective osmolality as body fluids (close to 285 milliosmolal [mOsm]). An example of an isotonic fluid is 0.9% sodium chloride. In contrast, a hypotonic solution has a lower osmolality than body fluids; an example of a hypotonic fluid is 0.45% sodium chloride. Finally, a hypertonic solution has an effective osmolality greater than that of body fluids; an example of a hypertonic fluid is 3% sodium chloride.

DIFFUSION

The continual movement of molecules among each other in liquids, or in gases, is called *diffusion*.[11] An example of diffusion is the exchange of oxygen and carbon dioxide (CO_2) between the alveoli and capillaries.

FILTRATION

Filtration is the transfer of water and dissolved substances from a region of high pressure to a region of low pressure; the force behind it is hydrostatic pressure.

An example of filtration is the passage of water and electrolytes from the arterial capillary bed to the interstitial fluid; in this instance, the hydrostatic pressure is furnished by the pumping action of the heart.

SODIUM–POTASSIUM PUMP

The sodium concentration is greater in the ECF than in the ICF; therefore, there is a tendency for sodium to enter by diffusion. This tendency is offset by the *sodium–potassium pump*, which is located in the cell membrane and, in the presence of adenosine triphosphate (ATP), actively moves sodium from the cell into the ECF. Conversely, potassium is the predominant cation in the ICF; therefore, the high intracellular potassium concentration is maintained by pumping potassium into the cell. Active transport occurs to move other ions (such as calcium and hydrogen) from areas of lesser concentration to areas of greater concentration. By definition, active transport implies that energy expenditure must occur for the movement to occur against a concentration gradient.

ROUTES OF GAINS AND LOSSES

Water and electrolytes are gained in various ways. In healthy humans, fluids are gained by drinking and eating (much of solid food is actually fluid). In illness, fluids may be gained by the parenteral route (intravenously or subcutaneously) or by means of an enteral feeding tube in the stomach or intestine. Organs of fluid loss include the lungs, skin, GI tract, and kidneys. When fluid balance is critical, *all routes of gain* and *all routes of loss* must be recorded and the volumes compared. For critically ill patients, even small gains of fluid (such as that provided by humidifiers) must be considered.

LUNGS

The lungs normally eliminate water vapor (*insensible loss*) at a rate of 300 to 400 mL/day. The loss is much greater with increased respiratory rate, depth, or both. Losses from the lungs are dependent on external factors, such as humidity and oxygen concentration.

SKIN

Visible water and electrolyte loss through the skin occurs by sweating (*sensible perspiration*). Sweat is a hypotonic fluid containing several solutes; the chief ones are sodium, chloride, and potassium. Actual sweat losses vary according to environmental temperature, from 0 to 1,000 mL or more an hour. Significant sweat losses occur if the patient's body temperature exceeds 38.3°C (101°F) or if room temperature exceeds 32.2°C (90°F).

Continuous water loss by evaporation (about 600 mL/day) occurs through the skin as *insensible perspiration*, a nonvisible form of water loss. The presence of fever greatly increases insensible water loss through the lungs and the skin. Loss of the natural skin barrier in major burns also increases water loss by this route.

GASTROINTESTINAL TRACT

Each day, the healthy small intestine absorbs fluids that are ingested as well as those that are secreted into the GI tract. Thus, although in adults about 8 liters of fluid circulate through the GI system every 24 hours (the "GI circulation"), only about 100 to 200 mL is lost through the GI tract each day. Obviously, very large losses can be incurred from the GI tract if abnormal conditions occur such as diarrhea, fistulas, or vomiting. Diarrheal fluid losses tend to be isotonic with the ECF; however, diarrheal losses from the terminal part of the large intestine are hypotonic and reflect losses of free water.[12] Not only does vomiting cause fluid loss by the ejection of ingested and secreted fluids in the stomach and upper small intestine, it is usually associated with nausea that further limits oral intake of fluid.

KIDNEYS

Although losses from the lungs, skin, and GI tract are determined by changing environmental events, losses from the kidney can be regulated by homeostatic organs. As such, the kidneys play a crucial role in the regulation of ECF volume in healthy and disease states.

The usual urine volume in the adult is between 1 and 2 L/day. A general rule of thumb is about 1 mL of urine per kilogram of body weight per hour (1 mL/kg/hr), with boundaries of 0.5 to 2 mL/kg/hr.[13]

Table 2-1 shows that in a healthy adult the average 24-hour intake and output of water is about equal.

⬤ HOMEOSTATIC MECHANISMS

The body is equipped with homeostatic mechanisms to keep the composition and volume of body fluid within narrow limits of normal. Organs involved in this mechanism include the kidneys, lungs, heart, blood vessels, adrenal glands, parathyroid glands, and pituitary gland.

KIDNEYS

The kidneys are vital to the regulation of fluid and electrolyte balance. They normally filter 180 liters of plasma a day in a normal adult, while excreting only 1.8 liters of urine.[14] They act both autonomously and in response to blood-borne messengers, such as aldosterone and antidiuretic hormone (ADH).

Major functions of the kidneys in fluid balance homeostasis include:

- Regulation of ECF volume and osmolality by selective retention and excretion of water and electrolytes. The juxtaglomerular apparatus (JGA) located within the kidney monitors both renal perfusion and solute excretion. The JGA, made up of specialized renin-secreting cells in the afferent glomerular arteriole and highly differentiated cells in the distal tubule (macula densa), is stimulated to release renin when there is a decrease in wall tension in the afferent arteriole or a decrease in salt delivery to the macula densa.[15] Renin converts angiotensinogen to angiotensin I, which is further metabolized to angiotensin II. In addition to being a vasoconstrictor, angiotensin II is a potent antinatriuretic hormone (causing sodium to be retained by the kidney). Also, angiotensin II stimulates aldosterone secretion, which enhances sodium reabsorption in the distal tubule.
- Regulation of electrolyte levels in the ECF by selective retention and excretion. The quantity of solutes and water in urine are highly variable according to the intake of these substances. For example, a person who has ingested a large quantity of sodium will excrete more sodium than will an individual who has been on a low-sodium diet.
- Regulation of acid–base balance. The kidneys must excrete the 50 to 100 mEq of noncarbonic acid generated each day. In addition, they are responsible for reabsorbing virtually all of the filtered HCO_3^-.[16] (It

should be remembered that loss of HCO_3^- in the urine is equivalent to adding hydrogen ions [H^+] ions to the body.)

- Excretion of metabolic wastes (primarily acids) and toxic substances. Urine contains high concentrations of uncharged molecules, particularly urea (allowing metabolic end products to be excreted, rather than accumulating in the body).[17]

Renal failure results in multiple fluid and electrolyte problems (see Chapter 17).

HEART AND ATRIAL NATRIURETIC FACTOR

Plasma must reach the kidneys in sufficient volume to permit regulation of water and electrolytes. The pumping action of the heart provides circulation of blood through the kidneys under sufficient pressure for urine to form; of course, renal perfusion makes renal function possible.

A hormone known as atrial natriuretic factor (ANF) or atrial natriuretic peptide (ANP) is released in the right atrium. The primary stimulus for release of ANF is atrial distention, which is associated with an increased venous return that increases right atrial pressure and stretch. This hormone acts on the kidney to cause a diuresis of sodium and water, thereby decreasing the intravascular volume. In addition, ANF is a direct vasodilator, which lowers the systemic blood pressure.[18]

The clinical significance and pharmacological use of ANF is as yet unclear. For patients with congestive heart failure, the diuretic effect of ANF appears to be most beneficial in acute heart failure; however, the renal response to ANF appears to be blunted in patients with chronic congestive heart failure.[19]

LUNGS

The lungs are also vital in maintaining homeostasis. Alveolar ventilation is responsible for the daily elimination of about 13,000 mEq H^+, as opposed to only 40 to 80 mEq excreted daily by the kidneys.

Under control of the medulla, the lungs act promptly to correct metabolic acid–base disturbances by regulating the level of CO_2 (a potential acid) in the ECF. For example, to compensate for metabolic alkalosis, the lungs hypoventilate to retain CO_2; the increased acidity helps correct excess alkalinity of the body fluids. Just the opposite occurs with metabolic

acidosis; the lungs hyperventilate to remove CO_2, which helps decrease the excess acidity of body fluids.

Pulmonary dysfunction can produce a rapid change (matter of seconds) in the plasma H^+ concentration (acid–base balance). Hypoventilation causes respiratory acidosis; hyperventilation causes respiratory alkalosis. When the lungs are at fault, the kidneys must compensate for the pH disturbances. Acid–base regulation is discussed in depth in Chapter 9.

The lungs also remove about 300 mL of water daily through exhalation (insensible water loss) in the healthy adult. Abnormal conditions, such as hyperpnea or continuous coughing, increase this loss; mechanical ventilation with excessive moisture decreases the loss.

PITUITARY GLAND

Specialized cells located in the hypothalamus manufacture a substance known as *antidiuretic hormone* (ADH), which is stored in the posterior lobe of the pituitary gland and released as needed. ADH is sometimes referred to by its chemical name (arginine vasopressin [AVP]).[20] Because ADH makes the body retain water, it is sometimes referred to as the "water-conserving" hormone.

The amount of water retained or excreted by the kidneys is partially regulated by ADH, which attaches to specialized receptor sites in the collecting and distal renal tubules, causing decreased urine output and increased urine osmolality. Thus, as ADH secretion increases, renal water retention increases. The opposite occurs when ADH production is decreased; that is, urinary output of dilute urine is increased. Minor changes in body fluid osmolality constantly occur during normal living and lead to minor physiological changes in ADH production. A rising plasma osmolality, such as occurs with salt intake, increases ADH production and, therefore, water retention; a falling plasma osmolality, such as occurs with water intake, decreases ADH production and enhances water excretion (Fig. 1-8). Therefore, plasma osmolality and ADH are in constant interaction. In the presence of a falling blood volume, ADH secretion and subsequent water retention are stimulated by volume stimuli (probably arising from sensors in the heart and great vessels). Other stimuli for ADH secretion are hypotension and volume depletion.[21] ADH is rapidly released in response to physiological stimuli and begins to act within minutes; when its secretion is inhibited, the hormone is cleared from the circulation

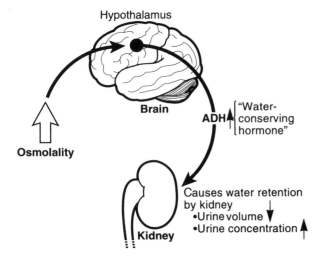

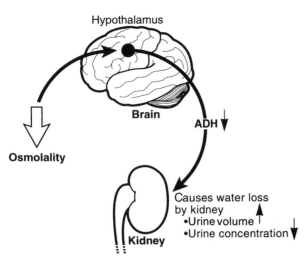

FIGURE 1-8. Effect of serum osmolality on ADH release and urine output. ADH, antidiuretic hormone.

quickly.[22] The half-life of ADH is about 10 minutes.[23]

The *syndrome of inappropriate antidiuretic hormone secretion* (SIADH) and *diabetes insipidus* (DI) are disorders of water balance caused by ADH disturbances at opposite ends of a continuum. In SIADH, excessive ADH secretion causes water retention. The opposite happens in DI, which is characterized by large urine volumes due to inadequate amounts of ADH. These pathological states are discussed further in chapters 4 and 19.

ADRENAL GLANDS

The primary adrenocortical hormone in the influence of fluid balance is *aldosterone*, a mineralocorticoid secreted by the outer zone of the adrenal cortex. This hormone acts chiefly on the distal tubules of the kidney to promote Na^+ reabsorption in exchange for K^+ and H^+ ions (which are excreted). Thus, aldosterone production causes sodium retention and expansion of the ECF, along with renal excretion of potassium. Occurrences that can stimulate aldosterone secretion include a decrease in the plasma sodium concentration or an increase in the potassium concentration. However, the primary regulator of aldosterone secretion appears to be angiotensin II, which is produced by the renin-angiotensin system. A decreased blood volume or flow activates this system and increases aldosterone secretion. The aldosterone, in turn, increases renal retention of sodium (along with water) to correct the volume deficit (Fig. 1-9). The opposite happens when a state of volume overexpansion exists.

Cortisol, another adrenocortical hormone, has only a fraction of the mineralocorticoid potency of aldosterone. However, secretion of cortisol in large quantities can produce sodium and fluid retention and potassium deficit.

PARATHYROID GLANDS

Most persons have four parathyroid glands (Fig. 1-10). These pea-sized glands, embedded in the corners of the thyroid gland, regulate calcium and phosphate balance by means of parathyroid hormone (PTH). Control of calcium ion concentration by PTH is largely due to this hormone's effect on bone resorption. The main function of PTH is to defend against hypocalcemia.[24] A decrease in calcium ion concentration stimulates PTH secretion, which then causes the release of calcium from the bones into the ECF. Conversely, when the extracellular calcium level is too high, PTH secretion is depressed so that almost no calcium is released from the bones. Long-term control of calcium ion concentration results from the effect of PTH on calcium reabsorption from the kidney tubules and calcium absorption from the gut through the GI mucosa. Both of these effects are significantly increased by PTH.

A reciprocal relationship exists between extracellular calcium and phosphate levels in that an elevation of

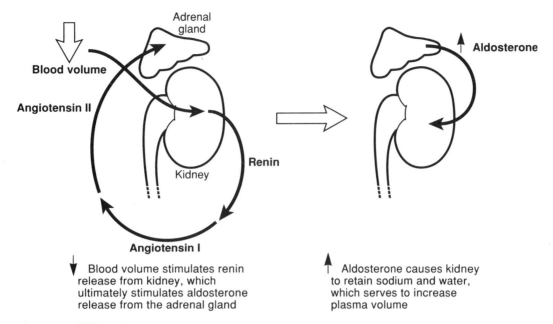

↓ Blood volume stimulates renin
release from kidney, which
ultimately stimulates aldosterone
release from the adrenal gland

↑ Aldosterone causes kidney
to retain sodium and water,
which serves to increase
plasma volume

FIGURE 1-9.   Effect of hypovolemia on the renin-angiotensin-aldosterone system.

one usually causes a depression of the other (Fig. 1-11). Thus, a high extracellular phosphate concentration causes a secondary depression of extracellular calcium; as a result, PTH release is stimulated (a condition often seen in renal failure).

Another hormone that bears consideration in the regulation of calcium is *calcitonin*, a substance secreted by the thyroid gland. The action of calcitonin on calcium is opposite to that of PTH; cal-

citonin reduces plasma calcium concentration. At high concentrations, calcitonin inhibits osteoclastic bone resorption.[25] Its effect on plasma calcium concentration is relatively stronger in children than in adults because the action of calcitonin involves bone remodeling, which is more rapid in children.[26] Pharmacological use of calcitonin in the treatment of hypercalcemia is discussed in Chapters 6 and 22.

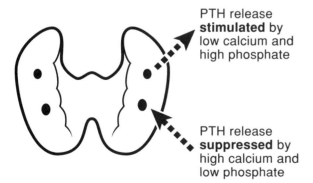

PTH release
stimulated by
low calcium and
high phosphate

PTH release
suppressed by
high calcium and
low phosphate

FIGURE 1-10.   Effect of serum calcium and phosphorus on PTH release. PTH, parathyroid hormone.

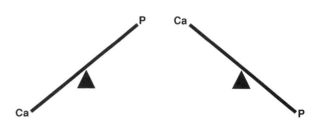

FIGURE 1-11.   Reciprocal relationship between calcium and phosphorus.

REFERENCES

1. Brensilver J, Goldberger E. *A Primer of Water, Electrolyte and Acid-Base Syndromes*, 8th ed. Philadelphia: FA Davis; 1996:4.
2. Narins R, ed. *Maxwell & Kleeman's Clinical Disorders of Fluid and Electrolyte Metabolism*, 5th ed. New York: McGraw-Hill; 1994:11.
3. Halperin M, Goldstein M. *Fluid, Electrolytes and Acid-Base Physiology*, 3rd ed. Philadelphia: WB Saunders; 1999:232.
4. Abelow B. *Understanding Acid-Base*. Baltimore, MD: Williams & Wilkins; 1998:10.
5. Guyton A, Hall J. *Human Physiology and Mechanisms of Disease*, 6th ed. Philadelphia: WB Saunders; 1997:14.
6. Halperin, Goldstein, p 228.
7. Smith K, Brain E. *Fluids and Electrolytes: A Conceptual Approach*, 2nd ed. New York: Churchill Livingstone; 1991:14.
8. Guyton A. *Textbook of Medical Physiology*, 8th ed. Philadelphia: WB Saunders; 1991:170.
9. Smith, Brain, p 18.
10. Smith, Brain, p 19.
11. Guyton, p 39.
12. Smith, Brain, p 4.
13. Pestana C. *Fluids and Electrolytes in the Surgical Patient*, 4th ed. Baltimore, MD: Williams & Wilkins; 1989:223.
14. Vander A. *Renal Physiology*, 5th ed. New York: McGraw Hill; 1995:19.
15. Szerlip H, Goldfarb S. *Workshops in Fluid and Electrolyte Disorders*. New York: Churchill Livingstone; 1993:3.
16. Rose B. *Clinical Physiology of Acid-Base and Electrolyte Disorders*, 4th ed. New York: McGraw-Hill; 1994:12.
17. Ibid, p 303.
18. Ibid, p 12.
19. Toto K. Endocrine physiology. In: Endocrine and Metabolic Disturbances in the Critically Ill. *Crit Care Nurs Clin North Am* December 1994:647.
20. Brensilver, Goldberger, p 17.
21. Fried L, Palevsky P. Hyponatremia and hypernatremia. *Med Clin North Am* 1997;81:585.
22. Kokko J, Tannen R. *Fluids and Electrolytes*, 3rd ed. Philadelphia: WB Saunders; 1996:67.
23. Czaczles J. Physiologic studies of antidiuretic hormone by its direct measurement in human plasma. *J Clin Invest* 1964; 43:1625.
24. Andreoli T, Carpenter C, Bennett J, Plum F. *Cecil Essentials of Medicine*, 4th ed. Philadelphia: WB Saunders; 1997:564.
25. Bell T. Diabetes insipidus. In: Endocrine and Metabolic Disturbances in the Critically Ill. *Crit Care Nurs Clin North Am* December 1994:676.
26. Narins, p 281.

Nursing Assessment

Nurses are responsible for monitoring patients for actual or potential fluid and electrolyte problems. It is logical for nurses to assume this vital role because they are directly responsible for hospitalized patients 24 hours a day and often they are the primary contact for patients both in extended-care facilities and the home setting. Monitoring for fluid balance disturbances involves more than simple observations and is based on an understanding of normal physiological mechanisms as well as the indicators of disrupted fluid balance. As with many conditions, a high level of suspicion is necessary to detect fluid and electrolyte problems. The suspicion that an electrolyte abnormality exists is strengthened by the presence of clinical features known to occur and often by the results of laboratory tests and electrocardiographic findings.

Nursing assessment of fluid balance requires a review of the patient's history and laboratory data, as well as careful clinical observation. In summary, the nurse must know "what to look for," "where and how often to look," and "when to expect certain changes as a result of interventions" (outcome criteria).

HISTORY

The following questions should be considered in the nursing history:

1. Is a disease process or injury state present that can disrupt fluid and electrolyte balance? (Examples might include diabetes mellitus, pancreatitis, and bowel obstruction.) In what type of imbalance(s) does this condition usually result?
2. Is the patient receiving any medication or treatment that can disrupt fluid and electrolyte balance? (Examples include steroids, diuretics, and total parenteral nutrition [TPN].) If so, how might this therapy upset fluid balance?
3. Is there an abnormal loss of body fluids and, if so, from what source? What types of imbalances are usually associated with the loss of these fluids?
4. Have any dietary restrictions (eg, a low-sodium diet) been imposed? If so, how might fluid balance be affected?
5. Has the patient taken adequate amounts of water and other nutrients orally or by some other route? If not, how long has the inadequate intake been present?

6. How does the total intake of fluids compare with the total output of fluid?

CLINICAL ASSESSMENT

After the history described above has been reviewed, the nurse should be able to identify potential problems related to fluid and electrolyte imbalances. At this point, a thorough nursing assessment is indicated. Of course, nursing assessment is not a one-time procedure but must be done at regular intervals to detect changes.

INSPECTION/EXAMINATION

Facial Appearance

An individual with a severe fluid volume deficit (FVD) has a pinched facial expression. A significant FVD causes decreased intraocular pressure; thus, the eyes appear sunken and feel soft to the touch.

Moisture in Oral Cavity

A dry mouth may be the result of FVD or of mouth breathing. If it is due to FVD, all of the oral tissues will be dry. In contrast, if the dryness is due to mouth breathing, the areas where the gums and cheek membranes meet will remain moist. Dry, sticky mucous membranes are noted with sodium excess (hypernatremia).

Thirst

Thirst is a subjective sensory symptom that has been defined as an awareness of the desire to drink. The thirst center is very sensitive to change in osmolality; an increase in osmolality of only 1% to 2% is sufficient to stimulate thirst.[1] An increased concentration of the extracellular fluid will osmotically pull fluid from the cells in the thirst control center and stimulate thirst. In general, any factor that causes intracellular dehydration will cause the sensation of thirst. The value of thirst is, of course, that it stimulates fluid intake and helps to dilute extracellular fluids and returns osmolality toward normal.[2]

It has been shown that drinking and the presence of water in the stomach of a person with thirst usually produces satiety (long before any significant absorption has occurred). Gastric distention is affected by the temperature and osmotic properties of the consumed liquids. For example, cold liquids tend to delay gastric emptying more than warm fluids; therefore, smaller volumes of cold liquids are required to achieve thirst satiation and small drinks of cold liquids are more likely to quench the thirst of patients on restricted fluid intake.[3]

The sense of thirst is so protective of the normal serum sodium level that hypernatremia virtually never occurs unless thirst is impaired or rendered ineffective because of unconsciousness or inaccessibility of water. In adults, hypernatremia is most often seen in persons older than 60 years of age, partially because age is associated with diminished osmotic stimulation of thirst.[4]

Thirst is prominent in patients who have increased water losses (such as occur in hyperglycemia, high fever, or diarrhea). An infant can be tested for thirst by offering water, although the presence of nausea may mask the symptom. Unfortunately, patients with altered states of consciousness do not experience normal thirst. Also, many patients are debilitated and unable to respond to thirst. It is no wonder that hypernatremia is a relatively common imbalance on neurologic units.

In addition to fluid volume changes, thirst can be affected by electrolyte balance. For example, thirst and polyuria are prominent and early signs of hypercalcemia. Also, long-standing hypokalemia can cause a type of diabetes insipidus and result in polyuria and thirst.

Tearing

Tearing is decreased in patients with FVD. This sign is one of four identified by Gorelick et al.[5] as being predictive of fluid volume deficit in children; the other three were prolonged capillary refill, dry mucous membranes, and an ill general appearance.

Tongue Turgor

In a healthy person, the tongue has one longitudinal furrow. In the person with FVD, additional longitudinal furrows are noted, and the tongue is smaller (due to fluid loss). Unlike skin turgor, tongue turgor is not appreciably affected by age and therefore is a useful assessment for all age groups. Sodium excess causes the tongue to appear red and swollen. Some authors believe that loss of tongue turgor is the most reliable physical sign of FVD.[6]

Filling of Neck Veins

The jugular veins provide a built-in manometer to follow the changes in central venous pressure (CVP). No invasive maneuvers are required and the procedure can be reliable when done correctly (Fig. 2-1). The vein on the right side is preferred for assessment because the right internal jugular vein is nearly a direct conduit to the right atrium. The left internal jugular vein is less desirable because the brachycephalic vein may be compressed by the aortic knob, resulting in false elevation of CVP.[7]

Changes in fluid volume are reflected by changes in neck vein filling, provided the patient is not in heart failure. Normally, with the patient supine, the external jugular veins fill to the anterior border of the sternocleidomastoid muscle. Flat neck veins in the supine position indicate a decreased plasma volume. With the patient positioned sitting at a 45° angle, the venous distentions normally should not extend higher than 2 cm above the sternal angle. Elevated venous pressure is indicated by neck veins distended from the top portion of the sternum to the angle of the jaw; this is often seen in severe heart failure.

To estimate jugular venous pressure, the nurse should:

1. Position the patient in a semi-Fowler's position (head of bed elevated to a 30° to 60° angle), keeping the neck straight.
2. Remove any of the patient's clothing that could constrict the neck or upper chest.

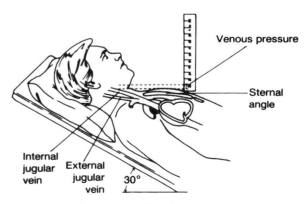

FIGURE 2-1. Assessment of jugular vein pulsations.

3. Provide adequate lighting to visualize effectively the external jugular veins on each side of the neck.
4. Measure the level to which the veins are distended on the neck above the sternal angle. The vertical distance between this point and the sternal angle is measured and reported as centimeters above or below the sternal angle.

Appearance and Temperature of Skin

Severe FVD causes the skin to be pale and cool because of peripheral vasoconstriction, which occurs to compensate for hypovolemia. Metabolic acidosis can cause warm, flushed skin due to peripheral vasodilation.

Skin Turgor

In a healthy person, pinched skin will immediately fall back to its normal position when released. This elastic property, referred to as turgor, partially depends on the interstitial fluid volume. In an individual with FVD, the skin flattens more slowly after the pinch is released and may remain elevated for several seconds.

Tissue turgor is best measured by pinching the skin over the sternum, in the inner aspects of the thighs, or on the forehead (Fig. 2-2), although some nurses prefer to test skin turgor in children over the abdominal area and on the medial aspects of the thighs.

Although the purpose of the skin turgor test is to measure only interstitial fluid volume, it also measures skin elasticity. It is common for persons older than 55 to 60 years of age to have reduced skin turgor because they have less skin elasticity relative to younger persons. Skin turgor may be difficult to assess in elderly patients or in those with recent weight loss and is not diagnostic in the absence of other signs of FVD.

In children, skin turgor begins to diminish after 3% to 5% of the body weight is lost. However, severe malnutrition, particularly in infants, can cause depressed skin turgor even in the absence of fluid depletion. Obese infants with FVD may have skin turgor that is deceptively normal. Infants with hypernatremia may have firm skin that feels thick.

Tissue turgor can vary with age, nutritional state, and even race or complexion. Observations are most meaningful if done sequentially before the development of a fluid balance abnormality.

Sunken Eyes

Sunken eyes (due to decreased intraocular fluid) are often observed in severe FVD and can be used in conjunction with other signs to help identify this condition. Sunken eyes is a valid indicator in both infants and elderly patients.[8,9]

Edema

Edema is defined as an excessive accumulation of interstitial fluid (the body fluid that bathes the cells). Edema usually does not become clinically apparent until the interstitial volume has increased by at least 2.5 to 3 liters.[10]

Causes of edema include:

- Increased capillary permeability, which allows fluid to leak into the interstitium (as in burns or localized trauma)

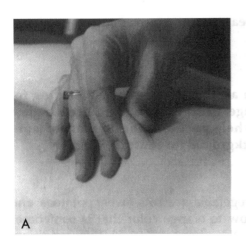
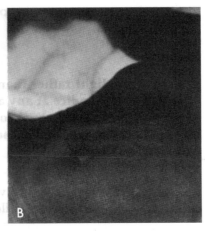

FIGURE 2-2. **(A)** Testing skin turgor on the abdomen of a well-hydrated infant. **(B)** Tenting of skin on the abdomen of a dehydrated patient.

- Increased capillary hydraulic pressure, which forces fluid into the interstitium (as in heart failure or venous obstruction)
- Decreased plasma oncotic pressure of hypoalbuminemia, which fosters the transfer of fluid into the interstitium, particularly when the plasma albumin level is less than 2 g/dL
- Lymphatic obstruction, which permits local edema (as in node enlargement of malignancy)[11]

Edema formation may be either localized (as in thrombophlebitis) or generalized (as in heart failure and the nephrotic syndrome). An excess of interstitial fluid accumulating predominantly in the lower extremities of ambulatory patients and in the presacral region of bedridden patients is referred to as *dependent edema*. *Generalized edema* is spread throughout the body and may accumulate in periorbital and scrotal regions because of the relatively lower tissue hydrostatic pressure in these regions. Edema related to salt retention is generally pitting and can be manifested by pressing one's finger into the soft tissues (Fig. 2-3). After the pressure is removed, the "pit" gradually disappears.

Overt edema is apparent only after 3 to 4 liters of fluid has accumulated.[12]

Describing peripheral edema by appearance is somewhat subjective. For example, it is sometimes indicated by using plus signs to represent the amount, ranging from 1+ to 4+, with 1+ indicating barely perceptible, 2+ and 3+ moderate, and 4+ severe edema. Measuring an extremity or body part with a millimeter tape in the same area each day is the most exact method.

There is little or no peripheral edema with only water retention (as occurs in excessive secretion of antidiuretic hormone [ADH]). Instead, there is cellular swelling that sometimes can be detected by pressing one's finger over the sternum (or other bony prominence) and producing a visible fingerprint.

Pulmonary Edema

Pulmonary edema results from excessive shifting of fluid from the vascular space into the pulmonary interstitium and air spaces. Cardiogenic pulmonary edema occurs when the pulmonary capillary pressure exceeds

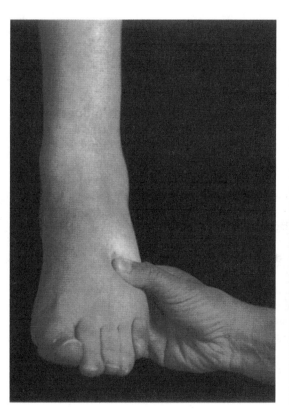
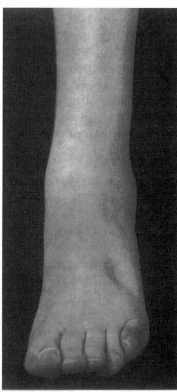

FIGURE 2-3. Pitting edema.

the forces that normally maintain fluid within the vascular space; these forces include serum oncotic pressure and interstitial hydrostatic pressure.[13] Accumulation of extravascular lung water (EVLW) affects pulmonary functioning and gas exchange. Clinical manifestations include dyspnea, anxiety, restlessness, wheezing, expectoration of pink frothy fluid, and use of accessory respiratory muscles.[14]

Capillary Refill

Capillary refill can be checked by applying pressure to a fingernail for 5 seconds and then releasing the pressure and noting how rapidly the normal color returns.[15] Color will return in less than 1 to 2 seconds in a healthy person. A delayed capillary refill could indicate constriction of the peripheral vessels, decreased cardiac output, or anemia. Other factors that reduce capillary refill time include cold temperatures and cigarette smoking.

Neuromuscular Irritability

It is sometimes necessary to assess patients for increased or decreased neuromuscular irritability, particularly when imbalances in calcium and magnesium are suspected.

The nurse may, as necessary, check for Chvostek's sign and Trousseau's sign; also, deep-tendon reflexes can be tested to monitor neuromuscular irritability.

To test Chvostek's sign, the facial nerve should be percussed about 2 cm anterior to the earlobe. A positive response shows a unilateral twitching of the facial muscles, including the eyelid and lips. Chvostek's sign is indicative of hypocalcemia or hypomagnesemia. However, it is not specific for these conditions because it is present in about 10% to 15% of healthy adults.[16]

To test for Trousseau's sign, place a blood pressure cuff on the arm and inflate above systolic pressure for 3 minutes. A positive reaction is the development of carpal spasm (Fig. 2-4). This hand cramp is characterized by the thumb and fifth finger approximating each other while fingers two to four are extended. Although more specific for hypocalcemia than is Chvostek's sign, it may be absent in some patients with this imbalance.[17]

The common deep-tendon reflexes include the biceps, triceps, brachioradialis, patellar, and Achilles

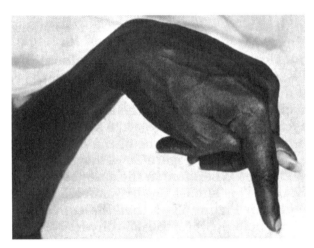

FIGURE 2-4.   Hypocalcemic tetany in the hand, called "carpopedal spasm." (Courtesy of Dr. Herbert Langford) (Guyton A, Hall J. *Human Physiology and Mechanisms of Disease*, 6th ed. Philadelphia: WB Saunders, 1997:636.)

reflexes. A deep-tendon reflex is elicited by briskly tapping a partially stretched tendon with a rubber percussion hammer, preferably over the tendon insertion of the muscle. The broad head of the hammer is used to stroke easily accessible tendons (eg, the Achilles) and the pointed end for less accessible tendons (eg, the biceps). The response in the prospective muscle is a sudden contraction. The muscle being tested should be slightly stretched (by the position of the limb), and the patient should be relaxed. With too little or too much muscle stretch the reflex cannot be elicited.

The reflexes are usually graded on a 0 to 4+ scale

0 = no response
1+ = somewhat diminished, but present
2+ = normal
3+ = brisker than average and possibly but not necessarily indicative of disease
4+ = hyperactive

Deep-tendon reflexes may be hyperactive in the presence of hypocalcemia, hypomagnesemia, hypernatremia, and alkalosis. They may be hypoactive in the presence of hypercalcemia, hypermagnesemia, hyponatremia, hypokalemia, and acidosis. Of course, many factors other than electrolyte disturbances can produce abnormalities in deep-tendon reflexes. As with most other signs, deep-tendon reflexes should be evaluated in light of other clinical signs, patient history, and laboratory data.

Other Signs

Other areas to consider in clinical assessment include changes in:

- Behavior
- Sensation
- Fatigue level

Because these changes are often vague, they are best evaluated in context with specific imbalances (see Chapters 3 through 9).

VITAL SIGNS AND HEMODYNAMICS

Body Temperature

Changes in body temperature as symptoms of fluid and electrolyte imbalances may include:

1. Elevation in body temperature in hypernatremia may occur due to excessive water loss.[18] The elevated body temperature is probably related to lack of available fluid for sweating. Also, dehydration probably has a direct effect on the hypothalamus.
2. In a cool room, a patient with an isotonic FVD may be slightly hypothermic (probably related to the decreased basal metabolic rate). After partial correction of the FVD, the temperature generally increases to an appropriate level. With moderate FVD, temperature taken rectally may be 36.1°C (97°F) to 37.2°C (99°F); with severe FVD, it may be 35°C (95°F) to 36.7°C (98°F).[19]

Changes in body temperature do not merely reflect fluid balance problems. Fever can *cause* fluid balance problems if not promptly recognized and treated. Fever causes an increase in metabolism rate and, as a result, in formed metabolic wastes, which require fluid to make a solution for renal excretion; therefore, fluid loss is increased. Fever also causes hyperpnea, an increase in breathing rate resulting in extra water vapor loss through the lungs. Because fever increases loss of body fluids, temperature elevations must be detected early and appropriate interventions taken.

A temperature elevation between 38.3°C (101°F) and 39.4°C (103°F) increases the 24-hour fluid requirements by at least 500 mL, and a temperature higher than 39.4°C (103°F) increases it by at least 1,000 mL.[20]

Pulse

Tachycardia is usually the earliest sign of the decreased vascular volume associated with FVD. It may also be associated with deficits of magnesium or potassium. Conversely, excesses of magnesium or potassium can cause decreased pulse rate. Irregular pulse rates also occur with potassium imbalances and magnesium deficit. Pulse volume is decreased in FVD and increased in fluid volume excess (FVE).

Respirations

Deep, rapid respirations may be a compensatory mechanism for metabolic acidosis or a primary disorder causing respiratory alkalosis. Slow, shallow respirations may be a compensatory mechanism for metabolic alkalosis or a primary disorder causing respiratory acidosis.

Weakness or paralysis of respiratory muscles is likely in severe hypokalemia or hyperkalemia and in severe magnesium excess (the respiratory center may be paralyzed at a serum magnesium level of 10–15 mEq/L). Moist rales, in the absence of cardiopulmonary disease, indicate FVE.

Blood Pressure

A sensitive method for detecting volume depletion is measurement of the blood pressure and pulse with the patient in a lying and then standing position. Standing from a supine position causes an abrupt drop in venous return, for which sympathetically mediated cardiovascular adjustments normally compensate. In the healthy individual, cardiac return is maintained by increased peripheral resistance and a slight increase in heart rate; systolic pressure falls only slightly and diastolic pressure may actually rise a few millimeters of mercury. In contrast, a fall in systolic pressure greater than 15 mm Hg or an increase in the pulse rate greater than 15 beats/min suggests intravascular volume deficit.[21] When hypovolemia is suspected, it is helpful to measure the blood pressure in three positions (supine, sitting, and standing); a repeat reading after 2 to 3 minutes may identify orthostatic hypotension missed by earlier readings.[22] Of course, conditions associated with autonomic neuropathy (such as diabetes) can also produce these orthostatic blood pressure and pulse changes, as can sympatholytic antihypertensive medications.

Hypotension may occur with magnesium excess, perhaps first occurring at a level of 3 to 5 mEq/L. Hypertension can occur with magnesium deficit and with FVE.

Nursing observations must be *interpreted*, using one's knowledge of the patient's history and pathophysiological condition to determine whether the information gained from the assessment suggests normal or abnormal signs or measurements, and to what degree. Then, the appropriate nursing action(s) must be determined. One must also know when medical intervention is required.

Central Venous Pressure

Central venous pressure refers to pressure in the right atrium or vena cava and provides information about the following parameters: blood volume, effectiveness of the heart's pumping action, and vascular tone. When CVP is measured with a water manometer, pressure in the right atrium is usually 0 to 4 cm of water and pressure in the vena cava is about 4 to 11 cm of water. When CVP is measured with a transducer system, the normal range is about 0 to 7 mm Hg. A *below normal* CVP may indicate:

- Decreased blood volume
- Drug-induced vasodilation (causing pooling of blood in peripheral veins)
- Sepsis inducted vasodilation
- Condition that reduces venous return to the heart

In contrast, an *above normal* CVP may indicate:

- Excessive blood volume
- Heart failure
- Vasoconstriction (causing the vascular bed to become smaller)
- Mechanical ventilation (which causes increased intrathoracic pressure)

More important than absolute values are the upward or downward trends; these trends are determined by taking frequent readings (often every 30–60 minutes). It is always important to evaluate the CVP in reference to other available clinical data such as:

- Blood pressure
- Pulse
- Respirations
- Breath and heart sounds
- Fluid intake
- Urinary output
- Neck vein distention

Example: A rise in CVP paralleling that of systolic blood pressure in a previously hypotensive patient is an indication of adequate fluid volume replacement. A low CVP persisting after fluid volume replacement may be a sign of continued occult bleeding.

In patients with normal cardiac function and relatively normal pulmonary function, the CVP remains an acceptable guide to blood volume.

Rate of Fluid Administration

Sometimes the rate of an infusion is titrated according to the patient's CVP; when this is necessary, the physician should designate the desired limits so that the nurse can adjust the flow rate accordingly. For example, in acute hypercalcemia, the physician may order isotonic saline at a rate of 250 mL/hr, provided that the CVP does not exceed 10 cm water. As long as urinary output remains adequate and the CVP does not change significantly, it can be assumed that the heart is accommodating the amount of fluid being administered.

Methods of Measuring Central Venous Pressure

The CVP can be measured with a water manometer or a pressure transducer system. The water manometer is most often used in the nonintensive care settings, whereas the pressure transducer system is usually used for patients in an intensive care unit.

Water Manometer. The manometer is a fluid-filled tube that relays the patient's pressure reading without the use of electrical equipment. It is connected to the patient's intravenous (IV) infusion system; in turn, this connects to the central venous catheter (Fig. 2-5).

Transducer System. A single transducer is connected to the central catheter lumen, which is connected to the monitor. The pressure is measured by the transducer and converted to a numerical value that is continuously displayed on the monitor (Fig. 2-6). (Halck et al.[23] reported a close linear correlation between CVP measurements performed with water manometrics and electric equipment.)

Nursing Considerations

1. Measure CVP with the patient lying flat in bed, if this position can be tolerated. If not, have the patient in the same position each time CVP is measured. Indicate the patient's position on the chart when recording the pressure. Place the zero point of the

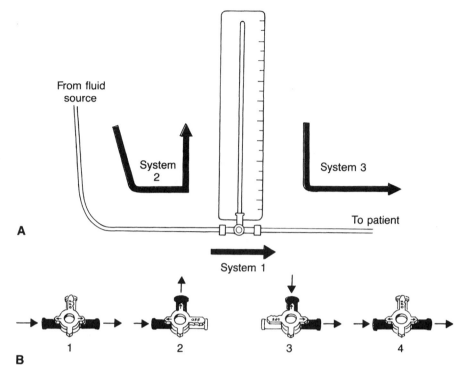

FIGURE 2-5. (A) Central venous pressure (CVP) water manometer system. System 1 allows for fluid administration. System 2 fills the manometer with fluid. System 3 allows the flow of fluid from the manometer to the patient and determines the CVP reading. (B) Steps in measuring central venous pressure. 1, Stopcock turned so that IV fluid flows to patient. 2, Stopcock in position to fill manometer with fluid. 3, Stopcock turned so that it is open from manometer to patient to obtain reading. 4, Stopcock returned to first position so that IV fluid flows to patient.

manometer at the level of the patient's right atrium. The point selected may be marked on the patient's side so that the zero mark may be used consistently.

2. Be aware that a slight fluctuation in the manometer occurs with respirations when the catheter is patent and properly positioned in the vena cava. The fluid level in the manometer falls with inspiration and rises on expiration; these changes correspond with changes in intrapulmonary pressure during breathing.

Pulmonary Artery and Pulmonary Artery Wedge Pressures

At times, CVP measurements are not adequate for evaluating the patient's clinical status or for determining proper flow rates. It may be necessary to use more invasive hemodynamic monitoring to adequately assess pressures in both sides of the heart in patients with acute cardiopulmonary decompensation.

The potential benefits for pulmonary artery catheter monitoring are:

- It affords a more accurate determination of the hemodynamic status of critically ill patients than is possible by clinical assessment of CVP alone.
- It can be helpful in assessing fluid status in patients with confusing clinical pictures, especially those for whom errors in fluid management and drug therapy have major consequences.

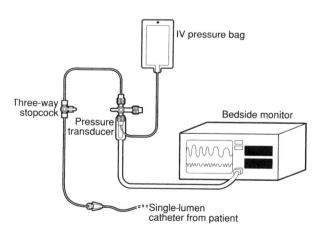

FIGURE 2-6. Transducer system. The transducer is an instrument that is used to sense physiological events and transform them into electrical signals. If central venous pressure is the only measure needed, a single lumen catheter may be used and connected to a water manometer or a transducer system. The transducer system is also used with pulmonary artery catheters.

The normal pulmonary artery pressure is 20 to 30 mm Hg; the normal diastolic pulmonary pressure is 8 to 15 mm Hg.[24]

URINE VOLUME AND CONCENTRATION

Urine Volume

The normal urinary output is about 1 mL/kg body weight/hr, with boundaries of 0.5 to 2 mL/kg/hr.[25] Table 2-1 shows that the usual urine volume in adults is about 1,500 mL/day (range, 1,000–2,000 mL/day). This is equivalent to 40 to 80 mL/hr in the typical adult. Urine volume in children is less and is dependent on age and weight.

During periods of stress, the 24-hour urine volume in the adult may diminish to 750 to 1,200 mL/day (or 30–50 mL/hr). Urine volume is somewhat less during periods of stress because of increased aldosterone and ADH secretion.

A low urine volume suggests FVD, and a high urine volume suggests FVE. Several factors can alter urinary volume, including:

- Amount of fluid intake
- Losses from skin, lungs, and gastrointestinal tract
- Amount of waste products for excretion. Urine volume is increased in conditions with high solute loads, such as diabetes mellitus, high-protein tube feedings, thyrotoxicosis, and fever.
- Renal concentrating ability. When concentrating ability is diminished, urine volume is increased to allow adequate solute excretion.
- Blood volume. Hypovolemia causes decreased renal perfusion and thus oliguria; hypervolemia causes increased urinary volume if the kidneys are functioning normally.

- Hormonal influences, primarily aldosterone and ADH

Nursing Considerations

1. Maintain input and output (I&O) records on all patients with real or potential fluid balance problems. Measure all fluid gains and losses according to routes.
2. Be alert for fluid intake greatly exceeding fluid output, or fluid output greatly exceeding fluid intake. Totals of I&O records for several consecutive days should be obtained for a clearer understanding of fluid balance status.
3. Be aware that the usual urine output in adults is 1 to 2 L/day (or about 750–1,200 mL/day during periods of stress).
4. Be aware that the usual urine output in adults is 40 to 80 mL/hr (or 30–50 mL/hr during periods of stress).
5. Use a device calibrated for small volumes of urine when hourly urine volumes must be measured (Fig. 2-7).
6. Be aware that patients taking in high-solute loads (as in high-protein tube feedings) need extra water to aid in solute elimination.
7. Be aware that individuals with diminished renal concentrating ability (such as the aged) need more fluid to excrete solutes than do those with normal renal function.
8. Be aware that a low urine volume with a high specific gravity (SG) indicates FVD.
9. Be aware that a low urine volume with a low SG is indicative of renal disease.
10. Evaluate I&O levels and urinary SG in relation to other clinical signs.

TABLE 2-1. Average Intake and Output in an Adult for a 24-hr Period

Intake		Output	
Oral liquids	1,300 mL	Urine	1,500 mL
Water in food	1,000 mL	Stool	200 mL
Water produced by metabolism	300 mL		
		Insensible:	
Total	2,600 mL	Lungs	300 mL
		Skin	600 mL
		Total	2,600 mL

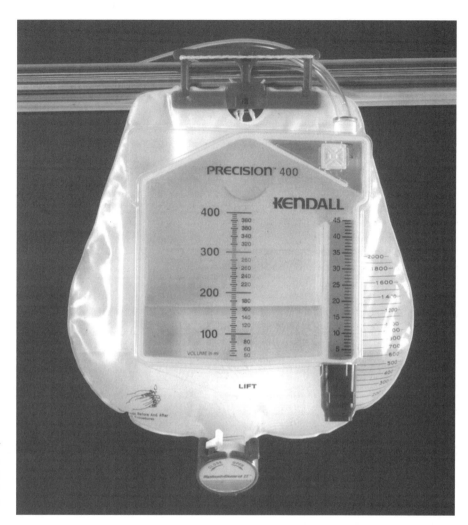

FIGURE 2-7. Device suitable for measuring small urine volume. Precision 400™ Urine Meter, Product, Code Number 2000. Kendall Healthcare Products, Mansfield, MA.

11. Be aware of common sources of errors in I&O measurements (see Clinical Tip: Overcoming Common Errors in Measuring Intake and Output).

Urine Concentration

Urinary SG measures the ability of the kidneys to concentrate urine. In this test, the concentration of urine is compared with the 1.000 SG of distilled water. Because urine contains electrolytes and other substances, its SG is greater than 1.000. The range of SG in urine is from 1.003 to 1.035; most random specimens are between 1.012 and 1.025. Typical urine osmolality (another measure of urine concentration) ranges from 500 to 800 mOsm/kg; extreme ranges are from 50 to 1,400 mOsm/kg.

Urinary SG is elevated when there is a FVD, as the healthy kidney seeks to retain needed fluid, thus excreting solutes in a small concentrated urine volume. However, one should be aware that heavy molecules not normally present in large quantities in urine can falsely affect SG readings. For example, glucose, albumin, or radiocontrast dyes will elevate urinary SG out of proportion to the actual concentration. Therefore, it is more accurate to measure urine osmolality in patients with glycosuria, proteinuria, or recent use of radiopaque dyes.

Specific gravity can be measured with a refractometer, a dipstick that has a reagent area for SG, or with a urinometer. Freshly voided urine specimens at room temperature are desirable for testing SG. Refrigerated samples may have falsely elevated readings, as may specimens exposed to excessive heat and dryness (a

CLINICAL TIP

Overcoming Common Errors in Measuring Intake and Output (I&O)

COMMON ERRORS	SUGGESTIONS
Errors Involving Both Intake and Output	1. A "measure intake–output" sign should be attached to the patient's bed to serve as a reminder.
Failure to communicate to the entire staff which patients require I&O measurement. (Body fluids are often discarded without being measured, and oral fluids are not recorded, merely because staff members are not aware of the patients on I&O.)	2. A list of all patients requiring I&O measurement should be posted in a convenient work area for quick reference. 3. An adequate patient report should be given to all personnel.
Failure to explain I&O to the patient and family. (Most patients will cooperate *if* they know what is expected of them.)	1. Both the patient and the family should receive a simple explanation of why I&O measurement is necessary. 2. Careful instructions are necessary to acquaint the patient and family with their role in helping to achieve an accurate I&O record.
Well-meaning intentions to record a drink of water or an emptied urinal at a later, more convenient time are often forgotten.	Measurements should be recorded at the time they are obtained.
Failure to measure fluids that can be directly measured because it takes less time to guess at their amounts	Measure *all* fluids amenable to direct measurement—guesses should be reserved for fluids that cannot be measured directly.
Errors Related to Intake	
Failure to designate the specific volume of glasses, cups, bowls, and other fluid containers used in the hospital. (Each person may ascribe a different volume to the same glass of water.)	The I&O form should list the volumes of glasses, cups, bowls, and other fluid containers used in the hospital.
Failure to obtain an adequate measuring device for small amounts of oral fluids. (Patients frequently drink small quantities of fluids; the amounts must be estimated unless a calibrated cup is available—frequent estimates increase the margin of error.)	Small calibrated paper cups should be kept at the bedside for such a purpose.
Failure to consider the volume of fluid displaced by ice in iced drinks frequently causes an overstatement of ingested oral fluids	Only small amounts of ice should be used for iced drinks so that the accurate amount of fluid ingested can be recorded.

CLINICAL TIP

Overcoming Common Errors in Measuring Intake and Output (I&O)—*cont'd*

COMMON ERRORS	SUGGESTIONS
Overstatement of fluid volume given as ice chips; note that the liquid volume of a glass of ice chips is only about half a glass	Record fluid intake from ice chips as about half of the ice chips volume (eg, an ounce of ice chips is about 15 mL water).
Failure to consider that parenteral fluid bottles are overfilled; a 1,000-mL bottle may actually contain 1,100 mL; a 500-mL bottle may contain 550 mL	Run excess fluid through tubing during set-up, or record actual volume infused.
Assuming that the contents of empty containers were drunk by the patient. (Patients sometimes give their coffee or juice to a visiting relative or other patients in the room; they may forget to tell the person checking the tray.)	The patient should be asked what fluids were drunk.

Errors Related to Output

Failure to estimate fluid lost as perspiration	1. An attempt should be made to describe the amount of clothing and bed linen saturated with perspiration—it has been estimated that one necessary bed change represents at least 1 L of lost fluid. 2. Some I&O records require the nurse to estimate perspiration as +, + +, + + +, or + + + + (+ represents sweating that is just visible, and + + + + represents profuse sweating).
Failure to estimate "uncaught" vomitus (Frequently, "uncaught" emesis is recorded merely as a lost specimen.)	The amount of fluid lost as vomitus should be estimated and recorded as an estimate—it is better to guess than to give no indication at all as to the amount.
Failure to estimate the amount of incontinent urine (I&O records often indicate the number of incontinent voidings but give no indication of the amounts; obviously, such records are of little value.)	The amount of incontinent urine should be estimated—it is helpful to note the amount of clothing and bed linen saturated with urine.
Failure to estimate fluid lost as liquid feces	1. The patient should be encouraged to use the bedpan or a measuring device over the toilet so that the fluid loss can be directly measured. 2. The amount of fluid lost in incontinent liquid stools should be estimated.
Failure to estimate fluid lost as wound exudate	1. The amount of drainage on a dressing should be measured and charted—this can be done by measuring the width of the stained area and determining the thickness of the dressing.

Continued

CLINICAL TIP

Overcoming Common Errors in Measuring Intake and Output (I&O)—*cont'd*

COMMON ERRORS	SUGGESTIONS
	2. If extreme measures are necessary, the dressing can be weighed before application and again when removed.
	3. If a fistula is present, a stoma bag should be applied to catch the drainage.
Failure to check a urinary catheter for patency when there is decreased drainage of urine. (It is sometimes too quickly assumed that decreased drainage from a catheter is due to decreased urine formation.)	Decreased drainage from a urinary catheter is an indication to check for patency before charting the absence of, or decrease in, urinary output.
Failure to obtain an adequate measuring device for hourly or more frequent checks on urinary output. (An error of even 10 mL could be significant when dealing with small amounts of urine.)	A collecting device calibrated to measure small amounts of urine should be used (see Fig. 2-7).
Failure to record the amount of solution used to irrigate tubes and the amount of fluid withdrawn during the irrigation	1. One method for dealing with this problem is to add the amount of irrigating solution to the intake column, and the amount of fluid withdrawn to the output column.
	2. Another method is to compare the amount of irrigating solution used with the amount of fluid withdrawn during the irrigation—if more fluid was put in than was taken out, the excess is added to the intake column; if more fluid was taken out than was put in, the excess is added to the output column.

result of evaporation). Ideally, urinary SG should be measured immediately after the specimen is collected; however, in some situations this is not possible.

To determine the variability in specimens tested immediately after voiding and at intervals up to 4 hours after voiding, a study of 20 ill infants with disposable diapers was conducted.[26] Urine was aspirated from each diaper immediately after voiding and tested with a refractometer. Subsequently, the diaper was folded, rolled, and taped so that the urine was not exposed to air, heat, or light. SG measurements of urine aspirated from each diaper at up to 4-hour intervals after voiding were not significantly different from those obtained at the time of urination.

INTAKE/OUTPUT AND BODY WEIGHT

Comparison of Intake and Output

Many serious fluid balance problems can be averted by maintaining a careful vigil on the patient's I&O and keeping accurate records. (Totals for several consecutive days should be compared.) If the total intake is substantially less than the total output, it is obvious that the patient is in danger of FVD. If the total intake is substantially more than the output, the patient is in danger of FVE (or, in the case of inappropriate secretion of ADH, water excess). To understand abnormal states better, it is helpful to review the 24-hour average I&O in a normal adult (see Table 2-1).

Balance of I&O is desirable only in steady-state conditions. In pathophysiological conditions, therapy is directed at promoting recovery. For example, in hypovolemic shock, as much as three times the volume of blood lost must be infused if the replacement fluids are crystalloids (such as isotonic saline or lactated Ringer's solution) to restore plasma volume to acceptable levels.[27]

It is important to initiate I&O records for any patient with a real or potential water and electrolyte problem: do not wait for an order from the physician.

1. Intake should include all fluids taken into the body (oral fluids, foods that are liquid at room temperature, IV fluids, subcutaneous fluids, fluids instilled into drainage tubes as irrigants, tube feeding solutions, water given through feeding tubes, and even enema solutions in patients requiring strict fluid intake recording, such as those in renal failure).
2. Output should include urine, vomitus, diarrhea, drainage from fistulas, and drainage from suction apparatus. Perspiration should be noted and its amount estimated. The presence of prolonged hyperventilation should also be noted because it is an important route of water vapor loss. Drainage from lesions (such as from large decubitus ulcers) should be noted and estimated.
3. The I&O record should include the time of day and the type of fluid gained and lost. This information is necessary in planning therapy.
4. The type of I&O record used often depends on the patient's condition. Patients with a severe fluid balance problem may require an hourly summary of their fluid gains and losses so that the fluctuating needs can be dealt with quickly. Many patients require only 8-hour summaries of their fluid gains and losses. A record suitable for this purpose, listing the volumes of containers used, should be available at the bedside.

Although it is not technically difficult to measure fluid I&O or to record the measurements, persistent effort is required to achieve an accurate account. Innumerable possibilities for error exist in the measurement and recording of fluid gains and losses; however, some errors occur much more frequently than others. Common errors and suggestions for overcoming them are shown in the Clinical Tip.

Pflaum[28] examined the accuracy of a routine I&O technique in a general hospital and found it lacking; when compared with measurement of body weight, the mean daily error was 800 mL. From these results, Pflaum concluded that measurement of I&O is of little value and that a more accurate indicator, body weight, should be adopted. Although it is generally recognized that I&O records are often sorely lacking, one should use I&O measurements *and* body weights to best evaluate a patient's fluid balance status. Unfortunately, body weight measurements are also often inaccurate. Kilfoy-Perez[29] reviewed the charts of 100 hospitalized patients on general medical divisions to compare acute fluid gains and losses to body weight changes. Only 52 of the 100 charts contained sufficient data to make these comparisons. Most of the 48 unusable charts were deficient in I&O recordings, but a few also lacked recordings of daily body weight measurements. Of the 52 usable records, a statistically significant, positive correlation was found between net differences in fluid and weight changes over a 48-hour period.

Body Weight Variations

Weighing patients with potential or actual fluid balance problems daily is of great clinical importance for the following reasons:

1. Accurate body weight measurements are usually easier to obtain than accurate fluid I&O measurements.
2. Rapid variations in weight, when measured correctly, reflect changes in body fluid volume.

When analyzing changes in a patient's weight, it is important to consider factors that may hinder the accuracy of weight measurement. For example, there may be errors in the weighing technique or in the recording of results, or the scales themselves may be faulty. A recent report, by means of a quality improvement program in which staff were held accountable for achieving accurate body weight measurements, showed a significant increase in both the number of weights performed as well as their accuracy; the improvements were attributed to use of written standards for the weighing procedure in addition to education programs on the topic.[30] Another recent study indicated that a small but significant percentage of scales in clinical use are inaccurate and imprecise to a clinically important degree.[31] The investigators perceived the problem to be related to breakage and wear rather than manufacturing defects. To minimize inaccuracies in weight measurements, medical institutions should test the accuracy of their clinical scales periodically. Before obtaining the patient's weight, it is helpful to test one's own weight on the scale to note any obvious discrepancy. Indicators of an inaccurate scale may include: one's own weight seems to be in error, a change greater than 1 lb occurs when one's weight is shifted on the scale's platform, the platform is wobbly, or other defects in the scale's structure are apparent.

The following practices should be followed in weighing patients:

1. Use the same scale each time because the variation among scales may be significant. Because this may present a problem when the patient is transferred from unit to unit, the need for accurate scales throughout an institution is obvious. This point emphasizes the need to test the accuracy of clinical scales routinely.
2. Measure weight in the morning before breakfast and after voiding.
3. Be sure the patient is wearing the same or similar clothing each time and that the clothing is dry.
4. If the patient is unable to stand for weighing on a small portable scale or a stand-on scale, use a sling-type scale. Wheelchair and under-bed scales are also commercially available.

Body weight as an index of fluid balance is based on the assumption that the patient's dry weight remains relatively stable. Over a short period (hour-to-hour), this assumption is valid, and changes in body weight reflect changes in body fluid volume rather than tissue mass changes. To assess these small hourly changes, it is necessary to use extremely accurate metabolic scales, which are not available on most patient care units.

Long-term (day-to-day) body weight variations reflect changes in tissue mass as well as body fluid volume. Thus, factors affecting tissue mass (caloric intake and metabolic status) must also be evaluated. Tissue loss occurs in catabolic states (such as severe stress) and tissue mass gain occurs in anabolic states. It is generally assumed that a relative deficit of 3,400 calories is needed to lose 1 lb of tissue mass; this deficit can be the result of inadequate caloric intake, increased metabolic rate, or both.

Body weight loss will occur when the total fluid intake is less than the total fluid output. In children, a rapid loss of 5% or less of total body weight indicates mild FVD, whereas between a 6% to 10% loss represents moderate FVD and a rapid loss of greater than 10% represents severe FVD.[32] Conversely, a rapid gain in body weight will occur when the total fluid intake is greater than the total fluid output.

A rapid body weight gain or loss of 1 kg (2.2 lb) is approximately equivalent to the gain or loss of 1 liter of fluid (or expressed another way, a gain or loss of 500 mL of fluid is equivalent to a gain or loss of 1 lb). A patient may have a severe FVD, although body weight is essentially unchanged or even increased, when there is a "third-space" shift of body fluid (see Chapter 3).

Bioelectrical impedance analysis (BIA) is sometimes used as a method to assess fluid balance. The principle of the BIA method is based on passing an imperceptible electrical current through the patient's body fluids (between surface electrodes applied to the patient's hand and foot). Adjacent electrodes measure the voltage drop across the body. Conductivity of the electrical current is far greater through the fat-free mass that contains most of the body's water than it is through fat (which is relatively anhydrous). Because bioelectrical conduction is related to water and its ionic distribution within the body, changes in body water or its electrolyte composition influence total body impedance. In a study in which researchers simultaneously measured fluid I&O and body weights, changes in the BIA readings correlated better with fluid I&O findings than did changes in body weight readings.[33] In summary, the researchers report that the speed and simplicity of this noninvasive bedside technique (which does not require active participation by the patient) and the information gained are the greatest assets of BIA.

EVALUATION OF LABORATORY DATA

Data from laboratory tests provide the nurse with valuable information about the patient's fluid and electrolyte status. However, it is important that specimens be collected properly to obtain valid results and that the findings be evaluated in light of the patient's history and clinical status. Treatment for an abnormality reported on an improperly performed laboratory test can be quite serious. For example, assume that the laboratory erroneously reports a serum potassium level of 8.0 mEq/L (due to an accidentally hemolyzed blood sample) in a patient with an actual serum potassium of 4.0 mEq/L. Initiation of aggressive treatment for nonexistent hyperkalemia could reduce the serum level to dangerously low levels. When in doubt, it is wise to confirm a grossly abnormal test result.

OBTAINING SPECIMENS

Peripheral Venous Blood Samples

Several general principles should be kept in mind when obtaining venous blood samples:

1. *Avoid drawing blood samples from a site above an infusing IV line.* Data indicate that specimens for serum biochemical and hematologic profiles should be drawn from the opposite arm or *below* the IV while it is infusing or out of the IV needle after the IV fluids have been stopped for 2 minutes.[34]
2. Take measures to prevent hemolysis of sample. This is particularly disruptive when the test is for serum potassium, magnesium, or phosphate levels. (Recall that these electrolytes are primarily found *intra*cellularly; rupture of the blood cells causes a falsely high reading of serum levels.) Measures to avoid hemolysis at the time of blood collection include[35]:
   - Allowing the alcohol applied to the skin to dry before performing the venipuncture
   - Avoiding overvigorous mixing of the blood in the collection tube
3. Avoid prolonged use of tight tourniquets and opening and closing of the patient's hand when drawing blood for potassium levels. Tight tourniquet application in combination with excessive arm exercise before venipuncture may cause a spurious elevation in potassium concentration.[36]
4. Repeated clenching and unclenching of the fist after the tourniquet has been applied is sometimes done in an attempt to make the veins more apparent; however, it may have a contributory role in artifactually elevating the plasma potassium concentration by as much as 1 to 2 mEq/L because exercise causes potassium to be released from the cells.[37]
5. Be aware that the blood-drawing procedure should be performed as skillfully and as atraumatically as possible. Watson et al.[38] suggest that when there is difficulty with phlebotomy, test results may show great variation and should be reviewed with care. The major cause of pseudohyperkalemia is mechanical trauma during venipuncture, resulting in the

release of potassium from red blood cells. (When this occurs, the serum will have a characteristic red tint as hemoglobin is also released.)[39]

Blood Sample Collection From Indwelling Catheters

Arterial and central venous catheters provide ready access to the patient's circulation and thus are used frequently in intensive care settings to collect blood samples. Although this is advantageous because it eliminates the need for numerous peripheral venipunctures, it can present a problem because blood specimens drawn from the catheters may be contaminated with whatever was administered through them. Therefore, the lines should be cleared before the collection of blood samples. A small volume of IV fluid (eg, 6 mL) is first withdrawn, and then a discard volume of blood (eg, 2–3 mL) is withdrawn before the actual sample is collected. The appropriate volumes to be discarded should be established by each laboratory.[40] A recent study showed that even small amounts of Ringer's lactate-containing solutions in catheters used for blood sampling to test for lactate may cause falsely elevated lactate results; the investigators emphasized that when blood specimens are drawn from indwelling lines, all IV solutions need to first be cleared from the line.[41]

Urine Samples

24-Hour Specimens

Because 24-hour urine specimens are often indicated in the measurement of urinary excretion of electrolytes, it is helpful to review the steps in the procedure:

1. Obtain a collection bottle from the laboratory; if a preservative is needed, it should be obtained with the bottle.
2. Follow directions from the laboratory with regard to any special preparation of the patient (eg, some tests may require dietary modifications or the withholding of certain drugs).
3. To begin collection, ask the patient to void and discard the specimen; note the exact time on the lab slip.
4. Save *all* urine for the next 24 hours and pour it into the collection bottle (omission of even one specimen invalidates the test).

5. Include a final voiding as close as possible to 24 hours after the initiation of the test (record exact finish time on the lab slip).
6. For infants, obtain specimens in pasted-on collection devices.
7. Be sure to explain the test to the patient and gain his or her cooperation. This is imperative for any successful 24-hour test (eg, patients who are using bedpans should be instructed to void before having a bowel movement, and not to place toilet paper in the collection container).
8. Remind the staff and patient (with signs) of the importance of saving all urine.

Single Urine Specimens

For a single urine specimen, the first voided morning specimen is ideal because of its greater concentration. However, a fresh specimen collected at any time is reliable for most purposes. To avoid false readings, the specimen must be collected in a clean container. Decomposition of urine begins within 30 minutes at room temperature and 4 hours at refrigeration.[42]

INTERPRETING TESTS USED TO MEASURE FLUID BALANCE

Blood and urine tests that can be used to assess fluid and electrolyte status are listed in Tables 2-2 and 2-3. Usual reference ranges for the tests and significance of variations are also included. Commonly used units of measures are reported with Système Internationale (SI) units in parentheses.

Laboratory reports in the chart should be reviewed at regular intervals to note the patient's current status and to detect trends in the data. Because normal ranges for laboratory tests vary slightly from institution to institution, it is necessary to evaluate results according to those listed by the laboratory performing the tests. Also, one must consider variables that can affect the results of specific tests.

TABLE 2-2.   Blood Tests Used to Evaluate Fluid and Electrolyte Status

Test	Usual Reference Range	Comments
Serum potassium	3.5–5.0 mEq/L (3.5–5.0 mmol/L)	Alterations in acid–base balance significantly affect potassium distribution: • Acidosis results in a shift of potassium out of the cells, causing serum potassium concentration to increase. • Alkalosis results in a shift of potassium into the cells, causing a decrease in serum potassium. • On the average, every 0.1-unit change in pH causes a reciprocal change of 0.5 mEq/L in plasma concentration.[43] There are a number of causes of factitious hyperkalemia: • Tight tourniquet around an exercising extremity (as in opening and closing the hand) can elevate potassium by shifting potassium from the cells to the serum. • Hemolysis of sample (as in traumatic venipuncture) releases potassium from blood cells into the serum, thus elevating the serum potassium level. • Leukocytosis in the range of 100,000/mm^3, as in leukemia, or platelet counts $> 400,000$/mm^3, as in thrombocytosis. (Leukocytes and platelets, which are rich in potassium, may release their large intracellular potassium stores during the clotting process.) In these conditions, there may be spurious elevations in the serum potassium concentration to as high as 9 mEq/L.[44]

TABLE 2-2.   Blood Tests Used to Evaluate Fluid and Electrolyte Status—*cont'd*

Test	Usual Reference Range	Comments
Serum sodium	135–145 mEq/L (135–145 mmol/L)	Serum sodium level is closely related to body water status: • For the adult, it can be roughly estimated that each 3–4-mEq elevation of serum sodium above normal range represents a deficit of about 1 L body water.[45] • An elevated plasma glucose level pulls water out of the cells into the extracellular fluid; by dilution, this lowers the plasma sodium concentration. In theory, every 62 mg/dL increment increase in plasma glucose will draw enough water out of the cells to dilute the plasma sodium concentration 1 mEq/L.[46] • The measured plasma sodium concentration may be artifactually reduced when marked hyperlipidemia is present.
Serum calcium	Total calcium: 8.9–10.3 mg/dL (2.23–2.57 mmol/L) Total calcium in serum is the sum of the ionized (47%) and nonionized (53%) components. The nonionized portion consists of calcium bound to albumin (40%) andthe portion (13%) chelated to anions (such as citrate andphosphate) Ionized calcium: 4.6–5.1 mg/dL (1.15–1.27 mmol/L)	Total calcium is the test performed in most clinical settings. To evaluate the actual calcium level, the clinician must first know the serum albumin level to apply the following rule: A fall in serum albumin of 1 g/dL decreases serum calcium about 0.8 mg/dL (0.2 mmol/L).[47] Hypocalcemia produced by hypoalbuminemia does not produce symptoms because the critical determinant of calcium action is the ionized fraction that remains unchanged.[48] Alkalosis lowers the ionized calcium level by increasing the binding of calcium to albumin. Other factors that can acutely lower ionized calcium are increased levels of lactate, bicarbonate, citrate, phosphate, and some substances in radiographic contrast media. Most laboratories have the capability to directly measure the ionized calcium level. This is desirable especially in critically ill patients, because it is the ionized level that is physiologically active and is clinically important.
Serum magnesium	1.3–2.1 mEq/L (0.65–1.05 mmol/L)	Hemolysis of the sample will invalidate the results by releasing magnesium from the red blood cells into the serum (recall that magnesium is primarily an intracellular ion).
Serum chloride	97–110 mEq/L (97–110 mmol/L)	• Less than normal concentration indicates hypochloremia (commonly associated with hypokalemia and metabolic alkalosis). • Greater than normal concentration indicates hyperchloremia, which may be associated with excessive administration of isotonic saline.

Continued

● **TABLE 2-2.** Blood Tests Used to Evaluate Fluid and Electrolyte Status—*cont'd*

Test	Usual Reference Range	Comments
Carbon dioxide content	22–31 mEq/L (22–31 mmol/L)	• This test measures total bicarbonate and carbonic acid in venous blood and is a general measure of the degree of alkalinity or acidity. (It should not be confused with the partial pressure of carbon dioxide, PCO_2, obtained from arterial blood gas analysis.) • A level below normal indicates metabolic acidosis. • In the absence of chronic obstructive pulmonary disease, an elevated level indicates metabolic alkalosis.
Serum phosphate	2.5–4.5 mg/dL (0.81–1.45 mmol/L)	• Hemolysis of the sample will invalidate the results by releasing phosphate from the red blood cells into the serum (recall that phosphate is primarily an intracellular ion). • Phosphate levels are evaluated in relation to calcium levels because there is an inverse relationship between the two (eg, an increased phosphorus level causes the calcium level to decrease). • Phosphate levels are normally higher in children than in adults. • Drugs containing high phosphate levels may temporarily increase the serum phosphate level for several hours after the dose. • Insulin promotes entry of extracellular phosphorus into cells. • Intravenous glucose running before or at the time of the test causes a lowered serum phosphorus level (due to carbohydrate metabolism).
Plasma ammonia	11–35 μmol/L (reported values vary according to laboratory)	• The body is less able to handle high ammonia levels when the serum potassium level is low or when alkalosis is present. • Ammonia level varies with protein intake and is affected by some antibiotics.
Serum osmolality	280–295 mOsm/kg Can be measured by lab or can be calculated by the following formula: $$pOsm = 2(Na) + \frac{G}{18} + \frac{BUN}{2.4}$$	• Serum osmolality is determined mainly by serum sodium concentration (recall that serum sodium makes up 90% of the osmotic pressure generated by plasma). • Finding is increased in dehydration (hypernatremia). • Finding is decreased in overhydration (hyponatremia). • Finding is increased in hyperglycemia and in presence of elevated blood urea nitrogen (BUN).
Anion gap	12 ± 2 mEq/L $AG = Na - (Cl + HCO_3)$	• Anion gap is useful in ascertaining cause of metabolic acidosis. • A level > 14 mEq/L indicates presence of excessive organic acid (as in diabetic ketoacidosis, lactic acidosis, uremic renal failure, and salicylate intoxication). • Normal anion gap acidosis may be due to diarrhea, ureterostomies, excessive chloride administration, and distal tubular acidosis.

TABLE 2-2. Blood Tests Used to Evaluate Fluid and Electrolyte Status—*cont'd*

Test	Usual Reference Range	Comments
BUN	8–25 mg/dL (2.9–8.9 mmol/L)	• Elevated BUN can be due to reduced renal blood flow secondary to fluid volume deficit (causing reduced urea clearance). • Excessive protein intake can elevate BUN by increasing urea production. • Increased catabolism due to trauma, starvation, bleeding into the intestines, or catabolic drugs can also increase the BUN by increasing urea production. • A low BUN is often associated with overhydration and may also be associated with low protein intake.
Creatinine	0.6–1.5 mg/dL (53–133 µmol/L)	• As an indicator of renal disease is more specific and sensitive than BUN because nonrenal causes of elevation are few. • In patients with large muscle mass of acromegaly, it may be slightly above normal. • A slightly elevated creatinine level may occur in severe fluid volume depletion, which results in a reduced glomerular filtration rate.
BUN/ creatinine ratio	10:1 (approximate)	This ratio is useful in evaluating hydration status: • When the ratio increases in favor of the BUN (ratio > 10:1), conditions such as hypovolemia, low perfusion pressures to the kidney, or increased protein metabolism may be present. • When the ratio is < 10:1, conditions such as low protein intake, hepatic insufficiency, or repeated dialysis may be present. • When both the BUN and creatinine level rise, maintaining the 10:1 ratio, the problem is likely intrinsic renal disease (although it may also be seen when fluid volume depletion results in reduction in the glomerular filtration rate).
Hematocrit (%)	Male: 44–52 Female: 39–47	• Hematocrit determines the percentage of red blood cells in plasma. • Changes are interpretable in terms of fluid balance only when no changes in the red blood cell mass (such as bleeding or hemolysis) are occurring. • Hematocrit is elevated in fluid volume deficit (because red blood cells are contained in a relatively smaller plasma fluid volume). • Hematocrit is decreased in fluid volume excess (because the red blood cells are contained in a relatively larger plasma fluid volume).

Continued

● **TABLE 2-2.** Blood Tests Used to Evaluate Fluid and Electrolyte Status—*cont'd*

Test	Usual Reference Range	Comments
Fasting plasma glucose	65–110 mg/dL (3.58–6.05 mmol/L)	A markedly elevated glucose level in bloodstream causes osmotic diuresis and resultant fluid volume deficit. • Results will be elevated above baseline if patient is receiving parenteral glucose (regardless of site from which the specimen is drawn).[49]
Plasma lactate (venous blood)	0.6–1.7 mEq/L (0.6–1.7 mmol/L)	• Lactic acidosis is considered to be present if the plasma lactate level is > 4–5 mEq/L in an acidemic patient.[50] • Most cases of lactic acidosis are due to marked tissue hypoperfusion. • Venous specimens are usually used for convenience, even though they may yield higher results than arterial specimens. Venous and arterial levels are virtually alike if the patient remains at complete bedrest before sample collection; hand clenching can significantly raise blood lactate levels.[51]
Albumin	3.5–4.8 g/dL (35–48 g/L)	• Decreased serum albumin level causes reduced colloidal osmotic pull in intravascular space, allowing fluid to shift to the interstitial space and produce edema. • It is important to know the albumin level when evaluating total calcium values.

● **TABLE 2-3.** Urine Tests Used to Evaluate Fluid and Electrolyte Status

Test	Usual Reference Range	Comments

Urinary sodium	No fixed normal values—kidneys vary rate of excretion to match dietary intake
	Sodium excretion in urine is usually 30–280 mmol/24 hr[52]
	Random specimen usually contains > 40 mEq/L[53]
		• Urinary sodium is helpful in assessing volume status, diagnosing hyponatremia and acute renal failure, and assessing dietary compliance in patients on sodium-restricted diets
		• < 20 mEq/L in hypovolemic states, reflecting renal sodium conservation to maintain blood volume.[54]
		• > 40 mEq/L in hypovolemic states associated with the following[5]
		  —Underlying renal disease
		  —Osmotic diuresis
		  —Hypoaldosteronism
		• > 40 mEq/L in SIADH*[56]
		• Important to record dietary intake during 24-hr period because measurement of urinary sodium without knowledge of dietary intake is of limited value.
		• Urinary sodium levels must be evaluated in light of total clinical picture.

TABLE 2-3. Urine Tests Used to Evaluate Fluid and Electrolyte Status *(Continued)*

Test	Usual Reference Range	Comments
Urinary potassium	No fixed normal values. Kidneys vary rate of excretion to match dietary intake and endogenous production Random specimen usually > 40 mEq/L[57] If potassium depletion occurs, urinary potassium excretion can fall to a minimum of 5–25 mEq/24 hr[58]	• Primary use of 24-hr urine measurement of potassium is to assess cause of hypokalemia. • Low value suggests nonrenal potassium loss (usually from the gastrointestinal tract) or diuretic use (if urine collected after diuretic effect has worn off). • In contrast, if > 25 mEq is excreted in the urine of a hypokalemic patient, there is at least a component of renal potassium wasting.[59]
Urinary chloride	110–250 mEq/24 hr (110–250 mmol/24 hr) Varies with salt intake	• Usually similar to that of sodium in hypovolemic states because sodium and chloride are generally reabsorbed together[60] • Helpful in differentiating between types of metabolic alkalosis[61] —< 25 mEq/L when metabolic alkalosis is due to vomiting, gastric suction, or diuretic use (late). —Usually > 40 mEq/L when metabolic alkalosis is due to mineralocorticoid excess, profound (< 2.0 mEq/L) hypokalemia, or early diuretic use.
Urinary calcium (quantitative)	100–300 mg/24 hr in adults (depends on dietary intake)[62]	• Increase in hypercalcemia associated with metastatic tumors • May be quite low when hypocalcemia present
Urinary specific gravity (SG)	Varies from 1.003 to 1.035[63] 1.016–1.022 (with normal fluid intake)[64]	• SG depends on the state of hydration and varies with the urine volume and solute load to be excreted. • SG is elevated in fluid volume deficit as the normal kidney seeks to retain needed fluid and thus excreted solutes in a small concentrated urine volume. • Urines < 1.007 SG are called hyposthenuria.[65] • SG fixed at 1.010 signals significant renal disease (isothenuria). • Heavy molecules such as glucose, albumin, or radiocontrast dyes will elevate SG out of proportion to the actual concentration. Thus, it is more accurate to measure urine osmolality in patients with glucosuria, proteinuria, or recent use of radiopaque dyes.
Urine osmolality	Maximally diluted and concentrated urine shows osmolalities between 50–1,400 mOsm/L[66] Correlates fairly well with urinary SG unless larger molecules (such as glucose or albumin) are present[67] SG 1.000 Osmolality 0 mOsm/L SG 1.010 Osmolality 350 mOsm/L	• Simultaneous measurement of serum and urine osmolality is a more accurate way to measure renal concentrating ability than is urinary SG.

Continued

● **TABLE 2-3.**   Urine Tests Used to Evaluate Fluid and Electrolyte Status *(Continued)*

Test	Usual Reference Range	Comments
	SG 1.020 Osmolality 700 mOsm/L SG 1.030 Osmolality 1,050 mOsm/L	
Urinary pH	4.6–8.0[68] (average is 6.0)	• Urine pH reflects serum pH and helps confirm the presence of acidosis or alkalosis (with the exception of paradoxical aciduria in hypokalemic alkalosis, alkaline urine due to urea-splitting infections, and alkaline urine in renal tubular acidosis). • Urine pH is increased with use of alkalinating agents such as sodium bicarbonate and potassium citrate. • Urine pH is decreased with the use of acidifying agents such as ascorbic acid, sodium acid phosphate, and methenamine mandelate. • Urine pH fluctuates throughout the day. • Specimen should be examined soon after collection because urine that is left standing too long becomes alkaline due to bacterial-induced splitting of urea into ammonia.

*SIADH, syndrome of inappropriate antidiuretic hormone secretion.

REFERENCES

1. Arieff A, Defronzo R, eds. *Fluid, Electrolyte, Acid–Base Disorders*, 2nd ed. New York: Churchill Livingstone; 1995:11.
2. Guyton A, Hall J. *Human Physiology and Mechanisms of Disease*, 6th ed. Philadelphia: WB Saunders; 1997:242.
3. Porth C. Physiology of thirst and drinking: Implications for nursing practice. *Heart Lung* 1992;21:273.
4. Phillips P, Bretherton M, Johnston C, Gray L. Reduced osmotic thirst in healthy elderly men. *Am J Physiol* 1991;261:R166.
5. Gorelick M, Shaw K, Murphy K. Validity and reliability of clinical signs in the diagnosis of dehydration [Abstr]. *Acad Emerg Med* 1996;3:395.
6. Lapides J, Bourne R, MacLean L. Clinical signs of dehydration and extracellular fluid loss. *JAMA* 1965;191:413.
7. Willis P. Inspection of the neck veins. *Heart Dis Stroke* 1994;3:9.
8. Duggan C, Refat M, Hashem M, et al. How valid are clinical signs of dehydration in infants? *J Pediatr Gastroenterol Nutr* 1996;22:56.
9. Gross C, Lindquist R, Woolley A, et al. Clinical indicators of dehydration severity in elderly patients. *J Emerg Med* 1992;10:257.
10. Rose B. *Clinical Physiology of Acid-Base and Electrolyte Disorders*, 4th ed. New York: McGraw-Hill; 1994:447.
11. Ibid, p 450.
12. Carey C, Lee H, Woeltje K. *The Washington Manual of Medical Therapeutics*, 29th ed. Philadelphia: Lippincott-Raven; 1998:41.
13. Ibid, p 119.
14. Ibid.
15. Sims L, D'Amico D, Stiesmeyer J, Webster J. *Health Assessment in Nursing*. Redwood City, CA: Addison-Wesley; 1995:467.
16. Arieff, Defronzo, p 115.
17. Ibid, p 455.
18. Schwartz S, Shires T, Spencer F. *Principles of Surgery*, 7th ed. Baltimore, MD: Williams & Wilkins; 1999:58.
19. Ibid.
20. Condon R, Nyhus L. *Manual of Surgical Therapeutics*, 9th ed. Boston: Little, Brown; 1996:200.
21. Kokko J, Tannen R. *Fluids and Electrolytes*, 3rd ed. Philadelphia: WB Saunders; 1996:4.
22. Bickley L. *A Guide to Physical Examination and History Taking*, 7th ed. Philadelphia: Lippincott, Williams & Wilkins; 1999:297.
23. Halck S et al. Reliability of central venous pressure measured by water column (Letter). *Crit Care Med* 1990;18:461.
24. Hudak C, Gallo B, Morton P. *Critical Care Nursing*, 7th ed. Philadelphia: Lippincott-Raven; 1998:235.
25. Pestana C. *Fluids and Electrolytes in the Surgical Patient*, 4th ed. Baltimore, MD: Williams & Wilkins; 1989:223.
26. Stebor A. Posturination time and specific gravity in infants' diapers. *Nurs Res* 1989;38(4):244.
27. Schwartz, p 107.
28. Pflaum S. Investigation of intake-output as a means of assessing body fluid balance. *Heart Lung* 1979;8:495.
29. Kilfoy-Perez L. Comparison of acute fluid gains and losses to body weight changes. Unpublished master's thesis, Saint Louis University School of Nursing, 1994.
30. Savage S, Wilkinson M. Patient weights: From physician complaints to improved nursing practice through quality improvement. *Gastroenterol Nurs* 1994;16(6):264.
31. Schlegal-Pratt K, Heizer W. The accuracy of scales used to weigh patients. *Nutr Clin Pract* 1990;5(6):254.

32. Kokko, Tannen, p 283.
33. Mequid M, Lukaski H, Tripp M, Rosenburg J, Parker F. Rapid bedside method to assess changes in postoperative fluid status with bioelectrical impedance analysis. *Surgery* 1992; 112:502.
34. Watson K, O'Kell R, Joyce J. Data regarding blood drawing sites in patients receiving intravenous fluids. *Am J Clin Pathol* 1983;79:119.
35. Henry J. *Clinical Diagnosis & Management by Laboratory Methods*, 19th ed. Philadelphia: WB Saunders; 1996:16.
36. Narins R, ed. *Clinical Disorders of Fluid and Electrolyte Metabolism*, 5th ed. New York: McGraw-Hill; 1994:707.
37. Rose, p 827.
38. Watson et al, p 119.
39. Rose, p 827.
40. Henry, p 19.
41. Jackson E et al. Effects of crystalloid solutions on circulating lactate concentrations: Part 1. Implications for the proper handling of blood specimens obtained from critically ill patients. *Crit Care Med* 1997;25(11):1840.
42. Lehmann C. *Saunders Manual of Clinical Laboratory Science.* Philadelphia: WB Saunders; 1998:777.
43. Condon, Nyhus, p 184.
44. Rose, p 827.
45. Condon, Nyhus, p 188.
46. Rose, p 668.
47. Carey et al, p 40.
48. Arieff, DeFronzo, p 448.
49. Watson et al, p 119.
50. Rose, p 555.
51. Henry, p 207.
52. Ibid, p 147.
53. Condon, Nyhus, p 196.
54. Rose, p 398.
55. Ibid.
56. Ibid, p 674.
57. Condon, Nyhus, p 196.
58. Rose, p 383.
59. Ibid.
60. Rose, p 490.
61. Ibid.
62. Henry, p 1455.
63. Ibid, p 144.
64. Ibid, p 1457.
65. Ibid, p 416.
66. Ibid, p 144.
67. Rose, p 648.
68. Henry, p 1456.

Overview of Fluid and Electrolyte Problems
Nursing Considerations

CHAPTER 3

Fluid Volume Imbalances

Fluid volume imbalances are commonly seen in nursing practice. Although they may occur alone, they most frequently occur in combination with other imbalances. Thus, events leading to fluid volume disturbances also frequently lead to electrolyte problems. For the purposes of this chapter, however, fluid volume imbalances are discussed in their "pure" form, that is, without the presence of other disturbances. The nurse can do much to prevent the occurrence of fluid volume imbalances or at least decrease their severity. This chapter describes assessment for fluid volume disturbances and explains rationales for nursing interventions.

● ISOTONIC FLUID VOLUME DEFICIT

Fluid volume deficit (FVD) results when water and electrolytes are lost in an isotonic fashion (Fig. 3-1). It should not be confused with the term *dehydration*, which refers to a loss of water alone (leaving the patient with sodium excess). FVD may occur alone or in combination with other imbalances. Unless other imbalances are present concurrently, serum electrolyte levels remain essentially unchanged.

ETIOLOGICAL FACTORS

Fluid volume deficit is almost always due to loss of body fluids and occurs more rapidly when coupled with decreased intake for any reason. It is possible to develop FVD solely on the basis of inadequate intake, provided the decreased intake is prolonged.

Losses of Gastrointestinal Fluids

Many liters of gastrointestinal (GI) secretions are produced each day; most of these secretions are reabsorbed in the ileum and proximal colon, leaving only about 150 mL of relatively electrolyte-free fluid to be excreted daily in the feces. When any abnormal route of loss is present, such as vomiting, diarrhea, GI suction, fistulas, or drainage tubes, it becomes evident how large losses can occur (resulting in FVD).

Fluids trapped in the GI tract, as is the case with intestinal obstruction, are physiologically outside the body (third-space effect). Indeed, any condition that interferes with the absorption of fluids from the GI tract can cause serious FVD.

Polyuria

Any condition that causes excessive urine formation can produce FVD. This situation is commonly seen in patients with profound hyperglycemia, as either diabetic ketoacidosis or nonketotic hyperosmolar syndrome. To excrete a large solute load, the kidneys must also excrete a large urine volume. Polyuria is also associated with a large solute load in patients receiving hyperosmolar tube feedings. No matter what the cause of the high solute load, absence of sufficient exogenous fluid to allow for excretion of the solute will cause fluid to be "pulled in" from the plasma, tissue space, and even from the cells to promote urinary excretion.

Fever

An elevated body temperature can cause FVD if extra fluids are not supplied as indicated. Fever causes an increase in metabolism and, as a result, in formed

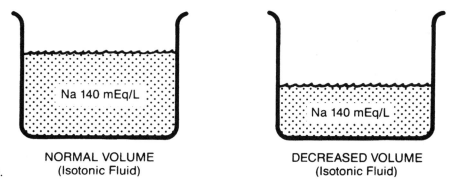

FIGURE 3-1.   Fluid volume deficit.

NORMAL VOLUME
(Isotonic Fluid)

DECREASED VOLUME
(Isotonic Fluid)

metabolic wastes that require fluid to make a solution for renal excretion; in this way, fluid loss is increased. Fever also causes hyperpnea, an increase in breathing resulting in extra water vapor loss through the lungs.

A temperature elevation between 38.3°C (101°F) and 39.4°C (103°F) generally increases the 24-hour fluid requirement in adults by at least 500 mL, and a temperature higher than 39.4°C (103°F) increases it by at least 1,000 mL.[1] A respiratory rate greater than 35/min further increases fluid needs.[2] Individual patients must be assessed clinically to determine precise fluid requirements.

Sweating

Recall that sweat is a hypotonic fluid containing primarily water, sodium, chloride, and potassium. Sweat can vary in volume from 0 to 1,000 mL/hr, or more. Thus, it is conceivable that a person can become volume depleted from severe perspiration in the absence of adequate fluid replacement. Frequently, a sodium imbalance is superimposed on the volume depletion (either hyponatremia if excessive water is ingested, or hypernatremia if no liquids are consumed).

Third-Space Fluid Losses

Because third-space fluid losses are unique in character, a separate section has been devoted to this subject immediately after the discussion of FVD.

Decreased Intake

Unfortunately, several circumstances can interfere with normal fluid intake. Among these are anorexia, nausea, and fatigue. Patients unable to swallow because of neurological impairment frequently have at least some degree of FVD. Others prone to this condition are patients who are reluctant to swallow because of oral or pharyngeal pain or those unable to gain access to fluids because of decreased mobility. Depression can be so severe as to interfere with normal fluid intake.

DEFINING CHARACTERISTICS

Fluid volume deficit can develop slowly or with great rapidity and can be mild, moderate, or severe, depending on the degree of fluid loss. Important characteristics of FVD are discussed below and listed in the Summary of Fluid Volume Deficit.

Weight Loss

Rapid weight loss reflects loss of body fluid because fluctuations in lean body mass do not occur quickly. For example, it has generally been assumed that it takes a caloric deficit of about 3,400 kcal to lose 1 lb (0.45 kg) of weight.[3] Theoretically, therefore, a typical adult on bedrest with a normal metabolism would have to take in zero calories to achieve a "real" weight loss of 1 lb in 2 days. On the other hand, 1 liter of fluid weighs about 2 lb; this amount of fluid can easily be lost in a short period. Indeed, some patients can quickly lose much more than this.

Decreased Skin and Tongue Turgor

In most healthy persons, pinched skin will immediately fall back to its original position when released. This elastic property, or turgor, is partially dependent on interstitial fluid volume. In a person with FVD, the skin may remain slightly elevated for many seconds after being pinched, indicating a deficit of fluid in the interstitial compartment (one segment of extracellular fluid [ECF]). It is important to remember that because tissue turgor also reflects the degree of skin elasticity, it is less valid as a sign of FVD in patients older than 55 to 60 years (because skin elasticity decreases with age). Although reduced skin turgor is an important finding, it is possible that turgor will appear normal in some individuals with fluid deficit (eg, this may occur when the deficit is mild or in obese patients with fat stores that interfere with turgor assessment).

In a person with FVD, the tongue is smaller and has additional longitudinal furrows, again reflecting loss of interstitial fluid. Fortunately, tongue turgor is not affected appreciably by age and thus is a useful assessment for all age groups. In a recent study of 55 emergency room patients, ranging in age from 61 to 98 years, tongue dryness and increased longitudinal tongue furrows were found to be good indicators of FVD (as were dry oral mucous membranes, sunken eyes, confusion, speech difficulty, and upper body muscle weakness).[4]

Decreased Moisture in Oral Cavity

A dry mouth may be due to FVD or to mouth breathing. If due to FVD, all of the oral tissues will be dry. In contrast, if the dryness is due to mouth breathing, the areas where the gums and cheek membranes meet will remain moist. If the serum sodium is elevated in conjunction with FVD, the mucous membranes will be dry and sticky.

Decreased Urinary Output

Decreased urinary output reflects inadequate perfusion of the kidney because there is not enough ECF to bring the requisite amount of plasma to the glomeruli. A urine volume less than 30 mL/hr in an adult is cause for concern if it persists. One must be constantly aware that persistent oliguria in the severely volume-depleted patient can result in renal tubular damage (discussed later in this chapter).

Increased Urinary Specific Gravity

Elevation of urinary specific gravity (SG) is a reflection of compensatory fluid conservation by the kidneys. Urinary SG can range from 1.003 to 1.035 in normal situations. Thus, a healthy renal response would be one toward the upper limits of normal.

Disrupted Blood Urea Nitrogen/Creatinine Ratio

The blood urea nitrogen (BUN) level rises slowly out of proportion to the serum creatinine with a long-standing FVD of sufficient magnitude to reduce glomerular filtration rate, thus interfering with clearance of nitrogenous wastes.

Changes in Vital Signs

Body temperature is subnormal (sometimes as low as 35°C [95°F]), due to decreased metabolism, unless infection is present. In contrast, note that body temperature is often elevated in patients with water deficit (hypernatremia), also referred to as dehydration.

Postural hypotension and increased pulse rate are signs of hypovolemia. On changing from a lying to an upright position, a drop in systolic pressure greater than 15 mm Hg or an increase in the pulse rate greater than 15 beats/min suggests intravascular volume deficit.[5] The blood pressure should be assessed immediately on assuming the erect position and again after 2 to 3 minutes (if indicated) to determine whether the pressure drop is sustained. Postural hypotension with dizziness strongly suggests hypovolemia in the absence of autonomic neuropathy or use of medications that are associated with postural hypotension (such as sympa-

tholytic drugs for hypertension).[6] As fluid volume depletion worsens, blood pressure becomes low in all positions due to loss of compensatory mechanisms. As always, the patient's baseline blood pressure should be used to assess the degree of blood pressure drop (not the commonly accepted "normal" value of 120/80 mm Hg). It is interesting to note that blood pressure measured by a sphygmomanometer (with auscultation or palpation) may reflect a lower pressure than is found if arterial pressure is being simultaneously measured with an intra-arterial catheter, because peripheral vasoconstriction leads to decreased intensity of Korotkoff sounds. Tachycardia occurs as the heart pumps faster to compensate for the decreased plasma volume.

Changes in Central Venous Pressure

The jugular veins provide a built-in manometer to detect changes in central venous pressure (CVP), and thus fluid volume status, and do not involve an invasive maneuver. Direct measurement of CVP is frequently performed in acutely ill patients and will reveal a reading less than normal in those with FVD (provided cardiopulmonary function is not impaired).

Decreased Capillary Refill

Peripheral blood flow is diminished as a compensatory reaction to FVD. Therefore, measuring the time it takes for capillaries to fill after compression is helpful in detecting the degree of fluid depletion. A study of this phenomenon was done in 30 healthy infants (2–24 months of age) and indicated that normal capillary refilling occurs in 0.81 ± 0.31 second (as measured in the fingernail bed after applying just the amount of pressure needed to blanch the nail bed).[7] The amount of time it took for capillary refilling to occur in 32 ill infants with diarrhea was also assessed and compared with laboratory indicators of fluid depletion. The investigators found that:

- A refill time less than 1.5 seconds suggested either a normal volume or a deficit of less than 50 mL/kg.
- A refill time of 1.5 to 3.0 seconds suggested a deficit between 50 and 100 mL/kg.
- A refill time of more than 3.0 seconds suggested a deficit greater than 100 mL/kg.

Another group of investigators studied an outpatient sample of 102 children under the age of 4 years and found that increased capillary refill time is a good indicator of fluid depletion (as is decreased skin turgor and increased thirst).[8]

Other Changes

Altered sensorium is the result of decreased cerebral perfusion, secondary to decreased blood volume. Cold extremities reflect peripheral vasoconstriction, which occurs to build up central blood volume. The hematocrit is elevated above baseline due to loss of intravascular fluid and subsequent concentration of the formed elements of blood.

TREATMENT

In planning fluid replacement for the patient with FVD, it is necessary to consider usual maintenance fluid volume requirements and other factors (such as fever) that can influence fluid needs. When the deficit is not severe, the oral route is preferred for replacement, provided the patient is able to drink. However, when fluid losses are acute, the intravenous (IV) route is required. Chapter 10 discusses formulas used in determining maintenance as well as replacement fluid requirements.

Isotonic electrolyte solutions (such as lactated Ringer's or 0.9% NaCl) are frequently used to treat the hypotensive patient with FVD because such fluids expand plasma volume. As soon as the patient becomes normotensive, a hypotonic electrolyte solution (such as 0.45% NaCl) is often used to provide both electrolytes and free water for renal excretion of metabolic wastes. These and additional fluids are discussed in Chapter 10.

If the patient with severe FVD is oliguric, it is necessary to determine whether the depressed renal function is the result of reduced renal blood flow secondary to FVD (prerenal azotemia) or, more seriously, to acute tubular necrosis due to prolonged FVD. The therapeutic test used in this situation is the fluid challenge test. Initial management of oliguria includes the administration of a fluid challenge (such as 500–1,000 mL 0.9% NaCl over 30–60 minutes) while carefully monitoring the cardiopulmonary status.[9] During the boluses, urine output should be monitored frequently, as should breath sounds. Diuretics should be avoided until the volume deficit has been corrected. For patients with congestive heart failure (CHF) or respiratory diseases, fluid management is often titrated according to CVP or pulmonary capillary wedge pressure values.

Prompt treatment of FVD is imperative to prevent the occurrence of renal damage. If FVD is allowed to progress to acute tubular necrosis, the patient will require strict renal management (see Chap. 17).

NURSING INTERVENTIONS

1. Assess for presence, or worsening, of FVD:
   - Measure and evaluate intake and output (I&O) at least at 8-hour intervals; sometimes hourly measurements are critical. For a valid picture of the patient's fluid balance status, compare the total I&O measurements for 2 or 3 consecutive days (see section on I&O in Chap. 2).
   - Monitor body weight daily. Consider factors necessary to obtain accurate readings (see Chap. 2). Remember that an acute weight loss of 1 lb represents a fluid loss of about 500 mL.
   - Monitor for postural hypotension (ie, a drop in the systolic reading greater than 15 mm Hg when the patient is moved from a lying to a sitting position).
   - Monitor for tachycardia (pulse increase greater than 15 beats/min) particularly when the patient is moved from a lying to a sitting position.
   - Monitor skin and tongue turgor (see Chap. 2).
   - Monitor the condition of mucous membranes. Remember that oral membranes will be dry in a mouth breather regardless of fluid status. When in doubt, run a finger over the gum folds to determine whether dryness is present; if it is, FVD is likely present.
   - Monitor concentration of urine; be aware that a low urinary SG in the presence of oliguria is a sign of renal disease. In a volume-depleted patient, the urinary SG should be more than 1.020 (indicating healthy renal conservation of fluid).
   - Monitor BUN/creatinine ratio. In FVD, BUN will elevate out of proportion to serum creatinine level (see Table 2-2).
   - Monitor CVP and pulmonary artery wedge pressures if devices are in use. CVP monitoring is discussed in Chapter 2.
   - Monitor body temperature; be aware that it will drop below normal when isotonic FVD is moderate or severe, unless infection is present. (Rectal temperatures of 35°C [95°F] have been observed in severe FVD.)
   - Monitor level of sensorium; expect that it will decrease as FVD progresses in severity.

2. Give oral fluids if indicated.
   - Consider the patient's preferences when offering fluids.
   - Consider the type of fluid the patient has lost. For example, select fluids containing sodium and potassium for a patient who has a FVD due to vomiting. Table 3-1 lists the electrolyte content of commonly available beverages. See Table 13-1 for a summary of the electrolyte content of selected body fluids.
   - If the patient is reluctant to drink because of oral discomfort, select fluids that are nonirritating to the mucosa, and provide frequent mouth care (offer saline gargles and apply lubricant to lips).

   - Offer fluids at frequent intervals.
   - Explain the need for fluid replacement and attempt to gain the patient's cooperation.
   - Administer medications as needed if nausea is present to provide relief before fluids are offered.
3. Consider the following interventions for patients with impaired swallowing:
   - Assess gag reflex and ability to swallow water before offering solid foods; have a suction apparatus on hand.
   - Position the patient upright with head and neck flexed slightly forward during feeding (tilting the head backward during swallowing predisposes to aspiration because this position opens the airway).

TABLE 3-1. Electrolyte Content of Selected Beverages

Beverage	Sodium (mg)	Potassium (mg)	Calcium (mg)	Magnesium (mg)	Phosphorus (mg)
Orange juice, canned 8 fl oz	5	436	20	27	35
Tomato juice, 6 fl oz	657	400	16	20	35
Cranberry juice cocktail, bottled, 6 fl oz	4	34	6	4	4
Prune juice, canned, 8 fl oz	10	707	31	36	64
Tea, instant powder, 1 tsp	1	46	0	3	3
Coffee, powdered instant, 1 round tsp	1	64	3	6	5
Pepsi Cola, 12 fl oz	35	10	–	–	53
Coca-Cola Classic, 8 fl oz	9	–	–	–	41
Sprite, 8 fl oz	23	0	–	–	0
Thirst Quencher, bottled, 8 fl oz	96	27	0	2	22
Kool-aid, mix, prepared with sugar & water, 8 fl oz	18	0	0	–	–
Milk, 2% fat, 8 fl oz	122	377	297	33	232
Beef broth/bouillon, 1 cup	782	130	14	5	31
Chicken broth, Swanson, 1 cup	1,000	–	0	–	–

From Pennington J. *Bowes and Church's Food Values of Portions Commonly Used*, 17th ed. Philadelphia: Lippincott-Raven; 1998.

- Provide thick fluids or semisolid foods (such as puddings or gelatin). These are more easily swallowed because of their consistency and weight than are thin liquids.[10]

4. If the patient is unable to eat and drink, discuss the possibility of tube feedings with the physician.

5. Consult with the physician for parenteral fluid directives if the patient is unable to consume fluids by the enteral route. This intervention is important to prevent renal damage related to prolonged FVD. Be aware that the IV route is favored in acute situations and when large volumes of fluid are needed.

6. Be aware that a carefully kept I&O record is necessary to determine the amount and type of fluids to be administered. Usually, abnormally lost fluids are replaced in the volume that has been lost.

7. Be familiar with the usual types of fluids used to treat FVD (review treatment section above and see Chap. 10).

8. Understand principles of the fluid challenge test and parameters for nursing assessment (see treatment section above).

9. Monitor response to fluid intake, either orally or parenterally. If therapy is adequate, one should observe the following:
   - Increased urinary volume toward 40 to 60 mL/hr in adults
   - If previously hypotensive, increased blood pressure toward normal
   - Return of pulse rate to baseline
   - Improved sensorium and sense of vitality
   - Improved skin and tongue turgor
   - Decreased dryness of oral mucosa
   - Increased CVP, toward normal
   - Improved wedge pressure readings
   - Normal, or no worse, breath sounds
   - Decreased urinary SG as urinary volume increases
   - Increased body weight, toward preillness level

10. Report inadequate response to fluid therapy to physician and seek appropriate fluid directives before renal damage occurs.

11. Monitor patients with tendency for abnormal fluid retention (such as renal or cardiac problems) for signs of overload during aggressive fluid replacement. A cardiac patient requiring fluid replacement for FVD often requires monitoring with pulmonary wedge pressures or CVP determinations during fluid replacement.

12. When administering fluids, either orally or parenterally, consider other illnesses that are occurring concurrently. For example, patients with the syndrome of inappropriate antidiuretic hormone secretion (SIADH), potential or actual increased intracranial pressure, renal failure, or preeclampsia require complex management. (These conditions are discussed in later chapters.)

13. Take safety precautions if altered sensorium is present.

14. Turn patient frequently and apply moisturizing agents to skin to avoid skin breakdown.

15. Give frequent oral care.

CASE STUDIES

● **3-1.** An 80-year-old man developed FVD as a result of overzealous diuretic use. After a 13-lb weight loss over 4 days, the CVP dropped to 1 cm water. Skin turgor over the sternum and medial aspect of the thigh was poor (when skin was pinched, it remained elevated for 6 seconds). Urine output was low at 20 mL/hr and the BUN was greatly elevated at 80 mg/dL (normal, 10–20 mg/dL). Body temperature was 36.3°C (97.4°F), pulse was 96 and weak in volume, and blood pressure was 140/90 mm Hg supine and 122/84 mm Hg in a sitting position.

COMMENTARY: This patient had lost 6 liters of fluid in a relatively short period; his CVP was far below the normal level of 4 to 11 cm water. His BUN was elevated; the urine volume was low, particularly for an elderly person. These factors, plus positional hypotension and increased pulse rate, were indicative of FVD. Note that the body temperature was not elevated, probably reflecting the slowed metabolic rate associated with FVD not complicated by infection.

● **3-2.** A 35-year-old woman developed FVD after 4 days of severe diarrhea and poor intake. She weighed 119 lb on admission (preillness weight, 128 lb). Her BUN was 40 mg/dL and serum creatinine was 1.3 mg/dL. Skin turgor was poor and urine output was 15 mL/hr (SG 1.030). Blood pressure was 120/80 mm Hg recumbent and fell to 98/60 mm Hg when erect. Pulse was 110, weak, and regular.

COMMENTARY: This patient lost 7% of her body weight in 4 days; her BUN was twice normal, whereas her serum creatinine was normal. Postural hypotension, poor turgor, and oliguria all point to FVD.

Summary of Fluid Volume Deficit

ETIOLOGICAL FACTORS

Loss of water and electrolytes, as in:
- Vomiting
- Diarrhea
- Excessive laxative use
- Fistulas
- GI suction
- Polyuria
- Fever
- Excessive sweating
- Third-space fluid shifts

Decreased intake, as in:
- Anorexia
- Nausea
- Inability to gain access to fluids
- Depression

DEFINING CHARACTERISTICS

Weight loss over short period (except in third-space losses)
- 2% (mild deficit, such as 2.4 lb loss in 120-lb person)
- 5% (moderate deficit, such as 6 lb loss in 120-lb person)
- ≥ 8% (severe deficit, such as 10 lb loss or more in 120-lb person)

Decreased skin and tongue turgor

Dry mucous membranes

Urine output < 30 mL/hr in adult

Postural hypotension (systolic pressure drops by more than 15 mm Hg when patient moves from lying to standing or sitting position)

Weak, rapid pulse

Slow capillary refill

Decreased body temperature, such as 95°–98° F (35°–36.7° C) unless infection is present

Central venous pressure < 4 cm water in vena cava

BUN elevated out of proportion to serum creatinine

Urinary specific gravity high

Hematocrit elevated

Flat neck veins in supine position

Marked oliguria, late

Altered sensorium

Cold extremities, late

⬤ THIRD-SPACING OF BODY FLUIDS

Third-spacing of body fluids is a unique situation leading to decreased intravascular volume and largely presenting with the same characteristics as those of FVD. However, because it is more difficult to diagnose than direct loss of body fluids, it is discussed separately. In addition, third-space fluid losses are discussed in the clinical chapters dealing with specific conditions associated with this phenomenon.

DEFINITION

Third-spacing refers to a shift of fluid from the vascular space into a portion of the body from which it is not easily exchanged with the rest of the ECF. This sequestration of fluid is the result of an alteration in capillary permeability secondary to injury, ischemia, or inflammation.[11] The trapped fluid, although still technically within the body, is essentially unavailable for functional use. Termed *nonfunctional* because it is not able to participate in the normal functions of the ECF compartment, the third-spaced fluid might just as well have been lost externally. Fluid can be sequestered from the intravascular space into body spaces (such as the pleural, peritoneal, pericardial, or joint cavities) or it can become trapped in the bowel by obstruction or in the interstitial space as edema after burns or other trauma. Furthermore, it can be trapped in inflamed tissue, as in peritonitis, pancreatitis, or fasciitis.

Major considerations in differentiating the FVD associated with third-spacing from that associated with fluid lost through vomiting or diarrhea are that (1) the latter fluid losses can be observed and measured, whereas the former cannot, and (2) decreased body weight does not occur in third-spacing as it does in actual fluid loss. Indeed, patients with third-spacing may gain weight as IV fluids are administered to replace the diminished intravascular volume.

PHASES OF THIRD-SPACE FLUID SHIFTS AND ASSOCIATED CLINICAL MANIFESTATIONS

Third-space fluid shifts occur in two phases. The first is described above and involves a shift of fluid from the intravascular space into a nonfunctional fluid space. Clinical manifestations expected with a significant shift of fluid are essentially those of FVD because, although the fluid is in the body, it is functionally unavailable for use. During this period, expect the following:

- Tachycardia and hypotension (effective blood volume is reduced as the fluid shifts out of the vascular space)
- Urine volume less than 30 mL/hr in the adult (decreased plasma volume causes a fall in renal perfusion and, therefore, less urine formation)
- High urinary SG and osmolality (renal attempt to conserve needed water)
- Elevated hematocrit (red blood cells become suspended in a smaller plasma volume as the fluid shifts out of the intravascular space)
- Postural hypotension
- Low CVP
- Poor skin and tongue turgor
- Insignificant body weight changes

During this phase, the body attempts to compensate for the third-space losses of ECF by renal conservation of sodium and water. As with any cause of FVD, it is important to correct the reduced plasma volume before

renal perfusion is compromised to the extent that acute tubular necrosis occurs.

After a variable number of days, the fluid shifts back to the vascular space and may impose a temporary hypervolemia. Resolution of the third-space is slower than its accumulation. In some instances the shift of fluid back to the intravascular space occurs within 48 to 72 hours. In others, it may not occur for 10 days or longer.[12] For example, fluid shifts from major burns or peritonitis are generally reversed within 2 to 3 days, whereas those associated with septic shock may not occur until the underlying cause of the sepsis is addressed.[13] As the extra fluid in the tissues or body spaces shifts back into the intravascular compartment, it is excreted through the kidneys. Excessive fluid administration during the period when fluid is shifting back into the bloodstream may cause circulatory overload, especially in patients with cardiac or renal failure. Assessment is primarily directed at detecting hypervolemia before serious effects occur. For example, observe for polyuria (hourly urine volume may be as high as 200 mL as the excess fluid is excreted), distended neck veins (a sign of fluid overload), moist lung sounds, shortness of breath, elevated CVP, and elevated systolic blood pressure.

PATHOPHYSIOLOGY OF CLINICAL SITUATIONS ASSOCIATED WITH THIRD-SPACE FLUID SHIFTS

Sequestration of fluids (third-spacing) is at least partially the result of altered capillary permeability; therefore, the leaked fluid stems from the vascular space (a compartment of the ECF). Understandably, then, the leaked fluid has the same composition as the ECF. Very large fluid shifts may occur in conditions associated with third-spacing. If there is no oral or IV intake of fluid, the effective circulating volume will decline to a point at which hypotension develops. If fluids are replaced to maintain the vascular volume, the ECF volume will expand and be reflected in weight gain. It is important to note that redistribution of fluid within the body does not appear as a decrease in the patient's weight, nor does it show up on the fluid I&O records; instead, these losses can be detected only by physiological changes in organ function. Not only does weight loss not occur during acute third-spacing, weight may actually be gained as fluid is infused to help compensate for the diminished vascular volume.

Because the exact mechanism of third-spacing varies somewhat with the specific cause, it is helpful to consider each separately.

Nonthermal Trauma and Surgery

Traumatic injury results in redistribution of intravascular fluid into the area of injury, thereby reducing the functional ECF volume. The volume of third-spacing varies with the severity of injury. For example, a patient with a fractured hip may lose 1,500 to 2,000 mL of blood into the tissues surrounding the injury site.[14] Although this fluid will eventually reabsorb (over a period of days or weeks), the deficit can cause an acute reduction in the vascular volume if it is not replaced.

Varying degrees of third-spacing occur in surgical procedures and are related to tissue manipulation and injury. The amount of fluid lost from the extracellular space varies with the extent and nature of the surgical undertaking. Minor operative procedures (such as appendectomy) are associated with considerably less fluid sequestration than are major operative procedures (such as extensive retroperitoneal dissection).[15] For example, a simple laparotomy with a total small bowel exploration can result in 700 mL of ECF distributional loss, whereas an extensive colon resection can cause as much as 2 to 3 liters of ECF to sequester into the peritoneal cavity in 2 to 4 hours.[16] After abdominal surgery, particularly pelvic surgery, fluid accumulates in the peritoneum, bowel wall, and other traumatized tissues. Formation of a third-space after nonthermal traumatic injury occurs immediately and is maximal by 5 to 6 hours.[17] In the surgical patient, it is difficult to assess fluid loss due to sequestration into the interstitial compartment. Such unrecognized deficits of ECF during the early postoperative period are manifested primarily as circulatory instability.[18]

Burns

Altered capillary permeability of burned tissue results in an exudation of plasma at the burn site. There is also an increase in fluid flux across capillaries in nonburned tissue that apparently results from hypoproteinemia rather than an alteration in capillary permeability. Formation of edema occurs primarily in the first 24 hours, with the greatest losses being incurred during the first 8 to 12 hours in mild to moderate burn injuries and 12 to 24 hours with extensive burn injuries.[19] See Chapter 15 for a discussion of fluid resuscitation in burned patients.

Intestinal Obstruction

Patients suffering from mechanical intestinal obstruction or adynamic ileus may sequester large quantities of ECF equal to many liters. In acute intestinal obstruction, as much as 6 liters or more can accumulate within the lumen and wall of the gut.[20] (See Chap. 13 for a more in-depth discussion of intestinal obstruction.)

Inflammation of Intra-abdominal Organs

Important third-space fluid losses can occur into the peritoneum, the bowel wall, and other tissues in the presence of inflammatory lesions of the intra-abdominal organs. The extent of these losses may not be fully appreciated unless one considers that the total area of the peritoneum is 1.8 m^2, which is almost equal to the body surface area of the skin.[21] A peritoneal thickness increase of only 1 mm can potentially sequester 18 liters of fluid.[22]

Sepsis

Sepsis produces a generalized capillary leak that produces a decrease in the functional ECF volume (while producing interstitial edema). As sepsis persists, protein malnutrition produces hypoproteinemia, which in turn may increase the formation of edema. Other toxic insults to the capillary endothelium (as may occur secondary to snakebites or after the administration of certain drugs, such as interleukin-2) may result in the "capillary leak" syndrome.[23] In these situations, edema forms at the expense of the intravascular volume.

Pancreatitis

In pancreatitis, inflammation and autodigestion by pancreatic enzymes lead to peripancreatic edema as well as fluid loss into the retroperitoneal tissue; a dramatic decrease in plasma volume causes systemic hypovolemia. Clinical signs of fluid loss include hypotension, tachycardia, oliguria, and increased hematocrit due to hemoconcentration. (In the presence of hemorrhagic pancreatitis, the hematocrit may drop rather than elevate.) See Chapter 20 for a more in-depth discussion of fluid and electrolyte problems associated with pancreatitis.

Ascites

The major difference between the fluid shifts described above and the development of ascites in hepatic cirrhosis is the rate of fluid accumulation. Although the above conditions are associated with fluid shifts that typically occur fairly rapidly, cirrhotic ascites develops relatively slowly, allowing time for renal sodium and water retention to replenish the effective circulating blood volume. As a result, patients with cirrhosis typically present with symptoms of edema instead of hypovolemia.[24] An exception could theoretically occur if rapid fluid removal by paracentesis resulted in a quick shift of fluid from the vascular space to the peritoneum (resulting in hypovolemia). Rarely, paracentesis of as little as 1,000 mL may lead to circulatory collapse, encephalopathy, and renal failure in patients with hepatic insufficiency.[25] However, recent studies suggest that large-volume paracentesis (4–6 liters) can be safely performed in selected patients, provided certain precautions are taken (see discussion of paracentesis in Chap. 21).

FLUID REPLACEMENT

Treatment is directed at correcting the cause of the third-space shift of body fluids. As is the case with any cause of FVD, the reduced plasma volume must be corrected before renal damage occurs.

Although the choice of a replacement fluid depends on the existence of concomitant electrolyte abnormalities, most third-space losses are properly replaced with a balanced salt solution such as lactated Ringer's solution. Attempts to correct the fluid deficit with hypotonic solutions (such as 5% dextrose in water or half-strength saline) may result in clinically significant hyponatremia. Any deficits in red blood cell concentration may require correction by the administration of packed cells to maintain optimal oxygen-carrying capacity of the blood. Large quantities of replacement fluids are often needed to maintain an effective circulating volume. Plasma or plasma substitutes may also be considered for use in addition to replacement electrolyte solutions for patients who have suffered protein loss (as may occur in burns or peritonitis).

Fluid replacement therapy must be tailored to the patient's response. For example, during the first phase, when fluid has shifted from the intravascular space, the aim of fluid therapy is to stabilize blood pressure and pulse and maintain an adequate urine volume (usually 30–50 mL/hr) in an adult.

FLUID VOLUME EXCESS

Fluid volume excess (FVE) is the result of the abnormal retention of water and sodium in about the same proportions in which they normally exist in the ECF (Fig. 3-2). It is always secondary to an increase in the total body sodium content, which, in turn, leads to an increase in total body water. Because there is isotonic retention of both substances, the serum sodium concentration remains essentially normal.

ETIOLOGICAL FACTORS

This imbalance may be caused by simple overloading with fluids or by diminished function of the homeostatic mechanisms responsible for regulating fluid balance. Etiological factors can include:

1. Compromised regulatory mechanisms, as in CHF, renal failure, cirrhosis of the liver, and steroid excess.
2. Overzealous administration of sodium-containing fluids, particularly to patients with impaired regulatory mechanisms. The commonly used isotonic fluids, 0.9% NaCl and lactated Ringer's solution, contain sizable amounts of sodium and, if used to excess, can easily exceed the tolerance of patients with impaired regulatory mechanisms. Note that 0.9% NaCl contains 154 mEq/L sodium and that lactated Ringer's has 130 mEq/L.
3. Excessive ingestion of sodium chloride or other sodium salts in the diet. See Table 3-3 for sodium content of compounds used to improve the texture or flavor of food or to extend freshness. Other "hidden" gains of sodium may result from the use of proprietary drugs such as Alka-Seltzer or the frequent use of hypertonic enemas (such as Fleet enema).

DEFINING CHARACTERISTICS

The defining characteristics of FVE are linked to an excess of fluid in the extracellular compartment and are listed in the Summary of Fluid Volume Excess.

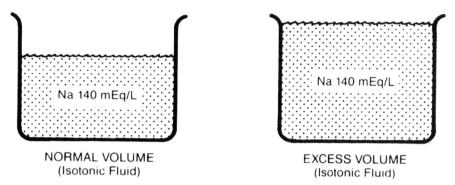

FIGURE 3-2. Fluid volume excess.

NORMAL VOLUME
(Isotonic Fluid)

EXCESS VOLUME
(Isotonic Fluid)

TREATMENT

When reversal of the primary problem is impossible, symptomatic treatment often consists of restriction of sodium and fluids and the administration of diuretics. In some conditions, only one of these therapies is necessary. Sodium-restricted diets and diuretic administration are discussed below, along with the effect of bedrest on mobilization of edematous fluid.

Sodium-Restricted Diets

Sodium content in foods may be expressed as grams of salt, milligrams of sodium, or milliequivalents of sodium. To understand conversions of grams of salt to grams of sodium, recall that sodium represents about 40% of the weight of salt (sodium chloride). Therefore, a gram of sodium chloride is equivalent to 0.4 g sodium. Dietary prescriptions are more sensibly stated in terms of sodium rather than salt content. A no-added-salt diet contains about 3 g sodium (132 mEq) per day; it is possible to restrict sodium intake to 2 g or even 1 g/day by limiting foods with high sodium content.[26] To convert milligrams of sodium to milliequivalents, divide the number of milligrams by 23 (the atomic weight of sodium); for example, 1,000 mg sodium is equivalent to about 43 mEq sodium.

The typical American diet contains about 10 to 12 g salt (NaCl) a day (or 4–4.8 g sodium).[27] About one-third comes from the salt shaker, one-third from processed foods, and one-third from the food itself.[28] Recall that processed foods often have hidden sources of sodium in the form of preservatives, such as monosodium glutamate, baking powder, baking soda, brine, and disodium phosphate. Tables 3-1 and 3-2 list the sodium and potassium contents of some common

beverages and foods. Table 3-3 summarizes the sodium content of common food additives. These figures clearly indicate how plentiful sodium is in the average diet.

Sodium-restricted diets are commonly prescribed for patients with fluid excess problems, such as occur with CHF, hepatic failure with ascites, renal failure, and hypertension. Some patients do well with only mildly restricted diets, whereas others require severe restrictions. A mild sodium-restricted diet requires only light salting of food (about half the usual amount) in cooking and at the table, no addition of salt to foods that are already seasoned (such as canned foods and foods ready to cook or eat), and avoidance of foods that are high in sodium. Examples of such foods include salty snack foods, olives, pickles, and luncheon meats.

Patients should be made aware that most canned and ready-to-eat foods already have added salt and thus should be used only as their specific diets allow. Foods that may be used freely include most fresh vegetables and fruits and unprocessed cereals. Cooking from scratch is usually the best way to prepare low-sodium food, and several excellent cookbooks are available for this purpose. Low-sodium baking powder can be found in the dietetic section of many grocery stores, and low-sodium milk, milk products, and bakery goods are available in most large cities. Patients on sodium-restricted diets should also consider the sodium content in over-the-counter drugs. For example, one Alka-Seltzer tablet (without aspirin) contains 958 mg sodium bicarbonate.[29]

Because a substantial portion of sodium is ingested in the form of seasoning, use of substitute seasonings plays a major role in cutting sodium intake. Lemon juice, onion, and garlic are excellent substitute flavoring agents, although some patients prefer salt substitutes.

TABLE 3-2. Sodium, Potassium, and Caloric Content of Selected Fruits and Vegetables

Food	Sodium (mg)	Potassium (mg)	Calories
Fruits			
Apple, raw with skin, 1 medium	0	159	81
Apricots, raw, 3 medium	1	314	51
Banana, raw, 1 medium	1	451	105
Grapefruit, raw, white	0	175	39
Grapes, American, (slip skin), 1 cup	2	176	58
Raisins, golden seedless, 2/3 cup	12	746	302
Orange, navel, raw, 1 medium	1	233	60
Vegetables			
Carrot, raw, 1 medium	25	233	31
Lima beans, boiled, 1 cup	4	955	216
Potato, baked, without skin, 1	11	641	145
Tomato, green, raw, 1	16	251	30

From Pennington J. *Bowes and Church's Food Values of Portions Commonly Used,* 17th ed. Philadelphia: Lippincott-Raven; 1998.

Most salt substitutes contain potassium and should be used cautiously by those taking potassium-conserving diuretics (Table 3-4) and by those who have renal impairment. Salt substitutes containing ammonium chloride can be harmful to patients with liver damage. (Salt substitutes are discussed further in Chap. 5 and are listed in Table 5-3).

 TABLE 3-3. Sodium Content of Common Food Additives

Additive	Sodium Content
Salt	2,325 mg in 1 tsp
Soy sauce, Kikkoman	3,074 mg in 1/4 cup
Baking soda (sodium bicarbonate)	1,368 mg in 1 tsp
Baking powder, Calumet	100 mg in 1/4 tsp
Yellow mustard	63 mg in 1 tsp
Catsup	178 mg in 1 tbl
A1 Steak Sauce	280 mg in 1 tbl

From Pennington J. *Bowes and Church's Food Values of Portions Commonly Used,* 17th ed. Philadelphia: Lippincott-Raven; 1998.

Diuretics

Diuretics are commonly used drugs that promote increased urine flow. More specifically, they act by inhibiting salt and water reabsorption by the kidney tubules. By inducing a negative fluid balance, these medications are useful in the treatment of conditions associated with FVE.

For the most part, diuretics can be grouped into three major classes:

1. Loop diuretics (such as furosemide, bumetanide, and ethacrynic acid), which act in the thick ascending loop of Henle
2. Thiazide-type diuretics (such as chlorothiazide and hydrochlorothiazide), which act in the distal tubule and connecting segment
3. Potassium-sparing diuretics (such as amiloride, spironolactone, and triamterene), which act in the cortical collecting tube

Examples of other diuretics are acetazolamide, a carbonic anhydrase inhibitor, and mannitol, a nonreabsorbable polysaccharide that acts as an osmotic diuretic.

To achieve excretion of excess fluid, either a single diuretic (such as a thiazide) or a combination of agents may be selected (such as thiazide and spironolactone). The latter combination is particularly helpful in that

TABLE 3-4. Commonly Used Diuretic Agents

Drug	Comments
Thiazides Examples: chlorothiazide (Diuril), hydrochlorothiazide (HCTZ)	Act by inhibiting sodium reabsorption in the distal tubule and, to a lesser extent, the inner medullary collecting duct Cause loss of sodium, chloride, and potassium Decrease urinary calcium excretion and sometimes result in slightly elevated serum calcium level Potassium supplements or extra dietary potassium may be necessary when these agents are used routinely.
Loop diuretics Examples: furosemide (Lasix), ethacrynic acid (Edecrin), bumetanide (Bumex)	Powerful diuretics that act primarily in the thick segment of the medullary and cortical ascending limbs of Henle's loop Cause loss of sodium, chloride, and potassium Potassium supplements or extra dietary K may be necessary when these agents are used routinely. Increase urinary calcium excretion.
Potassium-conserving diuretics Examples: spironolactone (Aldactone), triamterene (Dyrenium), amiloride (Midamor)	Cause loss of sodium and chloride Conserve potassium Spironolactone inhibits action of aldosterone (Recall that the hormone aldosterone causes sodium retention and potassium excretion.) Triamterene acts on the distal renal tubule to depress the exchange of sodium Effect of amiloride apparently due to inhibition of sodium entry into the cell from luminal fluid These drugs reduce potassium excretion and may lead to hyperkalemia; thus, potassium supplements are contraindicated, as are salt substitutes containing potassium. Often combined with thiazides for effective diuresis; in this case, the hypokalemic tendency of the thiazides may offset the hyperkalemic tendency of triamterene and spironolactone (examples of such combinations are Dyazide and Aldactazide).

the two drugs have different sites of action and thus allow more effective control of FVE.

Diuretics may be given orally or parenterally, depending on the particular agent to be administered and the status of the patient. For example, patients with advanced CHF may have difficulty in absorbing orally administered furosemide (due to decreased intestinal perfusion and perhaps intestinal mucosal edema).[30] In this situation, removal of edema with IV furosemide therapy and stabilization of cardiac function may partially correct this absorptive defect, thereby allowing oral therapy to be reinstituted.

Diuretics can have undesirable side effects, such as:

- Extracellular fluid volume depletion
- Hyponatremia
- Alterations in potassium excretion (hypokalemia and hyperkalemia)
- Magnesium wasting
- Alterations in calcium excretion
- Acid–base disturbances

Extracellular Fluid Volume Depletion

Depletion of the ECF volume is a common complication of diuretic use, especially when the potent loop-acting diuretics are used. Although the duration of sodium loss with diuretic use is limited, some patients have a relatively large initial response and develop true volume depletion.[31] This complication is most likely to occur in patients who are concurrently losing fluids from other routes (as in vomiting or diarrhea) or who are unable to take in sufficient amounts of salt and water. Clinical signs of fluid volume depletion include weakness, malaise, muscle cramps, and postural dizziness. Reduction of the effective circulatory volume decreases renal perfusion and can lead to prerenal azotemia, manifested by an increase in the BUN and plasma creatinine concentrations. In general, volume depletion causes a greater rise in the BUN than in the plasma creatinine level. If the patient has an underlying renal insufficiency, the ECF deficit can lead to overt uremia. Most fluid and electrolyte complications associated with use of diuretics occur within the first several weeks of therapy, provided that drug dose, dietary intake, and renal function remain stable.[32]

Hyponatremia

Hyponatremia is seen relatively frequently in patients taking diuretics.[33] Almost all cases of hyponatremia associated with diuretic use are due to a thiazide-type diuretic (as opposed to loop diuretics).[34]

Depression of free water clearance may occur in patients taking routine doses of thiazide diuretics.[35] Excessive water intake is to be discouraged in patients taking these medications.

Hypokalemia

Urinary potassium losses are increased by the thiazide and loop diuretics, often leading to the development of hypokalemia. There is some controversy regarding the seriousness of mild hypokalemia (plasma potassium levels between 3.0 and 3.5 mEq/L). Some physicians view the problem as relatively benign, whereas others believe it increases coronary risk. Although the mechanism for such risk is not known, a possible factor is increased ventricular arrhythmias associated with hypokalemia or hypomagnesemia. Among the potential problems associated with potassium depletion are cardiac muscle irritability (particularly when the patient is also taking digitalis); defects in renal concentrating ability, perhaps leading to interstitial fibrosis; sluggish insulin release, leading to carbohydrate intolerance; and predisposition to rhabdomyolysis (due to decreased striated muscle blood flow).[36] Urinary potas-sium loss and potassium depletion are most pronounced in patients who take diuretics and ingest large loads of solute and water; these individuals may need supplemental intake of potassium chloride.[37] However, the most appropriate way to eliminate excessive urinary potassium wasting is through restriction of dietary sodium intake (to about 87 mEq/day).[38] Obviously, the smallest dosage of a diuretic necessary to achieve the desired degree of fluid excretion should be used. Recent studies have indicated that lower dosages of diuretics than are commonly used are capable of achieving the desired effects without producing problems. For example, as little as 12.5 mg hydrochlorothiazide or 15 mg chlorthalidone (a thiazide-type agent) produce as large an antihypertensive effect as large doses, with little or no change in plasma potassium concentrations.[39–41]

Hyperkalemia

The potassium-conserving diuretics (such as spironolactone, amiloride, and triamterene) reduce potassium secretion and, as a result, can cause hyperkalemia. To prevent this problem, these drugs should be used with great caution (if at all) in patients with renal failure or in those treated with a potassium supplement or an angiotensin-converting enzyme inhibitor (which also decreases potassium secretion, perhaps by decreasing aldosterone levels).[42,43]

Magnesium Wasting

Magnesium depletion can be induced by thiazide and loop diuretics when they are administered chronically.[44] Oddly, although magnesium depletion is fairly common, most of these losses come from cellular stores because the plasma magnesium concentration often remains within the normal range.[45] A potential problem is cellular magnesium deficit with the increased possibility of cardiac arrhythmias. Magnesium depletion can also contribute to the development of hypocalcemia by reducing parathormone secretion.

Alterations in Calcium Excretion

Thiazide diuretics decrease urinary calcium excretion with both short- and long-term use.[46] Because of decreased calcium excretion in the urine, long-term thiazide administration may lead to overt hypercalcemia.[47] Amiloride also decreases calcium excretion. Conversely, bumetanide, furosemide, and ethacrynic acid increase urinary calcium excretion and, therefore, are useful in the treatment of acute hypercalcemic conditions.

Metabolic Acid–Base Disturbances

Hypokalemia occurring with use of thiazide and loop diuretics is often accompanied by metabolic alkalosis. In contrast, the potassium-sparing diuretics can result in both hyperkalemia and metabolic acidosis.

Bedrest

Bedrest alone can induce a diuresis, particularly in cases of heart failure. Mobilization of edematous fluid by the supine position is probably related to diminished peripheral venous pooling and a resultant increase in the effective circulating blood volume, and thus in renal perfusion.[48] Metabolic requirements of peripheral tissues are usually decreased by bedrest so that, in patients with CHF, there is less demand placed on the weakened myocardium. This action can transfer as much as 400 to 500 mL of interstitial fluid into the central circulation over a few days.[49] Bedrest can cause a 40% increase in glomerular filtration rate and a doubling of urinary sodium excretion in response to diuretics.[50]

NURSING INTERVENTIONS

1. Assess for the presence, or worsening, of FVE:
   - Monitor I&O and evaluate at regular intervals for excessive fluid retention.
   - Monitor changes in body weight; be alert for acute weight gain.
   - Assess breath sounds at regular intervals for presence, or worsening, of rales.
   - Monitor degree of peripheral edema; look for edema in most dependent parts of body (feet and ankles in ambulatory patients, sacral region in bedridden patients). Check for pitting edema (see Fig. 2-3) and measure extent of edema with millimeter tape.
   - Monitor degree of distention of peripheral veins.
   - Monitor laboratory values (look for low BUN and hematocrit; however, realize that there may well be other causes for abnormalities in these values, such as low protein intake and anemia).
2. Encourage adherence to sodium-restricted diet, if prescribed. Assist dietitian in diet instruction. Review section on sodium-restricted diets under treatment.
3. Instruct patients requiring sodium restriction to avoid over-the-counter drugs without first checking with the health care adviser.
4. When fluid retention persists despite adherence to dietary sodium intake, consider hidden sources of sodium, such as water supply or use of water softeners.
5. When indicated, encourage rest periods. Lying down favors diuresis of edematous fluid (see the above discussion in section on bedrest).
6. Monitor the patient's response to diuretics. Discuss significant findings with physician.
7. Monitor rate of parenteral fluids and the patient's response. Discuss significant findings with physician.
8. Teach self-monitoring of weight and I&O measurements to patients with chronic fluid retention (such as those with CHF, renal disease, or cirrhosis of liver).
9. Monitor for worsening of underlying cause of FVE. See Chapters 16, 17, and 21 for specific interventions for patients with cirrhosis and renal and heart failure.
10. If dyspnea and orthopnea are present, position the patient in semi-Fowler's position to favor lung expansion.
11. Turn and position the patient frequently; be aware that edematous tissue is more prone to skin breakdown than is normal tissue.

CASE STUDIES

● **3-3.** A 70-year-old woman with CHF was admitted to an acute care facility. In addition to distended neck veins and pedal edema, pulmonary edema was present. The CVP was 20 cm water and the BUN was 8 mg/dL.
COMMENTARY: See Figures 2-1 and 2-3 for examples of distended neck veins and pitting edema. Note in this case study the relatively low BUN, especially for an elderly person (indicating plasma dilution). The CVP was greatly elevated because normal is 4 to 11 cm water.

● **3-4.** A 10-year-old girl was inadvertently given 3.5 liters isotonic saline (0.9% NaCl) for 3 days postoperatively. A gain of about 6 lb over the admission weight was noted. According to laboratory data, the BUN was 6 mg/dL on the third postoperative day.
COMMENTARY: This is an example of fluid overloading during a period in which the kidneys were

Summary of Fluid Volume Excess

ETIOLOGICAL FACTORS

Compromised regulatory mechanisms:
- Renal failure
- Congestive heart failure
- Cirrhosis of liver
- Cushing's syndrome

Overzealous administration of sodium-containing IV fluids

Excessive ingestion of sodium-containing substances in diet or sodium-containing medications

DEFINING CHARACTERISTICS

Weight gain over short period:
- 2% (mild excess, such as 2.4 lb in 120-lb person)
- 5% (moderate excess, such as 6 lb in 120-lb person)
- $\geq$ 8% (severe excess, such as 10 lb gain or greater in 120-lb person)

Peripheral edema (excess of fluid in interstitial space)

Distended neck veins

Distended peripheral veins

Slow-emptying peripheral veins

Central venous pressure >11 cm water in vena cava

Moist rales in lungs

Polyuria (if renal function is normal)

Ascites, pleural effusion (when fluid volume excess is severe, fluid transudates into body cavities)

Decreased blood urea nitrogen (due to plasma dilution)

Decreased hematocrit (also due to plasma dilution)

Bounding, full pulse

Pulmonary edema, if severe

---

less able to excrete the excess. In the early postoperative period there is a tendency to retain fluids because of increased secretion of adrenal hormones (stress reaction). Fluid overload was reflected by the weight gain and low BUN. A review of the I&O record would also have reflected the problem. Had the staff paid attention to the far greater intake than output, the problem could have been alleviated early.

REFERENCES

1. Condon R, Nyhus L, *Manual of Surgical Therapeutics*, 9th ed. Boston: Little, Brown; 1996:200.
2. Ibid.
3. Alpers D, Stenson W, Bier D. *Manual of Nutritional Therapeutics*, 3rd ed. Boston: Little, Brown; 1995:90.
4. Gross C, Lindquist R, Woolley A, et al. Clinical indicators of dehydration severity in elderly patients. *J Emergency Med* 1992;10:267.
5. Kokko J, Tannen R. *Fluids and Electrolytes*, 3rd ed. Philadelphia: WB Saunders; 1996:4.

6. Rose B. *Clinical Physiology of Acid-Base and Electrolyte Disorders*, 4th ed. New York: McGraw-Hill;, 1994:395.
7. Saavedra J, Harris G, Song L, Finberg L. Capillary refilling in the assessment of dehydration. *Am J Dis Child* 1991;145:296.
8. MacKenzie A, Barnes G, Shann F. Clinical signs of dehydration in children. *Lancet* 1989;2:504.
9. Carey C, Lee H, Woeltje K. *The Washington Manual of Medical Therapeutics*, 29th. Philadelphia: Lippincott-Raven; 1998: 229.
10. Gettrust K, Ryan S, Engleman D. *Applied Nursing Diagnoses: Guides for Comprehensive Care Planning*. New York: John Wiley & Sons; 1985:17.
11. Schwartz S, Shires T, Spencer F. *Principles of Surgery*, 7th ed. New York: McGraw-Hill; 1999:57.
12. Ibid.
13. Narins R, ed. *Maxwell & Kleeman's Clinical Disorders of Fluid and Electrolyte Metabolism*, 5th ed. New York: McGraw-Hill; 1994:1424.
14. Rose, p 392.
15. Schwartz, et al, p 67.
16. Vannata J, Fogelman M. *Moyer's Fluid Balance*, 4th ed. Chicago: Year Book Medical Publishers; 1988:152.
17. Ibid.
18. Schwartz et al, p 67.
19. Carrougher G. Burn Care and Therapy. St. Louis: Mosby; 1998:108.
20. Ibid.
21. Schwartz et al, p 67.
22. Ibid, p 1517.
23. Szerlip H, Goldfarb S. *Workshops in Fluid and Electrolyte Disorders*. New York: Churchill Livingstone; 1993:7.
24. Rose, p 392.
25. Carey et al, p 341.
26. Tierney L, McPhee, Papadakis M. *Current Medical Diagnosis & Treatment*. Stamford, CT: Appleton & Lange; 1999:1195.
27. Szerlip, Goldfarb, p 15.
28. Ibid.
29. Shannon M, Wilson B, Stang C. *Appleton & Lange's 1999 Drug Guide*. Stamford, CT: Appleton & Lange; 1999:1477.
30. Rose, p 434.
31. Ibid, p 427.
32. Narins, p 561.
33. Rose, p 431.
34. Ibid.
35. Ashraf N et al. Thiazide-induced hyponatremia associated with death or neurologic damage in outpatients. *Am J Med* 1981; 70:1163.
36. Narins, p 561.
37. Ibid, p 562.
38. Ibid.
39. Johnston G, Wilson R, McDermott B, et al. Low-dose cyclopenthiazide in the treatment of hypertension: A one-year community-based study. *Q J Med* 1991;78:135.
40. Dahlof B, Hansson L, Acosta J, et al. Controlled trial of enalapril and hydrochlorothiazide in 200 hypertensive patients. *Am J Hypertens* 1988;1:38.
41. McVeigh G, Galloway D, Johnston D. The case for low dose diuretics in hypertension: Comparison of low and conventional doses of cyclopenthiazide. *R Med J* 1988;297:95.
42. Rose, p 430.
43. Narins, p 562.
44. Ibid, p 563.
45. Rose, p 432.
46. Narins, p 563.
47. Ibid.
48. Ibid, p 548.
49. Ring-Larsen H et al. Diuretic treatment in decompensated cirrhosis and congestive heart failure: Effect of posture. *Br Med J Clinical Research Edition* 1986;292:1351.
50. Szerlip, Goldfarb, p 15.

CHAPTER 4

Sodium Imbalances

SODIUM BALANCE

Disturbances in sodium balance frequently occur in clinical practice and develop under circumstances varying from the simple to the complex. These imbalances and the nurse's role in their management are discussed in this chapter. First, however, some basic facts about the role of sodium in physiological activities are reviewed.

Sodium is the most plentiful electrolyte in the extracellular fluid (ECF), with a concentration ranging from 135 to 145 mEq/L. More than 95% of the body's physiologically active sodium is in the ECF. In contrast, the intracellular concentration of sodium is small. Maintenance of this asymmetrical distribution across cell membranes requires transporting sodium out of the cell against an electrochemical gradient by the adenosine triphosphatase pump.

The fact that sodium does not easily cross the cell wall membrane, in addition to being the dominant electrolyte in quantity, accounts for its primary role in controlling water distribution as well as ECF volume. In general, a loss or gain of sodium is accompanied by a loss or gain of water.

Extracellular sodium concentration has a profound effect on body cells. A low serum sodium level (*hyponatremia*) results in a relatively diluted ECF and allows water to be drawn into the cells. Conversely, a high serum sodium level (*hypernatremia*) results in a relatively concentrated ECF and allows water to be pulled out of cells (Fig. 4-1).

The salt intake per day in the healthy individual varies between 50 and 90 mEq (3–5 g) as sodium chloride (NaCl).[1] More than this amount is readily available in the diet, in 1 liter of lactated Ringer's solution or isotonic saline (0.9% NaCl), or in 2 liters of half-strength saline (0.45% NaCl) (Table 4-1). The sodium balance can be maintained in a healthy individual over a wide range of intakes because the normal kidney can conserve or excrete sodium as needed.[2]

HYPONATREMIA

DEFINITION

Hyponatremia is probably the most frequent electrolyte disorder in clinical practice and refers to a serum sodium level that is below normal (135 mEq/L). A low serum concentration does not necessarily mean that the total body sodium is less than normal. In fact, many patients have hyponatremia when there is an excess of total body sodium (as occurs with congestive heart failure or cirrhosis of the liver). When marked hyperlipidemia or hypoproteinemia is present, the serum sodium may appear to be lower than it actually is (pseudohyponatremia).[3] These artifactual readings are rarely problematic because most laboratories measure plasma sodium by ion-specific electrodes.[4]

Syndrome of inappropriate antidiuretic hormone secretion (SIADH) produces a special kind of hyponatremia that is associated with excessive water retention. In conditions producing SIADH, there is either too much antidiuretic hormone (ADH) released or the renal response to the hormone is intensified. Release of ADH is termed *inappropriate* because in normal situa-

HYPERNATREMIA   **HYPONATREMIA**

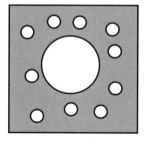

Normal cell size;
Normal serum Na
concentration

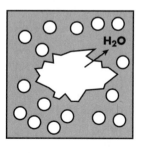

Cell shrinks
as H_2O is pulled
out of cell

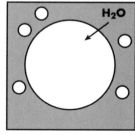

Cell swells
as H_2O is pulled
into cell

FIGURE 4-1. Effect of serum sodium level on cells.

TABLE 4-1. Approximate Sodium Content of Selected Parenteral Fluids

Parenteral Fluid	Sodium (mEq/L)
0.9% NaCl ("isotonic saline")	154
0.45% NaCl (half-strength saline)	77
0.33% NaCl	56
0.22% NaCl	38
0.11% NaCl	19
3% NaCl*	513
5% NaCl*	855
Lactated Ringer's solution	130

*Extremely hypertonic fluids.

tions a low serum sodium level would depress ADH activity.

PATHOPHYSIOLOGY

Hyponatremia may occur in four basic ways: (1) loss of sodium, as through the kidney, gastrointestinal (GI) tract, or skin; (2) gain of water, as in high ADH secretion; (3) shift of sodium into the cell, as may occur in potassium deficiency; and (4) shift of water from the cell to the ECF, as may occur in hyperglycemia or mannitol infusion.[5] For example, the serum sodium concentration may fall by about 1.6 mEq/L for each 100 mg/dL increase in glucose concentration.[6] A common imbalance, hyponatremia can range from mild to severe. When severe, it is often a marker of serious underlying disease. In addition, severe hyponatremia can itself cause major neurological damage and death. As noted in Figure 4-1, a decrease in the serum sodium concentration is expected to cause a shift of water from the ECF to the intracellular space, resulting in generalized cellular edema. Unlike other tissues, the brain's capacity to expand is limited by the bony cranium. Increased intracranial pressure resulting from brain edema may lead to herniation and death or irreversible brain damage.

As illustrated in Figure 4-2, hyponatremia can be superimposed on a normal fluid volume, on fluid volume deficit (FVD), or on fluid volume excess (FVE). Mechanisms accounting for hyponatremia coupled

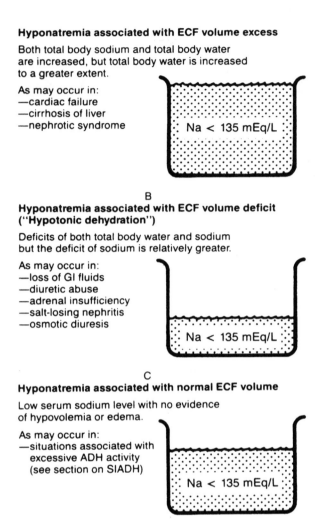

Hyponatremia associated with ECF volume excess

Both total body sodium and total body water are increased, but total body water is increased to a greater extent.

As may occur in:
—cardiac failure
—cirrhosis of liver
—nephrotic syndrome

Na < 135 mEq/L

B

Hyponatremia associated with ECF volume deficit ("Hypotonic dehydration")

Deficits of both total body water and sodium but the deficit of sodium is relatively greater.

As may occur in:
—loss of GI fluids
—diuretic abuse
—adrenal insufficiency
—salt-losing nephritis
—osmotic diuresis

Na < 135 mEq/L

C

Hyponatremia associated with normal ECF volume

Low serum sodium level with no evidence of hypovolemia or edema.

As may occur in:
—situations associated with excessive ADH activity (see section on SIADH)

Na < 135 mEq/L

FIGURE 4-2. Hyponatremic states.

with ECF volume excess in patients with cirrhosis of the liver and cardiac failure are described in Chapters 21 and 16, respectively. The effect of hyperglycemia on the serum sodium level is discussed in Chapter 18. In general, note that hyperglycemia promotes an osmotic gradient that causes water to move out of the cells into the ECF, thereby diluting the serum sodium level. For every 100 mg/dL rise in plasma glucose, the osmotic water shift dilutes the plasma sodium concentration by 1.3 to 1.6 mEq/L.[7]

ETIOLOGICAL FACTORS

Etiological factors associated with hyponatremia are listed in Table 4-2 and are briefly described below.

TABLE 4-2.   Etiological Factors Associated With Hyponatremia

- Use of thiazide diuretics, particularly in combination with low-salt diet, vomiting, diarrhea, or sweating
- Adrenal insufficiency
- Gastrointestinal fluid losses
- Heavy sweating
- Salt-losing nephritis
- Release of vasopressin (ADH) after anesthesia and surgery, especially when excessive sodium-free fluids administered IV
- Release of vasopressin (ADH) due to presence of nausea, especially when excessive sodium-free fluids administered IV
- Direct absorption of hypotonic irrigating fluids through veins during endometrial ablation or transurethral prostatectomy
- Drugs other than diuretics that have been reported to be associated with hyponatremia include:
    cyclophosphamide
    carbamazepine
    nonsteroidal anti-inflammatory drugs (NSAIDs)
    tricyclic antidepressants and selective serotonic reuptake inhibitors (SSRIs)
    oxytocin
    desmopressin acetate (DDAVP) to treat nocturnal enuresis
    chlorpropamide
    omeprazole
- Central nervous systems disorders such as:
    head trauma
    neoplasms
    vascular and infections disorders
(may cause hyponatremia by excessive ADH secretion, or by cerebral salt wasting, see Chapter 19)
- Compulsive water drinking (relatively common in psychiatric patients)
- Tumors associated with ectopic ADH production such as:
    oat-cell carcinoma of the lung
    carcinomas of the duodenum and pancreas
    Hodgkin's disease
    leukemia
    lymphoma
- Pulmonary disorders such as:
    pneumonia
    acute asthma
    acute respiratory failure
- Acquired immunodeficiency syndrome (for a variety of reasons, see text)

Gastrointestinal Fluid Losses

Gastric fluid loss by vomiting or gastric suction can predispose to hyponatremia by the direct loss of sodium. Gains of water can further dilute the serum sodium level. Nausea predisposes to water retention and as a result hyponatremia, because it

is a potent stimulus for the release of ADH. Despite this effect, however, hyponatremia is not likely to be severe without the intake of free water. When vomiting occurs at home, most patients greatly curtail oral intake and volume depletion usually occurs. In contrast, some patients who are vomiting may continue to drink while vomiting repeatedly and manage to absorb enough ingested water to develop hyponatremia while maintaining a near-normal plasma volume.[8] A case was recently reported in which a young previously healthy woman with severe vomiting and diarrhea associated with gastroenteritis drank copious amounts of water, causing her serum sodium concentration to drop to 106 mEq/L; this unfortunate scenario lead to her death.[9] In the hospital setting, the erroneous administration of excessive electrolyte-free solutions (such as 5% dextrose in water) can seriously dilute the serum sodium concentration.

Loss of intestinal fluid by diarrhea can result in an isotonic FVD, leaving the serum sodium within a normal range. The volume depletion induced by diarrhea can also serve as a stimulus for ADH release, leading to renal water retention and hyponatremia. The amount of oral or intravenous (IV) free-water intake frequently determines the severity of hyponatremia. At times, water loss through diarrhea can exceed sodium loss, leading to hypernatremia.

Adrenal Insufficiency

Hyponatremia is a common complication of adrenal insufficiency and is due to the effects of aldosterone and cortisol deficiencies. Lack of aldosterone increases renal sodium loss, and cortisol deficiency is associated with increased release of ADH (causing water retention). Replacement therapy usually includes a combination of glucocorticoids and mineralocorticoids; in mild cases, hydrocortisone alone may be adequate.

Sweating

Sweat is a hypotonic fluid with a sodium concentration of about 30 to 50 mEq/L.[10] Although sweat production is low in the basal state, it may exceed 1 to 2 L/hr in subjects exercising in a dry, hot climate.[11]

Salt-Losing Nephritis

Different kidney conditions can result in renal salt wasting. Among these are chronic interstitial nephropathy, medullary cystic disease, and polycystic kidney disease.[12] The degree of renal sodium wasting can range from mild to severe.

Drug-Induced Hyponatremia

Diuretics

A number of drugs can lead to hyponatremia. For example, hyponatremia is a fairly common and usually mild complication of diuretic therapy. However, severe hyponatremia may develop at times. Diuretic-induced severe hyponatremia is primarily a complication of thiazide-type drugs that apparently can cause excessive release of ADH.[13] Thiazide-induced hyponatremia most often affects women who are older than 70 years.[14] The majority of elderly women who develop symptomatic hyponatremia after being placed on thiazide diuretics will do so within 2 weeks from beginning the diuretic.[15] In a study of 64 patients admitted to hospitals for treatment of hyponatremia, thiazides were either the only cause or a major contributing factor to more than half of the cases.[16] In yet another study, thiazides were responsible for 94% of the 129 cases of diuretic-induced severe hyponatremia reported in the literature between 1962 and 1990.[17]

Antidepressants

Hyponatremia induced by antidepressants (such as tricyclic antidepressants and selective serotonin reuptake inhibitors [SSRIs]) is a relatively uncommon but potentially life-threatening adverse reaction and appears to be almost exclusively caused by SIADH.[18] Risks for hyponatremia during treatment with antidepressants seem to be highest in women, in the elderly, during the summer, and during the first weeks of treatment.[19] In a study reported by Bouman et al.[20] 4 of 32 elderly patients taking SSRIs developed symptomatic hyponatremia due to SIADH. An additional 4 patients developed symptomatic hyponatremia following the introduction of an SSRI although laboratory confirmation of SIADH was not established. Because symptoms of hyponatremia can mimic depression or psychosis, it is important to be aware of the possibility of this imbalance and to periodically monitor serum electrolytes. If hyponatremia is found, the medication should be discontinued until the imbalance is corrected.[21]

Antineoplastic Agents

Cyclophosphamide (Cytoxan) is an antineoplastic alkylating agent that can increase renal sensitivity to ADH and perhaps its release when given IV in high doses. Because a high fluid intake is generally prescribed to lessen the possibility of hemorrhagic cystitis, severe hyponatremia can result. Use of isotonic saline rather than water to maintain a high urine output can minimize this complication.[22] Vincristine is another antineoplastic drug that can cause hyponatremia, apparently by a neurotoxic effect on the hypothalamus, leading to an increased release of ADH.[23] Cisplatin is a widely used agent in cancer treatment and can lead to hyponatremia in 4% to 10% of cases due to salt wasting.[24]

Carbamazepine

Hyponatremia in psychiatric patients has been attributed to selected medications used to treat psychoses. For example, carbamazepine, used an an anticonvulsant, is a well-established cause of vasopressin release (which, of course, favors water retention). Hyponatremia associated with carbamazepine use is particularly common in psychiatric institutions among patients with polydipsia.[25] Up to 20% of patients receiving carbamazepine develop serum concentrations below 135 mEq/L.[26] Apparently, the hyponatremia caused by this drug is dose related.

Nonsteroidal Anti-inflammatory Drugs

The nonsteroidal anti-inflammatory drugs (NSAIDs) decrease renal water excretion because decreased synthesis of prostaglandins potentiates the action of ADH on the kidney. Despite this effect, hyponatremia due solely to these agents is uncommon.[27] Instead, NSAIDs tend to exacerbate the tendency toward hyponatremia in patients with other risk factors for hyponatremia.

Oxytocin

Oxytocin, like vasopressin (ADH), is synthesized in the hypothalamus and released by the pituitary gland. Although its primary effects are on uterine function and milk production, it also possesses significant antidiuretic activity. Administration of oxytocin to induce labor, therefore, can cause hyponatremia if improperly used. In the past, little attention was paid to the water-retentive capacity of oxytocin, and excessive fluid (usually in the form of 5% dextrose in water) was sometimes administered. Severe hyponatremia has developed in some cases after the infusion of less than 3 liters of fluid.[28] IV administration of oxytocin in dextrose and water to stimulate labor has resulted in water retention, severe hyponatremia, and seizures in both the mother and the fetus.[29] Safe guidelines for oxytocin administration are discussed in Chapter 23.

Desmopressin Acetate to Treat Nocturnal Enuresis

Intranasal desmopressin acetate (DDAVP) has been used extensively to treat conditions such as diabetes insipidus and nocturnal enuresis. The latter condition affects 5 to 7 million children in the United States.[30] Apparently a large proportion of patients with enuresis secrete too little ADH during the night, causing higher urine production during this time. This is counteracted by intranasal DDVAP. Although the medication has been safe and effective for many who are affected by enuresis, there is the potential for serious complications.[31] There have been reports of severe hyponatremia with seizures from the use of intranasal DDAVP; therefore, there is reason to use the least effective dosage to minimize this possibility. Some question the use of this agent to treat enuresis, particularly because the condition usually resolves spontaneously with age.[32] The problem of DDAVP-associated hyponatremia during the treatment of nocturnal enuresis is not limited to children. For example, a 29-year-old woman with a long history of nocturnal enuresis developed severe symptomatic hyponatremia shortly after beginning intranasal DDAVP use.[33] Monitoring electrolytes periodically may help prevent hyponatremia and its potentially serious sequelae.[34] The manufacturer recommends monitoring electrolyte levels at least once during intranasal DDAVP therapy if its use extends beyond 1 week; in addition, it is deemed prudent to monitor electrolytes in patients with intercurrent illnesses that might affect hydration status or alter drug absorption.[35] Also, providing patients and their families with a simple understanding of how DDAVP works and how they can minimize problems is essential. Avoiding extensive fluid intake in general and too much fluid near the dosing time are important factors.

Chlorpropamide

Chlorpropamide, an oral hypoglycemic agent, can induce SIADH by potentiating the effect of ADH on the kidney.[36] One study reported that 4% of patients in a clinical population receiving chlorpropamide were hyponatremic (suggesting excessive ADH effect).[37] This problem is most likely to occur in patients older than 60 years of age who are also taking a thiazide diuretic.[38] Second-generation sulfonyureas (glipizide and glyburide) promote water excretion and therefore are preferred in the treatment of type 2 diabetes, especially in patients with a history of congestive heart failure or hyponatremia.[39]

Omeprazole

Omeprazole, a proton pump inhibitor that decreases gastric acid secretion, has an overall low incidence of adverse effects. However, there have been case reports of hyponatremia associated with its use.[40] Although the mechanism of hyponatremia induced by omeprazole is not clear, it appears that an excessive loss of urinary sodium is more likely than water retention.[41]

Postoperative Hyponatremia

In a study of 1,088 postoperative patients, Chung et al.[42] reported a 4.4% incidence of hyponatremia (serum Na$^+$ < 130 mEq/L) within 1 week after surgery. Predisposing factors included a temporary increase in vasopressin release after anesthesia and the stress of surgery. Pain enhances the release of vasopressin by direct stimulation of the hypothalamus. Nausea, which is frequently present in postoperative patients, can increase vasopressin release by as much as 1,000-fold; the nausea does not have to be associated with vomiting.[43] Because of the tendency for hyponatremia in new postoperative patients, the excessive administration of electrolyte-free solutions during the first 2 to 4 postoperative days should be avoided. In fact, because elevated plasma levels of vasopressin are essentially a universal postoperative occurrence in the first few postoperative days, some researchers state that it may be important to avoid the use of any hypotonic IV solution in the immediate postoperative period.[44]

Direct absorption of hypotonic irrigating fluid through the veins during endometrial ablation or transurethral prostatectomy can also cause serious hyponatremia. Endometrial ablation is a relatively new procedure in which the lining of the uterus is ablated by a laser or similar device while an irrigating solution is usually continuously infused into the uterine cavity to facilitate surgical visualization and wash away operative debris. During transurethral resection of the prostate (TURP), the urologist must irrigate the prostatic bed with an electrolyte-free solution. If the procedure is prolonged or if the irrigating solution is introduced under pressure, large volumes of the fluid may be absorbed into the circulation. Thus, the fundamental pathology in the TURP syndrome is volume overload and dilutional hyponatremia.[45] In the past, distilled water was used but has been replaced by solutions containing isotonic or slightly hypotonic glycine, mannitol, or sorbitol.[46] Nonetheless, serum sodium concentration can still be lowered by the irrigating solution. Patients may develop symptoms during the surgical procedure itself; among these are tremulousness, hypothermia, or hypoxia; symptoms on awakening from anesthesia can include headache, nausea, and vomiting.[47] Specific side effects vary with the type of irrigant. Profound hyponatremia and a variety of other adverse neurological and cardiovascular events are reported to follow TURP in 1% to 7% of the patients.[48] Fluid overload with hyponatremia can also be a problem when electrolyte-free solutions are used for hysteroscopy. (See Chap. 14 for a more extensive discussion of these procedures.)

Deaths have occurred in young women who underwent relatively simple surgical procedures (such as hysterectomy or cholecystectomy) and then received excessive volumes of hypotonic fluids postoperatively. Postoperative hyponatremia is apparently a much more serious problem in menstruant women than in postmenopausal women or men. A recent report has indicated that although women and men are equally likely to develop hyponatremia and hyponatremic encephalopathy after surgery, menstruant women are about 25 times more likely to die or have permanent brain damage (compared with either men or postmenopausal women) if this condition develops.[49] The significantly higher mortality from postoperative hyponatremia in menstruant women may be due, at least in part, to physical factors that affect the ability of the brain to adapt to hyponatremia. Symptoms that should cause concern in these individuals include nausea and vomiting, headache, and other variable signs. In a study of 40 young women with hyponatremic encephalopathy, all experienced nausea and vomiting, 34 had headache, and some had other symptoms, including weakness, slurred speech, lethargy, confusion, disorientation, bizarre behavior, urinary incontinence, dyspnea, and decorticate posturing. Of the 40 women, 36 sustained an abrupt respiratory arrest postoperatively; at the time of respiratory arrest, the mean plasma sodium level was 113±1 mE/L (range, 91–128 mEq/L).[50] In summary, it is important to prevent this serious complication by avoiding the excessive use of electrolyte-free or hypotonic fluids in the immediate postoperative period. It is also important to detect developing hyponatremia and institute corrective measures before respiratory insufficiency occurs. Although early symptoms are somewhat nonspecific, the diagnosis can be easily established by measuring the plasma sodium level with virtually no risk to the patient and at minimal cost.[51]

Central Nervous System Disorders

Among the central nervous system (CNS) conditions that may be associated with hyponatremia are head trauma, neoplasms, and vascular and infectious disorders. Sometimes the hyponatremia is due to SIADH; other times, it may be due to cerebral salt wasting. See Chapter 19 for a more thorough discussion of this topic.

Tumors Associated with Ectopic ADH Production

Probably the most frequent cause of SIADH is oat-cell carcinoma of the lung. Other malignancies associated with this syndrome include carcinomas of the duodenum and pancreas, Hodgkin's disease, leukemia, and lymphoma. In some instances, malignant cells from patients with SIADH have been shown to synthesize and release a substance similar to native ADH ("ectopic ADH production"). In Chapter 22 SIADH in oncology patients is discussed further.

Compulsive Water Drinking

Excessive water intake is relatively common in psychiatric patients and can occasionally cause severe symptomatic hyponatremia. This syndrome is also referred to as "compulsive water drinking" or "self-induced water intoxication." The syndrome of psychosis, intermittent hyponatremia, and polydipsia is a potentially life-threatening problem. It has been suggested that up to 25% of patients with schizophrenia have polydipsia.[52] Dilutional hyponatremia is thought to occur when the rapid ingestion of voluminous quantities of water exceeds the excretory capacity of normally functioning kidneys. Because some of these patients appear to have an increased appetite for salt, they have been observed to self-medicate with table salt.[53] Patients who smoke may be more likely to be symptomatic because nicotine contributes to transient release of vasopressin, as may the psychosis itself.[54] In a recently reported study of 15 psychiatric patients with severe hyponatremia, all were heavy smokers.[55]

Pulmonary Disorders Associated With SIADH

Pulmonary disorders associated with hyponatremia include pneumonia, acute asthma, tuberculosis, acute respiratory failure, pneumothorax, and empyema.[56] The causes are not entirely clear, although increased production of AVP has been suggested. For example, mechanical ventilation, especially when combined with positive expiratory pressure, stimulates AVP release by impeding venous return, thus decreasing cardiac output.[57] Acute hypoxia and hypercapnia also stimulate AVP secretion.[58] Bioassays from tuberculous lung tissue have demonstrated ADH activity.[59]

Acquired Immunodeficiency Syndrome

Hyponatremia is very common in patients with acquired immunodeficiency syndrome (AIDS).[60] For example, Vitting et al.[61] reported that 56% of the patients with AIDS followed prospectively in their study were hyponatremic (mean serum sodium level, 126±4 mEq/L). In another study, Agarwal et al.[62] found that about 35% of 103 patients with AIDS admitted for opportunistic infections had serum sodium levels lower than or equal to 130 mEq/L. In a study of 86 children infected with human immunodeficiency virus-1, the incidence of hyponatremia was about 25%.[63] Although in some patients adrenal insufficiency and volume depletion (as from emesis or diarrhea) are responsible for hyponatremia, most patients appear to have SIADH. Conditions that may play a role in hyponatremia are *Pneumocystis carinii* pneumonia, malignancies, and CNS disease.[64] Hyponatremic states are aggravated by the excessive use of hypotonic fluids.

DEFINING CHARACTERISTICS

The defining characteristics of hyponatremia depend on its magnitude, rapidity of onset, and cause. In general, the lower the serum sodium level, the more likely symptoms are to be severe (Table 4-3). Another major factor is the rapidity of onset. For example, two patients having similar low serum sodium values may have greatly different symptoms if hyponatremia developed slowly in one and quickly in the other. In acute hyponatremia, symptoms develop at a higher rate than they do when hyponatremia is chronic, in which case, symptoms may not become evident until the serum sodium is quite low (eg, 110 mEq/L). Severity of symptoms may also vary with the cause. For example, acute water overloading is more likely to cause severe symptoms than is the chronic loss of sodium.

Hyponatremia causes cell hypo-osmolality, which in turn causes all of the clinical manifestations of hyponatremia.[65] Recall that cellular swelling occurs in

TABLE 4-3. Clinical Manifestations of Hyponatremia

Rapidity of Drop in Serum Sodium Concentration

Rapidity of development of hyponatremia has a major effect on symptom development. Slowly developing hyponatremia is better tolerated than is acutely developing hyponatremia. For example, patients with chronic hyponatremia may have few if any symptoms with serum sodium levels as low as 115 mEq/L.

Severity of Drop in Serum Sodium Concentration

Patients are often asymptomatic when the serum sodium level is > 125 mEq/L. However, when the sodium falls acutely to < 125 mEq/L, the following symptoms may occur:

20–125 mEq/L

Nausea

Malaise

115–120 mEq/L

Headache

Lethargy

Obtundation

< 110–115 mEq/L

Seizures

Coma

Because there is significant variability in patients, the figures are not necessarily precise. For example, women of childbearing age tend to be at much greater risk of developing severe neurological symptoms than men or postmenopausal women (presumably because of the effect of female hormones on the ability of the brain to adapt to osmotic changes). There are cases on record in which respiratory arrest has occurred in young women with serum sodium levels ≥ 125 mEq/L after acute water overloading in the early postoperative period.

Volume Status

Hyponatremia coupled with ECF volume depletion may produce added symptoms of weakness, fatigue, muscle cramps, and postural dizziness.

Hyponatremia due to SIADH does not produce significant peripheral edema (although water retention has occurred) because about two thirds of the retained water is located inside the cells.

Laboratory Data

By definition, serum sodium level is < 135 mEq/L.

Urinary sodium < 15 mEq/L indicates renal conservation of sodium and that loss of sodium is from a non-renal route.

Urinary sodium > 20 mEq/L in SIADH

ECF, extracellular fluid; SIADH, syndrome of inappropriate antidiuretic hormone secretion.

hyponatremia as the water from relatively dilute ECF is pulled into the cells. Placing a firm finger pressure over a bony prominence and observing for a fingerprint in the skin is a simple test sometimes done to demonstrate intracellular water excess.[66] Early manifestations of hyponatremia include those involving the GI system, such as nausea and abdominal cramps. However, most of the major manifestations of clinical hyponatremia are of a neuropsychiatric nature and are related to cellular swelling. Because the swollen brain has limited room for expansion within the skull, cerebral edema becomes a potentially lethal problem. Brain edema may be so severe that transtentorial herniation (heralded by respiratory arrest) occurs. In general, patients having acute decreases in serum sodium levels have higher mortality rates than do those with more slowly developing hyponatremia. Hyponatremia can reasonably be said to be acute when the serum sodium has fallen by more than 12 mmol/L/day and has been low for less than 48 hours.[67] Brain edema associated with hyponatremia can lead to devastating clinical entities, such as pulmonary edema, central diabetes insipidus, cerebral infarction, cortical blindness, persistent vegetative state, respiratory arrest and coma. Deaths and severe sequelae most commonly occur when the serum sodium level falls below 120 mmol/L and falls by more than 0.5 mmol/L/hr; the complications become even more common when the sodium level drops by more than 1 mmol/L/hr.[68]

Age and Gender Differences

There is a substantial interpatient difference in the susceptibility to symptoms from acute hyponatremia.[69] Perhaps because of differences in cerebral metabolism, women (especially premenopausal women) seem to be at substantially greater risk than men of developing severe neurological symptoms and irreversible brain damage. It is possible that sex hormones are responsible for this difference because there is no gender difference in the risk of symptomatic hyponatremia in prepubertal children.[70] Young women account for most of the reported cases of fatalities secondary to hyponatremia, presumably because their brains are less able to adapt to the effects of hyponatremia than are those of men or postmenopausal women. Because SIADH presents a unique set of circumstances, the clinical manifestations of this disorder are presented in Table 4-4.

TREATMENT

Water Restriction

In normovolemic patients with chronic asymptomatic hyponatremia, water restriction is generally recommended. If water restriction is unsuccessful in treating chronic hyponatremia, attempts may be made to increase water excretion. This may be achieved by using medications that interfere with urine concentration (such as demeclocycline or lithium). Even more effective is the administration of a loop diuretic (such as furosemide) in conjunction with increased sodium and potassium intake.[71]

Sodium Replacement

The obvious treatment for hyponatremia due to sodium loss is sodium replacement. This may be accomplished orally, by nasogastric tube, or by the par-

enteral route. For patients able to eat and drink, replacement is easily accomplished because sodium is plentiful in a normal diet. For those unable to take sodium orally or by gastric tube, the parenteral route is necessary. If the plasma volume is below normal, lactated Ringer's solution or isotonic saline (0.9% NaCl) may be prescribed. In the symptomatic patient with normal or excessive plasma volume, it may be necessary to cautiously administer a small volume of 3% or 5% NaCl (extremely dangerous fluids when used incorrectly). (See Table 4-1 for the sodium content of some parenteral fluids.)

The recommended speed and method of treatment of hyponatremia depend on the magnitude of symptoms, how long they have been present, and the status of the ECF volume. The goal of therapy in symptomatic hyponatremia is to reduce brain water and increase the plasma sodium level only to the point necessary to maintain normal respiration and keep the patient free of seizures and alert,[72] and at the same time prevent osmotic demyelination.

Too rapid a correction of hyponatremia, particularly when it has been present more than 48 hours, can result in an extremely serious condition referred to as "osmotic demyelination" or "central pontine myelinolysis." In this situation, it is thought that the rising serum sodium level causes water to be drawn from the brain across the blood–brain barrier, resulting in brain dehydration and injury.

There is disagreement as to what constitutes "too rapid" a correction of hyponatremia. Patients reported to be at greatest risk for osmotic demyelination associated with rapid sodium replacement have been hyponatremic for more than 48 hours, usually with very low serum sodium concentrations (< 110 mmol/L).[73] In most reported cases, correction of the hyponatremia has exceeded 12 mmol/L during any 24-hour period.[74]

Ayus and Arieff[75] argue that the judicious rapid correction of acute hyponatremia (that developing within 24–48 hours) is warranted to prevent seizures, cerebral herniation, respiratory arrest, and death.[76] They caution, however, that too rapid correction (defined as an increase of 25 mEq/L during the first 48 hours of treatment) may result in cerebral demyelination.[77]

It appears that a definitive recommendation for the treatment of severe hyponatremia cannot be made with certainty.[78] Rose[79] states that it seems advisable to raise the plasma sodium concentration in asymptomatic patients at a maximum average rate of 0.5 mEq/L/hr

TABLE 4-4.   Clinical Manifestations of SIADH

Water retention
- Intake of fluid greatly exceeds urinary output (as evidenced by I&O records)
- Acute weight gain (reflecting water retention)
- No significant peripheral edema (because water is primarily retained inside the cells, not in the interstitial space)
- Signs of cerebral edema (see neurological symptoms below)

Gastrointestinal symptoms
- Anorexia
- Nausea
- Vomiting
- Abdominal cramps

Neurological symptoms
- Lethargy
- Headaches
- Personality changes
- Seizures
- Pupillary changes
- Coma

Laboratory findings
- Hyponatremia
    Symptoms usually do not appear unless serum sodium is < 125 mEq/L
    Plasma osmolality below normal (reflecting low serum sodium level)
- Low BUN and creatinine
    Reflecting state of overhydration
- Urinary signs
    Urinary sodium > 20 mEq/L (as opposed to hyponatremia due primarily to sodium loss, where much lower sodium levels are expected due to renal conservation of the needed cation)
    Urinary SG > 1.012
    Urine osmolality is usually higher than plasma osmolality (urine contains important amounts of sodium; also, plasma is diluted with water)

BUN, blood urea nitrogen; I&O, intake and output; SG, specific gravity; SIADH, syndrome of inappropriate antidiuretic hormone secretion.

or 12 mEq/L/day. In contrast, for patients who already have severe neurological symptoms associated with hyponatremia, the risk of untreated hyponatremia and associated cerebral edema is greater than the potential harm of too rapid correction. In this situation, Rose states that hypertonic saline should be given to elevate the serum sodium level more quickly (1.5–2 mEq/L/hr for 3–4 hours or until the severe neurological symptoms abate); even then, the elevation in the plasma sodium concentration should not exceed 12 to 15 mEq/L/day.[80]

Management of SIADH

If the problem is SIADH, treatment is directed at eliminating the underlying cause if possible (eg, radiation therapy for a tumor secreting ectopic ADH-like substances or discontinuing a drug that increases ADH secretion). If this is not possible, alleviation of water overload by fluid restriction is indicated. Fluid is restricted to the extent that urinary and insensible losses induce a negative water balance (ie, fluid loss exceeds intake). Laboratory values and clinical status are used as guides for fluid restriction. The most important parameters are serum and urine electrolytes and osmolality, fluid intake and output, and body weight records.

For patients with mild hyponatremia, fluid restriction may be all that is needed. More severe cases may require the IV administration of a small amount of hypertonic saline (3% or 5% NaCl), in addition to fluid restriction, to provide sodium in a minimal fluid volume. Furosemide is often used in conjunction with hypertonic saline to promote water excretion and decrease the risk of FVE and its dangerous sequelae (such as pulmonary edema). Use of hypertonic saline alone elevates the serum sodium level only transiently because most of the administered sodium is rapidly lost in the urine. In contrast, furosemide causes loss of both water and sodium; however, when the sodium is given back as hypertonic saline, the result is a net removal of water.[81]

If the underlying cause of SIADH is chronic, as in patients with inoperable tumors producing ectopic ADH, other therapeutic measures must be considered. Although the mainstay of therapy in this setting is water restriction, it is not well tolerated by some patients over a prolonged period. For such patients, the administration of a variety of medications has been recommended. Among these are loop diuretics in conjunction with increased salt intake or other medications such as urea, demeclocycline, and lithium. In some patients, loop diuretics (such as furosemide) have been administered concomitantly with salt tablets to increase the serum sodium level when SIADH is present. Other patients have been placed on a high-salt, high-protein diet (the unused protein is excreted as urea) to increase renal solute load and increase urinary output.[82] Urea can also be given as a medication, usually in a dose ranging from 30 to 60 g/day.[83] Possible drawbacks to the use of urea are unpalatability and some GI discomfort. Demeclocycline and lithium carbonate block the action of ADH on the renal collecting duct, thereby causing increased urinary output (nephrogenic diabetes insipidus). The side effects of lithium limit its usefulness. In contrast, demeclocycline in a dose of 600 to 1,200 mg/day is usually well tolerated.[84] However, it has several disadvantages, including nephrotoxicity when hepatic function is impaired, delayed onset of action for several days, and persistent effect for several days after treatment has been discontinued.[85] The choice of agents in chronic SIADH depends partly on the urine osmolality of the individual patient.[86] Because arginine vasopressin (AVP, also called antidiuretic hormone or ADH) is inappropriately elevated in the majority of patients with hyponatremia, and because this leads to free water retention by stimulating V_2 receptors in the collecting ducts of the kidney, it is desirable to identify agents to counteract this action. Such an agent would ideally block the action of AVP on the kidney and thus produce free water loss. A nonpeptide AVP V_2 receptor antagonist has been described and recent studies have verified its efficacy in inducing free water diuresis.[87,88] V_2 receptor antagonists might be useful in the treatment of hyponatremia caused by SIADH, heart failure, cirrhosis, and the nephrotic syndrome.[89] These agents have not as yet been approved for routine clinical use but offer an exciting prospect for the treatment of hyponatremia.

NURSING INTERVENTIONS

1. Identify patients at risk for hyponatremia. As noted in Table 4-2, many common conditions can lower the serum sodium concentration.
   - Being aware of patients at risk for hyponatremia is crucial to monitoring for the occurrence of subtle early changes associated with this imbalance. A profound hyponatremia can be fatal if not detected early and treated appropriately.
2. Review medications the patient is receiving, noting those that predispose to hyponatremia (see Table 4-2).
3. Monitor fluid losses and gains for all patients at risk for hyponatremia. Look for loss of sodium-containing fluids (such as GI secretions or sweat), particularly in conjunction with a low-sodium diet or excessive water intake either orally or IV.
4. Monitor daily weights and note acute weight gains (reflecting excessive fluid retention).
5. Monitor laboratory data for serum sodium levels lower than normal.
6. Monitor for presence of GI symptoms, such as anorexia, nausea, vomiting, and abdominal cramping, because these may be early signs of hyponatremia. These symptoms must be evaluated in relation to other findings, such as fluid gains and losses, amount of sodium intake, and laboratory data.
7. Monitor for CNS changes, such as lethargy, confusion, muscular twitching, convulsions, and coma. Be aware that more severe neurological signs are associated with very low sodium levels that have fallen rapidly due to water overloading.

8. For patients able to consume a normal diet, encourage foods and fluids with a high sodium content. For example, a cup of beef broth/bouillion contains about 782 mg (34 mEq) of sodium and 6 oz of canned tomato juice contains about 657 mg (29 mEq) of sodium.[90] Sodium content of additional fluids can be found in Table 3-1.

9. When administering sodium-containing IV fluids to patients with cardiovascular disease, monitor especially closely for signs of circulatory overload. These include moist rales in the lungs (the greater the sodium concentration, the greater the risk).

Sodium content of some of the major IV fluids is listed in Table 4-1.

10. Avoid giving large water supplements to patients receiving isotonic tube feedings, particularly if routes of abnormal sodium loss are present or water is being retained abnormally (as in SIADH) (see Chap. 12).

11. Use extreme caution when administering hypertonic saline solutions (3% or 5% NaCl). Be aware that these fluids can be lethal if infused carelessly (see Clinical Tip: Nursing Considerations in Administration of Hypertonic Saline Solutions).

CLINICAL TIP

Nursing Considerations In Administration of Hypertonic Saline Solutions (3% and 5% NaCl)

Check the serum sodium level before administering these solutions and frequently thereafter.

Administer these solutions only in settings where the patient can be closely monitored:

Watch for signs of pulmonary edema and worsening of neurological signs. (Furosemide may be prescribed to promote water loss and prevent pulmonary edema.)

Use a volume-controlled apparatus to administer the fluid; maintain close vigilance on the device because none is foolproof.

Be aware that a definitive recommendation for the treatment of severe hyponatremia cannot be made with certainty. However, consider that factors affecting the rate of administration include (1) length of time the hyponatremia has been present, and (2) severity of symptoms.

For example sodium replacement should occur more slowly in patients who have had hyponatremia for greater than 48 hr (as opposed to < 48 hr); this is because these individuals are at increased risk for osmotic demyelination (also referred to as central pontine myelinolysis).

It appears that sodium replacement should occur more rapidly in patients with severe neurological symptoms and acute hyponatremia (hyponatremia present for < 48 hr); this is because the risk of untreated hyponatremia and associated cerebral edema is greater than the potential harm of too rapid correction of the plasma sodium level.

It seems advisable to raise the plasma sodium concentration in asymptomatic hyponatremic patients at a maximum rate of 0.5 mEq/L/hr or 12 mEq/L/day.[91]

According to Ayus and Arieff,[92] the judicious rapid correction of *acute* hyponatremia (that developing within 24–48 hr) is warranted to prevent seizures, cerebral herniation, respiratory arrest, and death. They caution, however, that too rapid correction (defined as more than 25 mEq/L during the first 48 hr of treatment) may result in cerebral demyelination.

According to Rose,[93] for patients who have severe neurological symptoms, hypertonic saline should be given to elevate the serum sodium level by 1.5 to 2 mEq/L/hr for 3 to 4 hr or until the severe neurological symptoms abate; even then, however, the elevation in the plasma sodium concentration should not exceed 12–15 mEq/L/day.

12. Be aware of the effect a low serum sodium level can have on patients receiving lithium. A low serum sodium level causes a relative increase in lithium retention and predisposes to toxicity. Because of this, decreased tolerance to lithium occurs in patients with protracted sweating and diarrhea. In such instances, supplemental salt and fluid should be administered. Because diuretics promote sodium loss, patients taking lithium should not use diuretics unless they are under close medical supervision. For all patients receiving lithium, an adequate salt intake should be ensured. The patient's food intake should be checked and the physician informed of anorexia (seek a dietary consultation if indicated).

13. To avoid serious sodium deficiency, instruct patients with adrenal insufficiency to:
    • Take steroid-replacement medications as prescribed.
    • Keep several days' dosage on their person when traveling.
    • Wear an identification bracelet stating need for steroids in case of emergency.
    • Seek consultation with a health care provider in times of excessive stress.

    • Monitor their weight and fluid intake and output (I&O) changes and report significant findings to the health care provider.
    • Increase dietary salt intake as indicated during presence of excessive sweating or diarrhea (or other causes of sodium loss).

14. Monitor patients with decreased adrenal function for signs of acute adrenocortical insufficiency (adrenal crisis) when they are exposed to severe stress (such as surgery, trauma, emotional upset, excessive heat, or prolonged medical illness). Look for extreme weakness, acute onset of nausea and vomiting, hypotension, confusion, and even shock.

Because SIADH requires special nursing management, clinical indicators of this condition are summarized in Table 4-4. A summary of factors to consider in assessment for SIADH is presented in Table 4-5, and nursing interventions are described in Table 4-6. Recovery from this dilutional state is usually rapid if the condition is recognized early and appropriate measures are initiated. The nurse plays a vital role in preventing serious consequences of this disorder.

 TABLE 4-5.   Nursing Assessment for SIADH

1. Identify patients at risk (such as those with excessive production of ADH by tumor, those with temporary excessive release of ADH following surgery, or those receiving drugs that potentiate ADH activity—see Table 4-2).
2. Maintain accurate I&O:
   • Look for fluid intake greatly exceeding output; I&O should be totaled and the overall picture observed for several consecutive days
3. Maintain daily body weight records:
   • Look for a sudden weight gain (recall that 1 L fluid weighs about 2.2 lb)
   • Although there will be an acute weight gain, do not expect to detect significant peripheral edema because most of the excess fluid will be retained inside the cells (not in the interstitial space)
4. Monitor serum sodium concentrations.
5. Observe for gastrointestinal symptoms, which usually occur early:
   • Be alert for anorexia, nausea, vomiting, and abdominal cramping.
6. Observe the neurological status carefully:
   • Be particularly alert for lethargy, headache, and personality changes (these symptoms occur relatively early—late neurological symptoms include seizures and coma)

ADH, antidiuretic hormone.

TABLE 4-6.   Nursing Interventions Related to Therapy for SIADH

1. Restrict fluids to the prescribed level:
   • Consider all routes of intake (eg, oral fluids, IV piggyback medications, "keep open" IV, flush fluids for enteral feeding tubes).
   • Space the allotted oral fluids over the 24-hr period to minimize thirst.
   • Place "fluid restriction" signs at the bedside.
   • Explain the need for water restriction to the patient and family.
   • Remove the water pitcher from the bedside.
2. Maintain an accurate I&O record and study its pattern:
   • A greater urinary output than fluid intake is desired because it indicates a negative water balance. (Remember, the excessive water load must be excreted before significant improvement occurs)
3. Maintain an accurate body weight record:
   • With proper therapy, expect to see an acute decline in body weight due to excretion of excess water. Recall that a liter of fluid is equivalent to 2.2 lb; for example, a weight loss of 6.6 lb over a period of 1 to 2 days indicates a loss of approximately 3 liters.
4. Assess neurological signs:
   • With appropriate therapy, an increased level of consciousness is hoped for; unfortunately, neurological damage induced by SIADH is not always reversible.
5. Monitor serum sodium levels:
   • With appropriate therapy, the sodium concentration should elevate slowly toward normal. It is important that the correction not take place too rapidly.
6. Administer hypertonic saline, when prescribed, with great caution.
   • Review the facts regarding administration of hypertonic saline (see the Clinical Tip.)

CASE STUDIES

● **4-1.** A 50-year-old man was started on hydrochlorothiazide and a low-sodium diet for the treatment of hypertension. After 2 weeks, he began to complain of weakness, abdominal cramping, leg cramps, and postural dizziness. On examination he was found to have decreased skin turgor and flat neck veins in the supine position. Laboratory data included:
Na = 118 mEq/L
K = 2.2 mEq/L
Cl = 66 mEq/L
Plasma osmolality = 240 mOsm/kg
COMMENTARY: This patient was obviously hyponatremic, as indicated by the low plasma sodium level and osmolality. In this instance, the hyponatremia was accompanied by decreased fluid volume (as evidenced by the decreased skin turgor and flat neck veins). In addition, the plasma potassium and chloride levels were quite low. Thiazide diuretics promote both sodium and

potassium excretion and predispose to hypochloremic alkalosis (metabolic alkalosis). Sodium loss, coupled with a low sodium intake, caused hyponatremia.

● **4-2.** A 40-year-old man with polycystic kidney disease developed nausea, vomiting, and diarrhea. He stopped eating but drank large quantities of water. Over a period of 4 days, he developed progressive lethargy and had a grand mal seizure. Laboratory data included:
Na = 108 mEq/L
Cl = 72 mEq/L
BUN = 142 mg/dL
Creatinine = 12 mg/dL
COMMENTARY: This patient lost sodium through vomiting and diarrhea and replaced only water. He continued to lose sodium through the kidneys because of his renal disease. The neurological symptoms were due to dilution of the already low

Summary of Hyponatremia

ETIOLOGICAL FACTORS

Loss of sodium
- Use of diuretics
- Loss of GI fluids
- Adrenal insufficiency
- Osmotic diuresis
- Salt-losing nephritis

Gains of water
- Excessive administration of D_5W
- Psychogenic polydipsia
- Excessive water administration with isotonic or hypotonic tube feedings

Disease states associated with SIADH
- Oat-cell carcinoma of lung
- Carcinoma of duodenum or pancreas
- Head trauma
- Stroke
- Pulmonary disorders (tuberculosis, pneumonia, asthma, respiratory failure)

Pharmacologic agents that may impair renal water excretion
- Chlorpropamide (Diabinese)
- Cyclophosphamide (Cytoxan)
- Vincristine (Oncovin)
- Thioridazine (Mellaril)
- Fluphenazine (Prolixin)
- Carbamazepine (Tegretol)
- Oxytocin (Pitocin)

DEFINING CHARACTERISTICS

Anorexia

Nausea

Vomiting

Lethargy

Confusion

Muscular twitching

Seizures

Coma

Respiratory arrest

Serum Na < 135 mEq/L

Serum osmolality < 285 mOsm/kg

Urinary Na level varies with cause of hyponatremia

serum sodium level by excessive water intake, resulting in brain swelling.

● **4-3.** A 58-year-old man with a history of inoperable oat-cell carcinoma of the lung was admitted to the hospital; according to his family, he had a 2-week history of progressive lethargy. Laboratory data included:

Plasma Na = 105 mEq/L
Urinary Na = 76 mEq/L
Cl = 72 mEq/L
Urinary osmolality = 800 mOsm/kg

COMMENTARY: The history of an oat-cell lung tumor strongly suggests the presence of ectopic ADH production. Lethargy is a prominent symptom of hyponatremia due to water excess. Laboratory data revealed an extremely low plasma sodium level. In contrast, note the relatively high urinary sodium level, indicating the kidneys' inability to retain sodium even though severe hyponatremia is present.

● **4-4.** After an automobile accident, a 30-year-old woman was admitted to the emergency department of a small suburban hospital. She had sustained facial fractures and a possible head injury (evidenced by temporary loss of consciousness at the accident scene). During the first 3 days of her hospitalization, she received an average of 4 liters of fluid daily (despite persistent low urinary output). She became increasingly lethargic and complained of headache and nausea. On the fourth day she had a grand mal seizure and was noted to have papilledema and Babinski's sign. At that time, her serum sodium level was 110 mEq/L. Despite intensive treatment, she died within a week. On autopsy, her brain was found to be swollen, and she weighed 10 lb more than when admitted (despite almost no caloric intake during her hospitalization).

COMMENTARY: Patients with head injuries (especially when facial injuries are also present) are at risk for SIADH and should be monitored closely for it. Care should be taken to avoid fluid overloading in patients with head injuries (see Chap. 19). Note that this patient did not have any concomitant injuries that necessitated large fluid volume replacement. Weight on autopsy was greater than on admission because water was abnormally retained in cells throughout her body. No peripheral edema was present because the excess water was retained intracellularly, not in the interstitial space. This patient's death could have been prevented had those providing care looked at the I&O record and paid attention to the obvious warning signs of SIADH. For example, despite an intake of 4,000 mL/day, she excreted less than 600 mL on most days. Nurses' notes made frequent mention of the presence of lethargy, nausea, abdominal cramping, and headache.

● **4-5.** A 23-year-old healthy woman (mother of two children) underwent an elective vaginal hysterectomy. Postoperatively, this 110-lb woman received 5% dextrose in 0.45% NaCl at a rate of 175 mL/hr for about 20 hours, even though her urinary output was less than 500 mL each shift. No abnormal routes of fluid loss were present. On the evening of her surgery, she complained of nausea and headache. In the early morning of the first postoperative day she was combative and disoriented. Two hours later, blood work revealed a serum sodium level of 126 mEq/L (no baseline sodium level was available because preoperative values were not obtained). One-half hour later, she was unresponsive to verbal stimuli. At this time, her serum sodium level was 122 mEq/L. Despite resuscitative efforts, she progressed on a downhill

course and subsequently died several weeks later without regaining consciousness.

COMMENTARY: Cerebral edema was apparent on autopsy. Apparently this patient suffered hyponatremic encephalopathy, resulting in respiratory arrest and her subsequent death. (See the discussion of postoperative hyponatremia in menstruant women in this chapter.) The cause of the hyponatremia was the greatly excessive administration of hypotonic fluid during a period when her ability to excrete fluid was limited (due to the effects of increased ADH activity in the postoperative period). Recall that ADH activity is increased for the first 2 to 4 postoperative days due to the stress of surgery, as well as the presence of pain and nausea. The I&O record showed a disproportionately large fluid intake/output ratio for all three shifts. In fact, from the time of her return from surgery to the catastrophic neurological event, this patient received about 3.5 liters of hypotonic fluid and excreted less than 1.5 liters of urine. The excess hypotonic fluid caused her serum sodium level to drop quickly, accounting for the severe neurological symptoms despite a serum sodium level of more than 120 mEq/L. This patient's death could have been easily prevented by the administration of an isotonic fluid (or at least by avoiding the greatly excessive rate of the hypotonic electrolyte fluid). Had her symptoms been recognized earlier, and the appropriate treatment instituted, the condition could likely have been safely reversed.

● HYPERNATREMIA

DEFINITION

Hypernatremia refers to a greater-than-normal serum sodium level, that is, a serum level greater than 145 mEq/L. The incidence of hypernatremia ranges from less than 1% to more than 3%.[94] In nonhospitalized patients, it is primarily a condition seen in the elderly; however, hospital-acquired hypernatremia occurs in patients of all ages. Mortality rates range from 40% to more than 60%; as in hyponatremia, the high mortality rate is influenced at least in part by the severity of the underlying disease.[95]

PATHOPHYSIOLOGY

Normally, the body defends itself against the development of hypernatremia by both increasing the release of ADH and stimulating thirst by the osmoreceptors in the hypothalamus.[96] Thus, when the serum sodium level begins to increase, the resultant retention of water and increased water intake lower the sodium concentration. Naturally, failure of these responses can lead to hypernatremia. Hypernatremia is virtually never seen in an alert patient with a normal thirst mechanism and access to water.

Causes of hypernatremia include a gain of sodium in excess of water, or a loss of water in excess of sodium. Disease states capable of causing a significant acute alteration in the serum sodium level frequently produce a concomitant change in the ECF volume. Thus, hypernatremia often occurs with either FVD or FVE. Figure 4-3 contains further explanations.

As noted in Figure 4-1, initially hypernatremia favors the shrinkage of cells as fluid is pulled away from them into the hypertonic ECF. It is this cellular dehydration in the brain that produces its contraction and is largely responsible for the neurological symptoms of hypernatremia. Contraction of the brain may cause mechanical traction on delicate cerebral vessels and produce vascular trauma. Autopsies on patients who died from hypernatremia have shown widespread cerebral vascular bleeding. For example, there can be rupture of bridging veins, causing subdural, subarachnoid, or intraparenchymal hemorrhage.[97]

The cerebral shrinking caused by hypernatremia is transient. Usually within a few hours, by means of complex mechanisms, the brain begins to adapt to the extracellular hyperosmolality by raising the amount of intracellular solutes and thereby minimizing its water loss. With increased intracellular solute, water movement back into the brain is initiated and the brain volume moves toward normal. This adaptation accounts for the relative absence of symptoms in patients with slow-developing high serum sodium levels (sometimes up to levels of 170–180 mEq/L).[98] Conversely, severe hypernatremia that develops over a period of less than 24 hours is often fatal.

ETIOLOGICAL FACTORS

Etiological factors associated with hypernatremia are listed in Table 4-7 and are briefly described below. In general, it should be noted that the etiology of hyper-

Hypernatremia associated with a near normal ECF volume

Loss of water causes elevation of serum sodium level; does not lead to volume contraction unless water losses are massive.

As may occur in:
—increased insensible water loss (as in hyperventilation)

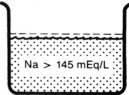

Hypernatremia associated with ECF volume deficit ("Hypertonic dehydration")

Losses of both sodium and water but relatively greater loss of water.

As may occur in:
—profuse sweating
—diarrhea, particularly in children
—aged individuals with poor water intake (recall that the aged kidney loses part of its ability to concentrate urine and thus cannot conserve water as it should)

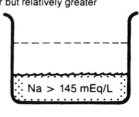

Hypernatremia associated with fluid volume excess

Gains of both sodium and water, but relatively greater gain of sodium.

As may occur:
—administration of hypertonic sodium solutions or substances (such as sodium bicarbonate in cardiac arrest)

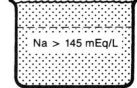

FIGURE 4-3.   Hypernatremic states.

natremia is quite different in children and in adults. For example, in infants the most common cause is diarrhea, whereas in the elderly, it is infirmity with inability to obtain sufficient free-water intake.

Water Deprivation

Hypernatremia may occur in any patient with a diminished mental status because the ability to perceive and respond to thirst is impaired. In adults, hypernatremia is most often seen in patients who are 65 years of age or older. Mortality rates in these patients are often reported to be in excess of 50%.[99] Not only are older persons at increased risk for illness and diminished mental status, increasing age is associated with lowered osmotic stimulation of thirst and decreased ability of the kidneys to conserve water in times of need. Infants,

TABLE 4-7.   Etiological Factors Associated With Hypernatremia

Deprivation of water, most common in unconscious or debilitated patients unable to perceive or respond to
  thirst (such as the elderly stroke patient)
Deprivation of water in infants, very young children, or retarded individuals unable to communicate thirst
Hypertonic tube feedings without adequate water supplements (see Chap. 12)
Greatly increased insensible water loss (as in hyperventilation or in extensive denuding effects of uncovered
  second- or third-degree burns)
Watery diarrhea
Ingestion of salt in unusual amounts (as in faulty preparation of oral electrolyte-replacement solutions)
Excessive parenteral administration of sodium-containing fluids
• Hypertonic saline (3% or 5% NaCl)
• Sodium bicarbonate ($NaHCO_3$) in cardiac arrest or treatment of lactic acidosis
• 0.9% NaCl (when primary fluid loss is water)
Diabetes insipidus if the patient does not experience, or cannot respond to, thirst; or if fluids are excessively
  restricted
Less common are heatstroke, near drowning in sea water (which contains a sodium concentration of about
  500 mEq/L), accidental introduction of hypertonic saline into maternal circulation during therapeutic
  abortion, and malfunction of either hemodialysis or peritoneal dialysis systems

because they are unable to ask for water, are also at
increased risk.

Insensible Water Loss

A typical adult with a normal body temperature will
lose about 1,000 mL of water per day through respiration and evaporation from the skin (insensible water
loss). When any condition is present that increases this
insensible water loss (such as fever, hyperventilation,
pulmonary infections, tracheostomy, exposure to hot
environmental temperatures, or massive burns), hypernatremia may result.

Watery Diarrhea

Gastrointestinal fluid losses are a major cause of hypernatremia in children and apparently result from a combination of hypotonic fluid loss in diarrheal stools,
increased insensible water loss associated with concomitant fever, and excessive sodium administration in
formulas or IV fluids. Fortunately, the incidence of this
imbalance has decreased in recent years because more
appropriate lower solute replacement fluids are used
(providing adequate amounts of free water). Loss of
hypotonic fluid in the stool of patients with end-stage

liver disease treated with lactulose may also result in
severe hypernatremia.[100]

Excessive Sodium Intake

Ingestion or IV infusion of too much salt can induce
hypernatremia. Acute or fatal hypernatremia due to
excessive sodium intake has been reported after the
accidental substitution of sodium chloride for sugar in
infant formulas. It can also result from improperly prepared oral electrolyte solutions (addition of too much
NaCl or $NaHCO_3$). Fatalities have resulted from the
administration of 5% NaCl solution instead of the
intended 5% dextrose solution because parenteral fluid
containers were not checked carefully. Other causes of
hypernatremia include excessive administration of
$NaHCO_3$ during cardiac arrest or in the treatment of
lactic acidosis. Elevated serum sodium levels can even
occur from the administration of an isotonic NaCl
solution (0.9% NaCl) if the patient's fluid deficit is primarily water.

Ingestion of sea water (which has a sodium concentration of 450–500 mEq/L) can lead to severe
hypernatremia.[101] Also, fatalities have been reported
with the accidental administration of hypertonic
salt solutions into the maternal circulation instead

of the amniotic cavity during therapeutic abortion attempts.[102]

Diabetes Insipidus

Diabetes insipidus (DI) is a disorder of water balance that is associated either with a lack of ADH or with an end-organ (kidney) resistance to the effects of ADH, leading to water diuresis. Hypernatremia will result if insufficient water is replaced either orally or IV. As a rule, however, the serum sodium level remains normal because the individual with DI experiences thirst and drinks sufficient fluid to replace the lost urine volume. The two types of DI are central and nephrogenic. Central DI (CDI) is sometimes referred to as neurogenic, and nephrogenic DI (NDI) is sometimes referred to as renal.

Central DI is due to a relative lack of ADH and is sometimes called vasopressin-sensitive DI because it responds favorably to ADH administration. This form of DI may occur after head trauma (particularly caused by fractures at the base of the skull or surgical procedures near the pituitary) or as a result of infection, primary tumor, or metastatic tumor. It may also be idiopathic; about 50% of the patients with CDI have no known underlying pathology.

Nephrogenic DI is due to failure of the kidney to respond to ADH, not to a deficit of the hormone. This condition is sometimes referred to as vasopressin-resistant DI because the administration of vasopressin does not relieve the disorder. It may occur as a rare genetic disorder or may be acquired. Acquired NDI is much more common and may be the result of electrolyte disorders (such as hypokalemia or hypercalcemia), chronic renal failure, or drugs such as lithium, demeclocycline, and methoxyflurane (a halogenated anesthetic).[103] Fortunately, the NDI caused by hypercalcemia and hypokalemia is usually reversible within 1 to 12 weeks after correction of the imbalance.[104]

DEFINING CHARACTERISTICS

Defining characteristics of hypernatremia are given in Table 4-8. When the patient is awake, thirst is the usual early sign of developing hypernatremia. It should be noted that thirst, by stimulating water intake, normally protects against hypernatremia. Thus, hypernatremia generally occurs in individuals either unable to perceive or unable to respond to thirst (eg, adults with an altered mental status or infants). An awake, alert patient with hypernatremia can be assumed to have a hypothalamic lesion affecting the thirst center.[105]

Like hyponatremia, the primary manifestations of hypernatremia are neurological in nature. The earliest signs are lethargy, weakness, and irritability. These symptoms can progress to twitching, seizures, coma, and death if the hypernatremia is severe. Although convulsions may occur from an acute, rapid increase of plasma sodium by 15 to 20 mEq/L within 24 hours or less, they usually occur with a sodium concentration greater than 160 mEq/L.[106] Presumably these symptoms are the consequence of cellular dehydration (resulting from pulling of fluid from the cells into the hyperosmotic ECF). If hypernatremia is severe, permanent brain damage can occur, especially in children. Brain damage is apparently due to subarachnoid hemorrhages that result from tearing of vessels during brain contraction. Because of rupture of cerebral vessels, a lumbar puncture may reveal blood in the cerebrospinal fluid. Symptoms in infants often include marked irritability and a high-pitched cry, with a depressed sensorium ranging from lethargy to frank coma. In adults, the symptoms of hypernatremia are often difficult to separate from those of the underlying pathology, which is often of a catastrophic nature.

As is the case with hyponatremia, the rapidity of onset is an important determinant of the severity of symptoms as well as the eventual outcome of hypernatremia. A high plasma sodium level that evolves over days to weeks is associated with minimal to mild neurological symptoms because the CNS cells have time to adapt to hyperosmolar changes.[107]

If the hypernatremia is accompanied by FVD, other symptoms such as postural hypotension may occur. Other physical signs of water deficit are dry, hot skin with decreased sweating; thick, rubbery-feeling skin; and fever of CNS origin.[108] Hypernatremia is the only state in which dry, sticky mucous membranes are characteristic.[109]

Diabetes Insipidus

The most prevalent signs of DI are polyuria and polydipsia. Depending on the severity of the disease, the degree of polyuria in DI can range from 3 to 20 liters in 24 hours. In complete CDI and NDI, the urinary specific gravity and osmolality are quite low (< 1.010 and 300 mOsm/L, respectively). In partial CDI and

TABLE 4-8. Defining Characteristics of Hypernatremia

Thirst (Note that thirst is so strong a defender of serum sodium in normal individuals that hypernatremia never occurs unless the person is rendered unconscious or is denied access to water; ill persons may have an impaired thirst mechanism.)

Elevated body temperature

Dry and sticky mucous membranes

Restlessness and weakness in moderate hypernatremia

Disorientation, delusions, and hallucinations in severe hypernatremia; or, patient may be lethargic when undisturbed and irritable and hyperreactive when stimulated

Lethargy, stupor, or coma (The level of consciousness depends not only on actual sodium levels, but on the rate of development of hypernatremia. For example, a patient may have a serum sodium level of 170 mEq/L and remain conscious if the imbalance developed slowly.)

Muscle irritability and convulsions

Signs of irritability and high-pitched cry in infants

Laboratory data:
- Serum sodium > 145 mEq/L
- Serum osmolality > 295 mOsm/kg
- Urinary SG > 1.015 as the kidneys attempt to conserve needed water, provided water loss is from a route *other* than the kidney (such as the GI tract, skin, or lungs). If the physiological defect involves water loss from the kidney (as occurs in complete diabetes insipidus), the urinary SG will be very low.

SG, specific gravity.

NDI, the urinary specific gravity and osmolality are somewhat higher (1.010–1.023 and 300–800 mOsm/L, respectively). This is because the patient has some remaining ability to concentrate urine. Clinical manifestations of DI are summarized in Table 4-9.

As a rule, the patient with an intact thirst mechanism will drink sufficient fluids to maintain the sodium balance (ie, an essentially normal serum sodium and serum osmolality). Unfortunately, the frequency of urination and drinking often interferes with other activities when the condition is severe.

If the patient is not able to perceive or respond to thirst or if parenteral fluid replacement is inadequate, polyuria will lead to severe dehydration (hypernatremia

 TABLE 4-9. Clinical Manifestations of Diabetes Insipidus (DI)

Excessive urinary output regardless of fluid intake:
- Urinary output usually ranges between 3 to 20 L/24 hr (depending on the severity of the pathologic process)
- Urinary output often exceeds 200 mL/hr
- In complete DI, urinary specific gravity < 1.010, urine osmolality < 300 mOsm/L
- In partial DI, urinary specific gravity and urinary osmolality are somewhat higher (such as 1.010–1.023 and 300–800 mOsm/L, respectively)
- Inability of kidneys to concentrate urine by fluid restriction (a common test for this disorder)

Intense thirst in the alert patient, resulting in an intake that corresponds to the urinary volume

Serum osmolality and sodium levels greater than normal if water intake does not match urinary losses (severe hypovolemia may occur with inadequate fluid intake)

and hyperosmolality of plasma) with weight loss, tachycardia, and even shock.

TREATMENT

Hypernatremia is treated either by the addition of water or by the removal of sodium, depending on the cause of the imbalance. If water loss is the cause, water needs to be added; if sodium excess is the cause, sodium needs to be removed. Too rapid a correction of hypernatremia can result in cerebral edema, seizures, permanent neurological damage, and death. The reasons for this is as follows. Hypernatremia initially pulls water from brain cells and produces brain contraction; however, after a few hours the brain begins to adapt by increasing the intracellular solute level.[110] Rapid lowering of the plasma sodium can render the plasma relatively hypo-osmotic to the brain cells and allow water to be pulled into the cells, producing cerebral edema. (Note that the blood–brain barrier prevents the intracellular solutes from being diluted at the same rate as the solute in the plasma.) To minimize the risk of complications, it is currently recommended that the plasma sodium concentration be gradually lowered to normal unless the patient has symptomatic hypernatremia.[111] In both children and adults, fluid therapy is administered such that normonatremia is achieved over a period of about 48 hours.[112] Because chronic hypernatremia is well tolerated, rapid correction offers no advantage and may be harmful because of the potential for causing brain edema. According to one group of investigators, chronic hypernatremia (defined as hypernatremia that has been present for 2 days) should not be corrected faster than 0.7 mEq/L/hr or about 10% of the serum sodium concentration per day.[113] In contrast, acute hypernatremia (present for < 12 hours) may be treated more rapidly.[114] In acute symptomatic hypernatremia, the serum sodium concentration may be reduced by 6 to 8 mEq/L in the first 3 to 4 hours, but thereafter the rate of decline should not be more than 1 mEq/L/hr.[115]

Standard formulas exist for calculating the degree of free-water deficit in hypernatremic patients. Generally, sufficient free water is given in the form of hypotonic fluids (ranging from 5% dextrose in water to 0.45% NaCl solution) to lower the plasma sodium level gradually over a period of about 48 hours.[116] Plasma electrolytes should be monitored at frequent intervals, such as every 2 hours.[117] Disease states that cause hypernatremia also often cause a decrease in the ECF volume.

In most cases, it may be safer to correct hypernatremia concomitantly with repletion of the volume deficit with half-strength saline (0.45% NaCl) or half-strength lactated Ringer's solution; this is because too rapid correction of the hyperosmolar ECF by 5% dextrose in water may cause convulsions and coma.[118] Patients who have sustained both water and· sodium losses and who show evidence of circulatory insufficiency may need to receive isotonic saline (0.9% NaCl) until they become hemodynamically stable; after stabilization, 0.45% NaCl may be infused.[119]

Diabetes Insipidus

The standard treatment of patients with complete CDI has been ADH replacement by means of vasopressin administration. Vasopressin may be administered in different forms, depending on the clinical situation.

Vasopressin (8-arginine vasopressin) is a short-acting aqueous ADH replacement possessing antidiuretic and pressor effects, which can be given subcutaneously, intramuscularly, or intranasally. This preparation is useful when a rapidly acting, short-duration ADH replacement is indicated, particularly after cranial surgery.[120] When a longer acting preparation is desirable, desmopressin (a synthetic analogue of vasopressin), may be used; this agent has a stronger antidiuretic effect than AVP but has negligible pressor activity.[121]

Until the polyuria is controlled by vasopressin therapy, careful attention must be paid to replacement of fluid (particularly if the patient has a decreased level of consciousness or other disturbances interfering with the perception of thirst or the ability to drink). However, it is important to recall that a potential complication of vasopressin therapy is water intoxication (excessive retention of water).

If the patient with CDI has some residual capacity to secrete ADH, drugs that increase the release of ADH or enhance its action on the kidney may be used instead of hormonal replacement therapy. Such drugs include chlorpropamide (Diabinese), an oral hypoglycemia agent, and carbamazepine (Tegretol), an anticonvulsant.

Paradoxically, thiazide diuretic agents are sometimes used to decrease the polyuria associated with both CDI and NDI.[122] It is believed that the thiazides act by decreasing the amount of sodium ions that reach the distal tubules of the kidneys. Patients taking thiazides for treatment of DI should be instructed to avoid liberal use of salt because it decreases the effectiveness of the drug.

NURSING INTERVENTIONS

1. Identify patients at risk for hypernatremia (review Table 4-7).
2. Monitor fluid losses and gains. Look for abnormal losses of water or low water intake, and for large gains of sodium as may occur with prescription drugs having a high sodium content. For example, 24 g of carbenicillin disodium (a possible daily dose) contains 142 mEq sodium.[123] Fleet enema solution also has a high sodium content, although it is not generally totally absorbed from the rectum.
3. Monitor for symptoms of hypernatremia (see Table 4-8). Evaluate these in relation to other factors in the patient's history.
4. Monitor serum sodium levels as frequently as indicated.
5. Prevent hypernatremia in debilitated patients unable to perceive or respond to thirst by offering them fluids at regular intervals. If fluid intake remains inadequate, consult with the physician to plan an alternate route for intake, either by tube feedings or by the parenteral route.
6. If tube feedings are used, give sufficient water to keep the serum sodium and the blood urea nitrogen (BUN) levels within normal limits (see Chap. 12).
7. Monitor the patient's response to corrective parenteral fluids by reviewing serial sodium levels and observing any changes in neurological signs. With gradual decrease in the serum sodium level, the neurological signs should improve, not worsen. Be aware that the serum sodium level should be decreased gradually (see Treatment section above and Case Study 4-2).
8. For patients with DI:
   - Monitor parameters outlined in Table 4-10.
   - Ensure that the alert patient with DI and an intact thirst mechanism is allowed to drink at will; also, ensure that this individual is near a bathroom because frequent voiding is anticipated until the condition is brought under control.
   - Ensure that the patient with a decreased level of consciousness or other disability interfering with drinking is given adequate fluid; if the patient is unable to take fluids orally, consult with the physician to obtain parenteral fluid orders.
   - Administer medications for DI with an understanding of their actions.
   - Be aware that a potential complication of vasopressin administration is water intoxication (excessive retention of water causing a low serum sodium level). This is particularly important because it is difficult to regulate vasopressin dosage in patients with rapidly fluctuating clinical states.
   - Educate patients regarding the proper use of prescribed medications and how to monitor and record fluctuations in their fluid I&O and body weight (see Summary of Hypernatremia).

CASE STUDIES

● **4-6.** An 80-year-old woman living in a nursing home had a stroke and developed aphasia and hemiplegia. Because of her neurological deficits, she required a great deal of assistance to eat and drink. Because of lack of attention from the staff, she ingested insufficient water and developed a serum sodium concentration of 188 mEq/L.

COMMENTARY: A serum sodium concentration greater than 150 mEq/L is virtually never seen in an alert patient with a normal thirst mechanism and access to water.[124] This hypernatremic patient represents a common problem (decreased awareness and inability to drink). One researcher stated that hypernatremic dehydration constitutes a "sentinel health event" in patients without documented rapid free-water loss. A sentinel health event is defined as an illness or death that should be preventable, given adequate care, or at least should cause those caring for the patient to ask why the event occurred.[125] In the absence of free-water loss, hypernatremic dehydration probably indicates fluid deprivation (a form of neglect).

● **4-7.** A 60-year old woman with a serum sodium level of 185 mEq/L was transferred from a nursing home to an acute care facility. Aggressive IV therapy with large volumes of 5% dextrose in water was instituted and her serum sodium dropped to 145 mEq/L in 5 hours. She became unresponsive; a lumbar puncture revealed an opening pressure of 32 cm water (normal is 10–20 cm water).

TABLE 4-10.   Assessment for Diabetes Insipidus (DI)

---

1. Be aware of patients at risk for DI
   Central DI
   • Head trauma (particularly with fractures at the base of the skull or surgical procedures near the pituitary)
   • Cerebral infections
   • Brain tumors
   Nephrogenic DI
   • Hypokalemia
   • Hypercalcemia
   • Certain drugs (such as lithium and demeclocycline)
2. Maintain an accurate I&O record for at-risk patients.
   • Look for a significantly greater output than intake (a danger signal of impending hypernatremia). Fortunately, many patients keep themselves "in balance" by drinking about as much as they urinate. It is helpful to calculate and record cumulative amounts for several days to obtain a more accurate account of the patient's fluid balance status, particularly if onset of polyuria was insidious.
3. Be alert for polyuria in at-risk patients.
   • It is frequently necessary to measure hourly urine volumes in such individuals to foster early detection. For example, a frequent directive in the care of postoperative neurosurgical patients is to report a urine volume > 200 mL in each of 2 consecutive hours or > 500 mL in a 2-hr period.
4. Monitor urinary SG in at-risk patients.
   • A persistently dilute urine is a hallmark of DI. (The SG may be as low as 1.005.)
5. Monitor serum sodium levels at least once a day (more often as indicated) in at-risk patients.
   • Look for hypernatremia (serum sodium >145 mEq/L). Once vasopressin therapy has been initiated, look for hyponatremia (a possible rebound effect).
6. Monitor body weights.
   • Look for weight loss paralleling polyuria. Maintaining a weight chart helps detect excessive fluid loss, particularly when I&O records are in doubt (as may occur in incontinent patients).

I&O, intake and output; SG, specific gravity.

COMMENTARY: This patient had been hypernatremic for some time, allowing her brain to adapt to the hyperosmolal state by increasing brain osmolality. (In hypernatremia, brain volume initially declines and then begins to adapt toward normal within several hours.)[126] Once this cerebral adaptation has occurred, any rapid lowering of the serum sodium level creates an osmotic gradient, allowing water to move into the brain, increasing brain size, and causing cerebral edema. This is precisely what happened in this patient; had the serum sodium been decreased gradually, the cerebral edema would not have occurred.

● **4-8.** Over a 16-hour period, a young child was inadvertently given 800 mL of 5% NaCl solution (containing 855 mEq/L of sodium) instead of the prescribed 5% dextrose in half-strength saline (containing 77 mEq/L of sodium). She developed lethargy, convulsions, and coma before the error was discovered. Despite resuscitative efforts, the child died.

COMMENTARY: Instead of a hypotonic sodium fluid, this child received a grossly hypertonic sodium solution, causing fatal brain damage. This terrible event would never have occurred had the fluid been checked properly before being administered.

Summary of Hypernatremia

ETIOLOGICAL FACTORS

Deprivation of water (most common in those unable to perceive or respond to thirst)

Increased insensible water loss (as in hyperventilation)

Watery diarrhea

Ingestion of salt in unusual amounts

Excessive parenteral administration of sodium-containing solutions
- Hypertonic saline (3% or 5% NaCl)
- Sodium bicarbonate
- Isotonic saline

Near drowning in sea water

Heatstroke

Diabetes insipidus if water intake is inadequate

DEFINING CHARACTERISTICS

Thirst usually occurs early

Dry, sticky mucous membranes

Fever may be present

Severe hypernatremia
- Disorientation
- Hallucinations
- Lethargy when undisturbed
- Irritability when stimulated
- Focal or grand mal seizures
- Coma

Serum sodium > 145 mEq/L

Serum osmolality > 295 mOsm/kg

Urinary SG > 1.015, provided water loss is from nonrenal route

For diabetes insipidus, see Table 4-10

● **4-9.** A 55-year-old comatose woman with a basal skull fracture was transferred to a medical center from a small suburban hospital. Her urine output was 200 mL/hr and her serum sodium level was 170 mEq/L. Urine osmolality was 80 mOsm/kg (extremely dilute, reflecting excessive water loss in the urine) and the serum osmolality was 360 mOsm/kg (reflecting hypernatremia). A diagnosis of central DI was made and vasopressin was administered. In 3 days the serum sodium level had fallen to 130 mEq/L.

COMMENTARY: This patient was not hydrated adequately at the onset and thus developed hypernatremia. The staff should have been alert for CDI because of the nature of the injury (basal skull fracture). Excessive use of vasopressin caused the development of hyponatremia.

● **4-10.** For the past 6 months a 65-year-old man had received diuretics to manage his hypertension. During a visit to his physician, he reported that he was more thirsty than usual and frequently had to get up at night to urinate (nocturia). Laboratory analysis found his serum potassium to be 2.4 mEq/L. He was hospitalized for evaluation; it was found that he could concentrate his urine to only 300 mOsm/kg on fluid restriction (instead of the expected 1,200–1,400 mOsm/kg in normal renal function). After correction of the hypokalemia, his renal concentrating ability and urine volume eventually returned to normal.

COMMENTARY: This patient had acquired NDI due to hypokalemia. Many patients with potassium depletion complain of polyuria; it is caused by a reduced ability to concentrate the urine due to decreased responsiveness to ADH. This resistance to ADH may be due to an interference with the generation and action of cyclic adenosine monophosphate.[127] Although the NDI associated with hypokalemia is usually reversible, recall that more severe changes are possible with prolonged hypokalemia. The serum sodium level was not elevated because the patient managed to drink sufficient fluids to match the increased output of dilute urine.

● **4-11.** A physician prescribed 20 mL of 0.9% NaCl to be administered over 30 minutes to a hypotensive newborn; instead of a vial of 0.9% NaCl, the nurse inadvertently obtained a vial of 14.6% NaCl.[128] (Unfortunately, the vial's label did not clearly warn that the solution was highly concentrated and required dilution.) Two doses were administered from the vial and the infant developed apnea and required intubation. Blood was drawn and showed a serum sodium level of 195 mEq/L.

COMMENTARY: The greatly elevated serum sodium level resulted in severe, permanent brain damage, requiring that the child be institutionalized. An important lesson to learn from the tragic event reported here is the need to carefully check all vials before administering any solution.

● **4-12.** A 70-year-old previously healthy woman suffered a stroke that rendered her partially paralyzed and unable to swallow normally. However, with assistance, she was able to consume fluids and nutrients without significant aspiration. The patient expressed a desire to be rehabilitated and tried to cooperate fully in her care. After treatment in an acute care facility, she was transferred to a skilled nursing facility for rehabilitation. While there, she did not receive adequate fluid or nutrients and lost over 7 lb; her serum sodium level increased from normal to 160 mEq/L and she had a sacral decubitus ulcer. From the skilled nursing home, she was transferred to a long-term care facility where the care was even worse. Over the course of several weeks, due to inadequate attention and assistance with drinking and eating, her serum sodium rose to 180 mEq/L. At no time while in either facility was the patient offered a feeding tube to assist in fluid and nutrient intake. When her neurological status deteriorated, her family insisted that she be readmitted to the acute care facility. Despite heroic efforts to correct her hypernatremia safely, the patient succumbed to her illness.

COMMENTARY: There was no excuse for the failure to provide adequate fluid and nutrients to this patient who wished to receive all needed therapeutic interventions. Another disturbing feature of this case was the frequent checking of a nursing diagnosis entitled "potential for inadequate fluid and nutrient intake due to swallowing deficit."

Other diagnoses checked off on a daily basis were "potential for skin breakdown due to incontinence" and "potential for electrolyte imbalances." Thus, while the staff indicated on the checklist that they were aware of potential problems, they did not take the necessary actions to prevent these serious problems nor did they recognize the problems in a timely fashion.

● SODIUM AND HEAT STRESS

Physiological disturbances related to heat stress range from mild to severe. This discussion describes the relationship between sodium and the major types of heat-related disorders.

HEAT SYNCOPE

Heat syncope is associated with postural hypotension, which occurs when blood is diverted to peripheral tissues for cooling. Diminished venous return to the heart and reduction of cardiac output lead to cerebral ischemia, which accounts for the syncope. This condition is most likely to occur in persons with deficiencies in salt and water, particularly if cardiovascular disease is present. Thus, patients receiving diuretics are at increased risk. Treatment other than rest in a cool environment generally is not needed.

HEAT EDEMA

Shortly after entering a hot climate, slight swelling of the hands and feet is common among individuals not accustomed to the heat. Most often occurring in women, the edema disappears as heat tolerance is gained. Likely causes are salt and water retention from salt supplementation, increased aldosterone production, and oliguria after heat-induced vasodilation.[129] Fortunately, this is a self-limiting condition that does not require treatment.

HEAT CRAMPS

As the name implies, *heat cramps* are characterized by painful muscle contractions in persons exposed to heat stress. More specifically, heat cramps are painful, intermittent contractions of skeletal muscles after strenuous activity in a hot environment. (Of interest, they most often occur in individuals in excellent physical condition who are accustomed to working in a hot environment. Such individuals are able to produce large quantities of sweat in response to strenuous exercise and heat stress.)

Precipitating factors are strenuous exercise, hemodilution (due to large water intake with no salt), and cooling of the muscle. Because individuals with heat cramps are hyponatremic, it is believed that the mechanism for heat cramp production is sodium depletion in the muscle. Typically, heat cramps occur toward the end of a strenuous period, after bathing in cool water.[130]

Ingestion of salt before or during exercise is usually an effective prophylaxis for heat cramps. To replace salt lost in sweat, salt can be added to foods as a seasoning or can be consumed in liquids having salt as a component. Once heat cramps have occurred, treatment involves salt ingestion, either orally or IV. For severe, unrelenting cramps, oral or IV salt solutions quickly relieve all signs.[131]

HEAT EXHAUSTION

Heat exhaustion is a common yet vague clinical entity. Although pure forms are uncommon, heat exhaustion can be divided into two major forms: (1) associated primarily with sodium depletion (hyponatremia) and (2) associated with dehydration (water deficit with hypernatremia).

Heat Exhaustion Due Primarily to Salt Depletion

Heat exhaustion due to salt depletion occurs when large volumes of sweat from heat-stressed individuals are replaced by adequate volumes of water but too little salt. This condition differs from heat cramps in two ways: (1) it tends to occur in individuals who are not accustomed to heat stress, and (2) it involves systemic effects beyond skeletal muscle cramps. Among these are fatigue, weakness, giddiness, frontal headache, anorexia, nausea, vomiting, and diarrhea.[132] Because water is consumed to replace the lost sweat, marked weight loss may not occur. Treatment consists of administering salted liquids by mouth. If necessary, isotonic saline (0.9% NaCl) may be given IV.

Heat Exhaustion Due to Water Depletion

This form of heat exhaustion is caused when sweat losses are not replaced by the individual working under heat stress, resulting in a negative water balance. As a rule, this set of circumstances is experienced by individuals for whom the water supply is limited (eg, soldiers or laborers who are unable to gain access to water). Clinically, there is intense thirst, fatigue, weakness, discomfort, and impaired judgment.[133] Body temperature is almost always elevated, although not to the level associated with heatstroke. The person with heat exhaustion due to water depletion usually has a temperature that is normal or lower than 39°C (102°F), whereas the person with heatstroke usually has a much higher temperature. Left untreated, heat exhaustion may terminate in heatstroke.[134]

Treatment consists of water replacement. However, rapid correction of severe hypernatremia must be guarded against to avoid initiating convulsive seizures. It has been recommended that the serum osmolality be decreased at a rate no faster than 2 to 4 mOsm/hr.[135] If possible, water should be given orally. However, if the patient is vomiting or unconscious, the solution of choice is 5% dextrose in water; when the serum sodium has fallen to 150 mEq/L, hypotonic saline (0.45% NaCl) can be substituted for water.[136]

HEATSTROKE

Heatstroke is likely with elevation of body temperature beyond a critical point (106°–108°F).[137] Symptoms include delirium, dizziness, abdominal distress, and eventually loss of consciousness. Symptoms are related in part to reduced circulatory volume brought about by excessive sweating. Others are directly related to the effects of hyperthermia on the brain and other body tissues. Autopsies on individuals who died from heatstroke have shown hemorrhages and parenchymatous cellular degeneration throughout the body.

Two forms of heatstroke are often described, classic and exercise-induced. *Classic heatstroke* occurs primarily in invalids or in the elderly during a sustained heat wave. In contrast, *exertion-induced heatstroke* usually occurs in well-conditioned athletes or workers whose physical means to dissipate heat are exceeded by endogenous heat production. Examples include football players, marathon runners, and military recruits.

Most important in the treatment of heatstroke is lowering body temperature to a safe level. Among the methods used are cold water immersion with skin massage,[138] compressed air/warm water sprays,[139] and strategically placed ice packs.[140] It has been suggested that effective body cooling may occur with water having a temperature of 15° to 16°C (59°–61°F).[141]

Placement of IV lines and tracheal intubation are necessary, as is placement of a rectal thermistor to measure core temperature. Hypotension is likely to be present as blood is shunted to the periphery for cooling. Excessive fluid replacement should be guarded against because pulmonary edema could result as cooling promotes return of peripheral blood to the central circulation. Sodium levels are variable and often depend on conditions leading to heatstroke. The most important laboratory measurements at time of admission are arterial blood gases, serum electrolyte concentrations, and complete blood count. Treatment is based on results and other clinical findings.

PREVENTIVE MEASURES AND RATIONALES

Heat disorders can often be prevented, or at least minimized, by some relatively simple measures.

1. Before engaging in sustained strenuous activity, undergo acclimatization to a hot environment.
   - Exposure to heat for several hours each day while performing physical activity will increase tolerance to heat in 1 to 2 weeks.[142] Acclimatized individuals attain an increased maximum rate of sweating, increased plasma volume, and decreased loss of salt in the sweat and urine. The latter two effects are related to an increased production of aldosterone. (Although the sodium content of sweat in these individuals is less than that in nonacclimatized persons, it can still be the source of significant sodium loss.)
2. To offset the body's loss of water and salt in sweat, drink cool liquids at regular intervals while undergoing heat stress.
   - First, consider fluids that are inappropriate for replacing losses. Alcohol is certainly contraindicated because it has diuretic effects but, more important, because it can alter judgment about heat exposure. Furthermore, a brief period of moderate or heavy alcohol intake often appears to cause loss of acclimatization.[143] Coffee and tea are not recommended for sole use in fluid replacement because these beverages have diuretic properties and predispose to further fluid loss.
   - Depending on individual need, fluid replacement can be in the form of water, NaCl solution, or a balanced electrolyte solution. *Water is often sufficient* when the subject has taken in a normal diet supplying ample sodium, potassium, and other electrolytes. However, sustained losses of sweat necessitate electrolyte replacement in addition to water. It is important for athletes to ensure adequate sodium intake during heavy exercise.[144] Care must be taken to avoid excessive salt and insufficient water intake because this practice predisposes to water-depletion heat exhaustion that can culminate in heatstroke.[145]
   - A few oral electrolyte-rehydrating fluids are available commercially and usually contain varying quantities of carbohydrates in the form of simple sugars or glucose polymers. Advantages of carbohydrates in replacement fluids are improved endurance during strenuous exertion (due to muscle glycogen sparing) and pleasant taste (perhaps ensuring that they will be consumed in greater quantity than plain water or electrolyte solutions).[146] It is thought that an athlete's performance is improved with the ingestion of about 60 g carbohydrate per hour during exercise.[147]

To compare the effects of drinking distilled water versus drinking a carbohydrate-electrolyte solution* on physiological disturbances during prolonged strenuous exercise in the heat, Carter and Gisolfi[148] studied seven men during and after vigorous bouts of cycle exercise. They concluded that the carbohydrate-electrolyte beverage used in their study maintained plasma volume at a level higher than water during exercise, supplied an energy source, and rehydrated subjects faster than water during recovery.

   - The number of people participating in marathons and triathlons has greatly increased over the past decade. Electrolyte disturbances are more likely to occur during events that last a prolonged period in the heat. During triathlon events in high environmental temperatures, vol-

---

*Composed of 4.85% polycose, 2.65% fructose, 9.2 mM Na, 5.0 mM K, 2.1 mM Ca, 2.1 mM Mg, 9.6 mM Cl, 250 mOsm/L.

ume depletion and hyponatremia are likely if the athlete replaces sweat losses with water (although in inadequate amounts) but no salt. As Hiller[149] reported, it is common for endurance athletes to be both volume depleted and hyponatremic after races, such as triathlons, lasting longer than 8 hours. In these situations, the exercise-induced hyponatremia is a combination of massive unreplaced sodium losses associated with partially replaced massive water losses. Hiller[150] recommends that endurance athletes practice programmed replacement of hourly fluid losses (such as 500 mL of fluid for each 1-lb weight loss), and that they use some form of sodium replacement during events lasting longer than 4 hours. He further recommends that they prepare by increasing their salt intake during the period before the event during which they become acclimatized. If sodium-containing fluids are needed to treat athletes after the events, 5% dextrose in normal saline may be used for races lasting longer than 4 hours and 5% dextrose in either normal or half-normal saline for events lasting less than 4 hours.[151]

3. Strenuous activity on hot days should be curtailed as much as possible.
   - Periods of prolonged exercise, such as training programs or athletic events, should take place during the cooler parts of the day (before 8 AM and after 5 PM). Care should be taken to avoid direct solar heat radiation during the hottest hours of the day (11 AM to 2 PM).

4. When possible, loose, porous clothing should be worn to allow for heat dissipation.
   - A hat and light-colored clothing are helpful in decreasing the amount of heat absorbed from direct sunlight, although workers in specific jobs may need different types of clothing. For example, those working with radiant heat should wear reflective garments. Unfortunately, the nature of some work requires that special protective clothing be worn, further predisposing to heat injury. For example, welders and others exposed to sparks should wear self-extinguishing materials like "green cotton," that is, cotton treated with flame retardant.[152]
   - Firefighters must wear heavy protective clothing (often rubberized) that predisposes them to

increased heat stress. Engaging in strenuous activity while dressed in impervious plastic sweat clothing is potentially disastrous. The belief that this activity can safely result in weight loss in overweight athletes is erroneous.

5. During extreme high temperatures, individuals without air conditioners or fans should make use of "cooling centers" that are usually available in most communities.
   - Unfortunately, many elderly inner city residents are hesitant to leave their homes for cooling centers during heat waves because of a fear of burglaries or vandalism.

6. Adequate fluids should be provided for confused or otherwise debilitated patients unable to respond to thirst.

7. Coaches and trainers in athletic programs and supervisors in the workplace should be aware of the warning signs of heat disorders and the measures to deal with them.

8. Participants and planners of competitive sports events should consider the following points:
   - Competitors should train in the heat before the big event to promote acclimatization.
   - Competitors should avoid fluid restriction before the start of the event. Pre-event dehydration results in a reduction of the body's sweating and, therefore, cooling abilities.
   - Fluid stations should be readily available at strategic locations to allow the competitors to replace needed fluids.
   - Competitors and race officials should be aware that events lasting longer than 4 hours are more likely to produce fluid and electrolyte problems than are those lasting less than 4 hours.
   - Trained spotters should be placed at regular intervals during the event to identify competitors with early signs of heat injury. Cooling and fluid replacement should be initiated on the spot. Athletes should use the "buddy system" and assume mutual responsibility for each other's well-being during the event.

9. Because children are less efficient thermoregulators than adults, they are at increased risk for heat illness. Like adults, children should undergo a period of acclimatization before indulging in heavy exercise in hot temperatures and should modify their physical activity in the face of high

ambient temperature and humidity. Although they may benefit from drinking carbohydrate-electrolyte-containing solutions, for the majority of young athletes, cold water remains the preferred choice for fluid replacement during exercise.[153]

REFERENCES

1. Schwartz S, ed. *Principles of Surgery*, 7th ed. New York: McGraw-Hill; 1999:56.
2. Narins R, ed. *Clinical Disorders of Fluid and Electrolyte Metabolism*, 5th ed. New York: McGraw-Hill; 1994:1196.
3. Ibid, p 591.
4. Kovacs L, Robertson G. Disorders of water balance-hyponatremia and hypernatremia. *Baillieres Clin Endocrinol Metab* 1992;6(1):107.
5. Oh M, Carroll H. Disorders of sodium metabolism: Hypernatremia and hyponatremia. *Crit Care Med* 1992;20(1):94.
6. Fried L, Palevsky P. Hyponatremia and hypernatremia. *Med Clin North Am* 1997;81(3)585.
7. Narins, p 592.
8. Ibid, p 595.
9. Sjoblom E, Hajer J, Ludwings S, et al. Fatal hyponatremic brain edema due to common gastroenteritis with accidental water intoxication. *Intensive Care Med* 1997;23:348.
10. Rose B. *Clinical Physiology of Acid-Base and Electrolyte Disorders*, 4th ed. New York: McGraw-Hill; 1994:391.
11. Ibid.
12. Narins, p 595.
13. Arieff A, DeFronzo R. *Fluid, Electrolyte, Acid-Base Disorders*, 2nd ed. New York: Churchill Livingstone; 1995:174.
14. Tierney L, McPhee S, Papadakis M. *Medical Diagnosis & Treatment*, 38th ed. Stamford, CT: Appleton & Lange; 1999: 842.
15. Lauriat S, Berl T. The hyponatremic patient: Practical focus on therapy. *J Am Soc Nephrol* 1997; 1599 (Volume 8).
16. Sterns R. Severe symptomatic hyponatremia, treatment and outcome: A study of 64 cases. *Ann Intern Med* 1987;107:656.
17. Sonnenblick M, Friedlander Y, Rosen A. Diuretic-induced severe hyponatremia: Review and analysis of 129 reported patients. *Chest* 1993;103:602.
18. Spigset O, Hedenmalm K. Hyponatremia in relation to treatment with antidepressants: A survey of reports in the World Health Organization data base for spontaneous reporting of adverse drug reactions. *Pharmacotherapy* 1997;17(2):348.
19. Ibid.
20. Bouman W, Pinner G, Johnson . Incidence of selective serotonin reuptake inhibitor (SSRI) induced hyponatremia due to the syndrome of inappropriate antidiuretic hormone (SIADH) secretion in the elderly. *Int J Geriatr Psychiatry* 1998;13:12.
21. Sharma H, Pompei P. Antidepressant-induced hyponatremia in the aged. *Drugs Aging* 1996;8(5):430.
22. Rose, p 662.
23. Kokko J, Tannen R. *Fluids and Electrolytes*, 3rd ed. Philadelphia: WB Saunders; 1996:86.
24. Peyrade F, Tailan B, Lebrun C, et al. Hyponatremia during treatment with cisplatin. *Presse Med* 1997;26:1523.
25. Narins, p 598.
26. Lahr M. Hyponatremia during carbamazepine therapy. *Clin Pharmacol Ther* 1985;37:693.
27. Rose, p 662.
28. Narins, p 597.
29. Rose, p 663.
30. Nelson W, Behrman R, Kliegman R, Arvin A. *Nelson Textbook of Pediatrics*, Philadelphia: WB Saunders; 1996:79.
31. Donoghue M, Latimer E, Pillsbury H, et al. Hyponatremic seizure in a child using desmopressin for nocturnal enuresis. *Arch Pediatr Adolesc Med* 1998;152:290.
32. Bloom D. The American experience with desmopressin. *Clin Pediatr* 1993;July (special issue):28.
33. Bernstein S, Williford S. Intranasal desmopressin-associated hyponatremia: A case report and literature review. *J Fam Pract* 1997;44(2):208.
34. Ibid.
35. Donoghue, p 292.
36. Rose, p 662.
37. Weissman P, Shenkman L, Gregerman R. Chlorpropamide hyponatremia: Drug-induced inappropriate antidiuretic hormone activity. *New England J of Med* 284(2):65.
38. Kadowaki T, Hagura R, Kajinuma H, et al. Chlorpropamide-induced hyponatremia: Incidence and risk factors. *Diabetes Care* 1983;5:468.
39. Arieff & DeFronzo, p 274.
40. Durst R, Pipek R, Levy Y. Hyponatremia caused by omeprazole treatment. *Am J Med* 1994;97:400.
41. Shiba S, Suguira K, Ebata A, et al. Hyponatremia with consciousness disturbance caused by omeprazole administration. *Dig Dis Sci* 1996;41:1617.
42. Chung. Postoperative hyponatremia. *Arch Intern Med* 1986; 146:333.
43. Narins, p 599.
44. Ayus C, Wheeler J, Arieff A. Postoperative hyponatremic encephalopathy in menstruant women. *Ann Intern Med* 1992; 117:891.
45. Ellis R, Carmichael J. Hyponatremia and volume overload as a complication of transurethral resection of the prostate. *J Fam Pract* 1991;33(1):89.
46. Narins, p 1419.
47. Tierney et al, p 841.
48. Narins, p 1419.
49. Ayus et al, p 893.
50. Ibid.
51. Ibid.
52. Verghese C, Leon J, Josiassen R. Problems and progress in the diagnosis and treatment of polydipsia and hyponatremia. *Schizophr Bull* 1996;22:455.
53. Shutty M, Leadbetter R. Salt appetite with psychosis, intermittent hyponatremia and polydipsia. *Am J Psychiatry* 1993;150:4.
54. Arieff A, DeFronzo, p 275.
55. Ellinas P, Rosner F, Jauma J. Symptomatic hyponatremia associated with psychoses, medications, and smoking. *J Nat Med Assoc* 1993;85:135.

56. Rose, p 662.
57. Narins, p 559.
58. Brown R. Disorders of water and sodium balance. *Postgrad Med* 1993;93:227.
59. Narins, p 598.
60. Glassock R et al. Human immunodeficiency virus (HIV) and the kidney. *Ann Intern Med* 1990;112:35.
61. Vitting et al. Frequency of hyponatremia and nonosmolar vasopressin release in the acquired immunodeficiency syndrome. *JAMA* 1990;263:973.
62. Agarwal et al. Hyponatremia in patients with the acquired immunodeficiency syndrome. *Nephron* 1989;53:317.
63. Tolaymat A, Al-Mousily F. Hyponatremia in pediatric patients with HIV-1 infection. *South Med J* 1995;88:1039.
64. Rose, p 661.
65. Oh, Carroll, p 94.
66. Pemberton L, Pemberton D. *Treatment of Water, Electrolyte & Acid-Base Disorders in the Surgical Patient.* New York: McGraw-Hill; 1994:77.
67. Narins, p 599.
68. Ibid.
69. Rose, p 671.
70. Arieff A, Ayus J, Fraser C. Hyponatremia and death or permanent brain damage in children. *Br Med J* 1992;304:1218.
71. Chernow B, ed. *The Pharmacologic Approach to the Critically Ill Patient,* 3rd ed. Baltimore, MD: Williams & Wilkins; 1994:560.
72. Ayus J, Arieff A. Symptomatic hyponatremia: Correcting sodium deficits safely. *J Crit Illness* 1990;5:905.
73. Brunner J et al. Central pontine myelinolysis and pontine lesions after rapid correction of hyponatremia: A prospective magnetic resonance imaging study. *Ann Neurol* 1990;27:61.
74. Narins, p 601.
75. Ayus J, Arieff A. Symptomatic hyponatremia: Making the diagnosis rapidly. *J Crit Illness* 1990;5:846.
76. Ayus J, Arieff A. Symptomatic hyponatremia: Correcting sodium deficits safely. *J Crit Illness* 1990;5:905.
77. Ibid.
78. Rose, p 678.
79. Ibid.
80. Ibid.
81. Chernow, p 959.
82. Rose, p 684.
83. Ibid.
84. Narins, p 606.
85. Ibid.
86. Rose, p 684.
87. Yamamura Y, Ogawa H, Yamashita H, et al. Characterization of a novel aquaretic agent OPC-31260, as an orally effective, nonpeptide V2 receptor antagonist. *Br J Pharmacol* 1992;105:787.
88. Saito T, Ishikawa S, Abe K, et al. Acute aquaresis by the nonpeptide arginine vasopressin (AVP) antagonist OPC-31260 improves hyponatremia in patients with syndrome of inappropriate secretion of antidiuretic hormone (SIADH). *J Clin Endocrinol Metab* 1997;82:1054.
89. Kitiyakara C, Wilcox C. Vasopressin V2 receptor antagonists: Panaceas for hyponatremia? *Curr Opin Nephrol Hypertens* 1997; 6:461.
90. Pennington J. *Bowes and Church's Food Values of Portions Commonly Used,* 17th ed. Philadelphia: Lippincott-Raven; 1998:140, 258.
91. Rose, p 678.
92. Ayus, Arieff, p 906.
93. Rose, p 678.
94. Palevsky P. Hypernatremia. *Semin Nephrol* 1998;18:20.
95. Ibid.
96. Rose, p 263.
97. Mochuria R, Schexnayder S, Glasier C. Fatal cerebral edema and intracranial hemorrhage associated with hypernatremic dehydration. *Pediatr Radiol* 1997;27:784.
98. Rose, p 711.
99. Mandal A, Saklayen M, Hillman N, et al. Predictive factors for high mortality in hypernatremic patients. *Am J Emerg Med* 1997;15:130.
100. Narins, p 1525.
101. Ellis R. Severe hypernatremia from sea water ingestion during near-drowning in a hurricane. *West J Med* 1997;167:430.
102. Narins, p 1525.
103. Ibid, p 636.
104. Rose, p 704.
105. Ibid, p 712.
106. Pemberton, p 101.
107. Ibid.
108. Ibid, p 102.
109. Schwartz, p 66.
110. Rose, p 710.
111. Ibid, p 721.
112. Narins, p 1529.
113. Oh, Carroll, p 94.
114. Ibid.
115. Chernow, p 960.
116. Narins, p 1529.
117. Ibid.
118. Schwartz p 76.
119. Votey S, Peters A, Hoffman J. Disorders of water metabolism: Hyponatremia and hypernatremia. *Emerg Med Clin North Am* 1989;7:749.
120. Bell T. Diabetes insipidus: In: Endocrine and Metabolic Disturbances in the Critically Ill. *Crit Care Nurs Clin N Am* December 1994:682.
121. Ibid.
122. Oh, Carroll, p 94.
123. Brensilver J, Goldberger E. *A Primer of Water, Electrolyte, and Acid-Base Syndromes,* 8th ed. Philadelphia: Lea & Febiger; 1996:102.
124. Rose, p 697.
125. Himmelstein D, Jones A, Woolhander S. Hypernatremic dehydration in nursing home patients: An indicator of neglect. *J Am Geriatr Soc* 1983;31:466.
126. Rose, p 710.
127. Ibid, p 704.
128. Cohen M. Sodium chloride vial concentration above 0.9% should make you nervous. *Intravenous Nurses Society Newsline* 1994;15:8, 10.
129. Ibid.
130. Narins, p 1559.
131. Ibid, p 1560.
132. Ibid.
133. Ibid.
134. Ibid.
135. Ibid, p 1561.
136. Ibid.
137. Guyton A, Hall J. *Human Physiology and Mechanisms of Disease.* Philadelphia: WB Saunders; 1997:581.
138. Costrini A. Emergency treatment of exertional heatstroke and comparison of whole body cooling techniques. *Med Sci Sports Exerc* 1990;22(1):15.
139. Wyndham C, Strydom B, Cooke H. Methods of cooling subjects with hyperpyrexia. *J Appl Physiol* 1959;14:771.
140. Kielblock A, VanRensberg J, Franz R. Body cooling as a method for reducing hyperpyrexia. *S Afr Med J* 1986;69:378.

141. Magazinik A et al. Tap water, an efficient method for cooling heatstroke victims-A model in dogs. *Aviat Space Environ Med* 1980;5:864.
142. Guyton, Hall, p 698.
143. Narins, p 1526.
144. Murray R. Rehydration strategies—balancing substrate, fluid, and electrolyte provision. *Int J Sports Med* 1998;19:S133.
145. Narins, p 1567.
146. Convertino V, Armstrong L, Coyle E, et al. American College of Sports Medicine position stand: Electrolyte and fluid replacement. *Med Sci Sports Exerc* 1996;82:i.
147. Murray, S135.
148. Carter J, Gisolfi C. Fluid replacement during and after exercise in the heat. *Med Sci Sports Exerc* 1989;21:532.
149. Hiller W. Dehydration and hyponatremia during triathlons. *Med Sci Sports Exerc* 1989;21:S219.
150. Ibid.
151. Ibid.
152. Eisma T. Cool under fire: Wearers of heat-protective clothing must avoid heat stress. *Occup Health Saf* 1989;November:26.
153. Squire D. Heat illness: Fluid and electrolyte issues for pediatric and adolescent athletes. *Pediatr Clin North Am* 1990; 37:1085.

Potassium Imbalances

Disturbances in potassium balance are common because they are associated with a number of disease and injury states. Unfortunately, they may also be induced by the administration of a variety of medications as well as by therapies such as hyperalimentation and chemotherapy as well as by a variety of medications (Table 5-1).

It is important to review some pertinent facts about potassium before proceeding to discussions of hypokalemia and hyperkalemia.

● POTASSIUM BALANCE

Potassium is the major *intracellular* electrolyte; in fact, 98% of the body's potassium is inside the cells. The remaining 2% is in the extracellular fluid (ECF): this 2% is important in neuromuscular function. For example, alterations in plasma potassium concentrations can significantly affect myocardial irritability and rhythm. Changes in the electrocardiogram (ECG) associated with serum potassium level variations are illustrated in Figure 5-1.

Normal renal function is necessary for maintenance of potassium balance because 80% of the potassium excreted daily from the body is by way of the kidneys. The other 20% is lost through the bowel (15%) and sweat glands (5%).[1]

Potassium must be replaced daily, either enterally or parenterally; about 40 to 50 mEq/day suffices in the adult if no abnormal losses are occurring. Dietary intake in the average adult is 50 to 100 mEq/day.[2] Because potassium is plentiful in the normal diet (in

● TABLE 5-1. Examples of Medications Associated With Potassium Imbalances

Hypokalemia	Hyperkalemia
Potassium-losing diuretics	Potassium-sparing diuretics
Acetazolamide	Amiloride
Bumetanide	Spironolactone
Chlorothalidone	Triamterene
Ethacrynic acid	Potassium supplements
Furosemide	Potassium chloride
Hydrochlorothiazide	Potassium citrate
Metolazone	Potassium gluconate
β_2-Adrenergic agonists	Angiotensin-converting enzyme inhibitors
Albuterol	Amiodipine
Dobutamine	Captopril
Tocolytic agents	Enalapril
Ritodrine	Lisinopril
Terbutaline	β blockers
Drugs associated with magnesium depletion	Metoprolol
Aminoglycosides	Penbutolol
Amphotericin B	Propranolol
Cisplatin	Nonsteroidal anti-inflammatory drugs
Others	Aspirin
Overdose of insulin	Ibuprofen
Overdose of verapamil	Indomethacin
Mineralocorticoids	Ketorolac
Fludrocortisone	Naproxen
Cathartics	Piroxicam
	Heparin
	Trimethoprim/sulfamethoxazole
	Cyclosporine

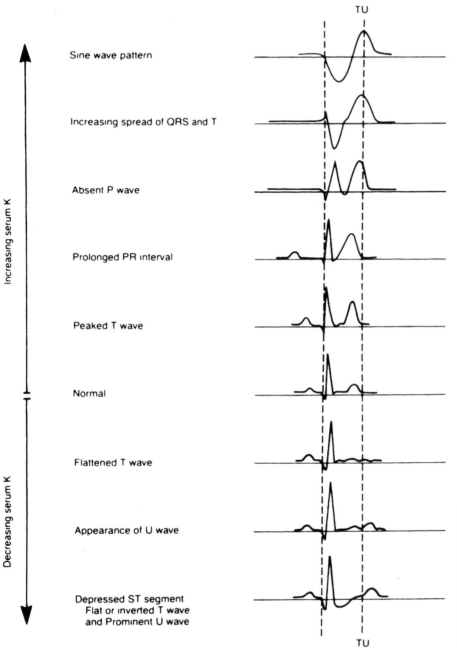

FIGURE 5-1. ECG manifestations of hypokalemia and hyperkalemia. Either extreme in the serum potassium level may lead to ventricular fibrillation; ventricular standstill or complete heart block is more common in hyperkalemia. (From Zull D. Disorders of potassium metabolism. *Emerg Med Clin North Am* 1989; 7:783.

meat, fruits, and some vegetables), poor dietary intake rarely causes hypokalemia; however, it contributes to other causes of hypokalemia.

Potassium is constantly moving in and out of cells according to the body's needs, under the influence of the sodium–potassium pump. For example, alterations in acid–base balance can have a significant effect on potassium distribution: potassium ions move into the cells when alkalosis is present and out of the cells when acidosis occurs. In the presence of acid–base disturbances, the plasma potassium level may not reflect the true status of total body potassium stores. Refer to Chapter 9 for a more thorough discussion of the effect of acidemia and alkalemia on plasma potassium concentration.

HYPOKALEMIA

Most laboratories list the normal plasma potassium range as 3.5 to 5.0 mEq/L. *Hypokalemia* refers to a below-normal serum potassium concentration. Mild hypokalemia is arbitrarily defined as ranging between 3.0 and 3.5 mEq/L. This degree of potassium depletion is usually well tolerated in the absence of digitalis therapy or severe hepatic disease. Moderate hypokalemia is arbitrarily said to range between 2.5 and 3.0 mEq/L, whereas severe hypokalemia is generally defined as less than 2.5 mEq/L.[3] Hypokalemia usually indicates a real deficit in total potassium stores; however, it may occur in patients having normal potassium stores when alkalosis is present (because alkalosis causes a temporary shift of serum potassium into the cells). Hypokalemia is a common disturbance with a number of etiologies. Frequently, a combination of factors predisposes to hypokalemia.

ETIOLOGICAL FACTORS

Renal Losses

Potassium-losing diuretics, such as the thiazides, furosemide, and ethacrynic acid, are commonly associated with hypokalemia, particularly when given in high doses to patients with poor potassium intake.

As many as 50% of patients receiving potassium-losing diuretics may develop serum potassium levels less than 3.5 mEq/L.[4] Diuretics may also induce intravascular volume contraction, which in turn stimulates aldosterone secretion, which adds to the renal loss of potassium. Diuretic-induced hypokalemia is usually (but not always) associated with a mild-to-moderate metabolic alkalosis.[5]

Aldosterone (a mineralocorticoid) is perhaps the most important hormone regulating total body potassium homeostasis. Excess aldosterone production enhances renal potassium wasting and thus commonly leads to hypokalemia. Although primary hyperaldosteronism (due to adrenal adenomas and adrenal hyperplasia) is relatively rare, secondary hyperaldosteronism is a common occurrence in patients with cirrhosis, nephrotic syndrome, congestive heart failure, and malignant hypertension.

High serum glucocorticoid levels, as occur in Cushing's syndrome, or excessive steroid administration, for conditions such as arthritis or asthma, can cause potassium depletion.

Renal potassium wasting may also be caused by certain medications, such as amphotericin B, gentamicin, and cisplatin.[6] In fact, hypokalemia due to increased urinary losses occurs in up to half of the patients receiving amphotericin B.[7] Also implicated as potential causes of hypokalemia are some of the penicillin derivatives (including sodium penicillin, ampicillin, carbenicillin, oxacillin, nafcillin, and ticaricillin).[8] Aminoglycosides can cause hypokalemia either in the presence or absence of overt nephrotoxicity.[9]

Chronic ingestion of licorice as candy or in certain chewing tobaccos can produce hypokalemia; this is because licorice contains glycyrrhizic acid, a substance that has mineralocorticoid activity (which favors potassium loss). A 55-year-old woman developed a serum potassium concentration of 2.0 mEq/L following the habitual ingestion of 1 kg licorice candy per week.[10]

Although the mechanism is poorly understood, hypomagnesemia from any cause can lead to potassium depletion. When this is the case, correction of the hypokalemia requires the restoration of magnesium balance.[11]

The osmotic diuresis associated with glucosuria causes real potassium wasting, which is presumably associated with increased fluid delivery to the distal tubular potassium secretory site.

Gastrointestinal Losses

Gastrointestinal (GI) losses of potassium are a common cause of potassium depletion. Vomiting and gastric suction frequently lead to hypokalemia, partly because of actual potassium loss in gastric fluid, but largely because of increased renal potassium loss associated with metabolic alkalosis. (Recall that loss of acidic gastric fluid causes metabolic alkalosis; then, the kidneys attempt to conserve hydrogen ions to correct the pH disturbances. In this process, potassium ions are lost in greater amounts.)

Relatively large amounts of potassium are contained in intestinal fluids; for example, diarrheal fluid may contain as much as 30 mEq/L. Therefore, potassium deficit occurs frequently with diarrhea, prolonged intestinal suction, recent ileostomy, and villous adenoma. A dramatic cause of diarrheal potassium loss occurs with villous adenomas, with which up to 1 to 3 liters of potassium-rich fluid (as high as 80 mEq/L) may be lost.[12]

Shift Into Cells

In alkalosis, hydrogen ions shift out of the cells to help correct the pH defect; potassium ions from the ECF move into the cells to maintain electroneutrality. (See Chap. 9 for a more thorough discussion of the effects of alkalemia on plasma potassium concentration.)

Entry of potassium into skeletal muscle and hepatic cells is promoted by insulin; thus, patients with persistent insulin hypersecretion may experience hypokalemia. This is often seen in individuals receiving high-carbohydrate parenteral fluids (as in hyperalimentation). Later in the chapter insulin administration is discussed as a therapeutic measure for temporary relief of life-threatening hyperkalemia.

Catecholamines promote potassium entry into the cells. Therefore, transient hypokalemia can be induced when epinephrine release is enhanced by the stress of an acute illness, such as an episode of coronary ischemia, acute head trauma, and postcardiopulmonary resuscitation.

Similarly, the plasma potassium concentration can fall by 0.5 to 1 mEq/L after the administration of a β-adrenergic agonist (such as albuterol or dobutamine) to treat asthma or heart failure.[13] Hypokalemia is a well known side effect of overdosage with albuterol and other β-adrenergic agonists; however, cases have also been reported after normal doses.[14] The hypokalemia associated with these drugs is sustained for up to 4 hours.[15]

Ritodrine and terbutaline are inhibitors of uterine contraction; these drugs can reduce serum potassium to as low as 2.5 mEq/L after 4 to 6 hours of intravenous (IV) administration.[16]

Hypothermia stimulates the cellular uptake of extracellular potassium; this hypokalemic effect is reversible on rewarming.[17] If the hypokalemia is treated with vigorous potassium replacement, "overshoot" hyperkalemia may occur. If irreversible tissue necrosis occurs during a period of profound hypothermia (as in patients who are essentially dead after accidental hypothermia), a plasma potassium concentration of more than 10 to 20 mEq/L may be found.[18]

Hypokalemic periodic paralysis is a rare disorder that is characterized by intermittent muscle weakness following an intracellular influx of potassium; it may be familial (through an autosomal dominant inheritance pattern) or acquired (associated with thyrotoxicosis) and is predominantly seen in men.[19] Muscle weakness may be so pronounced that the patient is temporarily paralyzed. Without interventions, the paralytic attacks last 7 to 14 days.

Sweat Losses

Potassium deficit related to heavy perspiration is most likely to occur in persons who are acclimated to heat, because sweat glands in these individuals tend to excrete more potassium than in those who are not acclimated to heat stress. The mechanism involved is presumably the result of an aldosterone-related effect attempting to conserve sodium (the primary electrolyte in sweat). Sweat losses exceeding 10 L/day have been reported in individuals exercising in a hot climate.

POOR INTAKE

Patients unable or unwilling to eat a normal diet for a prolonged period are candidates for hypokalemia. However, strict fasting usually induces only a moderate depletion of total body potassium if normal homeostatic mechanisms are present. Usually poor intake is coupled with other problems in individuals with low serum potassium levels. For example, in addition to poor intake, individuals with anorexia nervosa frequently abuse diuretics and laxatives and induce vomiting to maintain a low body weight. Alcoholics frequently have other factors predisposing to hypokalemia (such as vomiting, diarrhea, and magnesium deficiency). Refeeding a malnourished patient can lead to serious hypokalemia if inadequate potassium is supplied because insulin release is stimulated by the feeding and promotes anabolism with entry of potassium into the cells.

There is considerable variation in potassium intake, depending on individual preferences. African Americans tend to consume less dietary potassium, which may lead to a state of physiological potassium deficiency and contribute to the incidence of hypertension in this population.[20]

DEFINING CHARACTERISTICS

Because potassium is the major cation in intracellular fluid (ICF), it is understandable that potassium deficit can result in widespread derangements in normal physiological functioning. Some of the more common changes are discussed below. It must be remembered that severe hypokalemia can result in death from cardiac or respiratory arrest. Clinical signs are usually not present until the potassium level falls below 3.0 mEq/L. Among the exceptions are patients with even mild hypokalemia who are receiving digitalis (predisposing them to a greater chance for dysrhythmias) and patients with hepatic failure (who are more prone to hepatic encephalopathy because of increased ammonia production). Hypokalemia is rarely suspected on the basis of clinical presentation alone; the diagnosis is usually made by measurement of the serum potassium level.[21]

Cardiovascular Effects

The major cardiac effects of hypokalemia include abnormalities of electrophysiology and contractility. The most important cardiac derangement associated with hypokalemia is the potential for a variety of atrial and ventricular arrhythmias, particularly in patients with ischemic myocardial disease and those receiving digitalis preparations. Because hypokalemia is associated with increased binding of digitalis to Na^+-K^+-adenosine triphosphatase (ATPase), cardiac sensitivity to digitalis preparations is heightened by hypokalemia.[22] In many instances, hypokalemia and hypomagnesemia occur together; the most serious consequence of this combination of imbalances is increased cardiac irritability and risk for arrhythmias. In patients without underlying heart disease, abnormalities in cardiac conduction are unusual, even when the serum potassium concentration is less than 3 mEq/L.[23]

Still another cardiovascular effect of hypokalemia is its potential relationship with hypertension. A recent meta-analysis concluded that a low potassium intake may play an important role in the genesis of hypertension.[24] The antihypertensive effect of increased potassium intake appears to include enhanced sodium excretion, direct vasodilation, and lower cardiovascular reactivity to norepinephrine or angiotensin II.[25]

Muscular Changes

Potassium levels less than 3.0 mEq/L may be associated with muscular weakness and adynamic ileus. At least two mechanisms are involved; the first involves changes in the resting membrane potential and the other has to do with altered operation of intracellular enzymes. Hypokalemia can hyperpolarize skeletal muscle cells, interfering with their ability to develop the depolarization necessary for muscle contraction. Muscle weakness does not usually start until the

plasma potassium concentration is less than 2.5 mEq/L; the lower extremities are usually involved first (particularly the quadriceps).[16] Later, in severe cases, the muscles of the trunk and upper extremities are involved, eventually causing death from respiratory failure if the condition is not corrected. Symptoms, such as anorexia, nausea, vomiting, prolonged gastric emptying, gaseous distention, and paralytic ileus, are due to weakness of the smooth muscles of the GI tract and impairment of the response to parasympathetic stimulation.

Hypokalemia can reduce blood flow to skeletal muscles; this in turn can predispose to *rhabdomyolysis* (disintegration of striated muscle fibers with excretion of myoglobin in the urine). The effects of the muscle ischemia are made worse by exercising because hypokalemia blocks the vasodilation that normally occurs during exercise. Rhabdomyolysis is usually only seen when the plasma potassium level is less than 2.5 mEq/L.[27]

Renal Changes

Prolonged potassium depletion can lead to inability to maximally concentrate urine. This, in turn, results in dilute urine, polyuria, nocturia, and polydipsia. The reduced ability to concentrate urine is the result of a decreased responsiveness to antidiuretic hormone (ADH).[28] The resistance to ADH appears to be due to interference with the generation and action of cyclic adenosine monophosphate.[29] The polyuria associated with hypokalemia is usually mild, averaging 2 to 3 L/day.[30]

Hormonal Changes

Hypokalemia impairs both insulin release and end-organ sensitivity to insulin; therefore, it contributes to worsening hyperglycemia in diabetic patients.[31] For this reason, control of hypokalemia is especially desirable in patients with diabetes mellitus.

TREATMENT

The best treatment for hypokalemia is prevention. For patients at risk, a diet with ample potassium content should be provided. Table 5-2 lists some foods with high potassium content. However, once hypokalemia has developed, dietary potassium intake may be ineffective replacement because most potassium in foods is

TABLE 5-2. Some Foods With High Potassium Content

Food	Potassium (mg)	Potassium (mEq)
Apricots, raw, 3 medium	313	8.0
Bananas, raw, 1 medium	451	11.6
Cantaloupe, raw, 1 cup pieces	494	12.7
Dates, dried, 10	541	13.9
Orange, 1 medium	250	6.4
Raisins, dried, seedless, 2/3 cup	751	19.3
Carrot, raw, 1 medium	233	6.0
Potato, baked, without skin, 1 medium	610	15.6
Tomato, red, raw, 1	273	7.0
Apricot nectar, canned, 8 fl oz	286	7.3
Orange juice, canned, 8 fl oz	436	11.2
Milk, 1% fat, 8 fl oz	381	9.8

From Pennington J. *Bowes and Church's Food Values of Portions Commonly Used*, 17th ed. Philadelphia: Lippincott-Raven; 1998.

complexed to anions that metabolize into bicarbonate.[32] For example, potassium-rich foods such as orange juice or bananas contain phosphate and citrate rather than chloride and therefore are less likely to correct hypokalemia associated with metabolic alkalosis. Therefore, patients with significant hypokalemia associated with metabolic alkalosis should be given potassium chloride (KCl).[33] Because KCl is efficiently absorbed through the GI tract, no more solution should be given orally than would be given IV over 2 to 3 hours.[34] When dietary intake is inadequate, the physician may prescribe one of the commercially prepared potassium substitutes (available in liquids, effervescent tablets, capsules, or slow-release tablets) (see Clinical Tip: Nursing Considerations in Administer-ing Oral Potassium Supplements). Also available for potassium supplementation are potassium-containing salt substitutes (which usually contain between 50 and 65 mEq potassium per level teaspoon) (Table 5-3).[40] When possible, treatment of hypokalemia by oral replacement is favored because this route allows the serum potassium to rise slowly in equilibration with the intracellular compartment.

Usual maintenance requirements for potassium are 40 to 60 mEq/day in patients with no abnormal routes of potassium loss or other above-average needs for replacement (such as hyperalimentation). When potassium cannot be consumed in adequate amounts in the diet, and when oral potassium supplements are not feasible, the IV route is indicated for replacement. The IV

TABLE 5-3. Potassium and Sodium Content of Some Salt Substitutes and Seasoning Agents

Preparation	Potassium (mg/tsp)	Sodium (mg/tsp)
Morton salt substitute	2,400 (62 mEq)	—
Morton seasoned salt substitute	1,920 (49 mEq)	—
Morton Lite salt	1,400 (36 mEq)	1,120 (49 mEq)
Morton Nature's Seasons	1,520 (39 mEq)	12 (0.5 mEq)
Mrs Dash, salt-free, original	40 (1 mEq)	—
Morton iodized table salt	—	2,360 (103 mEq)

From Pennington J. *Bowes and Church's Food Values of Portions Commonly Used*, 17th ed. Philadelphia: Lippincott-Raven; 1998:279.

route is mandatory for patients with severe hypokalemia (such as < 2.5 mEq/L) (see Clinical Tip: Nursing Considerations in Administering Potassium Intravenously).

Although KCl is usually used to replace potassium deficits, the physician may prescribe potassium acetate or potassium phosphate. Potassium acetate can be used to treat patients with potassium loss associated with metabolic acidosis (as in renal tubular acidosis and potassium-losing nephritis); the acetate is metabolized to bicarbonate and helps correct the acidosis. Potassium phosphate is used when the patient has deficits of both potassium and phosphate.

Factors such as shifting of potassium in and out of the cells make it difficult to precisely identify the amount of potassium needed to correct potassium deficit by assessing plasma potassium levels. However,

in general, when the plasma potassium level falls from 4.0 to 3.0 mEq/L, there is apparently a deficit of 200 to 400 mEq potassium.[53] An additional deficit of 200 to 400 mEq potassium will lower the plasma potassium concentration to 2.0 mEq/L.[54]

As with other imbalances, the aim of treatment in hypokalemia is to get the patient out of danger, not to immediately correct the entire potassium deficit. A case described by Rose[55] dramatically makes this point. A patient with profound hypokalemia had flaccid paralysis; when 80 mEq potassium was administered over 15 minutes, the ECG changed from one typical of hypokalemia to one characteristic of severe hyperkalemia. It must be remembered that the administered potassium needs time to equilibrate with cellular stores; it may take days to totally correct the entire potassium deficit.

CLINICAL TIP

Nursing Considerations in Administering Oral Potassium Supplements

1. The most common adverse reactions to oral potassium salts are nausea, vomiting, abdominal discomfort, and diarrhea. To help minimize GI irritation, administer potassium supplements immediately after meals or with food.

2. Hyperkalemia can result from oral overdosage, just as it can from intravenous (IV) overdosage. Therefore, care should be taken to administer the intended dose. Because numerous forms of potassium supplements are available commercially, with widely variable concentrations, it is important to check the physician's order carefully against the preparation's label (some trade names are quite similar).

3. A single oral dose of potassium should probably not exceed the hourly IV dose (used in more life-threatening situations).[35] The ingestion of >160 mEq can produce a potentially fatal increase in the serum potassium concentration to >8.0 mEq/L, even when normal renal function is present.[36]

4. Potassium supplements are contraindicated in patients receiving potassium-sparing diuretics (ie, spironolactone [Aldactone], triamterene [Dyrenium], and amiloride [Midamor]).

5. Dosages of potassium supplements need to be decreased (or perhaps even discontinued) if the patient begins to use generous portions of potassium-containing salt substitutes.

6. Slow-release tablets should be administered with a full glass of water to help them dissolve in the GI tract. Observe patients taking slow-release KCl tablets for GI bleeding because these tablets may cause intestinal and gastric ulceration. These tablets should not be used if a patient has an obstruction of any part of the GI tract; in addition, they should be used with caution, if at all, if a patient has a history of a peptic ulcer.[37]

7. Do not crush potassium tablets unless the manufacturer's directions specifically state that it is appropriate.

8. Effervescent potassium supplements should be dissolved in 3 to 8 oz of cold water, juice, or suitable beverage and consumed slowly.[38]

9. The majority of patients with hypokalemia have mild to moderate decreases in serum potassium levels (such as 3.0–3.5 mEq/L); this range is usually well tolerated in the absence of digitalis therapy or severe hepatic disease. Provided they can swallow, these patients can usually be treated with oral potassium supplements in the range of 60–80 mEq/day.[39]

In summary, potassium replacement is the cornerstone of therapy for hypokalemia. However, it is important to remember that, unfortunately, supplemental potassium administration is also the most common cause of severe hyperkalemia in hospitalized patients.[56] Conditions requiring emergent therapy are rare and most patients can be treated with oral therapy. When questions exist about the speed of GI tract absorption or the patient's ability to consume oral doses, the IV route is necessary. IV replacement can be given safely at a rate of 10 mEq KCl per hour. Giving 20 mEq/hr causes the serum potassium level to increase by an average of 0.25 mEq/L/hr.[57] Rates of up to 40 mEq/hr, given through a central catheter with continuous ECG monitoring, are sometimes deemed necessary.[58]

NURSING INTERVENTIONS

1. Be aware of patients at risk for hypokalemia and monitor for its occurrence (see Summary of Hypokalemia.) Because hypokalemia can be life-threatening, it is important to detect it early.
2. Assess digitalized patients at risk for hypo-kalemia especially closely for symptoms of digitalis toxicity because hypokalemia potentiates the action of digitalis. Be aware that the physician usually prefers to keep the serum potassium level in the high normal range in digitalized patients.
3. Take measures to prevent hypokalemia when possible.
   - Prevention may take the form of encouraging extra potassium intake for at-risk patients (when the diet allows). Some foods high in potassium (and relatively low in sodium) are listed in Table 5-2. Of course, one must always consider dietary restrictions imposed by other conditions (such as diabetes mellitus or obesity).
   - When hypokalemia is due to abuse of laxatives or diuretics, education of the patient may help alleviate the problem. Part of the nursing history and assessment should be directed at identifying problems amenable to prevention through education.
4. Keep in mind the points summarized in Clinical Tip: Nursing Considerations in Administering Oral Potassium Supplements when administering potassium supplements.
5. Educate patients regarding the use of salt substitutes, keeping the following facts in mind:

- Salt substitutes may contain from 50 to 60 mEq potassium per teaspoon. Although they are often viewed as helpful for those taking potassium-losing diuretics (such as furosemide or thiazides), they can be dangerous for patients taking potassium-conserving diuretics (such as spironolactone, triamterene, and amiloride).
- As with any potassium-containing substance, there is a danger of hyperkalemia with excessive use, particularly if renal function is impaired or the patient is taking pharmacological potassium supplements.
6. Be thoroughly familiar with the nursing considerations involved with administering potassium IV (see Clinical Tip: Nursing Considerations in Administering Potassium Intravenously).

CASE STUDIES

● **5-1.** A 40-year-old woman was admitted to the hospital with complaints of progressive muscle weakness. She had been taking a thiazide diuretic for several weeks and had recently developed vomiting and diarrhea. Postural hypotension was present (110/70 mm Hg when supine and 90/60 mm Hg when upright). Skin turgor was reduced. Laboratory data included:

Plasma K = 2 mEq/L
HCO_3 = 40 mEq/L
Cl = 70 mEq/L

COMMENTARY: This patient had increased losses of potassium from the GI tract as well as in the urine. Her major presenting symptom, diffuse progressive muscle weakness, is common in hypokalemia. In addition to hypokalemia, signs of fluid volume deficit were present (reduced skin turgor and postural hypotension). Recall that postural hypotension can also be a sign of hypokalemia. On questioning, it was found that she was taking a friend's diuretic to induce weight loss. Note the presence of hypochloremic alkalosis (below-normal chloride and greatly elevated bicarbonate).

● **5-2.** A 65-year-old man with a draining intestinal fistula was receiving a total parenteral nutrition (TPN) solution at the rate of 120 mL/hr. The total potassium intake was 100 mEq/day. On a routine ECG, flattened T waves, ST segment depression, and arrhythmias were detected. A

CLINICAL TIP

Nursing Considerations in Administering Potassium Intravenously

1. No matter how low the serum potassium level is, concentrated potassium solutions from ampules should *never* be directly administered into a vein.

   Human subjects do not have the ability to adapt rapidly to a potassium load and will develop hyperkalemia and cardiac arrest, resulting in death.[41] Unfortunately, cases have been reported in which this has occurred following the accidental injection of undiluted potassium chloride (KCl) injections.

   To minimize the potential for this error, most hospitals have removed KCl for injection concentrate from nursing units.[42]

   Potassium solutions in commonly used strengths (such as 20 or 40 mEq/L) are available in premixed form from manufacturers; also, hospital pharmacies often provide nursing units with minibags containing more concentrated solutions as needed (such as 10 or 20 mEq/100 mL)

2. The appropriate dilution of KCl solutions depends on the amount of fluid the patient can tolerate, the site of administration (peripheral or central vein), and the patient's tolerance at the infusion site.

FLUID TOLERANCE

As a general rule, potassium should be diluted to the maximal point without exceeding the patient's tolerance for fluid. For example, if 80 mEq KCl is required in 24 hours, and the fluid intake for that period is 2,000 mL, the 80 mEq KCl should be divided equally between the 2 liters of fluid (ie, 40 mEq/L).

However, if a patient requires more potassium than can be administered at "typical" dilutions, it becomes necessary to administer more concentrated solutions. See below.

SITE

Peripheral Vein. A typical concentration of potassium for peripheral veins is 20 to 40 mEq/L.[43] The most frequently recommended maximal concentration of KCl in a peripheral vein is 40 mEq/L because higher concentrations are very irritating, resulting in pain and sclerosis of veins.[44,45]

Central Vein. The maximal recommended concentration in a central vein is variably defined as 140 mEq/L (14 mEq/100 mL) to 200 mEq/L (20 mEq/100 mL).[46] Unlike peripheral veins, central veins have a large blood flow, thereby allowing dilution of the irritating potassium solution. Although some authors have expressed concern that administering concentrated potassium solutions through central veins near the myocardium could cause dysrhythmias, this was not shown to be problem in a study of 495 sets of KCl infusions administered to a population in a medical intensive care unit.[47]

TOLERANCE FOR PAIN AT INFUSION SITE

Administration of KCl in a peripheral vein at a concentration of > 40 mEq/L is often associated with discomfort that increases as the concentration of KCl increases. Pain is more likely if the patient already has phlebitis associated with prolonged intravenous (IV) cannulation at the site and other irritating medications are also administered. The following steps are helpful in minimizing pain associated with the administration of KCl solutions:

A. Dilute the KCl as much as possible.

B. If a central line is in place, consider using this site for the infusion because rapid blood flow will dilute the KCl solution.

Continued

CLINICAL TIP

Nursing Considerations in Administering Potassium Intravenously—*cont'd*

C. If necessary, discuss with the physician the use of a small volume of lidocaine (either as a bolus through the IV device before the infusion or added to the solution) to minimize pain. Several studies have indicated that this method is of some benefit in alleviating pain associated with concentrated KCl solutions in peripheral veins:

In a double-blind study of 28 subjects, researchers evaluated the effectiveness of a pretreatment IV bolus dose of 3 mL lignocaine (versus a placebo bolus dose of 3 mL of 0.9% NaCl) at the infusion site in alleviating pain associated with the administration of concentrated KCl solutions (20 mEq/100 mL) over a 2-hour period. They concluded that pain at the IV site was significantly reduced in the group that received the lignocaine bolus dose.[48]

In an earlier study, the effect of lidocaine in alleviating pain induced by IV KCl administration was evaluated in six healthy volunteers.[49] Each subject received KCl in a concentration of 200 mEq/L (10 mEq KCl in 50 ml D_5w) in both arms. One of the infusions had 10 mg lidocaine added (although the subject was not told which infusion contained the lidocaine). The solutions were infused over 1 hour and each person was asked to rate the degree of pain in each arm on a 7-point scale (1 = mild, 7 = severe). Pain was significantly less in the arm with the lidocaine (mean, 3.17) than in the arm without lidocaine (mean, 6.17). It is worth noting, however, that pain was still at least moderate in the group receiving the lidocaine.

3. Rate of administration is dependent on the urgency for potassium replacement:

In usual situations, potassium is administered at a rate not exceeding 10 mEq/hr. In the presence of mild to moderate hypokalemia, it is safer to administer potassium at a rate no faster than 10 to 20 mEq/hr. Rates > 40 mEq/hr are not recommended because of the possibility of producing transient hyperkalemia and arrhythmias.[50] However, as much as 40 to 100 mEq/hr have reportedly been given to patients with paralysis or life-threatening arrhythmias.[51] Rapid potassium administration is potentially dangerous even in severely potassium-depleted patients and should be used only in life-threatening situations—ECG monitoring is essential in this setting.

4. Because potassium is primarily eliminated through the kidneys, it is important to monitor carefully the rate of urinary output. When giving potassium, a urine output > 30 mL/hr is recommended to avoid producing transient hyperkalemia.[52] If potassium replacement is needed in oliguric patients, the amount is reduced according to the level of renal function.

5. Because dextrose administered concurrently with potassium can cause a transient shift of potassium into the cells, urgent potassium replacement for severely hypokalemic patients is usually accomplished with a nondextrose solution (such as 0.9% NaCl).

6. Protocols for the safe administration of potassium solutions in specific institutions/agencies should be jointly written by nurses, physicians, and pharmacists. Such protocols are immensely helpful in preventing problems with potassium infusions. General precautions include:

A. Limit the amount of potassium available in a single container (such as 20 mEq/100 mL of solution) to avoid accidental overinfusion.

B. Use an infusion pump to control the flow rate, and carefully monitor the rate to be sure that the pump does not malfunction. (Also, remember that KCl inadvertently administered into subcutaneous tissue is extremely injurious and needs to be detected early; pumps will continue to infuse KCl, regardless of whether the cannula is in the vein or subcutaneous tissue).

C. When at all possible, KCl solutions should be mixed in the hospital pharmacy. If required to mix these solutions on a nursing unit, the medicine port of the plastic container should be squeezed while in the upright position and then the container should be inverted and agitated to thoroughly mix the medication with the IV fluid. Never add KCl to a hanging container.

blood sample was then drawn that revealed a plasma potassium level of 2.5 mEq/L. The rate of TPN infusion was tapered promptly, the serum glucose levels were monitored closely, and an IV infusion of KCl was initiated in a peripheral vein at the rate of 10 mEq/hr. After alleviation of the signs of hypokalemia, the TPN infusion was slowly reinstituted with adequate potassium added.

COMMENTARY: Potassium requirements in the patient receiving TPN are variable, ranging between 18 and 80 mEq/L of solution administered.[59] Most often there is greater than usual potassium need because, during nutritional repletion, potassium will be deposited in the newly syn-thesized cells, causing serum levels to fall abruptly if potassium is not supplied in sufficient amounts. This patient's needs were even greater than usual because intestinal fistulas result in significant potassium loss.

● **5-3.** A 31-year-old woman with a history of acute leukemia was admitted to an acute care facility with fever. On admission, her serum potassium level was 4.1 mEq/L. To deal with the infection, she was started on ticarcillin disodium, 3 g IV piggyback (IVPB) every 4 hours, and tobramycin, 90 mg, IVPB, every 8 hours. Isotonic saline was administered at a rate of 40 mL/hr. On the third day of hospitalization, her serum potassium fell to

Summary of Hypokalemia

ETIOLOGICAL FACTORS

Gastrointestinal Loss
• Diarrhea
• Laxative abuse
• Prolonged gastric suction
• Villous adenoma

Renal Loss
• Potassium-losing diuretics
• Hyperaldosteronism
• Sodium penicillin, carbenicillin, or amphotericin B
• Steroid administration
• Osmotic diuresis

Shift into Cells
• Alkalosis
• Excessive secretion or administration of insulin
• Hyperalimentation

Poor Intake
• Anorexia nervosa
• Alcoholism
• Debilitation

DEFINING CHARACTERISTICS

Skeletal Muscle
• Fatigue
• Weakness (initially most prominent in legs, especially the quadriceps, and then extending to the arms; involvement of respiratory muscles soon follows)
• Cramps
• Rhabdomyolysis

Cardiovascular System
• Increased sensitivity to digitalis
• ST segment depression
• Flattened T waves
• Ventricular arrhythmias
• Cardiac arrest

Gastrointestinal System
• Decreased bowel motility (intestinal ileus)

Renal System
• Impaired urinary concentrating ability when hypokalemia is prolonged, causing dilute urine, polyuria, nocturia, and polydipsia
• Increased ammonia production and H$^+$ excretion

Lab Data
• Serum potassium < 3.5 mEq/L.
• Often associated with alkalosis

2.8 mEq/L. She complained of weakness, fatigue, anorexia, and constipation. Potassium was replaced by the parenteral route until oral supplements could be tolerated.

COMMENTARY: Sodium penicillin is associated with increased renal losses of potassium, particularly when volume depletion is present.

● **5-4.**[60] A 42-year-old man with a history of untreated hypertension and alcohol abuse presented to the emergency department with a 1- to 2-month history of dyspnea, lower extremity swelling, and palpitations. His blood pressure was 199/108 and his lungs were clear. Blood work revealed:

Na = 137 mEq/L
K = 1.7 mEq/L
Cl = 87 mEq/L
HCO_3 = 39 mEq/L
Mg = 0.7 mEq/L

An ECG revealed sinus tachycardia, global ST segment depression, a prolonged QT interval, and a prominent U wave. He was admitted to the intensive care unit for cardiac monitoring; there he required more than 640 mEq KCl and 10 g $MgSO_4$ to correct the electrolyte disturbances.

Commentary: The etiology of the profound hypokalemia and hypomagnesemia was thought to be related to ethanol abuse.

● HYPERKALEMIA

Hyperkalemia refers to a greater than normal serum potassium concentration. It seldom occurs in patients with normal renal function. Apparently the incidence of hyperkalemia is twice as high in hospitalized adults older than 60 years of age than in younger hospitalized adults.[61] Like hypokalemia, hyperkalemia is often due to iatrogenic (treatment-induced) causes. Although less common than hypokalemia, it is often more dangerous because cardiac arrest is more frequently associated with high serum potassium levels.

ETIOLOGICAL FACTORS

Some of the causes of hyperkalemia are simple and straightforward (such as direct gain exceeding the kid-

ney's excretory rate). Others are related to shifts of potassium out of the cells into the plasma, or to decreased production of aldosterone, which causes potassium retention. Note the potassium-elevating influence exerted by several commonly used drugs, particularly when there are preexisting abnormalities in potassium metabolism.

Pseudohyperkalemia

A number of causes of factitious ("pseudo") hyperkalemia exist. When the blood sample is allowed to hemolyze, potassium leaks from ruptured erythrocytes into the serum. The most common cause of pseudohyperkalemia is hemolysis of the blood sample; the laboratory can detect this by a pink tinge to the plasma (caused by release of hemoglobin by the damaged red blood cells).[62] Other causes of pseudohyperkalemia include marked leukocytosis or thrombocytosis, drawing blood above a site where potassium is being infused, and obtaining a sample from an extremity in which repeated clenching and unclenching of the fist has been performed. Pseudohyperkalemia should be suspected when there is no apparent cause for elevated plasma potassium and there are no changes in muscle strength or on ECG tracings.[63]

Although the effect of fist clenching has been recognized for many years,[64] it continues to be a problem. Don et al.[65] reported a case in which a man was admitted for evaluation of hyperkalemia. Blood drawn from this individual in an outpatient setting (using a tourniquet with repeated fist clenching and unclenching) had a serum potassium concentration of 6.9 mmol/L. In the hospital, blood drawn from an indwelling catheter (without use of a tourniquet and fist clenching) had a normal value of 4.1 mmol/L. (It increased to 5.1 mmol/L within 1 minute after application of a tourniquet and repeated fist clenching.) The researchers concluded that it is advisable to avoid fist clenching altogether when obtaining samples for potassium testing and to rely on venous stasis alone, if needed, as an aid in performing phlebotomy.

Failure to be aware of factitious causes of hyperkalemia can result in aggressive treatment of the nonexistent hyperkalemia with serious lowering of serum potassium levels. Some clinicians favor withholding treatment for elevated serum potassium levels in stable patients until a confirmatory ECG can be obtained. Although absence of ECG evidence for hyperkalemia is usually consistent with a factitious reading, it does not necessarily preclude the presence of hyperkalemia. That is, although ECG abnormalities are typically present, they may be absent in nearly half of patients with elevated serum potassium levels.[66] Moderate levels of hyperkalemia are more difficult to detect by ECG than are severe potassium elevations. A study of 220 ECGs performed on patients at risk for hyperkalemia indicated that ECG interpretations made by two physicians were not especially good predictors of hyperkalemia; this caused the researchers to caution that it is prudent to delay treatment for hyperkalemia in stable patients until confirmatory serum values can be obtained to confirm the presence of hyperkalemia.[67]

Decreased Renal Excretion

A major cause of hyperkalemia is decreased renal excretion of potassium. This is understandable when one considers that the kidney is the major route of potassium excretion. Significant hyperkalemia, therefore, is commonly seen in untreated patients with renal failure, particularly when potassium is being liberated from cells during infectious processes or exogenous sources of potassium are excessive (as in diet or medications).

A deficiency of adrenal steroids causes sodium loss and potassium retention; thus, hypoaldosteronism and Addison's disease predispose to hyperkalemia. Between 40% and 65% of patients with chronic adrenal insufficiency manifest hyperkalemia on initial diagnosis.[68] Hyporeninemic hypoaldosteronism (type IV renal tubular acidosis) is a common renal cause of hyperkalemia. This condition is usually seen in elderly persons with mild renal insufficiency, many of whom are diabetic as well.[69]

Potassium-conserving diuretics, such as spironolactone (Aldactone), triamterene (Dyrenium), and amiloride (Midamor), are commonly implicated as causes of hyperkalemia (particularly when there is renal dysfunction, potassium supplementation, or concomitant use of other drugs predisposing to potassium retention). Serious and even fatal complications have been associated with these drugs.[70]

Trimethoprim (an antimicrobial) can impair renal excretion of potassium; therefore, when given in high doses to patients with acquired immunodeficiency syndrome (AIDS) with *Pneumocystis carinii* pneumonia, it can produce hyperkalemia.[71] In a recent study, hyperkalemia occurred in 20% to 53% of patients with AIDS while they were receiving high doses of trimethoprim in combination with sulfamethoxazole or dapsone for the treatment of *P. carinii* pneumonia.[72]

Hyperkalemia occurs with a variety of nonsteroidal anti-inflammatory drugs (NSAIDs) in association with renal insufficiency. Apparently the hyperkalemia is related to reduced plasma and urinary aldosterone levels.[73]

High Potassium Intake

Although sustained hyperkalemia is rarely observed after potassium ingestion in individuals with normal renal function, it can occur with massive oral potassium ingestion or by rapid IV potassium administration.

A case was reported in which a young physician took potassium in the form of a potassium-containing salt substitute to ward off hypokalemia after diuretic use and a bout of diarrhea.[74] On admission to a hospital, her plasma potassium concentration was 8.4 mmol/L. An ECG revealed signs of severe hyperkalemia (peaked T waves, absent P wave, and a broadened QRS complex). She experienced cardiorespiratory arrest and was resuscitated. After treatment, the hyperkalemia resolved; however, posthypoxic brain damage occurred.

Although excessive potassium intake by the oral route is less dangerous than the IV route (because GI absorption may be limited by either vomiting or diarrhea from the large potassium load), the above case illustrates that care is required with potassium administration in all situations. Cases are on record in which both intentional and accidental oral potassium overdosages have resulted in fatalities.[75,76]

Although potassium-containing salt substitutes are often recommended for patients requiring sodium restriction, they are contraindicated for patients on potassium-restricted diets or those with renal disease who have diminished capacity to excrete potassium. Note in Table 5-3 that the potassium content in most salt substitutes is quite high.

Because it is possible to exceed the renal tolerance of any patient with rapid IV potassium administration, extreme caution is required when administering potassium solutions (see Clinical Tip: Nursing Considerations in Administering Potassium Intravenously). The serum concentration of potassium increases as storage time of blood increases; therefore, aged blood should not be given to patients with impaired renal function (see Chap. 10).

In a patient with renal failure, the potassium content in tube feedings may be sufficient to cause hyperkalemia, as may IV hyperalimentation solutions containing usually recommended potassium concentrations.

Shift of Potassium out of Cells

Shifting of potassium out of the cells into the ECF is influenced by many factors, such as tissue injury, lysis of malignant cells during chemotherapy, catabolism, and acidemia. For example, an elevated plasma potassium concentration should be anticipated when extensive tissue trauma has occurred, as can happen in crushing injuries or severe infections. Similarly, it can occur with lysis of malignant cells after administration of chemotherapy, particularly in lymphomas, leukemia, and myeloma. Starvation also causes cellular breakdown and release of potassium into the extracellular space.

Potassium leaks out of the cells in acidosis as hydrogen ions enter the cells to help correct the acidic extracellular pH. However, evidence suggests that the extent of potassium shifting from the cells that occurs in acidemia is greatly influenced by the cause of the acidemia. More shifting is associated with metabolic acidosis due to the accumulation of nonorganic acids (as occurs in diarrhea and renal failure) than in metabolic acidosis due to organic acids (such as lactic acidosis or ketoacidosis). Respiratory acidosis has less effect on potassium shifting than does metabolic acidosis. (The reader is referred to Chap. 9 for a more thorough discussion of this topic.)

β-Adrenergic blockers (such as propranolol) increase the risk of hyperkalemia by interfering with entry of potassium into the cells. The increase in plasma potassium concentration is usually modest (0.2–0.5 mEq/L) and corrects on discontinuation of the drug.[77] Dangerous hyperkalemia is rarely due to β-blockers alone,[78] but these blockers can exacerbate hyperkalemia in patients with other risk factors.[79] For example, dialysis patients treated with propranolol (Inderal) exhibit an increase of about 1.0 mEq/L in predialysis serum potassium levels.[80] Digoxin has produced fatal hyperkalemia when taken in large amounts.[81] Although digitalis toxicity is aggravated by hypokalemia, severe digitalis intoxication poisons the Na^+–K^+–ATPase pump, resulting in potassium release from the cells and hyperkalemia.[82]

Other Causes

Lisonipril ace inhibitor aldosterone

One study found captopril (an angiotensin-converting enzyme inhibitor) to be one of the drugs most frequently implicated in producing hyperkalemia.[83] Significant hyperkalemia has been reported in association with captopril in patients with renal insufficiency, presumably due to the inhibitory effect of the drug on aldosterone secretion.[84]

Cyclosporin can cause hyperkalemia through a combination of mechanisms. For example, it can decrease potassium excretion, decrease prostaglandin production, and lower plasma renin and aldosterone levels.[85] Cyclosporin-induced hyperkalemia does not seem to be related either to dosage or duration of therapy.[86]

Because chronic heparin administration blocks a step in aldosterone synthesis, occasionally it can cause hyperkalemia.[87] Elevated serum potassium levels have been produced with heparin doses of 20,000 units/day.[88] Yet there are infrequent reports of heparin-induced hyperkalemia, despite widespread use of this drug.[89] However, in one study, heparin usage was present in a substantial percentage of patients having other conditions favoring hyperkalemia.[90]

Trimethoprim-sulfamethoxazole can cause hyperkalemia, especially when renal insufficiency is present; apparently it does so by its amiloride-like action.[91] Over half of inpatients receiving this drug have potassium levels over 5 mEq/L, and 20% have potassium levels greater than 5.5 mEq/L.[92]

DEFINING CHARACTERISTICS

Hyperkalemia can cause a variety of adverse effects; most are related to the effects of potassium on cellular membrane potential. By far the most prominent effect of hyperkalemia is on the myocardium.

Cardiac Effects

As the plasma potassium concentration is increased, disturbances in cardiac conduction occur. The earliest changes, often appearing at a serum potassium level greater than 6 mEq/L, are peaked narrow T waves and a shortened QT interval. If the serum potassium level continues to rise, the PR interval becomes prolonged and is followed by disappearance of the P waves. Finally, there is decomposition and prolongation of the QRS complex. Ventricular arrhythmias and cardiac arrest may occur at any point in this progression.

rate, may cause atri-
epolarization.[93] Fac-
of hyperkalemia are
els, as well as acido-
oncentration. These
ncreased serum cal-
infusion is an emer-
lemia. Medications
nia include pro-
n.[94]

he heart becomes
d strength of con-
ber of active mus-
l effects of hyper-
when the serum

nsitive to hyper-
s and even paral-
in muscle. Typi-
r until the plasma
han <u>8 mEq/L</u>.[95]
is first affect the
trunk and upper
also weakened by
eath may be <u>car-</u>

ausea, intermit-
occur in hyper-
been attributed

d Drugs

tment may be
m and discon-
hyperkalemia
potassium sup-
lt substitutes).
fect to hyper-
l β-adrenergic
...... (See previous discussion of possible etiological factors for hyperkalemia.)

Methods to Promote Potassium Excretion

Sodium Polystyrene Sulfonate

Sodium polystyrene sulfonate is a cation exchange resin that can be given orally or rectally to remove potassium from the body by exchanging sodium for potassium in the intestinal tract. Because there is a 2-mEq sodium load accompanying the removal of each milliequivalent of potassium, the patient's tolerance for sodium must be considered.[97] For example, severe congestive heart failure limits the amount of resin that can be safely administered. Although it is an effective method for managing developing hyperkalemia because of its relatively slow onset, it should not be the sole treatment for severe hyperkalemia.

When given orally, it is usually administered with an osmotic agent (such as sorbitol) to prevent constipation. If the oral route cannot be used, the drug can be given by enema and retained for a period of at least 30 to 60 minutes. Each enema can lower the plasma potassium concentration by as much as 0.5 to 1.0 mEq/L.[98]

Dialysis

Dialysis can remove potassium effectively but should be reserved for patients in whom more conservative methods do not suffice. Although peritoneal dialysis can be started relatively quickly, it is not as effective as hemodialysis. For example, using 2-liter exchanges cycled every 45 minutes, peritoneal dialysis can remove 10 to 15 mEq/hr of potassium, as compared to 25 to 30 mEq/hr for hemodialysis.[99] A major limitation of hemodialysis is the time needed to prepare the patient for the procedure.

Diuretics

In patients with normal renal function, diuretics (such as furosemide, 40–80 mg IV, or ethacrynic acid, 50–100 mg IV) have been effective in promoting potassium excretion and decreasing the total body potassium level.[100] These agents are most likely to be used in patients with chronic hyperkalemia due to hypoaldosteronism or heart failure.[101] Loop diuretics are of limited value in patients with severely impaired glomerular filtration rates.

Emergency Measures

Three generally accepted stop-gap measures for treating severe hyperkalemia include IV administration of

(1) calcium gluconate, (2) sodium bicarbonate, and (3) insulin and hypertonic dextrose. These methods and use of a selective β_2-adrenergic agonist are briefly described below.

Calcium Gluconate

The IV administration of calcium gluconate immediately antagonizes the effects of hyperkalemia on the myocardial conduction system and on myocardial repolarization.[102] This protective effect begins within 1 or 2 minutes but lasts only about 30 to 60 minutes. However, this action allows time for one of the measures described below (administration of either insulin and hypertonic dextrose or sodium bicarbonate) to force serum potassium into the cells. The usual dose is 10 mL of a 10% calcium gluconate solution administered slowly over 2 to 3 minutes under ECG monitoring.[103] Calcium should be used only when absolutely necessary in patients taking digitalis because hypercalcemia potentiates the toxic effects of digitalis on the myocardium. If calcium must be given to patients receiving digitalis, it should be added to 100 mL of 5% aqueous dextrose solution (D_5W) and infused slowly over 20 to 30 minutes.[104]

Sodium Bicarbonate

Sodium bicarbonate infusion temporarily shifts potassium into the cells and is especially helpful if the patient has metabolic acidosis. The typical dose is a 50-mEq bolus of $NaHCO_3$ infused slowly over 5 minutes.[105] The onset of action is about 5 to 10 minutes and the effect lasts for about 2 hours.[106] Possible problems associated with this treatment include expansion of the ECF and precipitation of congestive heart failure in patients with cardiac disease, as well as precipitation of tetany in patients with preexisting hypocalcemia.

Insulin and Glucose

Intravenous insulin stimulates potassium uptake by the cells, thereby reducing the plasma potassium concentration. A usual prescription is 10 units regular insulin with 50 g glucose given over 60 minutes[107] (eg, this could be accomplished by adding 10 units regular insulin to 500 mL of a 10% glucose solution). The typical onset of insulin's hypokalemic action is about 30 minutes, and the effects may last for up to 4 to 6 hours.

β_2-Adrenergic Agonists

Similar to insulin, the β_2-adrenergic agonists temporarily force potassium into the cells.[108] The most frequently used agent for this purpose is albuterol; as a rule, the dose for lowering the plasma potassium concentration is significantly greater than the dose used for treating asthma.[109] In the nebulized form, albuterol (10–20 mg in 4 mL normal saline, inhaled over 10 minutes) lowers the plasma potassium concentration for up to 2 to 4 hours. Because of reports of ventricular arrhythmias with the use of β_2-agonists, it has been suggested that these agents be used only when other approaches to control hyperkalemia have been unsuccessful.[110] β_2-Adrenergic agonists should not be used in patients with active coronary disease.[111]

NURSING INTERVENTIONS

1. Be aware of patients at risk for hyperkalemia and monitor for its occurrence (see Summary of Hyperkalemia). Because hyperkalemia is life-threatening, it is imperative to detect it early.
2. Take measures to prevent hyperkalemia when possible by following guidelines for administering potassium safely, both orally and IV (see Clinical Tip: Nursing Considerations in Administering Oral Potassium Supplements and Clinical Tip: Nursing Considerations in Administering Potassium Intravenously).
3. Avoid administration of potassium-conserving diuretics, potassium supplements, or salt substitutes to patients with poor renal function.
4. Caution patients to use salt substitutes sparingly if they are taking other supplementary forms of potassium or are taking potassium-conserving diuretics (such as spironolactone, triamterene, and amiloride).
5. Caution hyperkalemic patients to avoid foods high in potassium content. These include chocolate, coffee, cocoa, tea, dried fruits, dried beans, whole-grain breads, and milk desserts.[112] Meat and eggs also contain substantial amounts of potassium (review Table 5-2). (Foods with minimal potassium content include butter, margarine, cranberry juice or sauce, ginger ale, gumdrops or jellybeans, lollipops, root beer, sugar, or honey.)[113]
6. To avoid false reports of hyperkalemia, take the following precautions:

- Avoid prolonged use of a tourniquet while drawing blood sample.
- Do not allow patient to exercise extremity immediately before drawing blood sample.
- Take blood sample to the laboratory as soon as possible (serum must be separated from cells within 1 hour after collection).
- Avoid drawing blood specimen from a site above an infusion of potassium solution (or any solution for that matter). See section on obtaining blood samples in Chapter 2.

7. Be familiar with usual treatment regimens for hyperkalemia.

CASE STUDIES

● **5-4.** A 60-year-old man visited his family physician complaining of chronic tiredness and

increased skin pigmentation. On examination, his blood pressure was low (98/60 mm Hg). Blood tests revealed a plasma potassium level of 6.8 mEq/L and a plasma sodium level of 132 mEq/L. The blood urea nitrogen (BUN) was 20 mg/dL and the serum creatinine was 1.2 mg/dL.

COMMENTARY: This patient was diagnosed as having adrenal insufficiency. Recall that aldosterone regulates sodium and potassium balance by causing sodium retention and potassium excretion. Thus, a deficit of aldosterone results in potassium retention and elevation of the plasma potassium level. Note that the patient has normal renal function, as evidenced by the BUN and creatinine levels. Increased skin pigmentation is common in adrenal insufficiency.

● **5-5.** A 30-year-old man with chronic renal failure developed vomiting and diarrhea. Because

[handwritten margin notes: Salt Substitutes = KCl   Starvation = Release of K into ECS or ECF]

Summary of Hyperkalemia

ETIOLOGICAL FACTORS

Pseudohyperkalemia
- Prolonged tight application of tourniquet; fist clenching and unclenching immediately before or during blood drawing
- Hemolysis of blood sample
- Leukocytosis
- Thrombocytosis

Decreased Potassium Excretion
- Oliguric renal failure
- Potassium-conserving diuretics
- Hypoaldosteronism

High Potassium Intake
- Improper use of oral potassium supplements
- Excessive use of salt substitutes
- Rapid IV potassium administration
- Rapid transfusion of aged blood

Shift of Potassium out of Cells
- Acidosis
- Tissue damage, as in crushing injuries
- Malignant cell lysis after chemotherapy

DEFINING CHARACTERISTICS

Neuromuscular Effects
- Vague muscular weakness
- Flaccid muscle paralysis (first noticed in legs, later in arms and trunk; respiratory muscles and muscles supplied by cranial nerves are usually spared)
- Paresthesias of face, tongue, feet, and hands

Cardiovascular System
- Tall, peaked T waves
- Widened QRS complex progressing to sine waves
- Ventricular arrhythmias
- Cardiac arrest

Gastrointestinal System
- Nausea
- Intermittent intestinal colic or diarrhea

Laboratory Data
- Serum potassium > 5.0 mEq/L
- Often associated with acidosis

he became very weak, his family brought him to the emergency room. In addition to severe muscle weakness, he had decreased skin turgor. An ECG revealed tall, peaked T waves and widening of the QRS complex. Blood tests revealed a plasma potassium level of 9.4 mEq/L and a creatinine level of 2.9 mg/dL.

COMMENTARY: Due to fluid volume depletion after the bout of vomiting and diarrhea, this patient developed decreased renal perfusion and a reduced ability to excrete potassium. Because of the life-threatening situation (evidenced by the high plasma potassium level and the ECG changes), he was treated with calcium gluconate and sodium bicarbonate. A dextrose and saline solution was administered to achieve volume replacement. After volume repletion, kidney perfusion improved and the patient was again able to excrete potassium. Remember that patients with chronic renal failure can become seriously ill when volume depletion and thus decreased renal perfusion occur.

● **5-6.** A 65-year-old woman was admitted to the emergency room complaining of abdominal cramping and numbness in her extremities. Laboratory data revealed a BUN of 96 mg/dL and a creatinine of 3.9 mg/dL. The serum potassium was 8.6 mEq/L. She was given a retention enema of Kayexalate (sodium polystyrene sulfonate) in 20% sorbitol. She received 50 mL of 50% dextrose and 10 units regular insulin IV. An infusion of 5% dextrose and 0.45% NaCl containing two ampules of sodium bicarbonate was started at a rate of 25 mL/hr. By the next day, the serum potassium level was reduced to 5.0 mEq/L.

COMMENTARY: Kayexalate is an ion-exchange resin that causes sodium to be exchanged for potassium in the intestine, resulting in potassium excretion by this route. Hypertonic dextrose and insulin favor cellular uptake of potassium, and sodium bicarbonate, by alkalinizing the plasma,

also causes potassium to shift temporarily into the cells.

● **5-7.**[114] A 75-year-old man with a history of coronary artery disease and myocardial infarction presented at cardiac rehabilitation with complaints of malaise, fatigue, agitation, dyspnea on exertion, and nausea with one episode of vomiting. (His medications included torsemide 60 mg od, spironolactone 25 mg od, Lanoxin 0.25 mg od, enalapril 10 mg od, and Coumadin 3 mg bid.) He was immediately admitted to the hospital where he was noted to have dry mucous membranes, sunken eyes, and a blood pressure of 112/64. The following laboratory results were obtained:

Na = 139 mEq/L
K = 6.4 mEq/L
Cl = 100 mEq/L
BUN = 74 mg/dL
Cr = 2.8 mg/dL

He was treated with 10% calcium gluconate IV and 30 g Kayexalate by mouth. Two hours after the Kayexalate was administered, his potassium level had decreased to 5.4 mEq/L. It was assumed that the acute renal failure was due to overdiuresis and possible nephrotoxic effects of enalapril (an angiotensin-converting enzyme [ACE] inhibitor). He was taken off the spironolactone (a potassium-sparing diuretic) and was slowly rehydrated with 0.9% NaCl (50 mL/hr) to correct the fluid volume depletion. The enalapril was discontinued and hydralazine was started at 25 mg every 6 hours and titrated up to 100 mg every 6 hours on discharge. On the day of discharge, his BUN was 45 mg/dL and the serum creatinine was 1.8 mg/dL.

COMMENTARY: Hyperkalemia is a relatively common imbalance in the elderly, and it is often related to prescribed medications (such as potassium-sparing diuretics and ACE inhibitors, as present in this case).

REFERENCES

1. Mandal A. Hypokalemia and hyperkalemia. *Med Clin North Am* 1997;81:611.
2. Schwartz S, ed. *Principles of Surgery*, 7th ed. New York: McGraw-Hill; 1999:63.
3. Latta K et al. Perturbations in potassium balance. *Clin Lab Med* 1993;13:149.
4. Bloomfield R, Wilson D, Buckalew V. The incidence of diuretic-induced hypokalemia in two distinct clinic settings. *J Clin Hypertens* 1986;2:331.
5. Gennari F. Hypokalemia. *N Engl J Med* 1998;339:451.
6. Narins R, ed. *Clinical Disorders of Fluid and Electrolyte Metabolism*, 5th ed. New York: McGraw-Hill; 1994:671.
7. Rose B. *Clinical Physiology of Acid-Base and Electrolyte Disorders*, 4th ed. New York: McGraw-Hill; 1994:797.
8. Narins, p 671.
9. Weiner I, Wingo C. Hypokalemia-consequences, causes and correction. *J Am Soc Nephrol* 1997;8:1179.
10. Chataway S, Mumford C, Ironside J. Self-induced myopathy. *Postgrad Med J* 1997;37:593.
11. McDonald R. Disorders of potassium balance. *Pediatr Ann* 1995;24:131.
12. Zull D. Disorders of potassium metabolism. *Emerg Med Clin North Am* 1989;7:771.
13. Rose, p 779.
14. Udezue E, D-Souza L, Mahajan M. Hypokalemia after normal doses of nebulized albuterol. *Am J Emerg Med* 1995;13:168.
15. Gennari, p 452.
16. Braden G, von Oeyen P, Germain M, et al. Ritodrine- and terbutaline-induced hypokalemia in preterm labor: Mechanisms and consequences. *Kidney Int* 1997;51:1867.
17. Pemberton L, Pemberton D. *Treatment of Water, Electrolyte, and Acid-Base Disorders in the Surgical Patient.* New York: McGraw-Hill; 1994:178.
18. Rose, p 782.
19. Anderson K. Hypokalemic periodic paralysis: A case study. *Am J Crit Care* 1998;7:236.
20. Zemel P, Gualdoni S, Sowers J. Racial differences in mineral intake in ambulatory normotensives and hypertensives. *Am J Hypertens* 1988;1:146S.
21. Gennari, p 452.
22. Chernow B, ed. *The Pharmacologic Approach to the Critically Ill Patient*, 3rd ed. Baltimore, MD: Williams & Wilkins; 1994:989.
23. Gennari, p 451.
24. Whelton P, He J, Cutler J, et al. Effects of oral potassium on blood pressure: Meta-analysis of randomized controlled clinical trials. *JAMA* 1997;277:1624.
25. Barri Y, Wingo C. The effects of potassium depletion and supplementation on blood pressure: A clinical review. *Am J Med Sci* 1997;314:3.
26. Rose, p 800.
27. Ibid, p 802.
28. Ibid, p 803.
29. Ibid.
30. Mujais S, Katz A. Potassium deficiency. In: Seldin D, Giebish G, eds. *The Kidney.* New York: Raven Press; 1992:2249.
31. Weiner, Wingo, p 1180.
32. Zull, p 785.
33. Ibid.
34. Ibid.
35. Szerlip H, Goldfarb S. *Workshops in Fluid and Electrolyte Disorders.* New York: Churchill Livingstone; 1993:93.
36. Rose, p 826.
37. Brensilver J, Goldberger E. *A Primer of Water, Electrolytes and Acid-Base Syndromes*, 8th ed. Philadelphia: Lea & Febiger; 1996:280.
38. Lacey R et al. *Drug Information Handbook*, 2nd ed. Hudson (Cleveland), Lexi-Comp, Inc., American Pharmaceutical Association; 1994:769.
39. Rose, p 811.
40. Rose, p, 810.
41. Mandal, p, 611.
42. Davis N. Med errors: Potassium perils. *Am J Nurs* 1995;95:14.
43. Pemberton, Pemberton, p 187.
44. Kokko, Tannen, p 134.
45. Carey C, Lee H, Woeltjek K. *The Washington Manual of Medical Therapeutics*, 29th ed. Philadelphia: Lippincott-Raven; 1998:50.
46. Kruse J, Carlson R. Rapid correction of hypokalemia using concentrated intravenous potassium chloride infusions. *Arch Intern Med* 1990;150:613.
47. Ibid.
48. Lim E et al. Efficacy of lignocaine in alleviating potassium chloride infusion pain. *Anesth Intensive Care* 1992;20:196.
49. Morril G, Katz M. The use of lidocaine to reduce the pain induced by potassium chloride infusion. *J Intravenous Nurs* 1988;11:105.
50. Pemberton, Pemberton, p 187.
51. Rose, p 811.
52. Pemberton, Pemberton, p 183.
53. Narins, p 682.
54. Rose, p 809.
55. Ibid.
56. Rimmer J, Horn J, Gennari J. Hyperkalemia as a complication of drug therapy. *Arch Intern Med* 1987;147:867.
57. Kruse, Carlson, p 615.
58. Weiner, Wingo, p 1185.
59. Zaloga G, ed. *Nutrition in Critical Care.* St. Louis: Mosby; 1994:387.
60. Dietz T, Bissett J, Talley J. The effects of hypokalemia on the heart. *J Ark Med Soc* 1997;94:79.
61. Kleinfeld M, Corcoran A. Hyperkalemia in the elderly. *Compr Ther* 1990;16:49.
62. Weiner I, Wingo C. Hyperkalemia: A potential silent killer. *J Am Soc Nephrol* 1998;9:1535.
63. Rose, p 817.
64. Skinner S. A cause of erroneous potassium levels. *Lancet* 1961;1:478.
65. Don BR et al. Pseudohyperkalemia caused fist clenching during phlebotomy. *N Engl J Med* 1990;322:1290.
66. Tierney L, McPhee S, Papadakis M. *Current Medical Diagnosis & Treatment*, 38th ed. Stamford, CT: Appleton & Lange, 1999:846.
67. Wrenn K et al. The ability of physicians to predict hyperkalemia from the ECG. *Ann Emerg Med* 1991;20:1229.
68. Kokko J, Tannen R. *Fluids and Electrolytes*, 3rd ed. Philadelphia: WB Saunders, 1996:164.
69. Zull, p 788.
70. Schwartz A, Cannon-Babb M. Hyperkalemia due to drugs in diabetic patients. *Am Fam Pract* 1989;39:225.
71. Choi M et al. Trimethoprim-induced hyperkalemia in a patient with AIDS. *N Engl J Med* 1993;328:703.
72. Medina I et al. Oral therapy for *Pneumocystis carinii* pneumonia in the acquired immunodeficiency syndrome—a controlled trial of trimethoprim-sulfamethoxazole versus trimethoprim-dapsone. *N Engl J Med* 1990;323:776.

73. Schwartz, Cannon-Bobb, p 225.
74. van der Loeff H, van Schijndel S, Thijs L. Cardiac arrest due to oral potassium intake. *Intensive Care Med* 1988;15:58.
75. Illingsworth R, Proudfoot A. Rapid poisoning with slow-release potassium. *Br Med J* 1980;281:485.
76. Wetli C, Davis J. Fatal hyperkalemia from accidental overdose of potassium chloride. *JAMA* 1978;240:1339.
77. Schwartz, Cannon-Bobb, p 227.
78. Zull, p 788.
79. Rimmer et al, p 869.
80. Kokko, Tannen, p 161.
81. Schwartz, Cannon-Bobb, p 228.
82. Zull, p 788.
83. Rimmer et al, p 869.
84. Ibid.
85. Kokko, Tannen, p 169.
86. Schwartz, Cannon-Bobb, p 229.
87. Zull, p 789.
88. Kokko, Tannen, p 169.
89. Ibid.
90. Rimmer et al, p 869.
91. Beck L. Changes in renal function with aging. *Clin Geriatr Med* 1998;14:199.
92. Tierney et al, p 846.
93. Huerta B, Lemberg L. Potassium imbalances in the coronary unit. *Heart Lung* 1985;14:193.
94. Ibid.
95. Rose, p 845.
96. Rimmer et al, p 869.
97. Brensilver, Goldberger, p 200.
98. Rose, p 851.
99. Kokko, Tannen, p 158.
100. Narins, p 738.
101. Rose, p 851.
102. Weiner, Wingo (1998), p 1539.
103. Rose, p 849.
104. Narins, p 736.
105. Ibid.
106. Ibid.
107. Ibid, p 737.
108. Rose, p 850.
109. Kupin W, Narins R. The hyperkalemia of renal failure: Pathophysiology, diagnosis and therapy. In: Bourke E et al, eds. *Moving Points in Nephrology. Contrib Nephrol* 1993;102:1.
110. Narins, p 738.
111. Rose, p 851.
112. Brensilver, Goldberger, p 247.
113. Ibid.
114. Weber L. Iatrogenic induced hyperkalemia in an eldery male: A case study. (Unpublished paper). Saint Louis University School of Nursing; 1998.

Calcium Imbalances

Because many factors affect calcium regulation, there are a multitude of causes of altered calcium balance. Both hypocalcemia and hypercalcemia are relatively common imbalances, particularly in the acutely ill patient. For example, in one study, 64% of the patients in the intensive care unit were found to be hypocalcemic.[1] The opposite imbalance, hypercalcemia, is often seen in patients with malignant disease. To facilitate understanding of calcium disturbances, a review of factors affecting calcium balance follows.

CALCIUM BALANCE

DISTRIBUTION AND FUNCTION

Over 99% of the body's calcium is concentrated in the skeletal system, where it is a major component of strong, durable bones and teeth. About 1% of skeletal calcium is rapidly exchangeable with blood calcium; the rest is more stable and only slowly exchanged. The small amount of calcium located outside the bone circulates in the serum partly bound to protein and partly ionized. Calcium exerts a sedative action on nerve cells and has a major role in the transmission of nerve impulses. It helps regulate muscle contraction and relaxation, including normal heartbeat. Calcium has a vital role in the cardiac action potential and is essential for cardiac pacemaker automaticity.[2] It is also involved in blood clotting and hormone secretion.

SERUM CONCENTRATION

The test most frequently performed in clinical settings to measure serum calcium is total calcium, with results normally ranging from 8.9 to 10.3 mg/dL. (This is roughly equivalent to 2.23 to 2.57 mmol/L.) The total calcium in serum is the sum of the ionized (47%) and nonionized (53%) calcium components. The nonionized portion consists of calcium bound to albumin (40%) and the portion chelated to anions (13%), which include citrate and phosphate. When serum albumin levels and pH are within normal ranges, readings from total calcium are generally not problematic. However, when the serum albumin level is abnormal, corrections must be made in the total serum calcium levels.

In the noncritically ill patient, it is estimated that a decrease in the serum albumin of 1.0 g/dL below normal will decrease the total calcium by 0.8 mg/dL. The following is a convenient formula by which to calculate the "corrected" calcium level when *hypo*albuminemia is present[3]:

$$\text{Corrected calcium} = \text{measured serum calcium} + 0.8\ (4.0 - \text{measured serum albumin})$$

For example, if the patient's serum albumin level is below normal by 1 g/dL (eg, 3.0 g/dL rather than 4.0 g/dL), the measured total serum calcium concentration of 8.0 mg/dL should be adjusted upward to 8.8 mg/dL. In this situation, the ionized calcium level would be estimated at about half of the adjusted value (4.4 mg/dL). The direct relationship between albumin and total calcium often leads clinicians to ignore a low total serum calcium level in the presence of a similarly low serum albumin level.

The amount of calcium that is in the ionized form is affected by plasma pH. For example, when the arterial pH increases (alkalosis), more calcium becomes bound to protein. Although the total serum calcium remains unchanged, the ionized portion decreases. Therefore, symptoms of hypocalcemia often occur in the presence of alkalosis. Acidosis (low pH) has the opposite effect; that is, less calcium is bound to protein and therefore, more exists in the ionized form. Signs of hypocalcemia will develop only rarely in the presence of acidosis, even when the total serum calcium level is lower than normal.

Direct measurement of ionized calcium by ion-selective electrodes is highly desirable, especially in critically ill patients, because it is the ionized calcium (normal 4.6–5.1 mg/dL) that is physiologically active and clinically important. It has been recommended that blood obtained for ionized calcium be drawn anaerobically with minimal use of heparin, placed on ice, and measured immediately (in a manner similar to that used for measurement of arterial blood gases).[4]

REGULATION

Many biochemical and hormonal factors act to maintain a normal calcium balance. Among the most important are parathyroid hormone (PTH), calcitonin, and calcitriol (an active metabolite of vitamin D). PTH promotes a transfer of calcium from the bone to plasma (raising the plasma calcium level). The bones and teeth are ready sources for replenishment of low plasma calcium levels. PTH also augments the intestinal absorption of calcium and enhances the net renal calcium reabsorption.

Calcitonin (produced by C cells in the thyroid as well as several other tissues) is a physiological antagonist of PTH. Calcitonin secretion is directly stimulated by a high serum calcium concentration. At high levels, calcitonin inhibits bone resorption; the resultant reduced flux of calcium from bone causes a reduction in the serum calcium level. Because high levels of calcitonin have a hypocalcemic effect, calcitonin is thought to play a role in protecting against acute hypercalcemia.[5] However, its effect is thought to be minor when compared to that of PTH and calcitriol.[6]

Calcitriol (1,25-dihydroxyvitamin D$_3$) is a hormone that increases the extracellular calcium concentration by three main actions:

1. It promotes calcium absorption from the intestine.
2. It enhances bone resorption of calcium.
3. It stimulates renal tubular reabsorption of calcium.

The daily recommended oral dietary intake of calcium is 1,000 to 1,500 mg.[6] About one-third to one-half of the ingested calcium is absorbed, primarily through the small intestine. Calcium is excreted by both the gastrointestinal (GI) and urinary tracts.

OSTEOPOROSIS

Osteoporosis is associated with prolonged low intake of calcium. It is characterized by loss of bone mass causing bones to become porous, brittle, and susceptible to fracture. In the United States, osteoporosis affects 20 million people and leads to over 1 million fractures each year, with annual cost of health care and lost productivity that exceeds $10 billion.[7] Although serum calcium levels are usually normal in these individuals, total body calcium stores are greatly diminished. Bone loss begins at an earlier age in women than in men and is accelerated by menopause. However, men also develop negative calcium balance in later years. A dual process is involved in osteoporosis: increased bone resorption and inadequate bone formation. Menopause leads to rapid bone loss in women because estrogen deficiency reduces calcium absorption and increases excretion; as a result, bone loss far outpaces bone deposition.

Risk of developing serious bone problems is greater in postmenopausal, physically inactive women who are elderly, thin and small-framed, and smokers, and those who have a diet deficient in calcium.[8] Inactivity pre-

disposes to bone loss by reducing the efficiency of calcium use. Conversely, regular physical exercise (such as running, walking, or bicycling) slows the rate of bone loss and improves calcium balance.

Considering the magnitude of the problems associated with osteoporosis, prevention is the only cost-effective approach. Some authors recommend that postmenopausal women consume between 1,000 and 1,500 mg calcium daily, either in the diet or from supplements; further, in the United States, the Recommended Dietary Allowance for calcium in adolescents and young adults is 1,500 mg/day.[9] A recent study has suggested another possible benefit of calcium supplementation; that is, subjects who received 1,200 mg elemental calcium (calcium carbonate 3 g) developed fewer recurrences of colorectal adenomas than did subjects who received a placebo.[10]

Also important in the prevention of osteoporosis is increased physical activity and the elimination of bone toxins (such as cigarettes and heavy alcohol ingestion). Estrogen replacement therapy prevents bone loss in estrogen-dependent women, regardless of when it is started; however, indications suggest that the benefits are greater if therapy is started early because bone loss is most rapid in the first years of menopause.[11] See Chapter 25 for further discussion of osteoporosis.

● HYPOCALCEMIA

Hypocalcemia is defined as a total serum calcium level of less than 8.9 mg/dL and an ionized calcium concentration of less than 4.6 mg/dL. Hypoalbuminemia is a common cause of a reduced total serum calcium concentration; however, this is sometimes referred to as "pseudohypocalcemia" because the ionized calcium remains normal despite a low total calcium level.[12] In this situation, the patient is asymptomatic and does not require treatment. On the other hand, an alkalotic patient often has a decreased ionized calcium level (and therefore is symptomatic) although the total serum calcium level is normal. Thus, when total serum calcium measurements are performed to assess calcium balance, the need to consider the results in relation to the serum albumin level as well as acid–base status is obvious. Conditions associated with hypocalcemia are briefly discussed below.

ETIOLOGICAL FACTORS

Surgical Hypoparathyroidism

Primary hypoparathyroidism causes hypocalcemia, as does surgical hypoparathyroidism; however, the latter is a more common cause. Hypocalcemia is usually seen when the operation involves removal of a parathyroid adenoma, total or near-total thyroidectomy, or bilateral neck surgery for cancer.[13] Hypocalcemia reportedly occurs in up to 70% of patients undergoing parathyroidectomy, particularly when a severe hyperparathyroid state was present before surgery.[14] Transient hypocalcemia reportedly occurs in 5% to 10% of patients undergoing thyroidectomy.[15] The hypocalcemia may occur immediately or 1 to 2 days postoperatively and usually lasts less than 5 days.[16]

The most likely mechanism for hypocalcemia after radical neck dissection is ischemia to the parathyroid tissue after dissection and hemostatic maneuvers. Intraoperative release of calcitonin has been suggested as a possible mechanism for hypocalcemia that complicates thyroid surgery.[17] It is also possible that trauma to the parathyroid glands does not allow PTH to increase as needed to elevate the low serum calcium level, thus contributing to the hypocalcemia. If permanent parathyroid damage has not occurred, parathyroid insufficiency resolves as edema at the surgical site lessens and revascularization occurs, allowing reestablishment of parathyroid gland integrity.

Permanent hypocalcemia associated with thyroid surgery is due to accidental removal of the parathyroid glands or to vascular necrosis.[18] Fortunately, permanent postsurgical hypoparathyroidism is relatively uncommon after thyroidectomy. For example, in a study of 1,071 consecutive patients who underwent total or subtotal thyroidectomy during 1990 and 1991, only 5 (0.5%) had persistent hypocalcemia 1 year after surgery.[19] Another retrospective study of 142 patients who underwent thyroidectomy reported that 15 (10.6%) had hypocalcemic symptoms plus a requirement for oral vitamin D or calcium 6 months after surgery.[20] The frequency of this complication is partially dependent on the technical skill of the surgeon; surgeons performing thyroidectomies and parathyroidectomies strive to preserve the blood supply to the parathyroid glands.[21,22] Extensive neck surgery (as in radical neck dissection for cancer) is more likely to be associated with permanent hypoparathyroidism than are less involved surgical maneuvers.

Most patients who develop hypocalcemia after neck surgery are asymptomatic; however, some may develop paresthesias, laryngeal spasm, or tetany.[23] It has been recommended that the serum ionized calcium level be checked every 12 hours after neck surgery (and more frequently if symptoms of hypocalcemia are present) until the serum ionized concentration begins to elevate, indicating recovery of the parathyroid glands.[24] With the emphasis on cost containment in the current health care environment, there is concern that patients who have undergone thyroid or parathyroid gland surgery may be discharged before postoperative hypocalcemia becomes manifest. A recent retrospective study of 197 patients who had undergone such operations indicated that early postoperative calcium levels give a good indication of whether or not hypocalcemia is likely to occur.[25] In the study, postoperative calcium levels were plotted as a function of time, and the slope between the first two postoperative calcium levels was examined. The results indicated that an initial upsloping postoperative calcium curve based on these two early postoperative calcium measurements is a strong predictor of a stable postoperative calcium level; conversely, a steeply downsloping initial calcium curve is worrisome for eventual hypocalcemia.[26]

Symptomatic patients should receive supplemental calcium to increase the serum calcium level to the low normal range. It is possible that postoperative hypoparathyroidism may manifest itself months to years after neck surgery; therefore, in at-risk patients serum ionized calcium levels should be monitored serially. It is also possible that stress can induce hypocalcemia in these individuals; therefore, critically ill patients with a history of neck surgery should have a serum calcium test performed.[27]

Acute Pancreatitis

Inflammation of the pancreas causes release of proteolytic and lipolytic enzymes; it is believed that calcium ions combine with the fatty acids released by lipolysis, forming soaps, and thus decreasing the serum calcium concentration. Some investigators have found that there is an inadequate PTH response to the hypocalcemia caused by acute pancreatitis.[28] In any event, hypocalcemia is a common problem, occurring in as many as 40% to 75% of patients with acute pancreatitis.[29] See Chapter 20 for a more extensive discussion of this topic.

Magnesium Abnormalities

The serum magnesium level influences both PTH secretion and action, and thus the serum calcium level. Severe hypomagnesemia (< 1 mg/dL) inhibits PTH secretion. One study reported that 22% of the patients with hypocalcemia in their sample also had hypomagnesemia.[30] Chronic hypomagnesemia associated with impaired PTH secretion and hypocalcemia can occur in malnourished alcoholics and in the renal magnesium-wasting associated with cisplatin therapy.[31] Hypomagnesemic hypocalcemia responds poorly to calcium therapy alone but does respond to magnesium replacement.[32]

Hyperphosphatemia

Hyperphosphatemia that develops rapidly is associated with hypocalcemia. This might be seen in patients who receive excessive hypertonic phosphate enemas. For example, according to a recent report, a 3-year-old girl developed severe hyperphosphatemia and hypocalcemia after the administration of three adult-sized hypertonic phosphate enemas.[33] Although severe hypocalcemia usually results from hyperphosphatemia, it is possible that the serum phosphorus and calcium concentrations may rise together if rapid bone breakdown is the basic cause.[34]

Alkalosis

Blood pH alters Ca^{++} binding to serum proteins. Alkalosis can induce a decreased ionized serum calcium concentration as a result of increased binding of Ca^{++} to albumin. Although the total calcium concentration remains normal in this situation, tetany (presumably caused by the fall in ionized calcium) can occur if the blood pH rises above 7.6.[35]

Inadequate Vitamin D

Inadequate consumption of vitamin D or insufficient exposure to the sun (ultraviolet radiation) can cause reduced calcium absorption and thus lead to hypocal-

cemia. Deficiency of vitamin D occurs in malabsorptive states, as described below.

Malabsorption Syndromes

Intestinal malabsorptive disorders are likely to lead to hypocalcemia by decreasing the absorption of vitamin D, bile salts, and calcium.[36] Hypocalcemia has been found in 7% of patients who have undergone partial gastrectomy with gastrojejunostomy.[37] It may also occur after ileal bypass in obese persons[38] and those with Crohn's disease, pancreatic insufficiency, and hepatobiliary disease.[39]

Infusion of Citrate in Blood Products

Decreases in ionized Ca^{++} values during blood transfusion correlate with speed of transfusion and circulating citrate levels.[40] Citrate is present in bank blood to act as an anticoagulant and to preserve the life of the blood. Usually the citrate in blood is rapidly metabolized by the liver and presents no problem for calcium balance. However, when blood is transfused faster than the excess citrate can be metabolized, hypocalcemia results. Recall that citrate is negatively charged and calcium is positively charged, resulting in an attraction between these ions. Therefore, transient hypocalcemia can occur with massive administration of citrated blood (as in exchange transfusions in neonates), as citrate combines with ionized calcium and temporarily removes it from the circulation (also referred to as chelation). Citrate metabolism is hindered in the presence of liver disease, shock, and hypothermia. Also at increased risk for citrate-induced ionized calcium deficit during massive transfusion are small children, elderly or osteoporotic patients, and those who have been bedridden for extended periods; all of these individuals tend to have inadequate stores of bone calcium and therefore are less able to compensate for declined ionized calcium levels. When citrate intoxication occurs, it may be manifested as circumoral paresthesias, muscle tremors, or tetany; it does not affect coagulation.[41]

The infusion of packed red blood cells (instead of whole blood) lowers the amount of citrate infused and thus decreases the already low risk for hypocalcemia after transfusions. However, there is sufficient citrate even in packed red blood cells to affect calcium balance. For example, Chernow et al.[42] reported a significant fall in total serum calcium (from 9.49 ± 0.11 to 7.6 ± 0.11 mg/dL) in 21 patients after transfusion with packed red blood cells. Two cases were recently reported in which the transfusion of small volumes of packed red blood cells was sufficient to precipitate symptomatic hypocalcemia.[43] Subsequent investigation revealed that both of the patients had preexisting, untreated, and asymptomatic hypocalcemia (one following partial thyroidectomy years earlier and the other with documented hypocalcemia but without a definitive cause).

Current recommendations suggest the administration of calcium only when patients develop symptomatic hypocalcemia because calcium infusion can be associated with ventricular dysrhythmias and thus should not be used indiscriminately.[44]

Hypocalcemia has also been observed during plasmapheresis.[45] Ordinarily the citrate anticoagulant used during apheresis procedures is considered a safe medication because it is rapidly metabolized by the donor; however, life-threatening hypocalcemia can occur if the infusion rate of the citrate is too fast. A case was reported in which citrate was inadvertently administered too rapidly to a 54-year-old woman due to malfunction of the anticoagulant line of an apheresis instrument.[46] Seven minutes into the procedure she developed muscle spasms, chest pain, and hypotension; her serum ionized calcium level was 0.64 mmol/L

(normal in the reporting laboratory was 1.18–1.38 mmol/L).

Drugs

Many medications can predispose to hypocalcemia. Some are listed in Table 6-1 with a brief description of the underlying mechanisms.

Alcoholism

The hypocalcemia associated with chronic alcoholism has numerous causes. Among these are the direct effect of ethanol, intestinal malabsorption, low levels of 25-hydroxyvitamin D_3, hypomagnesemia, hypoalbuminemia, respiratory and metabolic alkalosis, and pancreatitis.[47] The most significant of these is probably hypomagnesemia. Magnesium replacement increases responsiveness to PTH and correction of the hypocalcemia.

Neonatal Hypocalcemia

Two types of hypocalcemia can occur in newborn infants. The first develops early, during the first 3 days of life. This type is attributed to parathyroid immaturity or maternal hyperparathyroidism (or both), resulting in neonatal parathyroid gland suppression; it most often resolves within the first week of life.[48] Among

 TABLE 6-1.   Drugs With Calcium-Lowering Effects

Drug	Mechanism
Loop diuretics (such as furosemide)	Increases renal excretion of calcium
Anticonvulsants (especially Dilantin and phenobarbital)	Inhibits gastrointestinal calcium absorption and causes faulty vitamin D metabolism
Citrate-buffered blood and blood products	Presumably binds ionized Ca^{++} with citrate
Phosphates (orally, IV, or enema)	Phosphate combines with calcium
Mithramycin	Decreases calcium mobilization from bone
Calcitonin	Decreases calcium mobilization from bone
Drugs that loweri serum Mg level (such as cisplatin and gentamycin)	By inducing hypomagnesemia, may decrease calcium mobilization from bone
EDTA (disodium edetate)	Physically combines with calcium for excretion
Alcohol (chronic abuse)	Multiple factors (see text)
Certain radiographic contrast media	Those containing chelating agents combine with calcium

the predisposing factors for this condition are prematurity, maternal insulin-dependent diabetes mellitus, and asphyxia at birth. A second type of neonatal hypocalcemia occurs about 1 week after birth and is associated with hyperphosphatemia and hypomagnesemia. Hypocalcemia in infants with this "late-onset" condition can be caused by feeding milk with a high phosphorus level, leading to hyperphosphatemia and then to hypocalcemia. Low serum calcium levels can persist until the parathyroid glands function well enough to respond.[49]

Sepsis

The underlying basis for hypocalcemia in septic patients is unclear. It is postulated that calcium moves from the extracellular compartment into the cells and that the hormonal response to hypocalcemia is inadequate.[50] Possible causes for hypocalcemia in a group of patients with gram-negative sepsis described by Zaloga and Chernow[51] are acquired parathyroid gland insufficiency, dietary vitamin D deficiency, or renal hydroxylase insufficiency. Treatment of ionized hypocalcemia in sepsis is not recommended unless the patient is symptomatic because calcium administration appears to increase organ dysfunction.[52]

Other Factors

Medullary thyroid carcinoma may produce hypocalcemia if calcitonin (a calcium-lowering hormone) is secreted by the tumor. Conditions associated with low serum albumin levels (such as cirrhosis of the liver and the nephrotic syndrome) are frequently associated with a low total serum calcium concentration. Often, the ionized calcium concentration is normal and no symptoms of hypocalcemia appear.

Hypocalcemia was reported in 17.9% of 66 patients with acquired immunodeficiency syndrome.[53] The researchers postulated that intestinal malabsorption of vitamin D is the most likely cause of hypocalcemia in this patient population.

DEFINING CHARACTERISTICS

Clinical manifestations of hypocalcemia vary widely among patients and depend on severity, duration, and rate of development. The concurrent presence of hypomagnesemia and hypokalemia can potentiate the neurological and cardiac abnormalities associated with hypocalcemia.

Neuromuscular Manifestations

Tetany, the most characteristic manifestation of hypocalcemia, refers to the entire symptom complex induced by increased neural excitability. Findings may include sensations of tingling around the mouth (circumoral paresthesia) and in the hands and feet, as well as spasms of the muscles of the extremities and face. The increase in nerve membrane excitability causes fibers to discharge spontaneously, eliciting tetanic contractions. Although laryngeal spasms may occur, they only rarely result in asphyxia.[54]

When hypocalcemic patients lack overt signs of tetany, neuromuscular excitability (latent tetany) can be elicited in two ways. One involves placing a blood pressure cuff on the upper arm and inflating to above systolic pressure for about 3 minutes and observing for carpal spasm (Trousseau's sign, see Fig. 2-4). Trousseau's sign is not specific for hypocalcemia because it is negative in about 30% of individuals with latent tetany and positive for a small percentage of healthy individuals.[55] Another test involves tapping over the facial nerve just anterior to the ear and observing for ipsilateral facial muscle contraction (Chvostek's sign). This sign is also not specific for hypocalcemia because it may occur in some healthy adults.

Cardiovascular Manifestations

In some patients altered cardiovascular hemodynamics may be the most significant effect of hypocalcemia. This is understandable when considering the important role calcium ions play in the contraction of cardiac muscle. The cardiovascular effects of hypocalcemia include decreased myocardial contractility leading to a reduced cardiac output, hypotension that is refractory to fluids and vasoconstrictive agents, and decreased responsiveness to digitalis.[56] Dysrhythmias associated with hypocalcemia can range from bradycardia to ventricular tachycardia and asystole. Hypocalcemia prolongs the QT interval, predisposing the patient to life-threatening ventricular dysrhythmia. Often cardiac patients are already predisposed to both hypocalcemia and hypomagnesemia because they are taking potent loop diuretics.

Long-standing hypocalcemia can be complicated by reversible cardiomyopathy. For example, a 46-year-old woman with chronic severe hypocalcemia associated with untreated hypoparathyroidism developed severe heart dysfunction.[57] After the hypocalcemia was corrected, near-normal cardiac function returned within a few months. Similar cases have been reported by other authors.[58]

Central Nervous System Manifestations

Severe hypocalcemia can cause convulsions and, in fact, these may be the initial manifestation.[59] Hypocalcemia may also cause impaired higher cerebral function. For example, anxiety, depression, confusion, and frank psychoses may occur.

Other Changes

In chronic hypocalcemia, the skin may be dry and scaling, the nails brittle, and the hair dry and easily shed; cataracts are common. Chronic hypocalcemia in children can retard growth and lower the IQ.

TREATMENT

Treatment of hypocalcemia depends on the underlying cause, the magnitude of the serum calcium deficiency, and the severity of symptoms. Numerous etiological factors are associated with hypocalcemia. Ideally, treatment is directed at alleviating the cause. If this is impractical or ineffective, the following general measures should be considered.

Acute Hypocalcemia

Acute symptomatic hypocalcemia is a medical emergency, requiring prompt administration of intravenous (IV) calcium. Parenteral calcium salts include calcium gluconate, calcium chloride, and calcium gluceptate. Although calcium chloride produces a significantly higher ionized calcium than an equimolar amount of calcium gluconate, it is not used as often because it is more irritating to the vein and can cause tissue sloughing if allowed to infiltrate. Because calcium is very irritating, it should be administered through a central line whenever possible.[60] For symptoms of severe hypocalcemia in adults, 20 mL of 10% calcium gluconate (90 mg elemental calcium/10 mL), administered at a rate not exceeding 2 mL/min, may be prescribed.[61] This

may be followed by the infusion of 30 to 40 mL of 10% calcium gluconate in 500 or 1,000 mL of 5% aqueous dextrose (D_5W) or 0.9% NaCl over a 4-hour period.[62] (Calcium should not be mixed with any solution containing bicarbonate because of the possibility of precipitation.) Patients receiving digitalis should be monitored with an electrocardiogram (ECG) during the infusion because calcium administration may produce fatal arrhythmias if the infusion is given rapidly.[63] The serum calcium level should be monitored every 4 to 6 hours and the infusion rate adjusted to avoid recurrent symptomatic hypocalcemia.[64]

An infusion of calcium gluconate may be needed to correct postoperative symptomatic hypocalcemia in the first 24 to 48 hours after neck surgery (such as thyroidectomy, radical neck dissection, or parathyroidectomy). The flow rate is titrated according to clinical signs and serum calcium levels.

Chronic Hypocalcemia

When oral calcium supplements can be tolerated, the oral route is preferred over the IV route because it is safer. Oral calcium intake can be provided as either carbonate, gluconate, or lactate salts. In some cases, long-term management may require the use of vitamin D preparations. These should be used with caution if severe hyperphosphatemia is present because of the danger of calcium phosphate precipitation in the soft tissues. If hyperphosphatemia is present, oral phosphate-binding medications (such as aluminum hydroxide) may be indicated.

NURSING INTERVENTIONS

1. Be aware of patients at risk for hypocalcemia and monitor for its occurrence (see Summary of Hypocalcemia). Also, review previous sections for explanations of etiological factors and defining characteristics.
2. Be prepared to adopt seizure precautions when hypocalcemia is severe.
3. Monitor the condition of the airway closely because laryngeal stridor can occur.
4. Take safety precautions if confusion is present.
5. Be aware of factors related to the safe administration of calcium replacement salts (see Clinical Tip: Nursing Considerations in the Administration of IV Calcium).

CLINICAL TIP

Nursing Considerations in the Administration of IV Calcium

1. The dosage of calcium prescribed for a specific hypocalcemic patient depends on the severity of hypocalcemia, as well as its cause.

2. The most commonly prescribed calcium preparations for IV use are:
   Calcium Gluconate: 10 mL of a 10% solution contains 90 mg (4.5 mEq) of elemental Ca^{++} (suitable for either IV or IM use)
   Calcium Chloride: 10 mL of a 10% solution contains 270 mg (13.5 mEq) of elemental Ca^{++} (suitable only for IV use)

3. Calcium preparations may be given by slow IV push (if indicated) or may be added to compatible parenteral fluids (such as 500 mL to 1,000 mL of 0.9% NaCl, lactated Ringer's solution, or D_5W) for slow infusion.

4. Calcium preparations are irritating to veins. Although they may be given undiluted via IV push, it is preferable to dilute them first with isotonic saline.[65]

5. Calcium chloride is especially irritating to veins and may cause venous sclerosis; for this reason, administration through a central vein is recommended.[66] Because calcium gluconate is less irritating to veins, it is more frequently prescribed (although it contains only one-third as much elemental calcium as calcium chloride). If a peripheral administration site is necessary the largest available vein should be used.[67] Do not use small hand veins. Great care should be taken to avoid extravasation of calcium solutions (especially calcium chloride) because they can cause severe soft tissue damage.

6. Calcium preparations should not be administered with bicarbonate or phosphate because a precipitate will form.[68]

7. Calcium should be administered cautiously (with ECG monitoring) to patients taking digitalis because accidental hypercalcemia induced by too rapid infusion of calcium could precipitate digitalis toxicity.

8. Frequent monitoring of the patient's response to calcium replacement therapy is indicated. Serum calcium levels should be checked frequently (such as every 1–4 hours) and the dosage adjusted accordingly.[69] Adequacy of treatment can also be monitored by following Chvostek's and Trousseau's signs, the ECG, and hemodynamic parameters.[70]

6. Educate individuals in high-risk groups for osteoporosis (especially postmenopausal women not receiving estrogen therapy) about the need for adequate dietary calcium intake.
   • Most sources recommend that the calcium intake for older persons be 1,000 to 1,500 mg each day. The best way for healthy individuals to ensure an adequate calcium intake is to eat a wide variety of foods from the four food groups daily.
   • Calcium supplements may be necessary for individuals unable to consume sufficient calcium in their diets, such as those who do not tolerate milk or dairy products.
   • Individuals with a tendency to form renal stones should be encouraged to increase their fluid intake throughout the day and night. Fluids should be ingested during meals, several hours after meals, before bedtime, and during the night when awakened to void.

7. Inform individuals at risk for osteoporosis about the value of regular physical exercise in decreasing bone loss. Walking is tolerated well by all age groups and is an excellent form of exercise, as is bicycling. (See Chap. 25 for further discussion of exercise and osteoporosis.)

8. To prevent osteoporosis in later years, educate young women about the need for a normal diet ensuring adequate calcium intake. Discuss the calcium loss associated with the use of alcohol and nicotine. Smoking lowers estrogen levels and interferes with the body's absorption of calcium; women who smoke are at greater risk of developing osteoporosis.

Summary of Hypocalcemia

ETIOLOGICAL FACTORS

Surgical hypoparathyroidism (may follow thyroid surgery or radical neck surgery for cancer)

Primary hypoparathyroidism

Malabsorption

Acute pancreatitis

Excessive administration of citrated blood

Alkalotic states (causing decreased calcium ionization)

Hyperphosphatemia

Sepsis

Hypomagnesemia

Medullary carcinoma of thyroid

Hypoalbuminemia (as in cirrhosis, nephrotic syndrome, and starvation)

DEFINING CHARACTERISTICS

Neuromuscular
- Numbness, tingling of fingers, circumoral region, and toes
- Muscle cramps, which can progress to muscle spasms, tremor, and twitching
- Hyperactive deep-tendon reflexes
- Trousseau's sign
- Chvostek's sign
- Convulsions (usually generalized but may be focal)
- Spasm of laryngeal muscles

Cardiovascular
- Decreased myocardial contractility with a reduction in cardiac output
- ECG: Prolonged QT interval
- Arrhythmias, ranging from bradycardia to ventricular tachycardia and asystole

Mental
- Impaired higher cerebral functioning, such as depression, emotional instability, anxiety, or frank psychoses

Total serum calcium level below 8.9 mg/dL or ionized calcium level below 4.6 mg/dL.

CASE STUDIES

● **6-1.** A 46-year-old woman with end-stage renal disease was admitted with a secondary diagnosis of seizure activity and multi-infarct dementia. She required dialysis twice a week. On admission, laboratory data from a venous blood sample revealed the following:

Na = 138 mEq/L
BUN = 41 mg/dL
K = 5.8 mEq/L
Serum creatinine = 8.2 mg/dL
Total Ca = 7.0 mg/dL

Albumin = 3.0 g/dL
PO_4 = 7.1 mEq/L
HCO_3 = 13.5 mEq/L

COMMENTARY: Note the low total calcium level and the presence of hypoalbuminemia. With correction for the low serum albumin level, the serum calcium would be nearer to normal. (Recall that for every gram the serum albumin is below the normal level of 4 g/dL, 0.8 mg must be added to the reported calcium level; because the albumin level is 1 g below normal, 0.8 must be added to the reported calcium level, making it 7.8 mg/dL.)

Although the total calcium level was below normal, the ionized fraction of the calcium was normal; thus, symptoms of hypocalcemia were not present. Note that this patient has metabolic acidosis (evidenced by the low serum bicarbonate level); both hypoalbuminemia and acidosis favor increased calcium ionization. Rapid correction, or overcorrection, of acidosis in a renal patient predisposes to precipitation of hypocalcemic symptoms. Hyperphosphatemia was present, a major factor in explaining the hypocalcemia.

6-2. An hysterical young woman was admitted to the emergency department after an automobile accident in which she fractured her arm. She complained of circumoral paresthesia and then fainted. Arterial blood gas findings included a pH of 7.55 (alkalosis) and an arterial carbon dioxide pressure ($PaCO_2$) of 20 mm Hg (normal, 40 mm Hg).

COMMENTARY: Hyperventilation secondary to hysteria is a common cause of tetany in the hospital emergency department. In this situation, the tetany resulted from a reduction in the plasma ionized calcium level consequent to respiratory alkalosis. Fainting was due to cerebral ischemia caused by the low $PaCO_2$ (recall that a low $PaCO_2$ causes cerebral vasoconstriction). The total serum calcium level was probably normal, although the ionized fraction decreased. Correction of the hyperventilation (and thus of respiratory alkalosis) will restore the ionized calcium level to normal and alleviate symptoms.

● HYPERCALCEMIA

The prevalence of hypercalcemia in the hospital inpatient population ranges from 0.6% to 3.6%.[71] If allowed to become severe, hypercalcemia is associated with significant morbidity and mortality; therefore, it is important to detect this imbalance early.

ETIOLOGICAL FACTORS

Primarily hyperparathyroidism and malignancy account for more than 90% of the cases of hypercalcemia.[72] In contrast, causes such as thiazide diuretics, immobilization, lithium use, and vitamin D and A

intoxication account for only a small percentage of the cases.[73]

Malignancies

Hypercalcemia of malignancy reportedly occurs in about 10% to 20% of cancer patients during the course of their illness.[77] The hypercalcemia of malignancy may be related to direct bone destruction with release of calcium into the bloodstream or to the secretion of factor(s) by malignant cells that produce PTH-related peptide.[78] Malignancies most often associated with hypercalcemia include breast and lung cancers and hematologic malignancies such as multiple myeloma or lymphoma.[79] See Chapter 22 for a more thorough discussion of tumors associated with hypercalcemia.

Primary Hyperparathyroidism

Hypercalcemia caused by primary hyperparathyroidism results from increased PTH production, and about 75% of the cases are caused by single adenomas.[74] Often the patients are elderly women who have a benign adenoma of a single parathyroid gland.[75] Due to increased PTH production, hyperparathyroidism causes increased bony release of calcium, augmented intestinal calcium absorption, and renal reabsorption of calcium. Hypercalcemia also occurs in some hyperthyroid patients. When total serum calcium is measured, about 10% to 20% of hyperthyroid patients have elevated values; the percentage is even higher when ionized calcium is measured.[76]

Immobilization

Bone mineral is lost during immobilization, sometimes causing elevation of total calcium in the bloodstream. The hypercalcemia associated with immobilization is the result of an imbalance between the rates of bone formation and bone resorption. This process is more conspicuous in patients with Paget's disease or in those in whom bone turnover is increased (such as adolescents during a growth spurt). Factors leading to hypercalcemia during immobilization are still largely unexplained.

Drugs

A variety of drugs can elevate calcium levels; some of these are listed in Table 6-2. Thiazide-induced hyper-

TABLE 6-2. Drugs with Calcium-Elevating Effects

Drug	Mechanism
Thiazide diuretics	Decrease renal calcium excretion
Lithium	Decreases renal calcium excretion
Prolonged megadoses of vitamins A and D	Vitamin A likely increases calcium mobilization from bone; vitamin D increases gastrointestinal calcium absorption and mobilization of calcium from bone
Theophylline	Perhaps increases effect of endogenous parathyroid hormone
Milk with soluble alkali (especially calcium carbonate)	Multiple mechanisms

calcemia may be partially mediated by volume contraction that increases renal reabsorption of calcium; also, it is thought that thiazides have a direct effect on distal tubular calcium reabsorption.

Use of lithium to treat manic-depressive patients has been reported to cause hypercalcemia and high circulating immunoreactive PTH levels.[80] Too aggressive treatment of hypoparathyroidism, rickets, or osteomalacia with vitamin D is the most common cause of vitamin D intoxication and its associated hypercalcemia. Excessive vitamin A intake can increase bone resorption and lead to hypercalcemia; it appears that large doses of vitamin A increase bone resorption. The widespread use of vitamin A analogues to treat acne and other skin conditions has occasionally been associated with hypercalcemia.[81]

Milk-alkali syndrome can occur in patients with peptic ulcers treated for a prolonged period with milk and alkaline antacids, particularly calcium carbonate. Patients who take large quantities of calcium-containing antacids may present with marked hypercalcemia.[82] The milk-alkali syndrome should also be considered as a cause of hypercalcemia with the current popularity of calcium ingestion to prevent osteoporosis.[83]

Renal Transplantation

Hypercalcemia may occur after successful renal transplantation as a result of increased PTH production by hyperplastic parathyroid glands. As a rule, it disappears within 6 months after transplantation as the glands undergo involution. In the vast majority of patients, the hypercalcemia eventually remits spontaneously; however, in some patients it may persist for as long as 7 or 8 years after the transplant.[84] If the serum calcium is persistently greater than 12 mg/dL, parathyroidectomy may be considered.[85]

DEFINING CHARACTERISTICS

The magnitude of the serum calcium elevation and the length of time during which it developed have a major significance for clinical findings, as does the underlying cause of hypercalcemia. For example, acute hypercalcemia is more symptomatic than chronic hypercalcemia. Also, malignancies can present with severe hypercalcemia (serum calcium level 14 mg/dL) more commonly than other conditions.[86]

In some patients mild hypercalcemia is found on routine examinations; others may present in hypercalcemic crisis. Although there are no firm diagnostic criteria for hypercalcemic crisis, it is generally thought to represent the presence of volume depletion, neurological manifestations, and cardiac arrhythmias in a patient with a serum calcium level above 14 mg/dL. As a rule, symptoms of hypercalcemia are proportional to the serum calcium level, although this is not always the case.

Neuromuscular Changes

Hypercalcemia reduces neuromuscular excitability because it acts as a sedative at the myoneural junction.

Symptoms such as muscular weakness and depressed deep tendon reflexes may occur.

Gastrointestinal Symptoms

Constipation, anorexia, nausea, and vomiting are common symptoms of hypercalcemia. Constipation results from decreased GI motility caused by calcium's action on smooth muscle and nerve conduction, as well as from dehydration.[87] Delayed gastric emptying, nausea, and vomiting are also related to altered motility. Patients with hypercalcemia are predisposed to duodenal ulcer disease because of the increased gastric acid secretion, promoted by calcium on the parietal cells of the stomach. Pancreatitis is another potential complication of severe hypercalcemia and is probably related to calcium deposits in the pancreatic ducts.

Behavior Changes

Behavior changes may range from subtle alterations in personality to acute psychosis and may include confusion, impairment of memory, and bizarre behavior. Patients may become inattentive and lose the ability to concentrate; recent memory is affected more than is distant memory.[88] Other mental status changes sometimes seen in patients with hypercalcemia are lethargy or drowsiness, and psychiatric disturbances, such as irritability and depression; severe cases are associated with stupor or coma.[89] Although the cause of these symptoms is not known, it has been suggested that increased calcium in the cerebrospinal fluid is involved.[90] The more severe symptoms tend to occur when the serum calcium level is about 16 mg/dL or higher. In a study of eight hypercalcemic cancer inpatients during a period of 66 patient-days, Mahon[91] found that the most evident changes were those affecting mental status. For example, many subjects could not remember their home telephone numbers or perform simple mathematical computations. Some displayed inappropriate behaviors, such as pulling out a Foley catheter while the balloon was inflated. As serum calcium levels decreased toward normal, the mental symptoms gradually subsided.

Renal Changes

Disturbed renal tubular function produced by the hypercalcemia can cause polyuria and polydipsia. More specifically, this disturbed function is a form of nephrogenic diabetes insipidus that is usually reversible within 1 to 12 weeks after correction of the imbalance. The concentrating defect may become clinically apparent when the plasma calcium concentration exceeds 11 mg/dL.[92] Renal colic may occur as a result of kidney stones, which may form from the excess calcium presented to the kidneys for excretion. Calcium salts deposited in the kidney can cause renal failure.

Cardiovascular Changes

Calcium is important in cardiac function; it exerts a positive inotropic effect on the heart and reduces heart rate in a way similar to the effect of cardiac glycosides. Calcium administration to patients receiving digitalis must be done with extreme care because it can precipitate severe arrhythmias (with shortening of the QT interval on the ECG).

Hypercalcemia causes alterations in myocardial muscle function and rhythm disturbances. Bradycardia, first-, second-, and third-degree heart block, and bundle branch block may occur.[93] Hypercalcemia can also affect the systemic vasculature, perhaps leading to hypertension. The mechanism for the increase in blood pressure may be multifactorial. For example, serum levels of epinephrine and norepinephrine are higher in patients with hypercalcemia than in those with normocalcemia, and elevated renin activity has been reported in patients with primary hyperparathyroidism.[94]

TREATMENT

Treatment should be directed at correcting the underlying cause of hypercalcemia whenever possible. For example, primary hyperparathyroidism is definitively managed by parathyroidectomy; further, when hypercalcemia is caused by malignant disease, treatment needs to be directed at the underlying tumor.[95] When direct treatment of the underlying cause is not feasible, a number of medical treatments are available to treat severe symptomatic hypercalcemia. These attempt to reduce the serum calcium level by increasing urinary calcium excretion, inhibiting bone resorption, blocking intestinal calcium absorption, or enhancing formation of calcium complexes.

General Conservative Measures

When hypercalcemia is not life-threatening, treatment may be limited to simple actions such as a large fluid intake (unless contraindicated) and eliminating drugs that can contribute to hypercalcemia (such as thiazide diuretics, vitamin D preparations, or calcium-containing antacids). Whenever possible, the patient should be encouraged to be active, because immobility predisposes to hypercalcemia.

Fluid Replacement

Because most patients with severe hypercalcemia are volume depleted, isotonic saline (0.9% NaCl) may be ordered initially at a rate of 300 to 500 mL/hr until the intravascular volume has been partially corrected.[96] Volume expansion with isotonic saline dilutes the plasma calcium, increases the glomerular filtration rate, and increases renal calcium excretion. A dose of 4 to 5 liters of saline over 24 hours, or more if tolerated, may be given; the serum calcium level may fall by 2 to 3 mEq/L over 8 to 24 hours.[97] A slowed saline infusion is maintained to promote renal calcium excretion after volume replacement has been achieved. Isotonic saline is the fluid of choice because renal calcium excretion is directly associated with sodium excretion.[98]

Cardiovascular and renal function should be assessed before rapid saline infusion because fluid overload and congestive heart failure are potential complications. Furosemide should be used as necessary after the plasma volume has been expanded to prevent volume overload and to enhance calcium excretion. (The loop diuretics such as furosemide and ethacrynic acid facilitate sodium and calcium excretion; conversely, the thiazide diuretics should not be used because they interfere with calcium excretion and may worsen hypercalcemia.) It may be necessary to monitor the central venous pressure to detect fluid overload, particularly in the elderly or those with marginal cardiac reserve; at least, breath sounds should be monitored at regular intervals. Hourly intake and output records should be maintained. Losses of potassium and magnesium will result from the large urinary output, which must be corrected as indicated by laboratory data.

When the use of saline and furosemide is ineffective or contraindicated, different measures may be instituted. Among these are the administration of bisphosphonates, mithramycin, calcitonin, glucocorticoids, and phosphate salts. In some situations, either peritoneal dialysis or hemodialysis may be indicated.

Bisphosphonates

Bisphosphonates such as pamidronate and etidronate inhibit bone resorption and therefore can treat the hypercalcemia.[99] Bisphosphonates are the mainstay of treatment of the hypercalcemia of malignancy.[100] The dosage is determined by the severity of the hypercalcemia; for example, when the corrected serum calcium level is 12 to 13.5 mg/dL, the adult dose of pamidronate ranges between 15 and 90 mg in 1,000 mL 0.9% NaCl or D_5W infused IV over 4 to 24 hours.[101] Serum calcium levels may remain in the normal range for weeks to months after bisphosphonate therapy.[102]

Mithramycin

Mithramycin (an antineoplastic agent) lowers serum calcium by inhibiting bone resorption. In general, it is less effective and less well tolerated than pamidronate.[103] Because of the potential for nephrotoxicity and hepatotoxicity, the long-term use of mithramycin is limited; it should be avoided in patients with underlying renal or liver dysfunction. Mithramycin is generally reserved for use in patients who do not respond to bisphosphonates.[104] It has a relatively rapid onset of action and the serum calcium level may begin to drop as early as 12 hours after administration.[105] The serum calcium level may be normalized in 75% to 85% of patients and remain normal for 6 days to several weeks.[106]

Calcitonin

By inhibiting bone resorption, salmon calcitonin may temporarily lower the serum calcium level by 1 to 3 mg/dL within hours.[107] Calcitonin is a safe drug but its hypocalcemic effect is mild and many individuals become unresponsive to it after 6 to 10 days of treatment.[108] Side effects include nausea, vomiting, diarrhea, facial flushing, and, rarely, allergic reactions.

Glucocorticoids

Glucocorticoids can reduce the serum calcium level by inhibiting calcium absorption in the intestine and by inhibiting osteoclastic bone resorption. They are effective in reducing serum calcium in hypercalcemia due to sarcoidosis, vitamin D intoxication, multiple myeloma, or other hematologic malignancies.[109] Steroid therapy may be initiated with hydrocortisone, 5 mg/kg body weight per day for 2 to 3 days; later, the dose is reduced to a maintenance level.[110] A drawback of glucocorticoids is that clinically significant reductions in serum calcium may not occur for 5 to 10 days after therapy is initiated.[111] Because of the slow onset of action, glucocorticoids are combined with other therapeutic measures when used to treat patients with severe hypercalcemia. Possible complications associated with glucocorticoids include hyperglycemia and sodium and water retention.

Phosphate Salts

When ingested orally, phosphate produces a small reduction in the serum calcium level by inhibiting bone resorption, interfering with the GI absorption of calcium, and inhibiting renal synthesis of 1,25-dihydroxyvitamin D.[112] Because of its modest effect on the serum calcium level, oral phosphate use is limited to long-term treatment of mild hypercalcemia. Phosphate salts may be administered orally as Phospho-Soda or Neutra-Phos. It is important to remember that increasing the serum phosphate concentration alters the extracellular calcium–phosphate equilibrium to promote the formation of calcium–phosphate precipitates that are then deposited in various body tissues including bone, soft tissues, blood vessels, lung, myocardium, and kidneys. Because of the risk of soft tissue calcification, phosphate therapy should be limited primarily to patients with low serum phosphate levels (< 3.0 mg/dL) and adequate renal function. The IV administration of phosphate is associated with an even greater risk for the precipitation of calcium–phosphate complexes in vital organs. Thus, even though phosphate administered IV produces a rapid and marked reduction in the serum calcium level, it is rarely (if ever) used for this purpose; fortunately, equally potent and safer alternatives are available to treat serious hypercalcemia.[113]

NURSING INTERVENTIONS

1. Be aware of patients at risk for hypercalcemia and monitor for its presence. See Summary of Hypercalcemia and review above sections on etiological factors and defining characteristics.
2. Increase patient mobilization when feasible; recall that immobilization favors hypercalcemia. Hospitalized patients at risk for hypercalcemia should be ambulated as soon as possible; outpatients should be told the importance of frequently moving about.
3. Encourage the oral intake of sufficient fluids to keep the patient well hydrated. Sodium-containing fluids should be given, unless con-

traindicated by other conditions, because sodium favors calcium excretion. Always consider the patient's preferences when encouraging oral fluids. Patients at home should be instructed to drink 3 to 4 quarts of fluid per day, if possible.
4. Discourage excessive consumption of milk products and other high-calcium foods. Depending on the cause of hypercalcemia, dietary restrictions do not necessarily need to be stringent. Consult with physician and dietitian as indicated.
5. Encourage adequate bulk in the diet to offset the tendency to constipation.
6. Take safety precautions if confusion or other mental symptoms of hypercalcemia are present. Explain to the patient and family that the mental changes associated with hypercalcemia are reversible with treatment.
7. Be aware that cardiac arrest can occur in patients with severe hypercalcemia; be prepared to deal with this emergency situation.
8. Be aware that bones may fracture more easily in patients with chronic hypercalcemia because bone resorption has been excessive, weakening the bony structure. Transfer patients cautiously.
9. Educate home-bound oncology patients with a predisposition for hypercalcemia, as well as their families, regarding symptoms that occur with this condition. Instruct them to report symptoms to the health care providers before they become severe. In a study reported by Mahon,[114] constipation, confusion, anorexia, increasing bone pain, weight loss, and weakness were the symptoms that most frequently caused readmission of patients with cancer. In a study of 22 hospitalized and 18 ambulatory cancer patients, Coward[115] reported that 90% were unaware that hypercalcemia might be a complication of their cancer. Furthermore, only one of the patients knew the symptoms of cancer-induced hypercalcemia. Almost 70% of the patients did not recall being told of measures that might prevent hypercalcemia.
10. Be alert for signs of digitalis toxicity when hypercalcemia occurs in digitalized patients.
11. Be familiar with the treatment modalities for hypercalcemia and associated nursing functions (see treatment section in this chapter and in Chapter 22).

Summary of Hypercalcemia

ETIOLOGICAL FACTORS

Hyperparathyroidism

Malignant neoplastic disease (lung tumors, breast tumors, and multiple myeloma account for more than 50% of the cases)

Drugs
- Thiazide diuretics
- Excessive vitamin A or D
- Overuse of calcium supplements
- Overuse of calcium-containing antacids
- Lithium
- Theophylline

Prolonged immobilization

DEFINING CHARACTERISTICS

Neuromuscular
- Muscle weakness
- Decreased deep-tendon reflexes

Renal
- Polyuria (nephrogenic diabetes insipidus)
- Hypercalciuria, perhaps leading to renal stones

Gastrointestinal
- Anorexia
- Nausea
- Vomiting
- Constipation

Cardiovascular
- Arrhythmias
- Heart block
- ECG: Shortened QT interval
- Increased digitalis sensitivity
- Hypertension

Mental
- Impaired higher cerebral functioning, such as confusion, emotional instability, anxiety, frank psychoses, lethargy or coma

12. Help prevent formation of calcium renal stones in patients with long-standing hypercalcemia or immobilization by:
    - Forcing fluids to maintain a dilute urine, thus avoiding supersaturation of precipitates.
    - Encouraging fluids that yield an acid ash (such as prune or cranberry juice) because a urinary pH of less than 6.5 favors calcium solubility. (However, it is important to be aware that dietary modifications do not usually alter urinary pH significantly; therefore, pharmacological acidifying agents [such as ascorbic acid, potassium acid phosphate, or methionine] may be prescribed by the physician to ensure a uniformly low pH.)
    - Preventing urinary stasis by frequently turning the immobilized patient, elevating the head of the bed, and having the patient sit up if this can be tolerated.
    - Encouraging weight-bearing and ambulation as soon as possible.

CASE STUDIES

● **6-3.** A 47-year-old woman who appeared thin and dehydrated was admitted to the hospital with abdominal pain, weight loss, and a history of vomiting for 3 months.[116] Her body weight of 38 kg was only 84% of her ideal body weight; her midarm circumference was 60% of standard. A recent cholecystectomy for cholelithiasis provided no relief from her symptoms. On examination, a nodule was felt in the right lobe of the thyroid gland and was later found to be an adenoma. A serum calcium level was obtained and was found to be high (13.8 mg/dL). Skull x-rays revealed a typical pepper pot appearance suggestive of hyperparathyroidism. She was rehydrated with 0.9% NaCl solution; however, saline diuresis did not represent a long-term solution to this woman's problem of severe hypercalcemia. Thus, the right upper parathyroid gland was surgically removed. The postoperative period was complicated by severe hypocalcemia due to "hungry bone" syndrome. Among the symptoms were circumoral paresthesia, Chovstek's sign, and Trousseau's sign; fortunately, her ECG was normal. The hypocalcemia was managed by the IV administration of calcium gluconate and later by calcium carbonate tablets. At the time of discharge from the hospital, her calcium concentration had normalized to 8.7 mg/dL; several months after the procedure, all of her symptoms had disappeared.

COMMENTARY: This patient initially had hypercalcemia due to a parathyroid adenoma (one of the most common causes of hypercalcemia). She received the usual treatment for this disorder (rehydration with isotonic saline and surgical removal of the tumor). Although this would be expected to end her calcium problem, she later developed hypocalcemia due to the "hungry bone" syndrome. This occurred as the unmineralized bone from her previous long-standing hypercalcemia became recalcified; "bone hunger" has been observed after successful surgical treatment of primary hyperparathyroidism.[117] The severity of the hypocalcemia correlates with the severity of the bone disease before treatment.

● **6-4.** A 49-year-old woman with a history of breast cancer and metastases to the bone and liver was admitted to the hospital with polyuria and polydipsia; her total serum calcium level was 3.08 mmol/L (12.3 mg/dL).[118] A single IV infusion of pamidronate was administered. The serum calcium level returned to normal and did not change until 6 weeks later. Several subsequent recurrences of hypercalcemia were also treated with single infusions of pamidronate given in the outpatient department. The patient was able to continue receiving palliative therapy at home and finally died 6 months later from other complications.

COMMENTARY: The polyuria associated with hypercalcemia occurs as a result of a renal concentrating defect; although the precise cause of this abnormality is not certain, a defect in the action of antidiuretic hormone in the collecting duct and damage to the concentrating segments of the nephron play a role.[119] Provided the patient is not too nauseated to drink fluids, fluid intake will increase as the patient becomes more thirsty. Treatment of her intermittent bouts of hypercalcemia allowed the patient to be more comfortable during her remaining months of life.

● **6-5.** A 59-year-old woman with carcinoma of the left breast underwent a radical mastectomy and adjuvant chemotherapy.[120] She was later admitted to the hospital for management of hip pain, confusion, and hypercalcemia (corrected serum calcium, 15.2 mg/dL, or 3.80 mmol/L). Isotonic saline was administered IV and she was given 100 units calcitonin subcutaneously every 8 hours. She also received 60 mg pamidronate IV. The patient remained confused after the serum calcium level normalized. No further treatment was administered when the hypercalcemia recurred, and she died 1 month later from a pulmonary embolus.

COMMENTARY: Because hypercalcemia can impair mental function, it is not unusual to observe confusion in patients with hypercalcemia. However, the behavior changes usually gradually subside once the hypercalcemia is resolved. Therefore, it was concluded that the confusion was due to something other than hypercalcemia.

● **6-6.** A 50-year-old man with dysphagia due to an adenocarcinoma in the gastroesophageal junction became acutely confused and reported recent nausea, anorexia, and polyuria. Because of his nausea, he was unable to consume fluids; his skin turgor was poor and his mucous membranes were dry. The ionized serum calcium level was elevated (2.17 mmol/L or 8.7 mg/dL). Isotonic saline and a single dose of pamidronate were administered IV. The serum calcium level normalized within 3 days and his confusion improved. Later, the confusion returned and he was found to have multiple metastases to the lung, bone, and brain. After consultation with his family, treatment of hypercalcemia was withdrawn, and he was treated palliatively at home until he died 10 days later.

COMMENTARY: Nausea and vomiting are classic symptoms of hypercalcemic states, as is constipation. High serum calcium levels cause slowed GI motility and delayed gastric emptying; these conditions contribute to anorexia, nausea, and vomiting.[121] The polyuria associated with hypercalcemia is related to a renal concentrating defect; inability to replace the large urinary losses with increased oral fluid intake results in fluid volume depletion. Although this patient's confusion was partially alleviated by correction of the serum calcium level, other causes were present that caused it to recur (namely, metastases to the brain).

REFERENCES

1. Chernow B et al. Hypocalcemia in critically ill patients. *Crit Care Med* 1982;10:848.
2. Chernow B, ed. *The Pharmacologic Approach to the Critically Ill Patient*, 3rd ed. Baltimore, MD: Williams & Wilkins; 1994: 777.
3. Rude R. Hypocalcemia and hypoparathyroidism. *Curr Ther Endocrinol Metab* 1997;6:546.
4. Yucha C, Toto K. Calcium and phosphorus derangements. In: Endocrine and Metabolic Disturbances in the Critically Ill. *Crit Care Nurs Clin North Am* December 1994:749.
5. Narins R, ed. *Clinical Disorders of Fluid and Electrolyte Metabolism*, 5th ed. New York: McGraw Hill; 1994:282.
6. Chernow, p 779.
7. Andreoli T, Carpenter C, Bennett J, Plum F. *Cecil Essentials of Medicine*, 4th ed. Philadelphia: WB Saunders; 1997:577.
8. Orwoll E et al. Axial bone mass in older women. Study of osteoporotic fractures research group. *Ann Intern Med* 1996; 124(2):187.
9. Andreoli et al, p 581.
10. Baron J et al. Calcium supplements for the prevention of colorectal adenomas. *N Engl J Med* 1999;340(2):101.
11. Ibid.
12. Yucha, Toto, p 751.
13. Chernow, p 780.
14. Condon R, Nyhus L. *Manual of Surgical Therapeutics*, 9th ed. Boston: Little, Brown; 1996:274.
15. Ibid.
16. Chernow, p 780.
17. Narins, p 1025.
18. Bourrel C et al. Transient hypocalcemia after thyroidectomy. *Ann Otol Laryngol* 1993;102:496.
19. Pattou F, Combemale F, Fabre S. Hypocalcemia following thyroid surgery: Incidence and prediction of outcome. *World J Surg* 1998;22(7):718.
20. Burge M, Zeise T, Johnsen M, et al. Risks of complication following thyroidectomy. *J Gen Intern Med* 1998;13(1):24.
21. Narins, p 1025.
22. Pemberton L, Pemberton D. *Treatment of Water, Electrolyte, and Acid-Base Disorders in the Surgical Patient*. New York: McGraw-Hill; 1994:216.
23. Chernow, p 780.
24. Ibid.
25. Adams J, Andersen P, Everts E, et al. Early postoperative calcium levels as predictors of hypocalcemia. *Laryngoscope* 1998; 108:1829.
26. Ibid.
27. Ibid.
28. Narins, p 1484.
29. Ibid, p 1026.
30. Whong S. Predictors of clinical hypomagnesemia. *Arch Intern Med* 1984;144:1794.
31. Narins, p 277.
32. Chernow, p 781.
33. Helikson M, Parham W, Tobias J. Hypocalcemia and hyperphosphatemia after phosphate enema use in a child. *J Pediatr Surg* 1997;32:1244.
34. Ibid, p 1085.
35. Kokko J, Tannen R. *Fluids and Electrolytes*, 3rd ed. Philadelphia: WB Saunders, 1996:242.
36. Narins, p 1028.
37. Merideth S, Rosenberg I. Gastrointestinal-hepatic disorders and osteomalacia. *Clin Endocrinol Metab* 1980;9:131.
38. Pemberton, Pemberton, p 173.

39. Narins, p 1028.
40. Chernow, p 778.
41. Condon, Nyhus, p 264.
42. Chernow et al, p 851.
43. Niven M, Zohar M, Shimoni Z, et al. Symptomatic hypocalcemia precipitated by small-volume transfusion. *Ann Emerg Med* 1998;32(4):498.
44. Condon, Nyhus, p 264.
45. Narins, p 1092.
46. Uhl L, Maillet S, King S, et al. Unexpected citrate toxicity and severe hypocalcemia during apheresis. *Transfusion* 1997; 37:1063.
47. Narins, p 1029.
48. Chernow, p 781.
49. Narins, p 1026.
50. Narins, p 1483.
51. Zaloga G, Chernow B. Pathogen mechanisms for hypocalcemia during gram negative sepsis (Abstr). *Crit Care Med* 1986;14:405.
52. Lawler D. Hormonal response in sepsis. In: Sepsis. *Crit Care Nurs Clin North Am* September 1994:272.
53. Peter S. Disorders of serum calcium in acquired immunodeficiency syndrome. *J Natl Med Assoc* 1992;84:626.
54. Olinger M. Disorders of calcium and magnesium. *Emerg Med Clin North Am* 1989;7:800.
55. Narins, p 1030.
56. Yucha, Toto, p 753.
57. Rallidis L, Gregoropoulos P, Papasteriadis E. A case of severe hypocalcemia mimicking myocardial infarction. *Int J Cardiol* 1997;61:89.
58. Suzuki T, Ikeda U, Fujikawa H, et al. Hypocalcemic heart failure: A reversible form of heart muscle disease. *Clin Cardiol* 1997; 20:227.
59. Olinger, p 800.
60. Yucha, Toto, p 753.
61. Carey C, Lee H, Woeltzje K. *The Washington Manual of Medical Therapeutics*, 29th ed. Boston: Little, Brown; 1998:446.
62. Narins, p 1031.
63. Ibid.
64. Carey et al, p 446.
65. Shannon M, Wilson B, Stang C. *Appleton & Lange's 1999 Drug Guide*. Stamford, CT: Appleton & Lange; 1999:209.
66. Szerlip H, Goldfarb H. *Workshops in Fluid and Electrolyte Disorders*. New York: Churchill Livingstone; 1993:188.
67. Shannon et al, p 209.
68. Yucha, Toto, p 753.
69. Ibid, p 754.
70. Zaloga, Chernow, p 784.
71. Narins, p 1011.
72. Andreoli et al, p 565.
73. Yucha, Toto, p 756.
74. Narins, p 1014.
75. Bushinsky D, Monk R. Calcium. *Lancet* 1998;352(9124):306.
76. Ibid, p 1015.
77. Andreoli et al, p 567.
78. Bushinsky et al, p 308.
79. Goni M, Tolis G. Hypercalcemia of cancer: An update. *Anticancer Res* 1993;13:1155.
80. Ibid, p 1019.
81. Ibid, p 1015.
82. Olinger, p 805.
83. Tierney L, McPhee S, Pakadakis M. *Current Medical Diagnosis & Treatment*, 38th ed. Stamford, CT: Appleton & Lange, 1999:849.
84. Arieff A, DeFronzo R. *Fluid, Electrolyte, and Acid-Base Disorders*, 2nd ed. New York: Churchill Livingstone; 1995:453.

85. Narins, p 1015.
86. Edelson G, Kleerkoper M. Hypercalcemic crisis. *Med Clin North Am* 1995;79:79.
87. Ibid, p 1021.
88. Arieff, DeFronzo, p 544.
89. Kokko, Tannen, p 396.
90. Ibid, p 1020.
91. Mahon S. Symptoms as clues to calcium levels. *Am J Nurs* 1987;87:354.
92. Rose B. *Clinical Physiology of Acid-Base and Electrolyte Disorders*, 4th ed. New York: McGraw-Hill, 1994:704.
93. Yucha, Toto, p 756.
94. Narins, p 1020.
95. Kaye T. Hypercalcemia: How to pinpoint the cause and customize treatment. *Postgrad Med* 1995;97:153.
96. Carey et al, p 443.
97. Szerlip H, Goldfarb H. *Workshops in Fluid and Electrolyte Disorders*. New York: Churchill Livingstone, 1993:171.
98. Andreoli et al, p 569.
99. Ibid, p 1087.
100. Tierney et al, p 849.
101. Shannon et al, p 1059.
102. Andreoli et al, p 569.
103. Carey et al, p 443.
104. de Beur J, Levine M. Hypercalcemia. *Curr Ther Endocrinol Metab* 1997;6:551.
105. Ibid.
106. Ibid.
107. Carey et al, p 443.
108. Olinger, p 830.
109. Andreoli et al, p 569.
110. Narins, p 1023.
111. Carey et al, p 444.
112. de Beur et al, p 551.
113. Andreoli et al, p 569.
114. Mahon, p 354.
115. Coward D. Hypercalcemia knowledge assessment in patients at risk of developing cancer-induced hypercalcemia. *Oncol Nurs Forum* 1988;15:471.
116. Balan S, Sriram K, Jayanthi V. Metabolic management of hyper- and hypocalcemia. *Nutrition* 1995;11:159.
117. Arieff, DeFronzo, p 454.
118. Kovacs C, MacDonald S, Chik C, et al. Hypercalcemia of malignancy in the palliative care patient: A treatment strategy. *J Pain Symptom Manag* 1995;10:224.
119. Kokko, Tannen, p 396.
120. Kovacs et al, p 224.
121. Narins, p 1021.

CHAPTER 7

Magnesium Imbalances

● MAGNESIUM BALANCE

About two-thirds of the body's magnesium is located in the skeleton and one-third is in the intracellular fluid; only about 1% is in the extracellular fluid (0.3% in the serum).[1] The normal serum magnesium level can be expressed in milliequivalents per liter, millimoles per liter, or milligrams per deciliter (Table 7-1). About one-third of the magnesium in serum is bound to proteins; the rest is ionized.

FUNCTIONS

Magnesium is an important constituent of intracellular fluid where it affects a number of cellular and whole body functions.[2] It participates in more than 300 enzymatic reactions, especially those processes involving the production and utilization of adenosine triphosphate (ATP).[3] Extracellular magnesium is implicated in neuronal control, neuromuscular transmission, and cardiovascular tone.[4] Its high concentration in bone relates magnesium closely to calcium and phosphorus. However, because it is a major intracellular ion, it is also closely related to potassium.

HOMEOSTASIS

Magnesium balance depends on normal intake and renal excretion. The recommended daily allowance for magnesium is 300 mg for women and 350 mg for men; the average American dietary magnesium intake is about 500 mg/day.[5] Magnesium is plentiful in green vegetables, grains, nuts, and seafood. Dietary magnesium is absorbed primarily in the jejunum and ileum. Although little is known about the control of intestinal magnesium absorption, it is thought that it may be increased by parathyroid hormone and growth hormone.[6]

The kidneys are the primary route of magnesium excretion. Fortunately, the kidneys are capable of conserving magnesium efficiently in times of need and excreting it when it is not needed. For example, when magnesium deficiency is present, urinary excretion may fall to less than 1 mEq (0.5 mmol) per day.[7] Also, the kidneys are capable of excreting excess magnesium; therefore, sustained hypermagnesemia is difficult to maintain when normal renal function exists because renal magnesium excretion increases in proportion to the load presented to the kidney.[8]

LABORATORY ASSESSMENT

Assessment of magnesium status by routine laboratory assays is problematic. Although the serum concentration of magnesium is the test most available for clinical use, it is a relatively insensitive measure. This is because only a fraction (0.3%) of the body's total magnesium content is located in the serum. Whereas a less than normal serum magnesium level is most often indicative of total body magnesium deficiency, normal serum magnesium concentrations may exist in some individuals with magnesium deficiency. A high index of suspicion is required for patients whose clinical condition suggests magnesium depletion but whose serum magnesium is normal or only slightly reduced.[9] The serum magnesium level may not fall until several hours after the onset of an acute illness (such as myocardial infarction [MI]).[10]

Other more involved methods exist for evaluating magnesium status. Among these are measuring intracellular magnesium in red blood cells and white blood cells and measuring skeletal muscle magnesium. One group of investigators found that 47% of patients admitted to a respiratory intensive care unit had magnesium content in quadriceps muscle below the lower limit of normal; only 9.4% of the same population had subnormal serum magnesium concentrations.[11]

● **TABLE 7.1.** Normal Serum Magnesium Values

Expression of Measurement	Normal Range
Milliequivalents per 1,000 mL (mEq/L)	1.3–2.1
Millimoles per 1,000 mL (mmol/L)	0.65–1.1
Milligrams per 100 mL (mg/10 dL)	1.6–2.5

Another group of researchers found that 53% of 104 patients admitted to a coronary care unit had low magnesium content in blood mononuclear cells, but only 7.7% had below normal serum magnesium concentrations.[12] Another type of test involves measuring 24-hour urinary magnesium excretion. This is helpful because patients with magnesium deficiency can be expected to conserve magnesium, excreting less magnesium in the urine per day than individuals with a normal magnesium balance. Under normal circumstances, given average magnesium intake and total body stores, 24-hour urinary magnesium excretion ranges from 120 to 140 mg.[13] In the absence of agents or conditions that promote magnesium excretion, a 24-hour urinary magnesium excretion of less than 25 mg suggests magnesium deficiency.[14] A more elaborate test is the magnesium load test; this involves obtaining a 24-hour baseline urine magnesium determination, followed by the administration of 30 mmol magnesium sulfate in 500 mL of 5% aqueous dextrose (D_5W) over 12 hours; urine is collected for 24 hours from the beginning of the infusion.[15] Patients with normal total magnesium stores are expected to excrete 60% to 80% of the administered magnesium, whereas patients with magnesium deficiency will excrete less than 50%.

A curious relationship exists between magnesium and calcium; although low serum levels of these electrolytes produce similar effects (ie, increased neuromuscular irritability), their actions sometimes antagonize each other. For example, magnesium narcosis can be antagonized by parenteral calcium administration.

⬤ HYPOMAGNESEMIA

Hypomagnesemia (and possibly magnesium depletion) is a common clinical problem, both in ambulatory and hospitalized patients. For example, hypomagnesemia was present in 10.2% of 5,100 consecutive ambulatory and hospitalized patients in one study.[16] Much higher rates are observed in critically ill patients. A recent study found that 61% of patients admitted to two postoperative intensive care units had lower than normal serum magnesium levels.[17] Similarly, 65% of patients with normal renal function in a medical intensive care unit population had lower than normal serum magnesium levels.[18]

ETIOLOGICAL FACTORS

Gastrointestinal Losses

An important route for magnesium loss is the gastrointestinal (GI) tract. Losses may take the form of drainage from nasogastric suction, diarrhea, or fistulas. Because fluid from the lower GI tract is richer in magnesium (10–14 mEq/L) than is fluid from the upper tract (1–2 mEq/L), losses from diarrhea and intestinal fistulas are more likely to induce magnesium deficit than are those from gastric suction.[19] However, hypomagnesemia will occur in patients with prolonged nasogastric suction, especially if parenteral fluids are magnesium free.

Because the distal small bowel is the major site of magnesium absorption, any disruption in small bowel function (as occurs in intestinal resection or inflammatory bowel disease) can lead to hypomagnesemia. One study reported that 15 of 42 patients with malabsorption syndromes had subnormal serum magnesium levels;[20] the degree of hypomagnesemia showed a rough correlation with the degree of steatorrhea. In the presence of steatorrhea, it is believed that magnesium ions are excreted in the stool in the form of magnesium soaps. In another study, 50% of 191 patients developed hypomagnesemia in the first postoperative year after bowel resection for the treatment of morbid obesity.[21]

Alcoholism

Chronic alcoholism is the most common cause of hypomagnesemia in the United States. One study found that 30% of all alcoholics and 86% of patients with delirium tremens had hypomagnesemia during the first 1 to 2 days of hospitalization.[22] Although there are no convincing data to indicate that hypomagnesemia causes delirium tremens, it is likely that magnesium deficiency aggravates alcohol withdrawal.[23] For this reason, it is recommended that the serum magnesium level be measured every 2 or 3 days in hospitalized alcoholic patients undergoing withdrawal.[24] Although the serum magnesium level may be normal on admission, it can fall as a result of metabolic changes associated with therapy (such as the intracellular shift of magnesium associated with intravenous [IV] glucose administration).

Decreased dietary intake of magnesium is a major factor in the development of hypomagnesemia in alcoholics. Other factors include increased GI losses (due to episodic emesis and diarrhea) and intestinal malabsorption. In addition, alcohol ingestion is believed to increase magnesium excretion in the urine.

Refeeding After Starvation

In the catabolic state, the protein structure of cells is metabolized as energy sources; as a result, intracellular[25] ions are lost and total body concentrations of these ions (magnesium, potassium, and phosphate) are decreased. Conversely, during nutritional repletion, these electrolytes are taken from the serum and deposited into newly synthesized cells. Thus, if the enteral or parenteral feeding formula is deficient in magnesium content, serious hypomagnesemia will occur. Serum levels of these primarily intracellular ions should be measured at regular intervals during the administration of IV total parenteral nutrition (TPN) and even during enteral feedings, especially in patients who have undergone a period of starvation. See Chapters 11 and 12 for further discussions of this topic.

Drugs Disrupting Magnesium Homeostasis

The loop diuretics (furosemide, bumetanide, and ethacrynic acid) increase urinary magnesium excretion. Although the loop diuretics are the most potent magnesuric diuretics, long-term use of thiazide diuretics may also lead to mild hypomagnesemia.[26]

Although the exact mechanism is not clear, it has been demonstrated that aminoglycosides (such as gentamycin, tobramycin, and kanamycin) are associated with urinary magnesium wasting. For example, one study found that of 55 patients receiving aminoglycoside antibiotics, 38% developed hypomagnesemia associated with renal magnesium wasting.[27] Amphotericin B (an antifungal agent) can also cause hypomagnesemia.[28]

Cis-platinum (cisplatin) administration is associated with hypomagnesemia secondary to increased urinary excretion of magnesium. This potentially nephrotoxic chemotherapeutic agent appears to cause hypomagnesemia in a dose-related manner.[29] Cyclosporine usage in renal transplant patients may produce a significant drop in the serum magnesium concentration, presumably by increasing renal magnesium wasting.[30]

Citrate is a preservative added to collected blood to prolong its longevity. Rapid administration of citrated blood (eg, faster than 1.5 mL/kg/min) can temporarily decrease the ionized magnesium level because citrate chelates circulating magnesium ions (and calcium ions).[31] This is most likely to occur when citrate clearance is diminished by renal or hepatic disease or by hypothermia.[32]

Other Factors

Magnesium deficiency is often seen in patients with diabetic ketoacidosis. It is primarily the result of increased renal excretion of magnesium during osmotic diuresis (caused by the high glucose load) and of the shifting of magnesium into cells that occurs with insulin therapy (see Chap. 18).

Some causes of renal disease, such as glomerulonephritis, pyelonephritis, and renal tubular acidosis, may produce hypomagnesemia by impairing renal magnesium reabsorption. However, remember that with advanced renal disease (glomerular filtration rate [GFR] <10–25 mL/hr), hypermagnesemia usually results from impaired renal magnesium excretion.[33]

Pancreatitis may cause hypomagnesemia in much the same way that it causes hypocalcemia (see Chap. 20). In addition, any condition associated with hypercalcemia, such as excessive doses of vitamin D or calcium supplements, may result in renal magnesium loss.[34] It should be noted that magnesium and calcium share a common route of absorption in the intestinal tract and appear to have a mutually suppressive effect; thus, if calcium intake is unusually high, calcium will be absorbed in preference to magnesium, and vice versa.

Magnesium deficiency has also been described in burn patients and is possibly related to loss of magnesium during débridement and bathing of denuded skin. Other conditions believed to predispose to hypomagnesemia are sepsis and hypothermia.[35] Postoperative patients may have increased magnesium loss in the urine due to increased aldosterone release associated with stress from the operative procedure.[36]

Administration of magnesium-free, sodium-rich IV fluids to induce extracellular fluid expansion can cause hypomagnesemia. In fact, any condition predisposing to excessive calcium or sodium in the urine can augment renal excretion of magnesium because magnesium is normally reabsorbed in the kidney with calcium and sodium.[37]

DEFINING CHARACTERISTICS

Some of the effects of hypomagnesemia are directly caused by the low serum magnesium level, whereas others are due to secondary changes in potassium and calcium metabolism. Manifestations of magnesium deficiency do not usually occur until the serum magnesium level is less than 1 mEq/L. However, because the serum magnesium concentration may underestimate intracellular magnesium depletion, a high index of suspicion for magnesium deficiency is warranted.[38]

Neuromuscular Changes

Neuromuscular hyperexcitability with muscular weakness, tremors, and athetoid movements may be seen. Other manifestations may include tetany, generalized tonic-clonic or focal seizures, laryngeal stridor, and positive Chvostek's and Trousseau's signs. The neuromuscular symptoms of hypomagnesemia are similar to those occurring in hypocalcemia and result mainly from increased neuronal excitability. Because severe hypomagnesemia may ultimately result in hypocalcemia and hypokalemia, it is possible that the symptoms may be partly due to these disturbances. Vague but nonspecific GI symptoms have been described; for example, dysphagia may develop.

Cardiovascular Effects

Magnesium is important for normal cardiac function; therefore, it is understandable that hypomagnesemia is associated with a high frequency of cardiac arrhythmias and sudden death.[39] Because standard antiarrhythmic drugs and defibrillation may be ineffective in controlling ventricular arrhythmias associated with magnesium deficiency, refractory arrhythmias should be treated with IV magnesium salts. Intracellular magnesium depletion in the myocardium is even more likely to predispose to arrhythmias if hypokalemia is also present. Electrocardiographic (ECG) changes observed in hypomagnesemia include PR and QT interval prolongation, widened QRS complex, ST segment depression, and T wave inversion.[40]

Increased susceptibility to digitalis toxicity is associated with low serum magnesium levels.[41] An experiment with animals found that the uptake of digoxin by myocardial cells was enhanced by magnesium depletion.[42] One report indicated that hypomagnesemia was present twice as often in digitalis-toxic patients (21%) as in nontoxic patients (10%).[43] This is important because patients receiving digoxin are also likely to be on diuretic therapy, which predisposes to renal loss of magnesium.

Epidemiological studies suggest that populations having low dietary magnesium intake have a higher incidence of hypertension.[44] Disease entities such as diabetes mellitus and alcoholism are commonly associated with both hypomagnesemia and elevated blood pressure.[45] The relationship between magnesium deficiency and hypertension is not entirely clear.[46] Apparently hypomagnesemia has vasoconstrictive effects that can be reversed by the administration of magnesium. However, although diets rich in fruits and vegetables may help protect against stroke secondary to hypertension, pill supplementation of magnesium (and calcium and potassium) is of limited or unproved efficacy.[47]

Central Nervous System Changes

Because decreased serum magnesium increases irritability of nerve tissue, convulsions may occur. Disorientation is common. Other changes may include ataxia, vertigo, depression, and psychosis.

Metabolic Effects

Associated Imbalances

Hypomagnesemia may arise together with and contribute to the persistence of other imbalances, such as hypokalemia, hypocalcemia, and hypophosphatemia. Hypokalemia is a relatively common finding in hypomagnesemic patients because the kidneys are not able to conserve potassium when magnesium deficiency exists. This hypokalemia accompanying hypomagnesemia is often refractory to potassium replacement alone, requiring the replacement of both potassium and magnesium before correction of the imbalance can occur. The plasma magnesium concentration should always be measured in patients with otherwise unexplained hypokalemia.[48] It is likely that hypocalcemia and hypophosphatemia accompany hypomagnesemia because severe magnesium depletion interferes with the secretion of parathyroid hormone (PTH), which is needed to return calcium and phosphorus to normal ranges. A recent study of 35 adult patients who exhibited profound hypomagnesemia, hypokalemia, and hypocalcemia on admission found that alcoholism and cisplatin administration were the most common causes of this combination of electrolyte imbalances.[49]

Insulin Resistance

Magnesium influences peripheral tissue responsiveness to insulin and also affects insulin secretion by the pancreas.[50] Hypomagnesemia has been reported in a variety of settings involving insulin resistance.[51] However, the relationship between hypomagnesemia and insulin resistance is not clear.

TREATMENT

Magnesium replacement may be indicated even when the serum magnesium concentration is normal; this is because total body magnesium stores may be decreased despite normomagnesemia. Magnesium deficiency is treated by correcting the cause of the imbalance (when possible) and supplying magnesium to correct the deficit. Serum magnesium levels may normalize rather quickly, but sustained magnesium replacement for several days is usually needed to replace cellular magnesium deficits. Provided the patient is able to eat, dietary sources of magnesium should be encouraged; among these are green vegetables, seafood, nuts, and grains. When symptoms of hypomagnesemia are absent, it is best to administer magnesium orally to avoid causing abrupt increases in the plasma magnesium level.[52] Magnesium salts in tablet form (such as magnesium oxide) can be given orally to replace continuous excessive losses. Unfortunately, diarrhea is a side effect that can interfere with the usefulness of oral magnesium preparations.

Magnesium may be given IV or by deep intramuscular injection (although painful) when indicated. Parenteral magnesium is especially helpful in patients with symptomatic hypomagnesemia or malabsorption. Before magnesium administration, renal function should be assessed because the kidneys are primarily responsible for the elimination of magnesium. When renal function is impaired in those receiving magnesium, blood levels should be closely monitored. During parenteral magnesium replacement, serum magnesium levels should be monitored, as should deep-tendon reflexes. Marked depression of deep-tendon reflexes signals too high a serum magnesium level and is an indication that no further magnesium should be administered.[53] Reports of serum levels at which loss of the patellar reflex occurs are variable, but most agree that it is decreased at 4 to 6 mEq/L and is lost at a range of 6 to 10 mEq/L. Because deep-tendon reflexes disappear before respiratory paralysis and heart block occur, frequent assessment of deep-tendon reflexes is reasonable to help detect hypermagnesemia before it reaches a critical level.

Patients with severe hypomagnesemia (defined as <1 mg/dL) should receive special attention. For example, in the treatment of life-threatening arrhythmias, Zaloga and Chernow[54] recommend 1 to 2 g (8–16 mEq) of magnesium sulfate IV over 5 minutes (while ECG monitoring is continuously performed). They further recommend that this bolus dose be followed by an infusion of 1 to 2 g/hr of magnesium sulfate for the next few hours and then the dose be reduced to 0.5 to 1 g/hr as a maintenance infusion (provided renal function is normal).

Magnesium sulfate is available in 10%, 20%, and 50% solutions; 1 g magnesium sulfate is equivalent to 2 mL of a 50% solution, 5 mL of a 20% solution, and 10 mL of a 10% solution.[55] A report of severe hypermagnesemia resulting from improperly written or executed orders for IV magnesium sulfate pointed out the need for extreme caution in administering magnesium.[56] Three cases of severe hypermagnesemia were attributed to the inadvertent use of 50-mL vials of 50% magnesium sulfate. In two cases, the orders called for "one amp" of 50% magnesium sulfate by slow IV infusion. Although the prescriber intended that a 2-mL ampule be given, a 50-mL ampule was substituted. In the third case, the order was for a 50-mL vial of 50% dextrose. Instead, a 50-mL vial of magnesium sulfate was mistakenly used. The author emphasizes the need to recognize the potency of currently available electrolyte solutions and the importance of physicians writing precise orders pertaining to their use. Certainly orders containing terms such as "amp" or "vial" without further specification should not be written by physicians or accepted by nurses. The third case emphasizes the need to read product labels carefully before use. Never rely solely on the size, shape, or label design of the container for product identification. General nursing considerations related to administering of magnesium salts are listed in Clinical Tip: Nursing Considerations in Administering IV Magnesium.

CLINICAL TIP

Nursing Considerations in Administering IV Magnesium

1. The extent of magnesium replacement needed for specific hypomagnesemic patients may vary widely according to (a) the severity of the magnesium deficiency, and (b) the current level of renal function. Generally, the more severe the symptoms, the more aggressive the therapy must be.

2. Carefully check the order for IV magnesium. Be sure that it stipulates one of the following:
   A. Concentration of the solution to be administered (as well as the number of milliliters), fluid in which it is to be diluted, and the time frame over which it is to be given. For example: "Give 2 mL of 50% $MgSO_4$, diluted in 100 mL of 0.9% sodium chloride, over 1 hr."
   B. Number of grams of magnesium sulfate ($MgSO_4$) to be administered, along with the required dilution, and time frame over which it is to be administered. For example: "Give 1 g of $MgSO_4$, diluted in 100 mL of 0.9% sodium chloride, over 1 hr."
   Recall that $MgSO_4$ is available in concentrations of 10%, 20%, and 50%. One gram of $MgSO_4$ is contained in 10 mL of a 10% solution, 5 mL of a 20% solution, and 2 mL of a 50% solution. Obviously, serious errors can occur if the wrong concentration is used.

3. Never accept order for "amps" or "vials" without further specifications.

4. Use IV magnesium with great caution in patients with impaired renal function (as evidenced by an elevated serum creatinine level). Recall that the primary route of magnesium excretion is via the kidneys; thus, it is easy to induce hypermagnesemia when renal impairment is present. If magnesium replacement is required in a patient with renal impairment, the physician will probably reduce the dose to be administered by 25% to 50% of that needed for a patient with normal renal function.

5. Monitor urine output at regular intervals throughout the magnesium infusion. Therapy is generally not continued if urinary output is less than 100 mL every 4 hours.[57] An output less than this amount raises the question of adequate urinary elimination of magnesium.

6. Check deep-tendon reflexes (such as patellar "knee jerk") before each dose of magnesium, or periodically during continuous infusion of the drug. If reflexes are absent, do not give additional magnesium, and notify the physician. (Because deep-tendon reflexes are decreased before adverse respiratory and cardiac effects occur, the presence of knee jerks can usually be relied on to indicate that life-threatening hypermagnesemia is not present.)

7. Therapeutic doses of magnesium can produce flushing and sweating because magnesium acts peripherally to produce vasodilation. Inform the patient that this might occur to minimize concern.

8. Check blood pressure, pulse, and respirations every 15 minutes and monitor the serum magnesium level at regular intervals. Look for a sharp fall in blood pressure on respiratory distress; both are signs of hypermagnesemia. (This can be induced rather easily with improper doses of magnesium.) Patients receiving very aggressive magnesium therapy should receive close cardiac monitoring.

9. If the patient displays signs of severe hypermagnesemia, stop IV administration of magnesium and run in the IV solution from the primary line (as appropriate) to keep the vein open. Notify the physician and be prepared to administer artificial ventilation and IV calcium (if prescribed).

10. Because magnesium is primarily an intracellular ion, it may take several days to completely correct cellular deficits. Therefore, normal serum magnesium values do not necessarily imply that the magnesium depletion has been corrected.

OTHER CONDITIONS THAT MAY BENEFIT FROM MAGNESIUM ADMINISTRATION

Briefly described in Table 7-2 are rationales for using magnesium in the treatment of patients with eclampsia and MI. Less clear are the rationales for considering using magnesium supplementation for patients with hypertension, diabetes mellitus, and migraine headaches. A link between magnesium, hypertension, and diabetes mellitus seems established beyond a reasonable doubt.[64] It has also been suggested that magnesium administration may be helpful to some patients who suffer from migraine headaches.[65] Further clinical studies are indicated to document under what circumstances magnesium supplementation would be helpful for patients with hypertension, diabetes mellitus, and migraine headaches.

NURSING INTERVENTIONS

1. Be aware of patients at risk for hypomagnesemia and monitor for its presence. See Summary of

---

TABLE 7-2. Conditions That May Benefit From Magnesium Administration

Condition	Possible Rationale for Use
Severe preeclampsia/eclampsia	Prevent or control convulsions Lower blood pressure Inhibit uterine contractions (see Chap. 23 for a more thorough discussion of magnesium administration in this disorder.)
Myocardial infarction (MI)	Postulated that magnesium infusion decreases some arrhythmias and decreases the size of ischemic injury after an acute MI (presumably by acting as a coronary artery vasodilator, potential antithrombotic agent, and a calcium competitor). Magnesium is thought to possess a "cardioprotective" effect, although the mechanism is unknown.[58] Several large studies have shown conflicting results regarding the value of magnesium in reducing mortality following acute MI. A 1992 study (the LIMIT-2 trial) of over 2,000 patients with acute MIs showed a mortality decrease of 24% when magnesium was administered.[59] However, findings from a study of over 50,000 patients presented in late 1993 from the ISIS-4 Collaborative Group suggest there is no benefit from the routine use of magnesium in acute MI.[60] The 1997 Advanced Cardiac Life Support manual recommends administering magnesium if the serum magnesium level is < 1.4 mEq/L (0.7 mmol/L) or if hypomagnesemia is suspected on the basis of the patient's history (such as the presence of malnutrition or alcoholism).[61] For acute MI prophylaxis, the recommended dose is 1–2 g mixed in 50–100 mL D_5W over 5–60 minutes IV (followed with 0.5–1.0 g/hr up to 24 hours).[62] Clinical trials are underway to further evaluate the role of magnesium in treating acute MI. Currently, there is no routine indication for the administration of magnesium to patients with MI.[63]

Hypomagnesemia and review above sections for a discussion of etiological factors and defining characteristics.

2. Assess digitalized patients at risk for hypomagnesemia especially closely for symptoms of digitalis toxicity because a deficit of magnesium predisposes to toxicity.

3. Be prepared to take seizure precautions when hypomagnesemia is severe.

4. Monitor condition of airway because laryngeal stridor can occur.

5. Take safety precautions if confusion is present.

6. Be familiar with magnesium replacement salts and factors related to their safe administration. Review treatment section above and Clinical Tip: Nursing Considerations in Administering IV Magnesium.

7. Be aware that magnesium-depleted patients may experience difficulty in swallowing. (Dysphagia is probably related to the athetoid or choreiform movements associated with magnesium deficit.) If difficulty in swallowing is suspected, test the ability to swallow with water before offering oral medications.

8. When magnesium deficit is due to abuse of diuretics or laxatives, educating the patient may help alleviate the problem. Part of the nursing assessment should be directed toward identifying problems amenable to prevention through education.

9. Be aware that most commonly used IV fluids have either no magnesium or a relatively small amount. For example, D_5W, isotonic saline, and lactated Ringer's solution have no magnesium. Prolonged use of magnesium-free parenteral fluids with no oral intake of magnesium and abnormal losses of magnesium by the GI or renal route will eventually lead to hypomagnesemia. When indicated, discuss need for magnesium replacement with physician.

10. For patients experiencing abnormal magnesium losses who are able to consume a general diet, encourage the intake of magnesium-rich foods, such as green vegetables, meat, seafood, dairy products, and cereal.

CASE STUDIES

● **7-1.** A 65-year-old emaciated woman with carcinoma of the stomach was started on a TPN protocol because she was unable to eat or tolerate enteral tube feedings. On the seventh day, when electrolytes were checked for the first time, the serum magnesium was 0.8 mEq/L. She was lethargic and had coarse tremors, most notable in the arms. TPN was stopped and 12 mL of 50% magnesium sulfate was added to 1 liter of 10% glucose in water and infused over 3 hours. Additional magnesium was administered over the next 2 days. TPN was slowly restarted with adequate magnesium supplementation.

COMMENTARY: Serum electrolytes should be measured regularly during TPN. In fact, they should be measured daily for the first 5 days. The purpose is to detect abnormalities before they become severe. Requirements for the intracellular ions potassium, magnesium, and phosphate vary with calorie and nitrogen intake and the nutritional state of the patient. As the anabolic state is achieved with TPN, these ions are incorporated into the newly synthesized cells. In this way, extracellular deficits will develop if inadequate amounts are provided in the nutrient solution.

7-2. A 50-year-old man with a history of chronic alcoholism was admitted for treatment. He had been on a diet of only alcoholic beverages for a week and then stopped drinking for a few days. Because of nausea, he ate very little. On examination, he was noted to have hyperactive knee jerks. Laboratory findings included a serum magnesium level of 0.7 mEq/L.

COMMENTARY: Hypomagnesemia is a frequent occurrence in alcoholic patients. Contributing to poor dietary intake of magnesium as a major cause of magnesium deficiency is the increased renal loss of this electrolyte associated with excessive alcohol intake.

7-3. A 40-year-old man developed a high-output intestinal fistula after treatment for an intestinal obstruction. For 2 weeks he received only isotonic saline (0.9% NaCl) and 5% dextrose in water with added KCl. He developed choreiform movements of the arms and muscle twitching. In addition, he was noted to be confused. Laboratory findings included:

Serum Na = 140 mEq/L
K = 3.3 mEq/L
Mg = 0.7 mEq/L

Summary of Hypomagnesemia

ETIOLOGICAL FACTORS

Inadequate Intake
Prolonged administration of magnesium-
  free fluids
Starvation
Total parenteral nutrition without
  adequate magnesium supplementation
Chronic alcoholism

Increased Gastrointestinal Losses
Diarrhea
Laxative abuse
Fistulas
Prolonged nasogastric suction
Vomiting
Malabsor btion syndromes

Increased Renal Losses
Drugs
  Loop and thiazide diuretics
  Mannitol
  Cisplatin
  Cyclosporine
  Aminoglycosides
  Carbenicillin
  Amphotericin B
Diuresis
  Uncontrolled diabetes mellitus
  Hyperaldosteronism

Changes in Magnesium Distribution
Pancreatitis
Thermal injury
Drugs causing shift into cells
  Insulin
  Glucose
  Catecholamines
Citrate Chelation
  Citrated blood products
  Plasmapheresis

DEFINING CHARACTERISTICS

Neuromuscular
Muscle weakness
Muscle twitching, cramps
Paresthesias
Chvostek's sign
Trousseau's sign

Cardiovascular
Increased sensitivity to digitalis
Hypertension
Arrhythmias
  Premature ventricular contractions,
  ventricular fibrillation, torsades de pointes,
  atrial fibrillation, paroxysmal supraventric-
  ular tachycardia
Increased sensitivity to ischemic heart
  disease arrhythmias
Coronary artery spasm

ECG changes
  Prolonged QT and PR intervals,
  widened QRS complex, depressed ST
  segment

Metabolic
Hypocalcemia
Hypokalemia
Hypophosphatemia
Insulin resistance

Central Nervous System
Depression
Agitation
Confusion
Psychosis

Commentary: Although the serum sodium level is normal, the magnesium is far below normal and there is some degree of hypokalemia, despite addition of KCl to the IV fluids. Recall that intestinal fluid contains about 10 to 12 mEq/L of magnesium. These losses were not replaced because the IV fluids were magnesium free. With a negative magnesium balance, there is often a below-normal serum potassium, even with adequate intake.

HYPERMAGNESEMIA

Although hypermagnesemia is much less common than hypomagnesemia, it may occur more frequently than previously thought. In one study, as many as 86% of hypermagnesemic patients were not clinically identified.[66] Serum magnesium concentrations tend to be good predictors of magnesium excess. Most causes of hypermagnesemia are iatrogenic.

ETIOLOGICAL FACTORS

Renal Failure

Hypermagnesemia is most likely to occur in patients with renal insufficiency (especially if creatinine clearance is <30 mL/min).[67] This is understandable because magnesium is primarily excreted by the kidneys and, therefore, diminished renal function results in abnormal renal magnesium retention. The predisposition of patients with renal failure to hypermagnesemia is aggravated if they are given magnesium to control convulsions or if they inadvertently receive one of the many commercial antacids or laxatives containing variable amounts of magnesium salts (Table 7-3). Despite its relatively low prevalence (as compared to that of hypomagnesemia), hypermagnesemia probably occurs more frequently than it should because clinicians are often unaware of the magnesium content of various preparations.[68]

Renal patients may also receive an exogenous magnesium load during hemodialysis, because of either an inadvertent use of hard water or an error in manufacture of the concentrate used for preparing the dialysate.

Elderly persons are at greater risk for hypermagnesemia because they have age-related reduced renal function and tend to consume more magnesium-containing preparations (such as antacids or mineral

TABLE 7-3. Examples of Over-the-Counter Antacids and Laxatives That Contain Magnesium

Citrate of magnesia
Magnesium hydroxide
    Di-Gel Antacid/Anti-Gas Liquid (Schering-Plough Healthcare)
    Maalox Antacid/Anti-Gas Tablets (Novartis)
    Mylanta Maximum Strength Liquid (J&J, Merck Consumer)
    Phillips' Milk of Magnesia Liquid (Bayer Consumer)
    Rolaids Antacid Tablets (Warner-Lambert)
Magnesium carbonate
    Gaviscon Liquid Antacid (SmithKline Beecham)
    Maalox Heartburn Relief Suspension (Novartis)
    Marblen Tablets (Fleming)
Magnesium gluconate
    Magonate Liquid (Fleming)

supplements) than younger individuals. Also, the elderly may have GI disorders (eg, gastritis and colitis) that alter the GI mucosal barrier and thus increase absorption of magnesium.[69]

Magnesium Administration for Therapeutic Purposes

Just as conventional magnesium doses can cause hypermagnesemia in patients with renal impairment, overly vigorous treatment with magnesium salts can cause hypermagnesemia in patients with normal renal function. For example, a case was reported in which a massive dose of a seemingly harmless magnesium-containing cathartic resulted in profound hypermagnesemia (21.7 mg/dL, normal 1.6–2.5 mg/dL) and cardiopulmonary arrest in a patient with normal kidney function.[70]

Magnesium sulfate is sometimes administered to treat eclampsia or to delay delivery. In either case, excessive magnesium administration can cause both maternal and fetal hypermagnesemia. In a recent study of the use of magnesium sulfate as a tocolytic agent in 111 women, investigators reported that side effects were common but were rarely severe enough to cause cessation of therapy.[71] They cautioned that because 90% of parenterally administered magnesium sulfate is cleared by the maternal kidneys, the drug should be administered with extreme caution in women with impaired renal function.

It is possible to exceed the renal tolerance of patients with normal renal function if excessive magnesium is accidentally administered during treatment of symptomatic hypomagnesemia or when too much magnesium is added to parenteral nutrition fluids.

DEFINING CHARACTERISTICS

Because magnesium is not measured as routinely as most other electrolytes, one must maintain a high index of suspicion for hypermagnesemia in at-risk patients. The clinical manifestations of hypermagnesemia largely reflect the ion's action on the nervous and cardiovascular systems.

Hypermagnesemia diminishes neuromuscular transmission and can depress skeletal muscle function and cause neuromuscular blockade.[72] Hypocalcemia may accompany hypermagnesemia because the latter suppresses PTH secretion.

Cardiovascular effects of hypermagnesemia are related to its "calcium channel blocker" effect on cardiac conduction and smooth muscle of blood vessels.[73] Arrhythmias occurring with hypermagnesemia may include bradycardia, atrioventricular block, and asystole. Changes seen on ECG tracings may include shortening of the QT interval as well as T wave abnormalities and prolongation of the QRS and PR intervals. Hypotension tends to occur early in hypermagnesemia and is related to vasodilation.

The Summary of Hypermagnesemia lists some rough relationships between the serum levels of magnesium and expected symptoms. However, it should be emphasized that authorities do not agree on precise serum magnesium levels at which specific symptoms will occur. In fact, quite variable results may be found in the literature. This is largely because patients respond differently to elevated serum magnesium levels. There is agreement that deep-tendon reflexes are decreased at a level around 4 to 6 or 4 to 7 mEq/L.[74,75] There is also fair agreement that deep-tendon reflexes are absent when the serum magnesium level is between 6 and 10 mEq/L.[76,77] However, authors vary as to when cardiac arrest is expected; some indicate this will occur when the serum magnesium level exceeds 15 mEq/L,[78,79] whereas others indicate it will occur at

levels above 10 mEq/L.[80] It is also not entirely clear when respiratory muscle paralysis is likely; some indicate that respirations will decrease at a serum magnesium level of 9 mEq/L,[81] whereas others predict respiratory paralysis at levels at or approaching 10 mEq/L.[82,83] Fortunately, there is good agreement that deep-tendon reflexes will diminish and disappear well before respiratory paralysis or cardiac arrest. It is for this reason that deep-tendon reflexes are monitored closely during magnesium infusions to prevent potentially life-threatening outcomes.

Rizzo et al.[84] reported a case in which a 27-year-old diabetic woman was inadvertently given two 25-g bottles of magnesium sulfate over a 6-hour period for treatment of hypomagnesemia. (This occurred after an order was placed for "2 amps of magnesium sulfate" to be administered in 1 liter of IV fluids.) Profound hypermagnesemia (9.85 mmol/L) resulted and caused total neuromuscular blockade and a pseudocoma state that mimicked a midbrain syndrome. Fortunately, the patient eventually recovered although she received a greatly larger dose of magnesium than intended. (One gram of magnesium sulfate provides 97.6 mg, 4 mmol, or 8 mEq elemental magnesium.)[85]

TREATMENT

The best treatment for hypermagnesemia is prevention. This can be accomplished by avoiding administration of magnesium to patients with renal failure and by carefully administering magnesium salts to seriously ill patients.

In the presence of hypermagnesemia, any parenteral or oral magnesium salt should be discontinued. This may be all that is needed if the deep-tendon reflexes are still present. Neuromuscular and cardiac toxicity of hypermagnesemia can be antagonized transiently by the IV administration of 10 to 20 mL of 10% calcium gluconate over 10 minutes.[86] (Recall that calcium acts as a direct antagonist to magnesium.) Mechanical ventilation may be needed for patients with compromised respiratory function. A temporary pacemaker may be needed for bradyarrhythmias.[87] Dialysis (either peritoneal or hemodialysis) may be needed for treating hypermagnesemic renal failure patients.

NURSING INTERVENTIONS

1. Be aware of patients at risk for hypermagnesemia and assess for its presence. See Summary of Hyper-

magnesemia and preceding sections explaining etiological factors and defining characteristics.

When hypermagnesemia is suspected, assess the following parameters:

- Vital signs: Look for low blood pressure and shallow respirations with periods of apnea.
- Patellar reflexes: If absent, notify physician because this usually implies a serum magnesium level greater than 6 mEq/L. If allowed to progress, cardiac or respiratory arrest could occur.
- Level of consciousness: Look for drowsiness, lethargy, and coma.

2. Do not give magnesium-containing medications to patients with renal failure or compromised renal function. (Be particularly careful in following "standing orders" for bowel preparation for radiography because some of these include the use of magnesium citrate.)

3. Caution patients with renal disease to check with their health care providers before taking over-the-counter medications. See Table 7-3 for a list of some commonly used medications containing magnesium.

4. Be aware of factors related to safe parenteral administration of magnesium salts. Review Clinical Tip: Nursing Considerations in Administering IV Magnesium.

CASE STUDIES

● **7-4.** A 43-year-old woman was awaiting a kidney transplant when an order was written for a barium enema. Routine orders for bowel preparation in the institution included the administration of magnesium citrate as a laxative. Without considering the need to modify directives for a renal patient, the preparation was administered. Shortly after administration of magnesium citrate, the patient became very lethargic and developed muscular weakness.
COMMENTARY: Magnesium salts should never be given to patients with acute or chronic renal disease because diseased kidneys are incapable of eliminating magnesium. Blindly following standing orders caused serious problems for this patient.

Hemodialysis was performed on an emergency basis.

● **7-5.** A 62-year-old woman with chronic glomerulonephritis took Maalox (a magnesium-containing antacid) to alleviate gastric discomfort. She developed lethargy and difficulty in breathing. On admission to an acute care facility, her serum magnesium level was 7.8 mEq/L (normal, 1.5–2.5 mEq/L). Calcium gluconate, 10 mEq, was administered to alleviate respiratory depression. Hemodialysis was initiated.
COMMENTARY: Magnesium-containing medications are contraindicated in patients with acute or chronic renal disease. Part of patient education should be directed at the need to avoid such preparations.

● **7-6.** A 42-year-old schizophrenic woman was admitted to the emergency department with confusion, abdominal pain, vomiting, and constipation.[88] Before admission, she had been treated with milk of magnesia (30 mL) each night and Maalox (30 mL) three times daily. Her abdomen was distended and diffusely tender and she would respond only briefly to voice or painful stimuli. Her laboratory tests revealed:

Serum Mg = 9.1 mEq/L (normal, 1.3–2.0 mEq/L)
BUN = 16 mg/dL
Creatinine = 0.9 mg/dL

A laparotomy was performed and an adhesive band from a previous surgery was found to be compressing the sigmoid colon. Despite successful treatment of the hypermagnesemia with calcium, IV fluids, and furosemide, the patient died from cardiac problems on the second postoperative day.
COMMENTARY: This patient had normal renal function (as indicated by the serum creatinine and blood urea nitrogen values); however, she still developed serious hypermagnesemia following the excessive use of magnesium-containing medications. The authors who reported this case recommend frequent use of the laboratory to identify hypermagnesemia because it is often a clinically unexpected finding and responds well to early treatment.[89]

Summary of Hypermagnesemia

ETIOLOGICAL FACTORS

Acute and chronic renal failure (particularly when magnesium-containing medications are used)

Excessive magnesium administration during treatment of eclampsia or to delay labor (affects both mother and fetus)

Excessive doses of magnesium during treatment of hypomagnesemia

Excessive use of magnesium-containing antacids or laxatives by elderly persons (who have age-related decreased renal function)

Adrenal insufficiency

Hemodialysis with excessively hard water or with a dialysate high in magnesium content

DEFINING CHARACTERISTICS

Serum Magnesium Levels (mEq/L)*

3–5	Peripheral vasodilation with facial flushing, sense of warmth, and tendency for hypotension; nausea and vomiting
4–7	Drowsiness; decreased deep-tendon reflexes; muscle weakness
5–10	More severe hypotension and bradycardia
7–10	Loss of patellar reflex
10	Respiratory depression
10–15	Respiratory paralysis; coma
15–20	Cardiac arrest

*These are only general ranges; precise levels at which signs and symptoms are expected to develop are not uniformly defined. Reports in the literature vary widely in regard to symptoms and the level at which they appear (see text).

REFERENCES

1. Matz R. Magnesium deficiencies and therapeutic uses. *Hosp Pract* April 1993;30:79.
2. Kelepouris E, Agus Z. Hypomagnesemia: Renal magnesium handling. *Semin Nephrol* 1998;18:58.
3. Ahsan S. Metabolism of magnesium in health and disease. J Indian Med Assoc 1997;95:507.
4. Narins R, ed. *Maxwell & Kleeman's Clinical Disorders of Fluid and Electrolyte Metabolism*, 5th ed. New York: McGraw-Hill; 1994:373.
5. Matz, p 80.
6. Ibid.
7. Ibid.
8. Reinhart R. Magnesium deficiency: Recognition and treatment in the emergency medicine setting. *Am J Emerg Med* 1992;10:78.
9. Narins, p 1100.
10. Reinhart, p 78.
11. Fiaccadori E et al. Muscle and serum magnesium in pulmonary intensive care unit patients. *Crit Care Med* 1988;16:751.
12. Ryzen E et al. Low blood mononuclear cell magnesium in intensive cardiac care unit patients. *Am Heart J* 1986;111:475.
13. White J, Campbell K. Magnesium and diabetes: A review. *Ann Pharmacother* 1993;27:775.
14. Matz, p 80.
15. Zaloga G, Chernow B. Divalent ions: Calcium, magnesium, and phosphorus. In: Chernow B, ed. *The Pharmacologic Approach to the Critically Ill Patient*, 3rd ed. Baltimore, MD: Williams & Wilkins; 1994:794.
16. Jackson C, Meier D. Routine serum magnesium analysis: Correlation with clinical state in 5100 patients. *Ann Intern Med* 1968;69:743.
17. Chernow B et al. Hypomagnesemia in patients in postoperative intensive care. *Chest* 1989;95:391.
18. Ryzen E et al. Magnesium deficiency in a medical intensive care unit population. *Crit Care Med* 1985;13:19.
19. Chernow B et al. Hypomagnesemia: implications for the critical care specialist. *Crit Care Med* 1982;10:193.
20. Booth C et al. Incidence of hypomagnesemia in intestinal malabsorption. *Br Med J* 1963;2:141.
21. Hallberg D. Magnesium problems in gastroenterology. *Acta Med Scand* 1981;662:62.
22. Sullivan J et al. Magnesium metabolism in alcoholism. *Am J Clin Nutr* 1963;63:297.
23. Zaloga G, Chernow B. Magnesium metabolism in critical illness. *Crit Care Q* 1983;6:24.

24. Ibid.
25. Silberman H, Eisenberg D. *Parenteral and Enteral Nutrition for the Hospitalized Patient*, 2nd ed. East Norwalk, CT: Appleton & Lange; 1989:309.
26. Rose B. *Clinical Physiology of Acid-Base and Electrolyte Disorders*, 4th ed. New York: McGraw-Hill; 1994:431.
27. Zaloga G et al. Hypomagnesemia is a common complication of aminoglycoside therapy. *Clin Res* 1983;31:261A.
28. Narins, p 679.
29. Kokko H, Tannen R. *Fluids and Electrolytes*, 3rd ed. Philadelphia: WB Saunders; 1996:714.
30. Narins, p 1391.
31. Zaloga, Chernow, p 24.
32. Ibid.
33. Ibid.
34. Chernow et al, 1982, p 193.
35. Ibid.
36. Pemberton L, Pemberton D. *Treatment of Water, Electrolyte, and Acid-Base Disorders in the Surgical Patient*. New York: McGraw-Hill; 1994:244.
37. Chernow et al, 1982, p 193.
38. Olerich M, Rude R. Should we supplement magnesium in critically ill patients? *New Horizons* 1994;2:186.
39. Cummins R, ed. *Advanced Cardiac Life Support*. Dallas, TX: American Heart Association. 1997:7.
40. Chernow et al, 1982, p 194.
41. Whang R. Clinical disorders of magnesium metabolism. *Compr Ther* 1997;23:168.
42. Goldman RH et al. The effect on myocardial ^{3}H-digoxin of magnesium deficiency. *Proc Soc Exp Biol Med* 1971;136:747.
43. Beller et al. Correlation of serum magnesium levels and cardiac digitalis intoxication. *Am J Cardiol* 1974;33:225.
44. Kokko, Tannen, p 426.
45. Narins, p 1107.
46. Kokko, Tannen, p 426.
47. Tierney L, McPhee S, Papadakis M. *Current Medical Diagnosis & Treatment*, 38th ed. Stamford, CT: Appleton & Lange, 1999:10.
48. Szerlip H, Goldfarb S. *Workshops in Fluid and Electrolyte Disorders*. New York: Churchill Livingstone; 1994:92.
49. Elisaf M, Milionis H, Siamopoulos KC. Hypomagnesemic hypokalemia and hypocalcemia: Clinical and laboratory characteristics. *Miner Electrolyte Metab* 1997;23:105.
50. White, Campbell, p 777.
51. Matz, p 81.
52. Narins, p 1110.
53. Toto K, Yucha C. Magnesium. In: Endocrine and Metabolic Disturbances in the Critically Ill. *Crit Care Nurs Clin North Am* 1994;6:767.
54. Zaloga, Chernow, 1994, p. 794.
55. Toto, Yucha, p 775.
56. Hoffman RS et al. An amp by any other name: the hazards of intravenous magnesium dosing (Letter). *JAMA* 1989;261:557.
57. Shannon Metal, Appleton & Lange's 1999 Drug Guide. Stamford, CT; Appleton & Lange; 1999:837.
58. Cummins, p 1-55.
59. Woods K, Fletcher S, Roffe C, Haider Y. Intravenous magnesium sulphate in suspected acute myocardial infarction: Results of the second Leicester Intravenous Magnesium Intervention Trial (LIMIT-2). *Lancet* 1992;339:1553.
60. ISIS Collaborative Group. ISIS-4: A randomised study of intravenous magnesium in over 50,000 patients with suspected acute myocardial infarction [Abstract]. *Circulation* 1993; 88(suppl):1.
61. Cummins, p 1-58.
62. Ibid., p. 1–55.
63. Ibid, p 9-33.
64. Resnick L. Magnesium in the pathophysiology and treatment of hypertension and diabetes mellitus: Where are we in 1997? *Am J Hypertens* 1997;10:368.
65. Mauskop A, Altura B. Role of magnesium in the pathogenesis and treatment of migraines. *Clin Neurosci* 1998;5:24.
66. Rude R. Magnesium metabolism and deficiency. *Endocrinol Metab Clin North Am* 1993;22:377.
67. Toto, Yucha, p 779.
68. Kokko, Tannen, p 970.
69. Clark B, Brown R. Unsuspected morbid hypermagnesemia in elderly patients. *Am J Nephrol* 1992;12:336.
70. Qureshi T, Melonakos T. Acute hypermagnesemia after laxative abuse. *Ann Emerg Med* 1996;28:552.
71. Dudley D, Gagnon D, Varner M. Long-term tocolysis with intravenous magnesium sulfate. *Obstet Gynecol* 1989;73:373.
72. Zaloga, Chernow, 1994, p 796.
73. Toto, Yucha, p 779.
74. Arieff A, DeFronzo R. *Fluid, Electrolyte, and Acid-Base Disorders*, 2nd ed. New York: Churchill Livingstone, 1995:481.
75. Kokko, Tannen, p 434.
76. Arieff, DeFronzo, p 481.
77. Narins, p 1111.
78. Ibid.
79. Kokko, Tannen, p 434.
80. Arieff, DeFronzo, p 481.
81. Kokko, Tannen, p 434.
82. Arieff, DeFronzo, p 481.
83. Narins, p 1111.
84. Rizzo M et al. Hypermagnesemic pseudocoma. *Arch Intern Med* 1993;153:1130.
85. Narins, p 1110.
86. Carey C, Lee H, Woeltje K. *The Washington Manual of Medical Therapeutics*, 29th ed. Philadelphia: Lippincott-Raven; 1998: 449.
87. Ibid.
88. McLaughlin S, McKinney P. Antacid-induced hypermagnesemia in a patient with normal renal function and bowel obstruction. *Ann Pharmacother* 1998;32:312.
89. Ibid.

CHAPTER 8

Phosphorus Imbalances

● PHOSPHORUS BALANCE

Phosphorus is primarily an intracellular anion and is a critical constituent of all tissues of the human body. It is the source of the high-energy phosphate bonds of adenosine triphosphate (ATP), which fuels numerous processes (including muscle contractility, neuronal transmission, and electrolyte transport).[1] It is a vital component of many intracellular compounds and has an important role as an intracellular messenger. Phosphorus is essential to the function of muscle, red blood cells, and the nervous system and to the intermediary metabolism of carbohydrate, protein, and fat.

The normal serum phosphorus level in adults ranges from 2.5 to 4.5 mg/dL (0.81–1.45 mmol/L). Levels are greater in children, presumably because of the higher rate of skeletal growth. For example, the normal serum phosphorus concentration in a newborn is 4.2 to 9.0 mg/dL, it is 3.8 to 6.2 in a 1-year-old child, and 3.5 to 6.8 mg/dL in children 2 to 5 years of age.[2] Phosphorus circulates in the bloodstream in three major forms: protein bound (12%), complexed (33%), and ionized (55%); it is the ionized form that is physiologically active.[3] Most laboratories measure total phosphorus.

Serum levels may fluctuate throughout the day; for example, glucose intake, insulin administration, or hyperventilation can lower the serum phosphorus concentration by increasing cellular uptake. Because phosphorus is primarily an intracellular ion, serum levels may not always reflect the total body stores. That is, hypophosphatemia does not necessarily imply a total body phosphate depletion. Conversely, a normal serum phosphate level does not necessarily mean the total body phosphate stores are normal. Nonetheless, in clinical settings, measurement of the serum phosphate level is the most widely used measure of body phosphate stores.

The usual dietary intake of phosphate ranges between 800 and 1,200 mg/day.[4] Adequate dietary intake is ensured by a normal diet because phosphorus is plentiful in many foods, including red meat, fish, poultry, eggs, milk products, and legumes. Most ingested phosphate is absorbed in the jejunum. However, absorption can be impaired by certain medications (such as phosphate-binding antacids) or by malabsorptive disorders.

Maintenance of normal phosphate balance requires an efficient renal conservation mechanism because the kidneys are the major route of excretion of phosphorus, being responsible for about 90% of the phosphorus excreted daily. During times of low phosphate intake, the kidneys retain more phosphorus.

● HYPOPHOSPHATEMIA

Hypophosphatemia in an adult refers to a serum phosphorus concentration below the lower limit of normal (< 2.5 mg/dL); it is considered to be severe at a concentration of less than 1.0 mg/dL.[5] It may occur in the presence of total body phosphorus deficit or merely reflect a temporary shift of phosphorus into the cells. In a study of 208 consecutive patients admitted to a surgical intensive care unit, 60 (28.8%) had hypophosphatemia.[6] There are various reasons why hypophosphatemia is prevalent in this population. For example, patients in intensive care settings may be chronically malnourished as a result of their preadmission illness and, as a result, often receive total parenteral or aggressive enteral feedings to help correct their malnourished states; also, they may receive drugs that increase phosphate loss (such as loop diuretics). Stress may add to the problem by increasing catecholamine release that may, in turn, produce a shift of phosphate into the cells.

When doubt exists about the presence of phosphorus depletion, it is helpful to measure the urinary excretion of phosphorus. In patients with phosphorus depletion, the urinary phosphorus level drops markedly to less than 100 mg and often less than 50 mg/day.[7]

ETIOLOGICAL FACTORS

A wide variety of clinical disorders and therapeutic interventions can cause hypophosphatemia. These etiological factors are listed in the Summary of Hypophosphatemia and are discussed briefly below. Essentially, these factors fall into one of three categories: (1) shift of phosphate from the extracellular fluid (ECF) into the cells; (2) decreased absorption of phosphate from the gastrointestinal (GI) tract; and (3) increased renal phosphate losses.[8] Usually at least two, and often all three, of these mechanisms are present in a given situation.[9] Many of the precipitating causes are related to treatment. For example, Halevy and Bulvik[10] reported that medications contributed to hypophosphatemia in 82% of the patients in their study; among the implicated medications were intravenous (IV) glucose, antacids, anabolic steroids, and diuretics.

Refeeding Syndrome

The *refeeding syndrome* is also referred to as the *nutritional recovery syndrome*. It occurs when malnourished patients are started on an overly aggressive refeeding program (either orally, by feeding tube, or by the parenteral route). Even the consumption of calories in normally required amounts to patients with severe protein-calorie malnutrition can result in serious electrolyte imbalances; one of the most serious is hypophosphatemia. It more frequently occurs with total parenteral nutrition (TPN) and tube feedings than with oral feedings.

A chronically malnourished patient is usually in a catabolic state, causing muscle breakdown and depletion of intracellular phosphate stores. Despite this, the extracellular (serum) phosphate level remains relatively normal until a large glucose load is administered, as in TPN. Glucose administration causes the pancreas to release more insulin, which in turn promotes the transport of both glucose and phosphorus into the cells (primarily of the skeletal muscle and liver) as the patient becomes anabolic. The resultant increased intracellular phosphate requirements unmasks a state of severe intracellular phosphate depletion. This, in turn, leads to a reduced serum phosphate level if sufficient phosphate additives are not provided. The development of severe hypophosphatemia in malnourished patients receiving TPN without adequate phosphate replacement has been well documented and may occur within the first 24 hours, although it often becomes evident only after 2 to 3 days of treatment (see Case Study 8-1). A lesser effect is associated with oral glucose intake.

The refeeding syndrome can occur in a wide variety of patients (such as those with anorexia nervosa or alcoholism and elderly debilitated patients). It has also been observed in children. For example, a 3-year-old boy was admitted after having been starved by an abusive parent; he was started on a regular diet by mouth and consumed an average of 140 kcal/kg/day and rapidly gained weight.[11] On admission, the serum phosphorus concentration was normal for his age (7.0 mg/dL); however, on the 20th day, it was low for his age (2.8 mg/dL). Fortunately, his imbalance was relatively minor and was easily correctable with phosphate replacement.

Because insulin promotes glycolysis, it causes a shift of phosphorus into the cells. In a study reported by Van Landingham et al.,[12] hypophosphatemia was found in 30% of tube-fed patients. This usually occurred in patients who were treated with insulin for hyperglycemia and the condition was assumed to be secondary to intracellular transport of phosphate.

Alcoholism

A common cause of severe hypophosphatemia is alcoholism. In one study, hypophosphatemia was found in 30.4% of alcoholic patients admitted to medical services (as compared to only 1.8% of matched nonalcoholic patients).[13] Factors contributing to phosphate depletion in alcoholics include poor intake, vomiting, use of antacids, and diarrhea. The fact that some alcoholics develop phosphate depletion in the absence of these factors suggests the presence of other mechanisms, perhaps the effects of ethanol, magnesium deficiency, ketoacidosis, and hypocalcemia.[14]

Excessive Pharmacological Phosphate Binding

Excessive use of phosphate-binding antacids (such as those that are aluminum or magnesium based) may cause severe hypophosphatemia, particularly when there is poor dietary intake of phosphorus. In a study of 35 patients who underwent major hepatic surgery, the use of antacids was significantly higher in those with hypophosphatemia than in those without it.[15] In this study, antacids were usually given by nasogastric tube or orally in the form of 30 mL aluminum-containing antacids four times daily. Phosphate-binding antacids are more likely to produce hypophosphatemia when other conditions associated with this imbalance are present, such as diuretic therapy, renal tubular defects, or hyperparathyroidism.

Respiratory Alkalosis

Prolonged, intense hyperventilation can depress serum phosphorus to values in the vicinity of 0.5 mg/dL, presumably by inducing respiratory alkalosis. Clinical situations associated with respiratory alkalosis include gram-negative bacteremia, withdrawal from chronic alcoholism, heat stroke, acute salicylate poisoning, primary hyperventilation, and thyrotoxicosis. Hypophosphatemia associated with alkalosis is secondary to increased cellular phosphate uptake.

Diabetic Ketoacidosis

Patients with poorly controlled diabetes who have glycosuria, ketonuria, and polyuria lose phosphate excessively into the urine. Although patients with untreated ketoacidosis may have normal or slightly elevated serum phosphorus levels, administration of insulin and parenteral fluids quickly causes serum phosphorus levels to drop below normal (see Chap. 18).

Excessive Catecholamine Secretion

Epinephrine may be a key mediator of hypophosphatemia and may explain partially the hypophosphatemia of sepsis, myocardial infarction, and other conditions associated with epinephrine release.[16]

Thermal Burns

Hypophosphatemia is common in patients with extensive burns and usually appears within several days after injury. The mechanism by which it develops is not clear. Because burn patients often hyperventilate, it is possible that respiratory alkalosis occurs and results in acceleration of glycolysis causing hypophosphatemia. It has also been postulated that urinary loss of phosphate may occur during the diuresis of salt and water or that phosphorus may be taken up by the cells as the burned patient becomes anabolic.

Other Factors

A survey of 100 hypophosphatemic patients suggested that diuretics were the cause in 7%.[17] Other possible causes include GI malabsorption syndrome, vitamin D deficiency, acute gout (presumably due to pain-induced hyperventilation), hypokalemia, hypomagnesemia, and hypocalcemia. Hypomagnesemia fosters hypophosphatemia through increased urinary losses of phosphate. Hypocalcemia can cause phosphaturia through stimulation of parathyroid hormone release.[18]

Reversal of hypothermia causes a shift of phosphate into the cells and may cause hypophosphatemia.[19] Patients with panic disorders may have a significant incidence of hypophosphatemia, at least partly due to respiratory alkalosis.[20] Moderate (usually well tolerated) hypophosphatemia is also common after kidney transplant and is the result of renal phosphaturia, glucocorticoid therapy, persistent hyperparathyroidism, and use of antacids.[21] Low birth weight infants may develop hypophosphatemia when fed human milk rather than cow's milk.[22]

DEFINING CHARACTERISTICS

Most signs and symptoms of phosphorus deficiency apparently result from deficiency of ATP, 2,3-diphosphoglycerate (2,3-DPG), or both. Cellular energy resources are impaired by ATP deficiency and oxygen delivery to tissues by 2,3-DPG deficiency.

Central Nervous System Changes

Cellular deficiencies of ATP and 2,3-DPG can produce a wide range of neurological symptoms, which may include irritability, apprehension, weakness, numbness, paresthesias, ataxia, lack of coordination, confusion, unequal pupils, nystagmus, convulsive seizures, and coma.[23] The basic cause of these disturbances is not clear; possibly it is related to a decreased availability of phosphate that in turn causes reduced ATP synthesis in the brain.[24]

Hematological Changes

Hypophosphatemia affects all the blood cells, but changes in the red blood cells are most pronounced. A decline in 2,3-DPG levels in erythrocytes occurs in hypophosphatemia. Recall that 2,3-DPG is an enzyme in red blood cells that normally interacts with hemoglobin to promote the release of oxygen. Thus, low levels of 2,3-DPG may reduce the delivery of oxygen to peripheral tissues, resulting in tissue hypoxia. Hemolytic anemia may occur because the red cells are more fragile and easily destroyed as a result of low ATP levels. This circumstance is particularly significant in critically ill patients who cannot tolerate even modest decreases in oxygen delivery.

In laboratory animals, hypophosphatemia depresses the chemotactic and phagocytic activity of granulocytes. These abnormalities are apparently reversible with correction of the hypophosphatemia. It is thought that hypophosphatemia impairs granulocytic function by interfering with ATP synthesis. Obviously, patients with impaired leukocyte function are at greater risk of infection.

Skeletal Muscle Changes

Hypophosphatemia can decrease the strength of skeletal muscle and produce symptomatic muscle weakness.[27] Actual muscle damage may develop as the ATP level in the muscles declines. This is manifested clinically by muscle weakness, release of creatinine phosphokinase (CPK), and, at times, acute rhabdomyolysis (disintegration of striated muscle). Profound muscular weakness has been described in severely hypophosphatemic patients, as has muscular pain. Elevations in CPK levels have been reported in patients with serum phosphate concentrations less than 1 mg/dL for 1 to 2 days.[28] It is possible that muscle cell injury could be the result of disrupted functioning of chemical processes important in maintaining cellular membrane integrity.

Ventilatory Changes

Investigators have reported weakness of the chest muscle in hypophosphatemic patients.[29] Ventilatory muscle fatigue may arise from cellular depletion of ATP, impaired cellular oxygenation, and central respiratory depression. Respiratory failure is most likely to occur in patients with underlying lung disease. Varsano et al.[30] recommended that the possibility of hypophosphatemia be considered for each patient who develops acute ventilatory failure or presents a problem of respiratory weaning. In some cases, patients can be removed from the ventilator soon after phosphate repletion has been achieved.[31]

Cardiac Changes

Evidence indicates that severe hypophosphatemic patients have decreased cardiac contractility that can be corrected with phosphorus replacement.[32] A reversible congestive cardiomyopathy may occur.[33] Phosphate depletion may also be associated with a decreased sensitivity to inotropic and vasoconstrictive medications.[34] There may be an increased incidence of arrhythmias in hypophosphatemic patients.[35]

Other Factors

There are indications that phosphorus deficiency may produce an insulin-resistant state, resulting in hyperglycemia.[36] Prolonged and severe hypophosphatemia may also be accompanied by severe metabolic acidosis.

TREATM ENT

Mild to Moderate Hypophosphatemia

Treatment of hypophosphatemia varies with the cause and severity of the imbalance. If mild and asymptomatic, it may be managed adequately by treatment of the primary disorder.[37] Because phosphorus is plentiful

in the diet, improved nutrition may suffice. However, if hypophosphatemia is likely to persist, therapy may require oral supplementation. Neutra-Phos capsules (250 mg elemental phosphorus and 7 mEq each of sodium and potassium per capsule) or Neutra-Phos K (250 mg elemental phosphorus and 14 mEq potassium), or Fleet Phospho-Soda (815 mg elemental phosphorus and 33 mEq sodium per 5 mL) may be prescribed as needed.[38] Nausea and diarrhea are side effects that may limit dosage of these agents.

Severe Hypophosphatemia

Severe hypophosphatemia (<1 mg/dL) is dangerous and requires IV replacement because oral phosphate preparations, when given in large amounts, usually cause diarrhea. Two IV preparations are available (sodium phosphate and potassium phosphate).[39] If the patient is oliguric, sodium salts rather than potassium salts should be administered.[40] Dosage is guided by serial determinations of serum phosphate levels (such as every 6 hours) and clinical response. Zaloga and Chernow[41] recommend giving 0.6 mg/kg/hr if phosphate depletion is recent and uncomplicated; if it is prolonged and multifactorial, 0.9 mg/kg/hr is recommended. After the serum level rises above 2 mg/dL, enteral replacement should be started and carried out over 5 to 7 days to replace cellular phosphate deficits.[42] Possible dangers of IV phosphorus administration include hyperphosphatemia and hypocalcemia. Another consideration is that calcium and phosphate should not be administered in the same IV infusion because of the risk of precipitation.

Phosphorus replacement in patients receiving TPN is discussed in Chapter 11; replacement in patients with diabetic ketoacidosis is discussed in Chapter 18.

NURSING INTERVENTIONS

1. Identify patients at risk for hypophosphatemia. See the Summary of Hypophosphatemia and discussion of etiological factors.
   - Extremely malnourished patients being started on TPN or large caloric intake by tube feeding (refeeding syndrome) are particularly at risk.
   - Also at great risk are alcoholic patients undergoing withdrawal therapy and initial treatment with IV glucose fluids.
   - Similarly at great risk are patients with diabetic ketoacidosis during the early treatment period

with insulin and IV fluids. This is particularly true if serum phosphate levels were low on admission. Fortunately, low-dose insulin therapy has decreased the incidence of rapid phosphate cellular shifts during early treatment (see Chap. 18).

2. Monitor patients at risk for hypophosphatemia. See Summary of Hypophosphatemia and discussion of defining characteristics.
   - Monitor serum phosphate levels in patients at high risk. Notify physician when levels are low. Hypophosphatemia is profound when serum levels are less than 1.0 mg/dL.
   - Be alert for paresthesias, particularly about the mouth.
   - Be alert for muscle weakness and pain. Test hand grasp strength on a serial basis to monitor for muscle weakness. Monitor for changes in speech that may reflect muscular weakness.
   - Be alert for mental changes associated with hypophosphatemia, such as apprehension, confusion, delirium, and decreased level of consciousness.
   - Be alert for signs of cardiac and ventilatory failure in patients with severe hypophosphatemia.

3. Be aware that severely hypophosphatemic patients are thought to be at greater risk for infection because of changes in white blood cells. Take precautions to prevent infections (as in meticulous care of central lines for TPN patients).

4. Administer IV phosphate products cautiously and monitor clinical response as well as serum phosphate levels. Because it is possible to give too much phosphorus, monitor for signs of hyperphosphatemia and of the salt in which it is administered. For example, excessive administration of potassium phosphate could cause paresthesias of the extremities, flaccid paralysis, listlessness, confusion, weakness, arrhythmias, heart block, and electrocardiographic abnormalities. Serum potassium or sodium levels (depending on the replacement salt) should be monitored in addition to the serum phosphorus levels.

5. Be aware that a sudden increase in the serum phosphorus level during treatment can cause hypocalcemia. For this reason, serum calcium levels should be monitored. Watch for twitching around the mouth, laryngospasm, positive Chvostek's sign, and paresthesias.

6. Be aware of the need to introduce hyperalimentation gradually in patients who are malnourished.

Gradual introduction of the feeding solution is less apt to be associated with rapid shifts of phosphate into the cells. Frequently monitor rates of TPN flow.

7. Monitor for diarrhea in patients taking oral phosphorus supplements; consult with physician if it persists or becomes severe.

8. Mix powdered oral phosphorus supplements with chilled or iced water to make them more palatable. Also, palatability may be increased by refrigerating the solution made from the powder. (Any palatable juice or beverage may be used in place of water.)

CASE STUDIES

● **8-1.** A 40-year-old woman with a prolonged history of severe diarrhea, nausea, and anorexia was admitted. Two months earlier she had undergone a bilateral salpingo-oophorectomy for ovarian cancer and a radium implant. A 30-lb weight loss was sustained over the previous 4 months. Weight on admission was 88 lb. A retroperitoneal small bowel fistula was found and surgical repair of the fistula and a colostomy were performed. After she suffered a multitude of postoperative complications, TPN was begun. At this time, serum electrolytes were:

Na = 136 mEq/L
PO_4 = 3.4 mg/dL
Cl = 93 mEq/L
CO_2 content = 31 mEq/L
K = 3.6 mEq/L
Glucose = 128 mg/dL
Ca = 8.7 mg/dL
BUN = 8 mg/dL

Eight days later, her condition had markedly deteriorated. A glucose intolerance (blood glucose, 270 mg/dL) required the administration of regular insulin, 20 units, every 6 hours. Inflammation was noted at the central line insertion site. At this time, her serum phosphate level was 0.4 mg/dL (normal, 2.5–4.5 mg/dL). Assessment revealed slurred speech and drooping of the mouth and tongue. The patient appeared restless and anxious and complained of numbness all over.

Summary of Hypophosphatemia

ETIOLOGICAL FACTORS	DEFINING CHARACTERISTICS
Glucose/insulin administration	Paresthesias
Refeeding after starvation	Muscle weakness (perhaps manifested as decreased strength of hand grasp and difficulty speaking)
Hyperalimentation	
Alcohol withdrawal	
Diabetic ketoacidosis	Muscle pain and tenderness
Respiratory alkalosis	Mental changes, such as apprehension, confusion, delirium, and coma
Phosphate-binding antacids	
Recovery phase after severe burns	Decreased cardiac contractility
	Acute respiratory failure (related to chest muscle weakness)
	Seizures
	Decreased tissue oxygenation
	Serum phosphate <2.5 mg/dL

The next day, muscle twitching and gross abnormal movements were noted. She was unable to grasp objects with her hands and was too weak to raise her arms. She complained of pain whenever anything touched her skin. At this time, her serum phosphate level was 0.2 mg/dL. A nutritional consultation was made and IV phosphate administration was started.

Two days later her speech remained slurred, spastic movements continued, and intense sensitivity to touch remained. However, her glucose intolerance had improved. Slowly, over a period of days, her hand grasps became perceptibly stronger and the muscle pain diminished. Numbness eventually disappeared. Three weeks later, the patient was discharged with a serum phosphate level of 4.5 mg/dL.

COMMENTARY: The patient's initial laboratory work was essentially normal, even though she was greatly malnourished; this is not uncommon in starving patients. As is typical in such patients, overzealous refeeding can cause the nutritional recovery syndrome, especially when inadequate cellular electrolytes (such as phosphate) are added

to the TPN solution. Note that this patient's serum phosphorus concentration reached extremely low levels before it was noticed and treated. Typical signs of hypophosphatemia were present. Even after the serum phosphorus concentration was raised to normal levels, it took days for the clinical manifestations to begin to resolve (indicating sustained cellular deficits) and weeks for her to fully recover. This patient was allowed to become critically ill before the cause of her problem was diagnosed and treated.

● **8-2.**[43] A 50-year-old woman with a series of complications after gallbladder surgery received phosphate-binding antacids for epigastric burning. Oral intake was poor and enteral feedings were not tolerated; thus, she was treated with dextrose solutions for 5 days and later with TPN for 10 days. For the first 2 days, no phosphate was added to the TPN solution; after that, only 10 mmol/L was added. On transfer to another facility, the patient had slurred speech and difficulty swallowing. She complained of weakness, perioral paresthesia, and numbness and tinging of both hands. Although very weak, she could move all extremities against gravity with better strength distally; reflexes were absent with flexor plantar responses. Laboratory tests revealed serum phosphate levels ranging from 0.4 to 0.6 mg/dL (normal in the reporting laboratory was 2.4–4.4 mg/dL). After appropriate phosphate replacement, the patient showed marked improvement in 3 weeks.

COMMENTARY: In addition to receiving TPN with insufficient phosphate, this patient received phosphate-binding antacids. (See Chap. 11 for a discussion of the relationship between phosphate and TPN.) Fortunately, her symptoms responded to phosphate replacement over a period of weeks. It took that long to replace the large cellular deficits. The profound hypophosphatemic neuropathy observed in this patient was caused by decreased nerve oxygen and energy supply.[44] (Recall that hypophosphatemia causes a decrease in ATP and in 2,3-DPG in the red blood cells, which in turn increases red cell affinity for oxygen while diminishing tissue oxygen supply.)

HYPERPHOSPHATEMIA

Moderate hyperphosphatemia is present when the serum level is 4.6 to 6.0 mg/dL; severe hyperphosphatemia exists at a phosphorus level of more than 6.0 mg/dL.

ETIOLOGICAL FACTORS

Three basic mechanisms can lead to hyperphosphatemia: (1) reduced renal phosphate excretion; (2) shift of phosphorus from the intracellular space into the ECF; and (3) increased phosphate intake or absorption.

Decreased Renal Excretion of Phosphorus

An increase in the serum phosphorus concentration is observed in patients with chronic renal failure when the glomerular filtration rate (GFR) is 25 mL/min or less. Also, hyperphosphatemia is common in acute renal failure.

Shift of Intracellular Phosphate to Extracellular Fluid

Large quantities of phosphates may be released into the circulation when chemotherapy is administered for neoplastic conditions (particularly acute lymphoblastic leukemia and lymphoma) and are the result of cell destruction and liberation of intracellular phosphates ("tumor lysis"). Shift from the cellular space to the ECF can also occur when sepsis, severe hypothermia, and rhabdomyolysis are present.[45] Recall that muscle tissue contains the bulk of soft tissue phosphate. Therefore, necrosis of muscle is a potent cause of hyperphosphatemia. Situations associated with rhabdomyolysis include direct trauma, viral infections, and heat stroke.

High Phosphate Intake

It is possible to impose an excess phosphorus load if phosphate substances are administered incorrectly, whether IV, orally, or in the form of phosphate-containing enemas. Even when renal function is normal, it is possible to cause hyperphosphatemia when phosphate-containing solutions are administered too rapidly. Substantial absorption of phosphorus can occur from the large bowel when Fleet Phospho-Soda is given as an enema. This is especially problematic for patients who have slowed colonic motility or defects in the bowel mucosa. A case was recently reported in which a constipated geriatric patient received multiple Fleet's hypertonic sodium phosphate enemas (six over a 12-hour period), resulting in life-threatening hyperphosphatemia (22 mg/dL).[46] Use of laxatives containing sodium phosphate may also result in accidental phosphate poisoning. Fatal hyperphosphatemia (59.6 mg/dL), secondary to enteral administration of Fleet Phospho-Soda, was recently reported in a 64-year-old man with colonic ileus.[47] Blood transfusions can be a source of exogenous phosphorus because of leakage from the blood cells during storage.

Large intake of vitamin D, either therapeutic or self-administered, causes increased phosphorus absorption that, together with impaired renal function, can result in hyperphosphatemia.

Hyperphosphatemia may develop in infants fed cow's milk, which contains more phosphate than human milk. Patients taking large quantities of milk for peptic ulcer management may develop increased serum phosphorus levels.

DEFINING CHARACTERISTICS

The clinical signs of hyperphosphatemia are primarily the ones of hypocalcemia because it is induced as the elevated serum phosphate combines with ionized calcium. Insoluble calcium phosphate is formed when the calcium–phosphate product exceeds 75.[48]

Hypocalcemia and Tetany

Because of the reciprocal relationship between phosphorus and calcium, a high serum phosphorus level tends to cause a low calcium concentration in the serum. Tetany can result and present as sensations of tingling in the tips of the fingers and around the mouth. These sensations may increase in severity and spread proximally along the limbs and to the face and be followed by numbness. Muscle spasms and pain may occur. Symptoms of tetany are most likely to occur in patients who are hyperphosphatemic because of a high phosphate load, either exogenous or endogenous. Because patients with renal disease often have some degree of acidosis, they are less prone to develop symptoms of hypocalcemia because acidosis favors increased calcium ionization.

Soft Tissue Calcification

High levels of serum inorganic phosphate are harmful because they promote precipitation of calcium phosphate in nonosseous sites. One such site is the kidney, where precipitation of calcium phosphate can result in progressive renal impairment. Other sites include the heart, lungs, skin, and cornea. Calcification of soft tissue is seen primarily in patients with chronic renal failure and long-term serum phosphate elevation. An attempt is made to control the hyperphosphatemia and thus keep the calcium and phosphate product below 70 mg/dL. Recall that normal serum levels of calcium (8.9–10.3 mg/dL) and phosphate (2.5–4.5 mg/dL) have a product of about 30 to 40 mg/dL.

Other Effects

One effect of hyperphosphatemia is an increase in red blood cell 2,3-DPG levels. In patients with chronic renal failure, hyperphosphatemia helps protect against the adverse effects of anemia on tissue oxygenation.

TREATMENT

When possible, treatment is directed at the underlying disorder. If due to excessive phosphate administration in drugs or in milk, the disorder is rather easily remedied by eliminating the products. Dietary restriction of phosphorus intake is also indicated.

Phosphate-binding agents, such as calcium acetate (Phoslo), are frequently used to decrease the serum phosphate level in patients with renal disorders.

In acute hyperphosphatemia, IV infusions of saline may promote renal phosphate excretion, provided the patient has functional kidneys. It may be necessary to administer hypertonic dextrose in conjunction with regular insulin to temporarily drive phosphorus into the cells. Either hemodialysis or peritoneal dialysis may be needed for patients with compromised renal function.

NURSING INTERVENTIONS

1. Administer prescribed enteral and IV phosphate supplements cautiously and monitor serum phosphate levels periodically during their use.
2. Identify patients at risk for hyperphosphatemia and monitor for signs of tetany, such as tingling sensations in the fingertips and around the mouth, and presence of muscle cramps or positive Chvostek's and Trousseau's signs.
3. Instruct patients that improper use of phosphate-containing laxatives may result in acute phosphate poisoning.
4. Be aware that phosphate-containing enemas can result in hyperphosphatemia if not used judiciously, particularly in individuals with slow bowel emptying and mucosal defects that hasten absorption. Instruct patients accordingly. See the Summary of Hyperphosphatemia on page 155.

CASE STUDIES

● **8-3.**[49] An elderly woman was admitted to the hospital with abdominal pain and constipation that had been present for 5 days. Abdominal radiography revealed multiple fecal impactions. Over a period of 12 hours, six Fleet phosphosoda enemas were administered to attempt to correct the constipation; however, no relief was obtained. The patient's condition deteriorated and she had positive Chvostek's and Trousseau's signs. Blood tests revealed a serum phosphorus level of 22 mg/dL (normal, 2.5–4.5 mg/dL) and a total serum calcium level of 5.4 mg/dL (normal, 8.9–10.3 mg/dL). IV fluids were maintained using central venous monitoring and calcium gluconate was administered by continuous infusion. In the first 24 hours, 6.7 liters of fluids were administered. Within 24 hours, serum electrolyte levels returned to near normal values (phosphorus, 4.7 mg/dL; calcium, 9.3 mg/dL). The paralytic ileus resolved slowly, after the fecal impactions were manually removed, with the assistance of isotonic enemas. The patient was discharged to an extended care facility in 2 weeks.

COMMENTARY: Most cases of hyperphosphatemia due to phosphate enemas have occurred in young children. However, severe electrolyte abnormalities can also occur in adults, particularly when conditions are present that cause prolonged retention of the enema solution. In this case, paralytic ileus and fecal impaction promoted retention of the phosphate solution and precipitated the extreme hyperphosphatemia and hypocalcemia described. Both of these imbalances were directly caused by the retained hypertonic phosphate solution. The high phosphorus content of the enema, which was absorbed through the colon, caused a rise in the serum phosphorus level; the elevated serum phosphorus level caused a reciprocal drop in the serum calcium level. Elderly patients with atonic colons and poor renal function are particularly at risk. In these patients, use of enemas should be carefully supervised, and whenever possible, isotonic enemas should be used.

● **8-4.**[50] A 64-year-old man was to undergo a colostomy revision to correct an area of stenosis. The evening before surgery, a standard oral bowel preparation with 4 liters of polyethylene glycol solution was ordered along with maintenance IV fluids to prevent dehydration. However, it was discovered the next morning that the patient did not drink all of the lavage solution; therefore, an order was given for "Fleet's enemas" through the end colostomy "until clear." It was later discovered that a total of 11 sodium phosphate-based enema preparations (about 1,100 mL) had been adminis-

tered over a period of 2 hours. When being readied for transport to the operating room, the patient was confused, ashen, and very weak. His heart rate was 60 beats/min and he was tachypneic. He was immediately moved to the surgical intensive care unit where IV resuscitation and oxygen therapy were initiated. A series of tests (including serum electrolytes) were performed. Laboratory results revealed:

Sodium = 157 mEq/L
Potassium = 6.5 mEq/L
Phosphate = 10.4 mg/dL
Calcium = 4.4 mg/dL
Arterial blood gases:
pH = 6.94
HCO_3 = 6.9 mEq/L
$PaCO_2$ = 37 mm Hg
PaO_2 = 83 mm Hg

Despite vigorous attempts to correct the patient's severe metabolic disturbances, he died of shock and multisystem organ failure about 8 hours after the enemas were given.

COMMENTARY: This tragic case was due to an improperly written order and failure of the staff to consider the danger of administering large doses of sodium phosphate enemas to a patient unable to evacuate the solution normally. Although under normal circumstances the enema solution would be evacuated in 2 to 15 minutes resulting in minimal absorption from the bowel, the authors concluded that the stenotic colostomy prevented this from occurring in this patient. The 11 adult-sized enemas given to this patient resulted in a total dose of about 209 g sodium biphosphate, 77 g sodium phosphate, and 48.4 total g sodium over 2 hours.[51] Absorption of phosphate from the enema caused binding of serum calcium and ultimately resulted in hyperphosphatemia and hypocalcemia. This, in turn, led to severe cardiovascular collapse with hypoperfusion, metabolic acidosis, and finally multisystem organ failure. When the house staff and nursing personnel were interviewed, it was found that the term "Fleet's enema" was used variably to describe true sodium phosphate-based enema preparations, simple saline enemas, or as a generic term encompassing all types of enemas.[52] (This is not unlike calling all facial tissues "Kleenex" or all feeding tubes "Dobbhoff's.") Of course, referring to all enemas as "Fleet's enemas" should be avoided because there are vast differences between possible enema solutions. The authors of the article in which this case was reported emphasized the need for all health care personnel to be fully aware of the potential for clinically significant hyperphosphatemia and hypocalcemia with the use of sodium phosphate-based enema preparations. Indeed, the manufacturer of Fleet's enemas carefully explains the precautions needed to use their product safely.[53]

Summary of Hyperphosphatemia

ETIOLOGICAL FACTORS

Renal failure

Chemotherapy, particularly for acute lymphoblastic leukemia and lymphoma

Use of cow's milk in infants

Overzealous administration of phosphorous supplements, orally or IV

Excessive use of Fleet's phosphosoda as enema solution or laxative, particularly in children and individuals with slow bowel elimination

Large vitamin D intake (increases phosphorus absorption)

DEFINING CHARACTERISTICS

Short-term consequences; symptoms of tetany, such as tingling of fingertips and around mouth, numbness, and muscle spasms

Long-term consequences: precipitation of calcium phosphate in nonosseous sites, such as the kidney, heart, arteries, skin, or cornea

Serum phosphate >4.5 mg/dL

REFERENCES

1. Bugg N, Jones N. Hypophosphatemia. *Anaesthesia* 1998;53:895.
2. Worley G, Claerhout S, Combs S. Hypophosphatemia in malnourished children during refeeding. *Clin Pediatr* 1998;37:347.
3. Zaloga G, Chernow B. Divalent ions: Calcium, magnesium, and phosphorus. In: Chernow B, ed. *The Pharmacologic Approach to the Critically Ill Patient*, 3rd ed. Baltimore, MD: Williams & Wilkins; 1994:796.
4. Ibid, p 796.
5. Narins R, ed. *Clinical Disorders of Fluid and Electrolyte Metabolism*, 5th ed. New York: McGraw-Hill; 1994:1046.
6. Zazzo J, Troche G, Ruel P, et al. High incidence of hypophosphatemia in surgical intensive care patients: Efficacy of phosphorus therapy on myocardial function. *Intensive Care Med* 1995;21:826.
7. Pemberton L, Pemberton D. *Treatment of Water, Electrolyte, and Acid-Base Disorders in the Surgical Patient*. New York: McGraw-Hill; 1994:228.
8. Zaloga, Chernow, p 798.
9. Narins, p 1055.
10. Halevy J, Bulvik S. Severe hypophosphatemia in hospitalized patients. *Arch Intern Med* 1988;148:153.
11. Worley et al., p 350.
12. Van Landingham S et al. Metabolic abnormalities in patients supported with enteral tube feeding. *JPEN J Parenter Enteral Nutr* 1981;5:322.
13. Ryback R. Clinical relationship between serum phosphorus and other blood chemistry values in alcoholics. *Arch Intern med* 1980;140:673.
14. Knochel J. The pathophysiology and clinical characteristics of severe hypophosphatemia. *Ann Intern Med* 1977;137:205.
15. Buell J, Berger A, Plotkin J, et al. The clinical implications of hypophosphatemia following major hepatic resection or cryosurgery. *Arch Surg* 1998;133:757.
16. Narins, p 1053.
17. Juan D, Elrazak M. Hypophosphatemia in hospitalized patients. *JAMA* 1979;242:163.
18. Tucker S, Schimmel E. Postoperative hypophosphatemia: A multifactorial problem. *Nutr Rev* 1989;47:111.
19. Zaloga, Chernow, p 797.
20. Balon J et al. Relative hypophosphatemia in patients with panic disorders. *Arch Gen Psychiatry* 1988;45:294.
21. Zaloga, Chernow, p 798.
22. Narins, p 1054.
23. Narins, p 1070.

24. Ibid.
25. Larner A. Visual hallucinations (Letter). *J R Coll Physicians Lond* 1997;31:221.
26. Ibid.
27. Bugg, Jones, p 900.
28. Knochel, p 213.
29. Newman J. Acute respiratory failure associated with hypophosphatemia. *N Engl J Med* 1977;297:1101.
30. Varsano S et al. Hypophosphatemia as a reversible cause of refractory ventilatory failure. *Crit Care Med* 1983;11:908.
31. Narins, p 1068.
32. O'Connor L et al. Effect of hypophosphatemia in myocardial function in man. *N Engl J Med* 1977;291:901.
33. Peppers M et al. Hypophosphatemia and hyperphosphatemia. *Crit Care Clin North Am* 1991;7:201.
34. Narins, p 1068.
35. Venditti F et al. Hypophosphatemia and cardiac arrhythmias. *Miner Electrolyte Metab* 1987;13:19.
36. DeFronzo R, Lang R. Hypophosphatemia and glucose intolerance: Evidence for tissue insensitivity to insulin. *N Engl J Med* 1980;303:1259.
37. Carey C, Lee H, Woeltje K. *The Washington Manual of Medical Therapeutics*, 29th ed. Philadelphia: Lippincott-Raven; 1998:448.
38. Ibid.
39. Yucha C, Toto K. Calcium and phosphorus derangements. In Endocrine and Metabolic Disturbances in the Critically Ill. *Crit Care Nurs Clin North Am* December 1994:763.
40. Narins, p 1078.
41. Zaloga, Chernow, p 800.
42. Ibid.
43. Siddiqui M, Bertorini T. Hypophosphatemic-induced neuropathy: Clinical and electrophysiologic findings. *Muscle Nerve* 1998;21:650.
44. Ibid.
45. Zaloga, Chernow, p 800.
46. Korzets A et al. Life-threatening hyperphosphatemia and hypocalcemic tetany following the use of Fleet enemas. *J Am Geriatr Soc* 1992;40:620.
47. Fass R et al. Fatal hyperphosphatemia following Fleet phosphosoda in a patient with colonic ileus. *Am J Gastroenterol* 1993;88:929.
48. Zaloga, Chernow, p 801.
49. Korzets et al, p 620.
50. Pitcher D, Ford R, Nelson M et al. Fatal hypocalcemic, hyperphosphatemic, metabolic acidosis following sequential sodium phosphate-based enema administration. *Gastrointest Endosc* 1997;46:266.
51. Ibid.
52. Ibid.
53. *Physicians' Desk Reference*, 53rd ed. Montvale, NJ: Medical Economics; 1999:1012.

Acid–Base Imbalances

This chapter provides a basic explanation of the four acid–base imbalances: metabolic acidosis, metabolic alkalosis, respiratory acidosis, and respiratory alkalosis. Actually, it is common to further classify each of the respiratory imbalances as acute or chronic. In this sense, one might think of six possible acid–base imbalances.[1]

Etiological factors and defining characteristics of each of the imbalances are presented, followed by brief discussions of their treatment. For the nursing interventions used to deal with these disturbances, see the later chapters concerning specific situations associated with acid–base imbalances.

Before turning to a discussion of the acid–base disturbances, it is helpful to review how the body regulates the acid–base balance.

⬤ REGULATION OF ACID–BASE BALANCE

The body has the remarkable ability to maintain plasma pH within the narrow normal range of 7.35 to 7.45. It does so by means of chemical buffering mechanisms, by the kidneys, and by the lungs. The pH is defined as hydrogen ion concentration; the more hydrogen ions, the more acidic the solution. The pH range that is considered to be compatible with life (6.8–7.8) represents a 10-fold difference in hydrogen ion concentration in plasma.

It has been estimated that metabolism normally produces 13,000 mEq/day of hydrogen ions; less than 1% of this amount is excreted by the kidneys. Therefore, renal shutdown can be present for hours or days before life-threatening acid–base imbalance occurs, yet cessation of breathing for minutes produces critical acid–base changes.

CHEMICAL BUFFERING MECHANISMS

Chemical buffers are substances that prevent major changes in the pH of body fluids by removing or releasing hydrogen ions; they can act within a fraction of a second to prevent excessive changes in hydrogen ion concentration.

The body's major buffer system is the bicarbonate (HCO_3)-carbonic acid (H_2CO_3) buffer system. Normally, there are 20 parts bicarbonate to 1 part carbonic acid. If this ratio is upset, the pH will change. It is the ratio that is important in maintaining pH, not absolute values.

Example: In a healthy individual:

HCO_3, 24 mEq/L [20 parts]
(pH = 7.4)
H_2CO_3, 1.2 mEq/L [1 part]

In an individual with chronic obstructive lung disease, one might see:

HCO_3, 48mEq/L [20 parts]
(pH = 7.4)
H_2CO_3, 2.4 mEq/L [1 part]

Carbon dioxide (CO_2) is a potential acid. When CO_2 is dissolved in water, it becomes carbonic acid: $CO_2 + H_2O = H_2CO_3$. Thus, when CO_2 is increased, the carbonic acid content is also increased, and vice versa.

If either bicarbonate or carbonic acid is increased or decreased so that the 20:1 ratio is upset, acid–base imbalance results. Figure 9-1 demonstrates changes in plasma pH when the bicarbonate/carbonic acid ratio is altered.

Other less important buffer systems in the extracellular fluid (ECF) include the inorganic phosphates and the plasma proteins. Intracellular buffers include proteins, organic and inorganic phosphates, and, in red blood cells, hemoglobin.

KIDNEYS

The kidneys regulate the bicarbonate level in ECF; they are able to regenerate bicarbonate ions as well as reabsorb them from the renal tubular cells.

In the presence of respiratory acidosis, and most cases of metabolic acidosis, the kidneys excrete hydrogen ions and conserve bicarbonate ions to help restore balance. (The kidneys obviously cannot compensate for the metabolic acidosis created by renal failure.)

In the presence of respiratory and metabolic alkalosis, the kidneys retain hydrogen ions and excrete bicarbonate ions to help restore balance. Renal compensation for imbalances is slow (a matter of hours or days). Because of this slow compensation, respiratory imbalances are categorized as either acute or chronic. That is, acute respiratory imbalances exist with little compensation by the kidneys (due to their slow response); however, chronic respiratory imbalances have been present long enough for the kidneys to make compensatory changes.

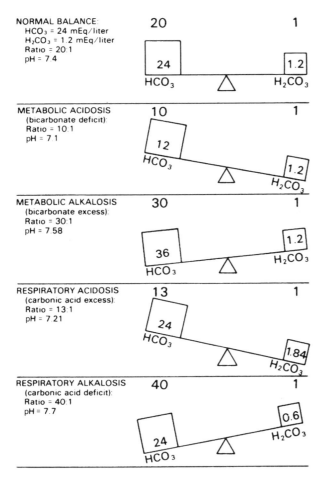

NORMAL BALANCE:
$HCO_3 = 24$ mEq/liter
$H_2CO_3 = 1.2$ mEq/liter
Ratio = 20:1
pH = 7.4

20   1

24   1.2
HCO_3 H_2CO_3

METABOLIC ACIDOSIS
(bicarbonate deficit):
Ratio = 10:1
pH = 7.1

10   1

12
HCO_3 1.2
              H_2CO_3

METABOLIC ALKALOSIS
(bicarbonate excess):
Ratio = 30:1
pH = 7.58

30   1

              1.2
36   H_2CO_3
HCO_3

RESPIRATORY ACIDOSIS
(carbonic acid excess):
Ratio = 13:1
pH = 7.21

13   1

24
HCO_3 1.84
              H_2CO_3

RESPIRATORY ALKALOSIS
(carbonic acid deficit):
Ratio = 40:1
pH = 7.7

40   1

              0.6
24   H_2CO_3
HCO_3

FIGURE 9-1.   Examples of pH changes with alterations in the bicarbonate:carbonic acid ratio.

LUNGS

In normal individuals, a rise in the arterial carbon dioxide ($PaCO_2$) concentration is a much more powerful stimulant to respiration than is a decreased arterial oxygen (PaO_2) concentration. The stimulatory effect of increased CO_2 reaches its peak within a few minutes; however, it gradually declines for the next 1 or 2 days to as little as 20% of the initial effect.[2] Therefore, after several days, elevation of blood CO_2 has only a weak effect as a respiratory stimulant. This is of significance in patients with chronic obstructive pulmonary disease (COPD); in these patients, the primary drive to ventilation is a depressed PaO_2.

Partial pressure of O_2 in arterial blood (PaO_2) influences respiration; however, decreased PaO_2 normally will not stimulate alveolar ventilation significantly until it falls to very low levels. For example, ventilation approximately doubles when the PaO_2 falls to 60 mm Hg and increases almost sixfold when it falls to 20 mm Hg.[3]

Also, the lungs compensate for metabolic disturbances by either conserving or retaining CO_2. Because they do this very quickly, it is not customary to classify the metabolic imbalances as acute or chronic.

1. In the presence of metabolic acidosis, respiration is increased, causing greater elimination of CO_2 (to lighten the acid load).
2. In the presence of metabolic alkalosis, respiration is decreased, causing CO_2 to be retained (increasing the acid load).

Faulty pulmonary function disrupts the acid–base balance. For example, hypoventilation due to emphysema causes excessive CO_2 retention and respiratory acidosis, whereas hyperventilation due to hysteria causes excessive elimination of CO_2 and respiratory alkalosis. Of course, the lungs are unable to compensate for metabolic pH disturbances when there is severe pulmonary dysfunction; in these instances, compensation must be accomplished solely by the kidneys.

● MEASUREMENT OF ACID–BASE BALANCE

Before discussing acid–base measurement, it is useful to review the definition of acid and base. Simply stated, an *acid* is a substance that can donate hydrogen ions. For example, H_2CO_3 (carbonic acid) yields H^+ (hydrogen ion) + HCO_3^- (bicarbonate). A *base* is a substance that can accept hydrogen ions (H^+). For example, $HCO_3^- + H^+$ yields H_2CO_3.

The best way to evaluate acid–base balance is to measure arterial blood gases (ABGs) (Table 9-1). The analysis of ABGs allows the sampling of blood that has come from various parts of the body (not just one extremity as is the case with venous blood). Also, arterial blood gives information as to how well the lungs are oxygenating the blood.

Note in Table 9-1 that only two of the listed measures are actually of gases ($PaCO_2$ and PaO_2). However, reporting the nonrespiratory component (bicarbonate) is essential to understanding the respiratory measures. In review, the $PaCO_2$ is controlled by the lungs and refers to the pressure exerted by dissolved CO_2 gas in

---

⬤ **TABLE 9-1.**   Arterial Blood Gases

Term	Normal Value	Definition-Implications
pH	7.35–7.45	Reflects H^+ concentration; acidity increases as H^+ concentration increases (pH value decreases as acidity increases) • pH < 7.35 (acidosis) • pH > 7.45 (alkalosis)
$PaCO_2$	35–45 mm Hg	Partial pressure of CO_2 in arterial blood • When < 35 mm Hg, hypocapnia is said to be present (respiratory alkalosis) • When > 45 mmHg, hypercapnia is said to be present (respiratory acidosis)
PaO_2	80–100 mm Hg	Partial pressure of O_2 in arterial blood
Standard HCO_3	22–26 mEq/ L	HCO_3 concentration in plasma of blood that has been equilibrated at a $PaCO_2$ of 40 mm Hg, and with O_2 to fully saturate the hemoglobin

---

arterial blood. Carbon dioxide should be considered as an acid substance because, when dissolved in water, it forms carbonic acid (H_2CO_3). The PaO_2 refers to the pressure exerted by dissolved oxygen in the blood.

In the evaluation of acid–base status using venous blood, the reporting of CO_2 content is often confusing. This measure is usually included with routine plasma electrolyte determinations in venous blood. Although listed on the laboratory sheet as "CO_2," it is actually a measure of the sum of bicarbonate (24 mEq/L) and dissolved CO_2 gas (1.2 mEq/L). Note the normal ratio of 20 parts HCO_3 to 1 part dissolved CO_2 gas. Thus, in normal situations, the CO_2 content should be 25.2 mEq/L.[4] Because CO_2 content primarily reflects the concentration of bicarbonate, it is largely a measure of the nonrespiratory (or metabolic) component of acid–base balance. Instead of merely using CO_2 as a term, it is important to clarify whether it refers to the gas ($PaCO_2$) or the "CO_2 content."

To ensure patient safety and accuracy, only clinicians specially instructed in drawing blood gas samples should perform this maneuver. Listed at the end of the chapter, after discussion of the four primary acid–base imbalances, are guidelines for interpreting blood gases (see Clinical Tip: Systematic Assessment of Arterial Blood Gases) and information regarding the calculation of expected compensatory changes (see Table 9-8).

⬤ EFFECT OF pH ON POTASSIUM BALANCE

Acid–base changes can produce concurrent changes in potassium distribution between cellular fluid and ECF. Generally, acidemia causes potassium to shift from the cells into the ECF and thus elevates plasma potassium concentration. Just the opposite occurs with alkalemia; that is, potassium shifts into the cells, thus lowering the plasma potassium concentration. In the past, it was thought that the inverse relationship between pH and plasma potassium concentration was so precise that it could be expressed in mathematical terms. However, the relationship between pH and plasma potassium concentration is more complex than was originally assumed.

ALKALEMIA

In alkalemic states, hydrogen ions (H^+) are released from the cellular buffers and move into the ECF to help correct the elevated pH. In turn, to preserve electroneutrality, extracellular potassium enters the cells. Although the effect of alkalemia itself is relatively small, hypokalemia is commonly present in patients with metabolic alkalosis. Partly this is because common causes of hypokalemia (such as potassium-losing diuretics and vomiting) also cause loss of hydrogen ions (thereby inducing alkalosis).[5] Apparently there is little change in plasma potassium concentration with respiratory alkalosis.[6]

ACIDEMIA

In acidemic states, hydrogen ions shift into the cells to help correct the low plasma pH; in turn, to preserve electroneutrality, cellular potassium moves from the cells into the ECF. Respiratory acidosis is a weaker stimulus for potassium shifting than is metabolic acidosis.

The cause of metabolic acidosis has an effect on the extent to which the plasma potassium concentration will elevate. For example, hyperkalemia typically occurs in untreated diabetic ketoacidosis, but it is due more to insulin lack and hyperosmolality than it is to acidemia.[7] In contrast, lactic acidosis typically does not cause hyperkalemia.[8] The plasma potassium concentration is usually *low* when metabolic acidosis is caused by diarrhea.[9] This is because the actual loss of potassium in the liquid stools predominates over the amount of potassium shifted from the cells into the ECF. The shift of cellular potassium to the bloodstream in a patient with diarrhea becomes clinically important because it may result in normokalemia (masking the true state of potassium deficit, perhaps leading to inadequate potassium replacement therapy).

⬤ METABOLIC ACIDOSIS

Metabolic acidosis (HCO_3 deficit) is a clinical disturbance characterized by a low pH (increased hydrogen concentration) and a low plasma bicarbonate concentration. It can be produced by a gain of hydrogen ion or a loss of bicarbonate. In compensation, the lungs hyperventilate to decrease the $PaCO_2$ concentration (movement in the same direction as the primary bicarbonate disturbance).

ANION GAP

Metabolic acidosis can be divided into two forms, depending on the values of the serum anion gap (AG):

Anion gap (AG) = $Na^+ - (Cl^- + HCO_3^-)$ = 12 ± 2 mEq/L.

As the equation demonstrates, sodium represents the major cation in body fluids, and chloride and bicarbonate represent the two major anions. Other anions in body fluid not accounted for in the equation include anionic proteins, phosphates, sulfates, and organic anions (such as ketones and lactic acid). Normally the sum of these unmeasured anions should be no greater than 12 ± 2 mEq/L.[10] However, in some situations, these anions are markedly increased and the AG is greater than expected. These situations are referred to as high AG metabolic acidosis. On the other hand, if the primary problem is direct loss of bicarbonate, gain of chloride, or decreased renal ammonia production, the AG will be within normal limits (12 ± 2 mEq/L). Table 9-2 lists causes of metabolic acidosis classified as either high or normal AG. Normal values for AG may vary according to the laboratory performing the assays; therefore, clinical laboratories need to establish the AG reference interval for the analyzer used in their laboratory.[11]

High Anion Gap Acidosis

The three most common disorders associated with high AG acidosis are lactic acidosis, ketoacidosis, and renal failure.[12] The next most frequent cause is the ingestion of toxins (especially methanol, ethylene gly-

---

⬤ **TABLE 9-2.** Causes of Metabolic Acidosis Classified as High Anion Gap or Normal Anion Gap

High Anion Gap (Gain of Unmeasured Anions)	Normal Anion Gap
Diabetic ketoacidosis	Diarrhea
Starvational ketoacidosis	Biliary or pancreatic
Alcoholic ketoacidosis	fistulas
Lactic acidosis	Excessive adminis-
Renal failure	tration of isotonic
Poisonings:	saline or ammo-
• Salicylate	nium chloride
• Ethylene glycol	Ureteroenterostomies
• Methyl alcohol	Renal tubular
	acidosis
	Acetazolamide
	(Diamox)

col, or salicylates). Although there are varied ranges in the AG with these causes, the largest gaps are caused by ketoacidosis, lactic acidosis, and methanol or ethylene glycol ingestion.[13]

Lactic Acidosis

Lactic acidosis is most commonly seen in patients with significant cardiopulmonary problems and sepsis.[14] When intracellular oxygen is not available, energy is produced by the anaerobic metabolic pathways, producing lactate and hydrogen ions (which in turn form lactic acid in the bloodstream). Accumulation of lactic acid produces a profound decrease in pH. Correlation of elevated lactate levels with mortality in critically ill patients is well established; for example, an arterial lactate level of greater than 10 mmol/L is associated with a 95% mortality rate.[15] The normal arterial lactate level is less than 2.5 mmol/L. Lactate is a credible clinical indicator of tissue hypoxia because it reflects anaerobic metabolism.

Example: The high AG in a patient with lactic acidosis:

Na = 131 mEq/L
HCO_3 = 9 mEq/L
Cl = 86 mEq/L
AG = $Na^+ - (HCO_3^- + Cl^-)$ 131 - (9 + 86) = 36 mEq/L (elevated above normal)

Ketoacidosis

Both glucose and oxygen are required for energy production in normal cellular metabolism, and insulin is required for transporting glucose across the cell wall. Lack of insulin leads to utilization of metabolic pathways that produce ketones (strong acids) rather than CO_2.[16] More specifically, diabetic ketoacidosis occurs in diabetic patients with a severe insulin deficiency coupled with excessive secretion of counterregulatory hormones. Due to insulin deficiency, lipolysis is increased, releasing free fatty acids that are delivered to the liver where they are converted to ketones. Accumulation of ketones (anions) causes a reciprocal decrease in bicarbonate and an increase in the AG.

Hepatic ketone production is a normal consequence of starvation; yet, the excess ketones are rarely a cause of severe acidosis in healthy nondiabetic persons. However, alcoholics who have gone on a recent drinking binge and are eating poorly may suffer significant ketoacidosis. Although ketosis is initiated by starvation, alcohol itself stimulates ketoacid production. Thus, alcoholic ketoacidosis can produce concentrations of ketones in the blood that are similar to those seen in severe diabetic ketoacidosis. Alcoholic ketoacidosis is reported to occur in two vastly different populations: chronic alcoholics and young children. In children, alcoholic ketoacidosis typically occurs when a small child who has fasted overnight awakens and samples an alcoholic drink left out by the parents the previous evening.[17]

Toxic Substances

Ingestion of toxic substances such as salicylates, ethylene glycol, and methanol produces metabolites that cause metabolic acidosis with a high AG. Excessive salicylate ingestion alters peripheral metabolism, causing overproduction of organic acids. Ethylene glycol is metabolized to glycolic acid and oxalic acids, and methanol is transformed to formaldehyde and formic acid.[18] Abnormal increases in these anions cause a reciprocal decrease in bicarbonate and elevation of the AG.

Renal Failure

Metabolic acidosis is a frequent complication of both acute and chronic renal failure. As the failing kidneys are unable to excrete phosphate, sulfate, and various other organic acids, these anions elevate in the bloodstream and cause a reciprocal drop in the serum bicarbonate level. Usually the AG does not rise appreciably until the glomerular filtration rate (GFR) has fallen to 20% of normal.[19]

Example: The high AG associated with chronic renal failure:

Na = 139 mEq/L
HCO_3 = 14 mEq/L
Cl = 105 mEq/L
AG = Na - (HCO_3 + Cl)
AG = 139 - (14 + 105) = 20 mEq/L (elevated above normal)

Normal Anion Gap Acidosis

The most frequent causes of normal AG acidosis are diarrhea and renal tubular acidosis. Although renal failure typically causes a high AG acidosis, it may also present with a normal AG when renal function is still good enough to allow the excretion of unmeasured anions.

Diarrhea

Diarrhea causes direct loss of bicarbonate in the stool, ECF volume depletion, and concentration of the remaining serum chloride, resulting in hyperchloremic acidosis. Because no change is caused in the "unmeasured" anions, the AG remains within normal limits. The same mechanism is seen in pancreatic and biliary fistulas, through which bicarbonate-rich fluid is lost in external drainage.

Excessive Chloride

Excessive infusion of chloride-containing fluids, such as isotonic sodium chloride (0.9% NaCl) or ammonium chloride, can cause hyperchloremic acidosis. Other causes include renal tubular acidosis and carbonic anhydrase inhibitors. Renal tubular acidosis exists in various forms and can be characterized by either bicarbonate loss in the urine or inability to generate new bicarbonate. As the plasma bicarbonate level decreases, the chloride level increases. Carbonic anhydrase inhibitors (such as acetazolamide) cause renal bicarbonate wasting.

Hyperchloremic acidosis often develops in patients with urinary diversion into the sigmoid colon. Apparently it is associated with bicarbonate secretion into the colon in exchange for the reabsorption of urinary chloride. The same changes may occur with urinary diversion to an ileal segment.

Example: The normal AG in a patient with ureterosigmoidostomy:

Na = 134 mEq/L
HCO_3 = 10 mEq/L
Cl = 115 mEq/L
$AG = Na - (HCO_3 + Cl)$
$134 - (10 + 115)$ = 9 mEq/L (normal AG; fall in HCO_3 is due to a reciprocal rise in Cl)

Decreased Anion Gap

Most often, a decreased AG is due to either severe dilution or hypoalbuminemia. Hypoalbuminemia is not a surprising cause because albumin accounts for most of the nonchloride or nonbicarbonate anions in the blood. A decreased AG may also be due to an increase in unmeasured cations (as in hyperkalemia, hypercalcemia, hypermagnesemia, or lithium intoxication).[20]

Expected blood gas changes for uncompensated, partly compensated, and completely compensated metabolic acidosis are presented in Table 9-3.

DEFINING CHARACTERISTICS

Both etiological factors and defining characteristics of metabolic acidosis are given in the Summary of Metabolic Acidosis. An example of blood gases in patients with metabolic acidosis is presented below.

Example: Patient with diabetic ketoacidosis:

pH = 7.05
HCO_3 = 5 mEq/L (primary disturbance is decreased bicarbonate level)
$PaCO_2$ = 12 mm Hg (represents compensatory hyperventilation to decrease CO_2)

 TABLE 9-3.   Expected Directional Changes in Blood Gases in Metabolic Acidosis

Imbalance	pH	HCO₃	PaCO₂
Uncompensated metabolic acidosis	↓	↓	N
Partly compensated metabolic acidosis	↓	↓	↓
Completely compensated metabolic acidosis	N	↓	↓

N, normal.

Acidemia depresses myocardial contractility, lowers the fibrillation threshold, and blunts the pressor response to catecholamines,[21] but it also enhances tissue oxygenation by shifting the oxyhemoglobin dissociation curve to the right.

TREATMENT

Because many conditions may lead to the development of metabolic acidosis, it is reasonable that treatment must vary, at least somewhat, according to the cause of the imbalance. For example, dialysis may be needed for the patient with extremely acidotic renal failure. Insulin administration and fluid replacement are frequently sufficient to correct even very low pH values in patients with ketoacidosis. The need for alkali therapy is influenced by the severity of acidosis. The precise level to which the pH must drop before alkali therapy is necessary is somewhat controversial. However, in the absence of clear evidence of harm, it is generally considered reasonable to judiciously administer bicarbonate to maintain a blood pH of 7.15 to 7.20 to mitigate the adverse hemodynamic effects of acidosis.[22] It is thought that correcting severe acidemia to a pH of 7.20 will decrease the risk for arrhythmias and enhance cardiac contractility.[23] Generally, there are three types of alkali that can be used for the treatment of metabolic acidosis: bicarbonate, salts of organic acids (such as lactate, acetate, and citrate) that are metabolized to bicarbonate, and tromethamine (THAM).[24] Sodium bicarbonate is most frequently used because it is effective immediately and requires no metabolic activation, unlike lactate, acetate, and citrate.[25] Care must be taken during bicarbonate administration to avoid overalkalinization of the plasma, which could result in cardiac arrhythmias and tetany. Thus, frequent monitoring of the acid–base status is warranted during treatment. The response to the administration of alkali partially depends on the cause of the metabolic acidosis. Refer to Chapter 18 for a discussion of the use of alkali in the treatment of ketoacidosis and to Chapter 16 for a discussion of the use of alkali during cardiac resuscitation.

Summary of Metabolic Acidosis (Base Bicarbonate Deficit)

ETIOLOGICAL FACTORS

Normal anion gap:
- Diarrhea
- Intestinal fistulas
- Ureterosigmoidostomy
- Acidifying drugs (such as ammonium chloride)
- Renal tubular acidosis

High anion gap:
- Diabetic ketoacidosis
- Starvational ketoacidosis
- Alcoholic ketoacidosis
- Lactic acidosis
- Renal failure
- Ingestion of toxins (such as salicylates, ethylene glycol, and methanol)

DEFINING CHARACTERISTICS

Headache

Confusion

Drowsiness

Increased respiratory rate and depth (may not become clinically evident until HCO_3 is quite low)

Nausea and vomiting

Peripheral vasodilatation (may be present, causing warm, flushed skin)

Decreased cardiac output when pH falls below 7.1

Arterial blood gases:
- Fall in pH (< 7.35)
- $HCO_3 < 22$ mEq/L (primary)
- $PaCO_2 < 35$ mm Hg (compensation by lungs)

METABOLIC ALKALOSIS

Metabolic alkalosis (HCO_3 excess) is a clinical disturbance characterized by a high pH (decreased hydrogen concentration) and a high plasma bicarbonate concentration. It can be produced by a gain of bicarbonate or a loss of hydrogen ion. In compensation, the lungs hypoventilate to increase the $PaCO_2$ concentration (movement in the same direction as the primary bicarbonate disturbance).

ETIOLOGICAL FACTORS

Probably the most common cause of metabolic alkalosis is vomiting or gastric suction (results in loss of hydrogen and chloride anions). Metabolic alkalosis occurs frequently in pyloric stenosis because only gastric fluid is lost in this disorder. Recall that gastric fluid usually has an acid pH (usually <4); loss of acidic fluid, of course, increases alkalinity of body fluids. (Vomiting related to other conditions sometimes involves loss of both gastric and alkaline upper small intestinal fluid. When this occurs, the severity of the pH change is tempered.)

Other factors predisposing to metabolic alkalosis include the loss of potassium, such as that caused by certain diuretics (eg, thiazides, furosemide, and ethacrynic acid) and the presence of excessive adrenal corticoid hormones (as in hyperaldosteronism and Cushing's syndrome). Hypokalemia produces alkalosis in two ways:

1. In the presence of hypokalemia, the kidneys conserve potassium and thus increase hydrogen ion excretion (recall that these ions compete for renal excretion).
2. Cellular potassium shifts out into the ECF in an attempt to maintain near-normal serum levels (as potassium leaves the cell, hydrogen must enter to maintain electroneutrality).

Excessive alkali ingestion, as in the use of bicarbonate-containing antacids (eg, Alka-Seltzer) can also cause metabolic alkalosis. Metabolic alkalosis due to high-dose sodium bicarbonate administration during cardiopulmonary resuscitation was a common finding a decade ago.[26]

Abrupt relief of chronically high CO_2 level in plasma (eg, assisted ventilation) results in a "lag period" before the chronically high serum bicarbonate level can be corrected by the kidneys.

DEFINING CHARACTERISTICS

Alkalosis is manifested primarily by symptoms related to decreased calcium ionization, such as tingling of the fingers and toes, dizziness, and hypertonic muscles. Respirations are depressed as a compensatory action by the lungs.

Arterial blood gases show an increased pH (>7.45) and an elevated bicarbonate level (>26 mEq/L), the primary disorder. To help temper the severity of the imbalance, compensatory hypoventilation occurs (elevating the $PaCO_2$) and is more pronounced in semiconscious, unconscious, or debilitated patients than in alert patients. Debilitated patients may develop marked hypoxemia as a result of hypoventilation.

Example: Patient with vomiting:

pH = 7.62
HCO_3 = 45 mEq/L (primary disturbance is high bicarbonate level)
$PaCO_2$ = 48 mm Hg (compensatory elevation in CO_2)

Other laboratory values are also disrupted in metabolic alkalosis. The serum potassium concentration is often, although not always, below 3.5 mEq/L. This is especially likely if the cause of the alkalosis is also associated with potassium loss (as in use of potassium-losing diuretics or vomiting). The serum chloride is relatively lower than sodium, as an elevation in the serum bicarbonate level causes the chloride level to drop. (Recall that as one anion increases, another tends to decrease to maintain electroneutrality.)

The ionized fraction of serum calcium decreases in the presence of alkalosis as more calcium combines with serum proteins. Because it is the ionized fraction of calcium that influences neuromuscular activity, it is understandable why symptoms of hypocalcemia are often the predominant ones of alkalosis.

Urinary chloride concentration is sometimes measured to determine the cause of metabolic alkalosis. It is usually less than 15 mEq/L when metabolic alkalosis is due to vomiting or gastric suction or prolonged diuretic use. Conversely, it is usually greater than 20 mEq/L when metabolic alkalosis is due to

TABLE 9-4. Expected Directional Changes in Blood Gases in Metabolic Alkalosis

Imbalance	pH	HCO₃	PaCO₂
Uncompensated (acute) metabolic alkalosis	↑	↑	N
Partly compensated (subacute) metabolic alkalosis	↑	↑	↑
Completely compensated (chronic) metabolic alkalosis	N	↑	↑

N, normal.

hyperaldosteronism, Cushing's syndrome, or profound potassium depletion (serum potassium <2.0 mEq/L).

Metabolic alkalosis can be acute or chronic. Expected directional changes in blood gases for uncompensated, partly compensated, and completely compensated metabolic alkalosis are listed in Table 9-4. The Summary of Metabolic Alkalosis lists the etiological factors and defining characteristics of metabolic alkalosis.

TREATMENT

Treatment is aimed at reversal of the underlying disorder. Sufficient chloride must be supplied for the kidney to absorb sodium with chloride (allowing the excretion of excess bicarbonate). Treatment also includes restoration of normal fluid volume by administration of sodium chloride fluids (because continued volume depletion serves to maintain the alkalosis).

Summary of Metabolic Alkalosis (Base Bicarbonate Excess)

ETIOLOGICAL FACTORS

Vomiting or gastric suction

Hypokalemia

Hyperaldosteronism

Cushing's syndrome

Potassium-losing diuretics (eg, thiazides, furosemide, ethacrynic acid)

Alkali ingestion (bicarbonate-containing antacids)

Parenteral NaHCO₃ administration for cardiopulmonary resuscitation

Abrupt relief of chronic respiratory acidosis

DEFINING CHARACTERISTICS

Those related to decreased calcium ionization, such as:
- Dizziness
- Tingling of fingers and toes
- Circumoral paresthesia
- Carpopedal spasm
- Hypertonic muscles

Depressed respiration (compensatory action by lungs)

Arterial blood gases:
- pH >7.45
- Bicarbonate >26 mEq/L (primary)
- PaCO₂ >45 mmHg (compensatory)

Serum Cl relatively lower than Na

RESPIRATORY ACIDOSIS

Respiratory acidosis (H_2CO_3 excess) can be either acute or chronic; the acute imbalance is particularly dangerous. When respiratory acidosis is acute, the bicarbonate level remains in the normal range because renal compensation is very slow. Therefore, the high $PaCO_2$ can quickly produce a sharp decrease in plasma pH. When respiratory acidosis is chronic, as in COPD, the kidneys compensate for the elevated $PaCO_2$ by increasing the bicarbonate level. (Compensatory renal bicarbonate generation takes several hours to days to develop.)

ETIOLOGICAL FACTORS

Respiratory acidosis is always due to inadequate excretion of CO_2 (inadequate ventilation), resulting in increased plasma CO_2 levels and therefore increased carbonic acid levels. In addition to an elevated $PaCO_2$ level, hypoventilation usually causes a decrease in PaO_2.

Acute respiratory acidosis is associated with certain emergency situations (such as acute pulmonary edema, aspiration of a foreign object, atelectasis, pneumothorax, overdosage of sedatives, and severe pneumonia). Chronic respiratory acidosis is associated with chronic situations such as emphysema, bronchiectasis, and bronchial asthma. Other etiological factors are listed in the Summary of Respiratory Acidosis.

DEFINING CHARACTERISTICS

Clinical signs vary between acute and chronic respiratory acidosis and are listed in the Summary of Respiratory Acidosis.

Acute Respiratory Acidosis

Sudden hypercapnia (elevated $PaCO_2$) can cause increased pulse and respiratory rate, increased blood pressure, mental cloudiness, and a feeling of fullness in the head ($PaCO_2$ causes cerebrovascular vasodilation and increased cerebral blood flow, particularly when more than 60 mm Hg).

Ventricular fibrillation may be the first sign of respiratory acidosis in the anesthetized patient. Respiratory acidosis may occur as soon as 15 minutes after the start of anesthesia and is most likely to occur in patients with chronic pulmonary disease. Changes in the ABGs occur immediately when ventilation is abruptly altered. The pH may reach a level of 7 or less in a few minutes. The $PaCO_2$ is greater than 45 mm Hg and may reach 120 mm Hg or higher. The bicarbonate is normal or only slightly elevated because there has been little time for renal compensation (an exception would be the patient with COPD who has a chronically elevated bicarbonate; in that situation, it would not be high enough to compensate for the sudden increase in $PaCO_2$). The PaO_2 is below normal when the patient is breathing room air and is the result of hypoventilation.

Example: Patient with acute respiratory acidosis:

pH = 7.26
$PaCO_2$ = 56 mm Hg (primary problem is high CO_2)
HCO_3 = 24 mEq/L (kidneys have not yet started to
   compensate by retaining bicarbonate)

Chronic Respiratory Acidosis

The patient with chronic respiratory acidosis may complain of weakness, dull headache, and the symptoms of the underlying disease process. The ABGs reveal a pH less than 7.35 or within the lower limit of normal (if complete compensation has occurred). The $PaCO_2$ is greater than 45 mm Hg (frequently between 50 and 60 mm Hg or greater). Patients with COPD who gradually accumulate CO_2 over a prolonged period (days to months) may not develop symptoms of hypercapnia (listed previously under Acute Respiratory Acidosis) because compensatory changes have had time to occur. For example, an emphysematous patient kept alive with oxygen therapy for more than 1 year was mentally alert although his $PaCO_2$ was 140 mm Hg. In the healthy person, a rapid rise in the $PaCO_2$ to 140 mm Hg would surely produce unconsciousness. The patient with chronic respiratory acidosis has had time for partial or complete renal compensation; therefore, the bicarbonate is above normal.

Example: Patient with chronic respiratory acidosis:

pH = 7.38
$PaCO_2$ = 76 mm Hg (primary disturbance is high
   CO_2)
HCO_3 = 42 mEq/L (kidneys have compensated by
   retaining bicarbonate)

Remember that when the $PaCO_2$ is chronically elevated above normal, the respiratory center becomes relatively insensitive to CO_2 as a respiratory stimulant, leaving hypoxemia as the major drive for respiration.

TABLE 9-5. Expected Directional Changes in Blood Gases in Respiratory Acidosis

Imbalance	pH	PaCO$_2$	HCO$_3$
Uncompensated respiratory acidosis (acute)	↓	↑	N
Partly compensated respiratory acidosis	↓	↑	↑
Completely compensated respiratory acidosis	N	↑	↑

N, normal

Excessive oxygen administration removes the stimulus of hypoxemia and the patient develops acute ventilatory failure unless the situation is quickly reversed.

Expected directional changes in blood gases in uncompensated, partly compensated, and completely compensated respiratory acidosis are listed in Table 9-5.

Summary of Respiratory Acidosis (Carbonic Acid Excess)

ETIOLOGICAL FACTORS

Acute respiratory acidosis:
- Acute pulmonary edema
- Aspiration of a foreign body
- Atelectasis
- Pneumothorax, hemothorax
- Overdosage of sedatives or anesthetic
- Position on operating table that interferes with respirations
- Cardiac arrest
- Severe pneumonia
- Laryngospasm
- Mechanical ventilation improperly regulated

Chronic respiratory acidosis:
- Emphysema
- Cystic fibrosis
- Advanced multiple sclerosis
- Bronchiectasis
- Bronchial asthma

Factors favoring hypoventilation:
- Obesity
- Tight abdominal binders or dressings
- Postoperative pain (as in high abdominal or chest incisions)
- Abdominal distention from cirrhosis or bowel obstruction

DEFINING CHARACTERISTICS

Acute respiratory acidosis:
- Feeling of fullness in the head (PaCO$_2$ causes cerebrovascular vasodilatation and increased cerebral blood flow, particularly when higher than 60 mm Hg)
- Mental cloudiness
- Dizziness
- Palpitations
- Muscular twitching
- Convulsions
- Warm, flushed skin
- Unconsciousness
- Ventricular fibrillation may be first sign in anesthetized patient (related to hyperkalemia)
- Arterial blood gases:
  —pH < 7.35
  —PaCO$_2$ > 45 mm Hg (primary)
  —HCO$_3$ normal or only slightly elevated

Chronic respiratory acidosis:
- Weakness
- Dull headache
- Symptoms of underlying disease process
- Arterial blood gases:
  —pH < 7.35 or within lower limits of normal
  —PaCO$_2$ > 45 mm Hg (primary)
  —HCO$_3$ > 26 mEq/L (compensatory)

TREATMENT

Treatment is directed at improving ventilation; exact measures vary with the cause of inadequate ventilation. Pharmacological agents are used as indicated. For example, bronchodilators help reduce bronchial spasm; antibiotics are used for respiratory infections. Pulmonary hygiene measures are used, when necessary, to rid the respiratory tract of mucus and purulent drainage. Adequate hydration (2–3 L/day) is indicated to keep the mucous membranes moist and thereby facilitate removal of secretions. Supplemental oxygen is used as necessary.

A mechanical respirator, used cautiously, may improve pulmonary ventilation. Remember that overzealous use of a mechanical respirator may cause such rapid excretion of CO_2 that the kidneys will be unable to eliminate excess bicarbonate with sufficient rapidity to prevent alkalosis and convulsions. For this reason, the elevated $PaCO_2$ must be decreased slowly.

RESPIRATORY ALKALOSIS

ETIOLOGICAL FACTORS AND DEFINING CHARACTERISTICS

Respiratory alkalosis (H_2CO_3 deficit) is always due to hyperventilation, which causes excessive "blowing off" of CO_2 and, hence, a decrease in plasma H_2CO_3 content. Etiological factors associated with respiratory alkalosis and defining characteristics are listed in the Summary of Respiratory Alkalosis.

As with respiratory acidosis, acute and chronic conditions can occur in respiratory alkalosis. In the acute state, the pH is elevated above normal as a result of a low $PaCO_2$ and a normal bicarbonate level. (Recall that the kidneys cannot alter the bicarbonate level quickly.)

Example: Patient with acute respiratory alkalosis:

pH = 7.52
$PaCO_2$ = 30 mm Hg (primary problem is low CO_2)
HCO_3 = 24 mEq/L (kidneys have not started compensatory change as yet)

In contrast, in chronic form, the kidneys have had time to lower the bicarbonate level.

Example: Patient with chronic respiratory alkalosis:

pH = 7.40
$PaCO_2$ = 30 mm Hg (primary problem is low CO_2)
HCO_3 = 18 mEq/L (compensatory decrease in bicarbonate)

Expected directional changes in blood gases in uncompensated, partly compensated, and completely compensated respiratory alkalosis are listed in Table 9-6.

TREATMENT

If the cause of respiratory alkalosis is anxiety, the patient should be made aware that the abnormal breathing practice is responsible for the symptoms accompanying this condition. Instructing the patient to breathe more slowly (to cause accumulation of CO_2) or to breathe into a closed system (such as a paper bag) is helpful. Usually a sedative is required to relieve hyperventilation in very anxious patients. (If alkalosis is severe enough to cause fainting, the increased ventilation will cease and respirations will revert to normal.) Treatment for other causes of respiratory alkalosis is directed at correcting the underlying problem.

TABLE 9-6. Expected Directional Changes in Arterial Blood Gases in Respiratory Alkalosis

Imbalance	pH	PaCO$_2$	HCO$_3$
Uncompensated respiratory alkalosis	↑	↓	N
Partly compensated respiratory alkalosis	↑	↓	↓
Completely compensated respiratory alkalosis	N	↓	↓

N, normal.

Summary of Respiratory Alkalosis (Carbonic Acid Deficit)

ETIOLOGICAL FACTORS

Extreme anxiety (most common cause)

High fever

Hypoxemia

Early salicylate intoxication (stimulates respiratory center)

Gram-negative bacteremia

Central nervous system lesions involving respiratory center

Pulmonary emboli

Thyrotoxicosis

Excessive ventilation by mechanical ventilators

Pregnancy (high progesterone level sensitizes the respiratory center to CO_2; physiological)

DEFINING CHARACTERISTICS

Lightheadedness (a low $PaCO_2$ causes cerebral vasoconstriction and thus decreased cerebral blood flow)

Inability to concentrate

Those of decreased calcium ionization (numbness and tingling of extremities and circumoral paresthesia; more likely to occur if respiratory alkalosis develops rapidly)

Hyperventilation syndrome:
• Tinnitus
• Palpitations
• Sweating
• Dry mouth
• Tremulousness
• Precordial pain (tightness)
• Nausea and vomiting
• Epigastric pain
• Blurred vision
• Convulsions and loss of consciousness (may be partly due to cerebral ischemia, caused by cerebral vasoconstriction)

Arterial blood gases:
• pH > 7.45
• $PaCO_2$ < 35 mm Hg (primary)
• HCO_3 < 22 mEq/L (compensatory)

MIXED ACID–BASE IMBALANCES

The preceding discussions have described single acid–base imbalances. These single imbalances do occur; however, one should be aware that in some clinical situations the patient may have two or more primary acid–base disturbances simultaneously. Some examples are given in Table 9-7 and at the end of the chapter. A number of steps and formulas are available to evaluate blood gas changes and determine whether they are purely compensatory in nature or represent a second primary imbalance. These are listed in Clinical Tip: Systematic Assessment of Arterial Blood Gases and Table 9-8.

SAMPLE MIXED ACID–BASE PROBLEMS

Use rules in Table 9-8 and Clinical Tip: Systematic Assessment of Arterial Blood Gases to analyze the following situations:

Respiratory Alkalosis Plus Metabolic Acidosis

Example: A patient has taken an overdose of aspirin. Recall that early in salicylate poisoning, the medulla is stimulated to produce hyperventilation (respiratory alkalosis results). Later, due to disrupted glucose metabolism, metabolic acidosis may result.

pH = 7.4
$PaCO_2$ = 18 mm Hg
HCO_3 = 16 mEq/L

TABLE 9-7. Examples of Combinations of Mixed Acid–Base Disorders

Metabolic acidosis/respiratory acidosis

Cardiopulmonary arrest

Hypoxemia produces lactic acidosis with decrease in HCO_3
Respiratory arrest causes CO_2 retention

Metabolic acidosis/respiratory alkalosis

Salicylate intoxication

Salicylate alters peripheral metabolism and causes overproduction of organic acids with resultant decrease in HCO_3
Salicylate stimulates respiratory center and causes decrease in CO_2

Metabolic acidosis/metabolic alkalosis

Renal failure with vomiting

Renal failure causes retention of acid metabolites with decrease in HCO_3
Vomiting causes loss of H^+ and Cl^- and thus increase in HCO_3

Metabolic alkalosis/respiratory alkalosis

Vomiting during pregnancy

Vomiting causes loss of H^+ and Cl^- and thus increase in HCO_3
Progesterone increase during pregnancy stimulates respirations and causes decrease in CO_2

Metabolic alkalosis/respiratory acidosis

Vomiting with COPD

Vomiting causes loss of H^+ and Cl^- and thus increase in HCO_3
COPD is associated with sustained elevation of CO_2

COPD, chronic obstructive pulmonary disease.

TABLE 9-8. Compensatory Changes Related to Primary Acid–Base Disturbances

Imbalance	Primary Change	Compensatory Change
Metabolic acidosis (base bicarbonate deficit)	HCO_3 decreased	$1.5(HCO_3) + 8 \pm 2$
Metabolic alkalosis (base bicarbonate excess)	HCO_3 increased	0.6 mm Hg increase in $PaCO_2$ for every 1 mEq/L rise in HCO_3
Respiratory acidosis (carbonic acid excess)		
• Acute	$PaCO_2$ increased	1.0 mEq/L increase in HCO_3 for every 10 mm Hg rise in $PaCO_2$
• Chronic	$PaCO_2$ increased	3.5 mEq/L increase in HCO_3 for every 10 mm Hg rise in $PaCO_2$
Respiratory alkalosis (carbonic acid deficit)		
• Acute	$PaCO_2$ decreased	2.0 mEq/L decrease in HCO_3 for every 10 mm Hg fall in $PaCO_2$
• Chronic	$PaCO_2$ decreased	5.0 mEq/L decrease in HCO_3 for every 10 mm Hg fall in $PaCO_2$

CLINICAL TIP

Systematic Assessment of Arterial Blood Gases

The following steps are recommended to evaluate arterial blood gas values. They are based on the assumption that the average values are

$$pH = 7.4$$
$$PaCO_2 = 40 \text{ mm Hg}$$
$$HCO_3 = 24 \text{ mEq/L}$$

I. *First,* look at the pH. It can be high, low, or normal as follows:

pH > 7.4 (alkalosis)
pH < 7.4 (acidosis)
pH = 7.4 (normal)

A normal pH may indicate perfectly normal blood gases, or it may be an indication of a compensated imbalance. A compensated imbalance is one in which the body has been able to correct the pH by either respiratory or metabolic changes (depending on the primary problem). For example, a patient with primary metabolic acidosis starts out with a low bicarbonate level but a normal carbon dioxide level. Soon afterward, the lungs try to compensate for the imbalance by exhaling large amounts or carbon dioxide (hyperventilation).

Another example, a patient with primary respiratory acidosis starts out with a high carbon dioxide level; soon afterward, the kidneys attempt to compensate by retaining bicarbonate. If the compensatory maneuver is able to restore the bicarbonate:carbonic acid ratio back to 20:1, full compensation (and thus normal pH) will be achieved.

II. *The next step is to determine the primary cause of the disturbance. This is done by evaluating the PaCO₂ and HCO₃ in relation to the pH.*

pH > 7.4 (alkalosis)

1. If the PaCO₂ is < 40 mm Hg, the primary disturbance is respiratory alkalosis. (This situation occurs when a patient hyperventilates and "blows off" too much carbon dioxide. Recall that carbon dioxide dissolved in water becomes carbonic acid, the acid side of the "carbonic acid:base bicarbonate" buffer system.)

2. If the HCO₃ is > 24 mEq/L, the primary disturbance is metabolic alkalosis. (This situation occurs when the body gains too much bicarbonate, an alkaline substance. Bicarbonate is the basic, or alkaline side of the "carbonic acid:ba se bicarbonate" buffer system.)

pH < 7.4 (acidosis)

1. If the PaCO₂ is > 40 mmHg, the primary disturbance is respiratory acidosis. (This situation occurs when a patient hypoventilates and thus retains too much carbon dioxide, an acidic substance.)

2. If the HCO₃ is < 24 mEq/L, the primary disturbance is metabolic acidosis. (This situation occurs when the body's bicarbonate level drops, either because of direct bicarbonate loss or because of gains of acids such as lactic acid or ketones.)

III. *The next step involves determining if compensation has begun.*

This is done by looking at the value other than the primary disorder. If it is moving in the same direction as the primary value, compensation is under way. Consider the following gases: Example:

	pH	PaCO₂	HCO₃
(1)	7.20	60 mm Hg	24 mEq/L
(2)	7.40	60 mm Hg	37 mEq/L

The first set (1) indicates acute respiratory acidosis without compensation (the PaCO₂ is high, the HCO₃ is normal). The second set (2) indicates chronic respiratory acidosis. Note that compensation has taken place; that is, the HCO₃ has elevated to an appropriate level to balance the high PaCO₂ and produce a normal pH.

Note in the above situation that the simultaneous appearance of respiratory alkalosis and metabolic acidosis has produced a normal pH. (This is not always the case; one imbalance may be stronger than the other and cause an abnormal pH in its favor.)

If the only problem in this situation were respiratory alkalosis, the HCO_3 would be expected to be about 20 mEq/L. Note that it is lower than expected (indicating metabolic acidosis). If the only problem were metabolic acidosis, the $PaCO_2$ would be expected to be about 32 mEq/L. Note that it is lower than expected (indicating respiratory alkalosis).

Respiratory Acidosis Plus Metabolic Acidosis

Example: A patient has lactic acidosis secondary to cardiac failure and hypercapnia secondary to pneumonia.

pH = 7.10
$PaCO_2$ = 50 mm Hg
HCO_3 = 15 mEq/L

Because both primary disturbances produce acidosis, the pH is quite low. If the only problem were acute respiratory acidosis, the HCO_3 level would increase to slightly above normal (instead, it has decreased). If the only problem were metabolic acidosis, the $PaCO_2$ would decrease (instead, it has increased).

REFERENCES

1. Schlichtig R, Grogono A, Severinghaus J. Human $PaCO_2$ and standard base excess for compensation for acid-base imbalances. *Crit Care Med* 1998;26:1173.
2. Guyton A, Hall J. *Textbook of Medical Physiology*, 9th ed. Philadelphia: WB Saunders; 1996:528.
3. Ibid, p 531.
4. Narins R. *Clinical Disorders of Fluid and Electrolyte Metabolism*, 5th ed. New York: McGraw-Hill; 1994:669.
5. Rose B. *Clinical Physiology of Acid-Base and Electrolyte Disorders*, 4th ed. New York: McGraw-Hill; 1994:778.
6. Ibid.
7. Ibid, p 512.
8. Narins, p 790.
9. Abelow B. *Understanding Acid-Base.* Baltimore, MD: Williams & Wilkins; 1998:299.
10. Narins, p 762.
11. Roberts W, Johnson R. The serum anion gap. Has the reference interval really fallen? *Arch Pathol Lab Med* 1997;121:568.
12. Abelow, p 229.
13. Ibid.
14. Shapiro B, Peruzzi W, Templin R. *Clinical Application of Blood Gases*, 5th ed. St. Louis: CV Mosby; 1994:238.
15. Ibid, p 173.
16. Ibid, p 238.
17. Hoffman R, Goldfrank L. Ethanol-associated metabolic disorders. *Endocrinol Metabol Emerg* 1989;7:943.
18. Kokko J, Tannen R. *Fluids and Electrolytes*, 3rd ed. Philadelphia: WB Saunders; 1996:225.
19. Halperin M, Goldstein M. *Fluid, Electrolyte, and Acid-Base Physiology*, 3rd ed. Philadelphia: WB Saunders; 1999:128.
20. Jurado R et al. Low anion gap. *South Med J* 1998;91:624.
21. Kearns T, Wolfson A. Metabolic acidosis. *Endocrinol Metab Emerg* 1989;7:823.
22. Epstein F. Protection of acid-base balance by pH regulation of acid production. *N Engl J Med* 1998;339:819.
23. Carey C, Lee H, Woeltje K. *The Washington Manual of Medical Therapeutics*, 29th ed. Philadelphia: Lippincott Raven, 1998:59.
24. Chernow B, ed. *The Pharmacologic Approach to the Critically Ill Patient*, 3rd ed. Baltimore, MD: Williams & Wilkins; 1994:965.
25. Pemberton L, Pemberton D. *Treatment of Water, Electrolyte, and Acid-Base Disorders in the Surgical Patient.* New York: McGraw-Hill; 1994:324.
26. Shapiro, p 240.

PRACTICE EXERCISES

Review the following situations and determine the primary acid–base problem as well as the compensatory change. Also determine whether the imbalance is compensated or uncompensated. Answers are provided below the exercises.

All values are arterial.

$PaCO_2$ (units in mm Hg; normal range 35–45 mm Hg)

    HCO_3 (units in mEq/L; normal range 22–26 mEq/L)

	#1	#2	#3	#4	#5	#6
pH	7.54	7.20	7.55	7.35	7.36	7.15
$PaCO_2$	29	34	58	95	25	80
HCO_3	24	15	49	49	15	28

#1. The pH is above normal (> 7.45); therefore, this is alkalosis. Two conditions can produce a high pH (one is a low $PaCO_2$ and the other is a high HCO_3).

The $PaCO_2$ is below the lower limit of normal and is the primary change.

The HCO_3 is unchanged (remember, the kidneys are slow to respond in compensation for respiratory problems). In time, the HCO_3 will decrease (following the direction of the primary problem).

Because the pH is not within the normal range, this imbalance is *uncompensated respiratory alkalosis*. One might see a set of blood gases like this in an anxious patient who is hyperventilating.

#2. The pH is below normal (< 7.35); therefore, this is acidosis. Two conditions can produce a low pH (one is a high $PaCO_2$ and the other is a low HCO_3).

The HCO_3 is below normal and is the primary change.

The $PaCO_2$ has started to decrease below normal and is a compensatory change (following the direction of the primary change).

Because the pH is not within the normal range, this imbalance is *uncompensated metabolic acidosis*. One might see a set of blood gases like this in a patient with diabetic ketoacidosis.

#3. The pH is above normal (> 7.45); therefore, this is alkalosis. Two conditions can produce a high pH (one is a low $PaCO_2$ and the other is a high HCO_3).

The HCO_3 is far above normal and is the primary change.

The $PaCO_2$ has increased above normal and is a compensatory change (following the direction of the primary change).

Because the pH is not within the normal range, this imbalance is *uncompensated metabolic alkalosis*. One might see a set of blood gases like this in a patient who has been vomiting.

#4. The pH is within the normal range, but just barely. Because it is closer to acidosis than to alkalosis, one would look for changes that would produce acidosis. Two conditions can produce a low pH (one is a high $PaCO_2$ and the other is a low HCO_3).

The $PaCO_2$ is far above normal and is the primary change.

The HCO_3 has increased dramatically to compensate for the very high $PaCO_2$ (following the direction of the primary change).

Because the pH is within the normal range, this imbalance is *compensated respiratory acidosis*. This set of blood gas values is often seen in patients with chronic obstructive pulmonary disease (COPD).

PRACTICE EXERCISES—*cont'd*

#5. The pH is within the normal range, but just barely. Because it is closer to acidosis than to alkalosis, one would look for changes that would produce acidosis. Two conditions can produce a low pH (one is a high $PaCO_2$ and the other is a low HCO_3).

The HCO_3 is far below normal and is the primary change.

The $PaCO_3$ has decreased to compensate for the low HCO_3 (following the direction of the primary change).

Because the pH is within the normal range, this imbalance is *compensated metabolic acidosis*. One might see a set of blood gases like this following diarrhea or in a patient with diabetic ketoacidosis or lactice acidosis.

#6. The pH is below the normal range (< 7.35); therefore, this is acidosis. Two conditions can produce a low pH (one is a high $PaCO_2$ and the other is a low HCO_3).

The $PaCO_2$ is far above normal and is the primary change.

The HCO_3 has increased slightly to help compensate for the high $PaCO_2$ (following the direction of the primary change). In time, the kidneys will retain even more HCO_3 to further compensate for the primary excessive retention of $PaCO_2$.

Because the pH is below the normal range, this imbalance is *uncompensated respiratory acidosis*. One might see a set of blood gases like this in a patient who is hypoventilating because of a respiratory depressant drug overdose.

#7. The following set of blood gases occurred in a patient with emphysema who recently developed an acute respiratory infection.

pH = 7.20
$PaCO_2$ = 55 mm Hg
HCO_3 = 20.5 mEq/L
PaO_2 = 55 mm Hg

This patient has two primary uncompensated imbalances; one is *respiratory acidosis* and the other is *metabolic acidosis*. If the only problem were respiratory acidosis (high $PaCO_2$), the HCO_3 would have elevated above normal. Instead, it decreased below normal. The cause of the metabolic acidosis is likely lactic acidosis, associated with the low PaO_2.

#8. The following set of blood gases were found in a young man admitted to the emergency department with Kussmaul breathing and an irregular pulse.

pH = 7.05
$PaCO_2$ = 15 mm Hg
HCO_3 = 6 mEq/L

This patient has *uncompensated metabolic acidosis* (note the extremely low HCO_3 level). The below normal $PaCO_2$ is due to compensatory hyperventilation. The expected $PaCO_2$ in this patient should be between 15 to 19 mm Hg, as calculated by the following formula:

Expected $PaCO_2$ = 1.5 (HCO_3) + 8 ± 2

#9. The following set of blood gases were found in a young woman who entered the emergency department with a broken ankle and multiple contusions.

pH = 7.55
$PaCO_2$ = 25 mm Hg
HCO_3 = 22 mEq/L

Continued

PRACTICE EXERCISES—*cont'd*

This patient has *uncompensated respiratory alkalosis* (as manifested by the below normal $PaCO_2$). In acute respiratory alkalosis, one would expect to see a 2.0 mEq/L decrease in the HCO_3 level for every 10 mm Hg decrease in the $PaCO_2$ level. This compensatory change has not been achieved as yet, but is underway.

#10. The following set of blood gases were found in a man who had been vomiting for several days.
   pH = 7.56
   $PaCO_2$ = 49 mm Hg
   HCO_3 = 40 mEq/L

This patient has *uncompensated metabolic alkalosis* (as manifested by the far above normal HCO_3 level). The expected compensatory change would be an increased $PaCO_2$ level (about 0.6 mm Hg for every 1 mEq/L rise in the HCO_3). This expected change is present.

Parenteral and Enteral Nutrition

Parenteral Fluids

The nurse's role in parenteral fluid therapy is crucial because it is the nurse who usually initiates fluids and, almost invariably, is responsible for monitoring the patient's response. One must be knowledgeable about the contents of parenteral fluids, their purposes, and the contraindications and complications associated with their uses.

Before discussing the types of parenteral fluids available and the factors to be considered with their administration, it is helpful to review some basic facts.

The three major purposes for parenteral fluid therapy are: (1) providing fluids to meet daily maintenance needs; (2) providing fluids to replace ongoing losses; and (3) providing electrolytes to correct any existing disturbances. Each of these purposes is briefly discussed.

⬤ PURPOSES OF FLUID THERAPY

PROVISION OF USUAL MAINTENANCE NEEDS

As noted in Table 2-1, the average healthy adult requires about 2,600 mL of fluid daily to replace fluid lost in urine, stool, exhalation, and radiation from the skin. Many patients require parenteral fluids for only a few days while they are temporarily unable to ingest food and fluid during a limited illness or after surgery. In these patients, the typical fluid prescription for maintenance needs ranges between 2,000 and 3,000 mL/day.

Of course, the body needs more than water for maintenance; electrolytes are also needed. The average adult needs 50 to 150 mEq sodium and 20 to 60 mEq potassium each day.[1] An example of a 24-hour fluid prescription to meet these needs is 2 liters of 0.45% NaCl with 20 mEq KCl added to each liter. Because each liter of 0.45% NaCl contains 77 mEq sodium, 2 liters would provide 154 mEq (easily meeting the daily sodium requirement of most adults). Addition of 20 mEq KCl to each liter of fluid would provide the typically needed 40 mEq potassium per day.

Because 0.45% NaCl is a hypotonic solution, it provides some free water to aid in the renal excretion of solutes. Free water can also be supplied in the form of 5% dextrose in water. Calories are needed in parenteral fluids to minimize protein catabolism and prevent ketosis of starvation. Thus, the above example would

more likely be 2 liters of 5% dextrose in 0.45% NaCl (rather than 0.45% NaCl alone). Because each liter of a 5% dextrose solution provides 50 g carbohydrate with about 170 calories, 2 liters would provide 100 g carbohydrate with 340 calories. Although this is a small fraction of the daily caloric need, it is far better than none in terms of warding off ketosis of starvation. As discussed in Chapter 11, sophisticated solutions are available to meet the nutritional needs of patients requiring prolonged parenteral therapy or of those needing a large caloric intake due to hypermetabolism (as occurs with trauma or burns).

Maintenance needs for sodium and potassium were discussed briefly. Remember that calcium, magnesium, and phosphorus may be necessary if parenteral therapy is prolonged.[2]

Although 2,000 to 3,000 mL water per day for the average healthy adult is a useful figure to keep in mind, it is important to realize that it may need to be adjusted downward for smaller adults. Furthermore, children need entirely different volumes based on their body size and age. To avoid the possibility of fluid volume error, some clinicians favor the use of fluid volume replacement based on body surface area.

This discussion of needed fluid volume is predicated on the assumption that the patient has normal renal function. If this is not the case, fluid volume as well as sodium and potassium replacement must be adjusted according to severity of the renal impairment. For example, a patient in oliguric renal failure might logically receive the same amount of fluid as the sum of urinary output and estimated insensible losses.

REPLACEMENT OF ABNORMAL FLUID LOSSES

If the patient is losing fluid by an abnormal route (such as gastric suction, vomiting, or diarrhea), more than maintenance fluids must be provided to prevent fluid volume deficit (FVD). In addition, the electrolyte content of the parenteral fluid will need to be modified to correct imbalances. The need for a carefully kept intake and output (I&O) record is evident to identify lost water and electrolytes. It is also important to record elevated body temperature because this increases fluid needs. Free water needs are increased in individuals with unusual insensible water losses, such as those who are hyperventilating or exposed to low environmental humidity. Water needs are also greater in patients with decreased renal concentrating ability because relatively more water is required to eliminate wastes. Finally, fluid requirements are greatly increased by shock, multiple trauma, and sepsis (either because of direct fluid loss or pooling of fluid in the capillaries or interstitial space). See Chapters 13 through 25 for discussion of fluid therapy in patients with specific clinical problems.

CORRECTION OF EXISTING ELECTROLYTE DISTURBANCES

Providing maintenance fluid and electrolytes is more complicated if the patient has electrolyte disturbances that need correction. The task becomes one of safely providing needed electrolytes in conjunction with maintenance needs. For discussion of fluid therapy for specific electrolyte disturbances, see Chapters 3 through 9.

⬤ ASSESSMENT OF PATIENTS RECEIVING PARENTERAL FLUID THERAPY

Before parenteral fluid therapy is initiated for a patient with a real or potential fluid balance problem, renal status must be evaluated. There is danger of causing other imbalances if the kidneys are not functioning adequately. For example, administration of potassium-containing fluids to a patient with inadequate renal function can induce serious hyperkalemia.

If the patient with a severe FVD is oliguric, it is necessary to determine if the depressed renal function is due to prerenal azotemia secondary to decreased renal perfusion or, more seriously, to actual renal parenchymal damage (acute tubular necrosis [ATN]) after prolonged untreated FVD. To differentiate between these conditions, a fluid load is infused over a short period and the patient is observed closely. If urine output improves, the problem was simple FVD; if urine flow is not reestablished, the problem is likely to be renal insufficiency. A fluid challenge test to distinguish simple FVD from a deficit complicated by ATN is described in Chapter 3. These two conditions must be differentiated because prompt treatment of prerenal azotemia can prevent ATN. Treatment of a patient with adequate renal function is simplified greatly. If sufficient water and electrolytes are provided, healthy kidneys can select needed substances and maintain normal fluid and electrolyte balance.

Although physicians are responsible for writing fluid orders, nurses share in the responsibility for safe fluid replacement therapy. A major nursing responsibility is the provision of precise I&O records and daily weight charts. The accuracy of this information is crucial to the correct formulation of fluid replacement regimens. In addition, nurses must share the responsibility for detecting undesirable trends in these data.

Parameters to be considered in assessment include:

- Comparison of I&O measurements
- Daily or more frequent body weights
- Vital signs
- Skin turgor
- Hemodynamic measurements (such as central venous pressure [CVP], pulmonary arterial pressure [PAP], pulmonary capillary wedge pressure [PCWP], cardiac output [CO])
- Urinary specific gravity
- Laboratory values

Refer to Chapter 2 for a review of these indices and to Chapters 13 through 25 which deal with specific clinical conditions. Chapters 3 through 9 also present specific information regarding assessment of patients receiving parenteral fluids.

Giving the right amount of fluid depends on calculating measurable fluid losses, estimating insensible and third-space losses, factoring in the functional ability of key homeostatic organs, and revising fluid prescriptions according to current indicators of the patient's fluid and electrolyte status. Standing fluid orders are never acceptable. For typical patients, fluid orders are readjusted every 24 hours. However, this is not sufficient for many critically ill patients whose fluid status is subject to rapid change. For these patients, it may be necessary to readjust fluid directives every 8 hours (or even more frequently).

⬤ WATER AND ELECTROLYTE SOLUTIONS

Table 1 lists some commercially available water and electrolyte solutions. Examples of these fluids are discussed.

DEXTROSE SOLUTIONS

Five percent dextrose in water (D_5W) is a roughly isotonic (278 mOsm/L) fluid given to provide free water. (Distilled water without additives cannot be infused intravenously [IV] because it would cause hemolysis of

TABLE 10-1 Contents of Selected Water and Electrolyte Solutions With Comments About Their Use

Solution	Comments
5% dextrose in water (D₅W): No electrolytes 50 g dextrose	Supplies about 170 cal/L and free water to aid in renal excretion of solutes Should not be used in excessive volumes in patients with increased antidiuretic hormone activity or to replace fluids in hypovolemic patients
0.9% NaCl (isotonic saline): Na⁺ 154 mEq/L Cl⁻ 154 mEq/L	Isotonic fluid commonly used to expand the extracellular fluid in presence of hypovolemia Because of relatively high chloride content, it can be used to treat mild metabolic alkalosis
0.45% NaCl (½-strength saline): Na⁺ 77 mEq/L Cl⁻ 77 mEq/L	A hypotonic solution that provides Na⁺, Cl⁻, and free water (Na⁺ and Cl⁻ provided in fluid allow kidneys to select and retain needed amounts) Free-water desirable as aid to kidney s in elimination of solutes
0.33% NaCl (1/3-strength saline): Na⁺ 56 mEq/L Cl⁻ 56 mEq/L	A hypotonic solution that provides Na⁺, Cl⁻, and free water Often used to treat hypernatremia (because this solution contains a small amount of Na⁺, it dilutes the plasma sodium while not allowing it to drop too rapidly)
3% NaCl: Na⁺ 513 mEq/L Cl⁻ 513 mEq/L	Grossly hypertonic solutions used only to treat severe hyponatremia See Clinical Tip: Nursing Considerations in Administration of Hypertonic Saline Solutions (3% and 5% NaCl) in Chapter 4 for summary of important nursing considerations in administration
5% NaCl: Na⁺ 855 mEq/L Cl⁻ 855 mEq/L	Dangerous solutions
Lactated Ringer's solution: Na⁺ 130 mEq/L K⁺ 4 mEq/L Ca²⁺ 3 mEq/L Cl⁻ 109 mEq/L Lactate (metabolized to bicarbonate) 28 mEq/L	A roughly isotonic solution that contains multiple electrolytes in about the same concentrations as found in plasma (Note that this solution is lacking in Mg and PO₄.) Used in the treatment of hypovolemia, burns, and fluid lost as bile or diarrhea Useful in treating mild metabolic acidosis
Sodium lactate solution, 1/6 M: Na⁺ 167 mEq/L Cl⁻ 167 mEq/L	A roughly isotonic solution used to correct severe metabolic acidosis (Lactate is metabolized to bicarbonate in 1–2 hr by the liver.) Not used in patients with liver disease (lactate cannot be converted to bicarbonate in such individuals), also not used in patients with oxygen lack (unable to adequately convert lactate to bicarbonate)
Sodium bicarbonate, 5% Na⁺ 595 mEq/L Cl⁻ 595 mEq/L	A very hypertonic solution used to correct severe metabolic acidosis Should be cautiously administered at a slow rate, under careful volume control Should be administered only with extreme caution to salt-retaining patients (eg, those with cardiac, renal, or liver damage)
Ammonium chloride, 2.14%	Acidifying solution used to correct severe metabolic alkalosis Due to high ammonium content, must be administered cautiously to patients with compromised hepatic function
Potassium chloride, 0.15% K⁺ 20 mEq/L Cl⁻ 20 mEq/L	Premixed potassium chloride solution
Potassium chloride, 0.30% K⁺ 40 mEq/L Cl⁻ 40 mEq/L	Premixed potassium chloride solution

red blood cells as it entered the vein.) The dextrose in D_5W is metabolized to carbon dioxide and water, leaving a solution physiologically equivalent to distilled water but without the hemolysis. Water given IV as D_5W is distributed evenly into every body compartment. For each liter of free water given IV, no more than 100 mL remains in the intravascular space after 1 hour.[3] Thus, D_5W is used to replace deficits of total body water but is never used alone to expand the extracellular fluid (ECF) volume. Too much D_5W can seriously dilute serum sodium, especially in a patient who has excess antidiuretic hormone activity.

Dextrose and water solutions are also available in 2.5%, 10%, 20%, and 50% concentrations. Theoretically, because each gram of carbohydrate supplies 4 calories, the 50 g in 1 liter of D_5W should supply 200 calories. However, because dextrose in parenteral solution provides only 3.4 calories per gram, 1 liter of D_5W provides 170 calories and 1 liter of $D_{10}W$ provides 340 calories. Although 50 or 100 g dextrose is a small portion of an adult's daily caloric requirements, either amount is often enough to stave off the ketosis of starvation, which is the reason dextrose is often added to electrolyte solutions until the patient can assume oral intake. (Electrolyte solutions without added nutrients have essentially no calories.) Examples of dextrose and electrolyte solutions are 5% dextrose in 0.9% NaCl, 5% dextrose in 0.45% NaCl, and 5% dextrose in lactated Ringer's solution. As discussed in Chapter 11, a typical total parenteral nutrition (TPN) solution for central vein administration consists of 500 mL of 50% dextrose mixed with 500 mL amino acid solution (for a net 25% dextrose solution). Because concentrated solutions of dextrose can cause hyperglycemia and osmotic diuresis, they must be infused slowly.

SODIUM CHLORIDE SOLUTIONS

Isotonic Saline

Also called normal saline, 1 liter of isotonic saline (0.9% NaCl) contains 154 mEq sodium and 154 mEq chloride. Total cations (Na^+) and anions (Cl^-) amount to 308 mEq/L, an isotonic concentration. Solutions are considered roughly isotonic if the total electrolyte content (ie, anions plus cations) approximates 310 mEq/L, hypotonic if the total is less than 250 mEq/L, and hypertonic if electrolyte content exceeds 376 mEq/L. (These are arbitrary figures but are useful as a basis for comparing solutions.)

When infused IV, isotonic saline is distributed in the ECF compartment; none enters the intracellular fluid (ICF). One liter of isotonic saline adds 1 liter to the ECF, theoretically expanding the plasma volume in the average adult by one-fourth of a liter and the interstitial volume by three-fourths of a liter 1 hour after administration.[4] In the critically ill or injured patient, only one-fifth or less of the volume may remain in the circulation 1 to 2 hours after infusion.[5]

The ECF normally contains 140 mEq sodium and 103 mEq chloride per liter, amounts that are smaller and in different proportions from those in 0.9% NaCl (isotonic saline). The greater amount of chloride than normally present in plasma imposes an excess chloride load on the kidney and could result in hyperchloremic metabolic acidosis. However, this excess of chloride makes isotonic saline an ideal fluid for patients with FVD coexisting with hyponatremia, hypochloremia, and metabolic alkalosis (such as patients with excessive vomiting or gastric suction loss). Because of its high sodium content, however, the solution is used cautiously in patients whose renal or other regulatory mechanisms are compromised.

Half-Strength Saline (0.45% NaCl)

As its name implies, 1 liter of half-strength saline provides half the electrolytes found in 1 liter of isotonic saline, therefore, 77 mEq each of sodium and chloride. If this hypotonic solution is understood as a mixture of 500 mL isotonic saline and 500 mL free water, it is obvious why it is a good choice to provide some sodium to adjust serum levels plus free water to replace insensible losses. It is frequently used as a basic fluid for maintenance needs. It is also used to treat hypovolemic patients who have hypernatremia, that is, those who have a greater water deficit than solute deficit.

Other even more hypotonic NaCl solutions are available commercially. Examples are 0.11% NaCl (furnishing about 19 mEq/L each of sodium and chloride), 0.2% (34 mEq/L of each), 0.225% (39 mEq/L of each), and 0.33% (56 mEq/L of each). Excessive use of these hypotonic solutions can cause dilutional hyponatremia, especially in people who tend to retain water.

Hypertonic Saline

On relatively rare occasions, 3% or 5% NaCl (hypertonic saline solutions) is used to treat severe symptomatic hyponatremia. Small volumes are infused slowly and with great caution to avoid inducing a severe volume overload, along with pulmonary edema. Patients with cardiovascular compromise or severe volume overload may need a diuretic to help remove hypotonic fluid as soon as the concentrated saline solution is infused. Hypertonic saline should be used only in settings where the patient can be closely monitored because it requires frequent assessment for pulmonary edema, worsening neurological signs, and serum sodium levels. The 3% solution provides 513 mEq/L each of sodium and chloride and the 5% solution provides 855 mEq/L of each. The reader is referred to Clinical Tip: Nursing Considerations in Administration of Hypertonic Saline Solutions (3% and 5% NaCl) in Chapter 4 for a summary of important nursing aspects.

Clinical and experimental studies have indicated that a 7.5% NaCl solution is useful in the resuscitation of hemorrhagic shock and burns. This hypertonic fluid provides resuscitation with less volume than do isotonic crystalloids (such as isotonic saline or lactated Ringer's solution). After infusion, hypertonic saline pulls fluid away from the intracellular into the extracellular space. Apparently this action provides about 7 mL free water for every 1 mL hypertonic saline administered.[6] Resuscitation with 200 mL hypertonic saline (7.5% NaCl) expands the extracellular space by 1,600 mL (the 200 mL infused plus 1,400 mL pulled from the cellular space).[7] To keep the fluid within the intravascular space, the hypertonic saline has usually been added to a hyperoncotic agent (such as 6% dextran) in clinical trials. Patients resuscitated with hypertonic saline solution require careful monitoring of serum electrolytes to prevent serious hypernatremia and hyperosmolar coma.[8] Although resuscitation with hypertonic saline results in a more rapid elevation of blood pressure in the first few minutes after administration as well as a lower water load than equivalent resuscitation with isotonic saline or lactated Ringer's solution, no differences in survival rates have been clearly demonstrated.[9]

BALANCED ELECTROLYTE SOLUTIONS

The most frequently prescribed balanced solution, lactated Ringer's, carries the same name regardless of the commercial supplier. One liter of this commonly used fluid provides 130 mEq sodium, 4 mEq potassium, 3 mEq calcium, 28 mEq lactate, and 109 mEq chloride. Lactated Ringer's solution contains 137 mEq/L each

of cations and anions, for a total concentration of 274 mEq/L. It behaves similarly to isotonic saline in terms of expanding the ECF volume.

Considered a near-physiological solution, the electrolyte content of lactated Ringer's solution is similar to that of plasma. It is often used to correct isotonic FVDs (as in hypovolemia due to third-space fluid shift after major trauma or surgery). Because each liter of lactated Ringer's solution contains 28 mEq lactate that normally is quickly metabolized into bicarbonate, the solution can be used to treat many forms of metabolic acidosis. The lactate load in lactated Ringer's solution apparently does not potentiate the lactic acidosis associated with hemorrhagic shock.[10] Isotonic saline is preferred for the treatment of hyponatremia and hypercalcemia because isotonic saline contains more sodium (154 mEq/L, as opposed to 130 mEq/L in lactated Ringer's solution). Although isotonic saline (0.9% NaCl) and lactated Ringer's solution are apparently equivalent in the treatment of moderate hemorrhage, lactated Ringer's is thought to be superior to isotonic saline (0.9% NaCl) for the treatment of massive hemorrhage.[11] (Because isotonic saline contains 154 mEq chloride per liter, it is possible that the excessive use of isotonic saline could cause hyperchloremic acidosis.)

Numerous other balanced electrolyte solutions are available commercially in a wide array of electrolyte combinations. Some solutions are designed for maintenance needs, whereas others are formulated to replace specific body fluids. Each manufacturer usually affixes its own trade name to these solutions, making it necessary to refer to the label to review the specific content. It is common to refer to these fluids by the number of cations in the solution. For example, a liter of electrolyte #48 contains 25 mEq sodium, 20 mEq potassium, and 3 mEq calcium; and a liter of electrolyte #75 contains 40 mEq sodium and 35 mEq potassium. Of course, each solution must contain an equal number of anions; in the case of these two fluids, it is a varying combination of chloride, phosphate, and a bicarbonate precursor.

POTASSIUM SOLUTIONS

Premixed potassium-replacement solutions are available in a variety of strengths furnishing from 10 to 40 mEq potassium per liter. Concentrated potassium solutions are available in ampules for addition to parenteral fluids (such as D_5W, 0.9% NaCl, or 0.45% NaCl). Of course, concentrated solutions from ampules are *not* meant for direct IV injection because they would cause fatal cardiac arrhythmias. See Clinical Tip: Nursing Considerations in Administering Potassium Intravenously in Chapter 5 for a list of critical points in administering potassium IV.

MAGNESIUM ADMINISTRATION

Magnesium is not present in most routine IV solutions. However, it is found in some of the commercially available balanced electrolyte solutions (see Table 10-1). Magnesium is also available in concentrated form in ampules for addition to parenteral fluids when deemed necessary. Refer to Clinical Tip: Nursing Considerations in Administering IV Magnesium in Chapter 7 for a review of nursing considerations in administering IV magnesium solutions.

CALCIUM ADMINISTRATION

Calcium is not present in most routine IV solutions; however, it is found in some balanced electrolyte solutions (see Table 10-1). Calcium is also available in concentrated form in ampules for addition to parenteral fluids as deemed necessary. Refer to the Clinical Tips in Chapter 6 for a review of nursing considerations in administering IV calcium solutions.

SOLUTIONS TO CORRECT ACID–BASE DISORDERS

Alkalinizing Solutions

Alkalinizing solutions (such as sodium lactate or sodium bicarbonate) are available to correct severe metabolic acidosis. Sodium bicarbonate is available as a 5% solution, furnishing 595 mEq/L each of sodium and bicarbonate.[12] Some clinicians elect to mix their own solutions by adding a concentrated $NaHCO_3$ solution (44.6 mEq/50-mL ampule) to existing parenteral fluids. Sodium bicarbonate should not be added to lactated Ringer's solution or any other calcium-containing fluid because calcium and bicarbonate combine to form the insoluble salt, calcium chloride.[13] As described in Chapter 9, controversy exists about when bicarbonate replacement is indicated in the treatment of acidosis. However, because severe acidosis can cause myocardial depression, it is generally considered prudent to keep the blood pH above 7.1 to 7.2.[14] Bicarbonate therapy must be instituted cautiously because

overalkalinization can induce tetany, seizures, and cardiac arrhythmias. The use of sodium bicarbonate during cardiorespiratory arrest is discussed in Chapter 16.

Acidifying Solutions

When metabolic alkalosis is due to chloride deficiency, the use of isotonic saline (0.9% NaCl) may suffice as treatment. If hypokalemia is a contributing factor, the administration of potassium chloride is indicated.

If sodium chloride and potassium chloride solutions are unable to correct the metabolic alkalosis, consideration is given to using ammonium chloride (NH_4Cl) as an acidifying salt. However, NH_4Cl should be avoided in patients with impaired hepatic function because it might cause hepatic coma.[15] Frequent monitoring of blood gases, pH, and serum electrolytes is indicated for patients receiving treatment for severe alkalosis.

⬤ COLLOIDS

In addition to the water and electrolyte solutions described previously, occasionally patients with fluid and electrolyte disturbances may require treatment with colloids. Colloid solutions contain substances of high molecular weight that do not readily migrate across capillary walls.[16] By increasing the osmotic pressure within the bloodstream, colloids draw fluid in from other compartments to increase the vascular volume. Examples of colloids are albumin, hetastarch, and dextran.

ALBUMIN

Albumin provides about 80% of the plasma colloid osmotic pressure (COP) in healthy adults. Albumin for therapeutic uses is prepared from donor plasma; there is no risk for hepatitis with albumin or any known risk for AIDS.[17] Normal human serum albumin (NHSA) is available as either 5% or 25% solutions. Five percent albumin solution is osmotically and oncotically equivalent to plasma; 25% albumin solution is hyperoncotic. The sodium content of albumin preparations is 145 ± 15 mEq/L.

The major clinical use of albumin is as a plasma volume expander in the treatment of shock caused by blood or plasma loss. Both 25% albumin (100 mL) and 5% albumin (500 mL) preparations cause the intravascular volume to expand by an equivalent amount

(400–500 mL).[18] The use of the 25% albumin is particularly helpful in patients with clinical evidence of both edema and hypovolemia.

Albumin may be useful in treating burns and third-space fluid shifts caused by acute peritonitis, intestinal obstruction, or radical surgical procedures. It is also prescribed for acute volume depletion associated with paracentesis, dialysis, or overaggressive diuresis in patients with chronic diseases such as cirrhosis and nephrotic syndrome.

Albumin will not correct chronic hypoalbuminemia caused by malnutrition, cirrhosis, or nephrotic syndrome and should not be used for this purpose. In these situations, the decreased albumin level reflects basic underlying problems that need to be corrected. Using albumin as a source of nutritional protein is not only inefficient, it is expensive; nutritional repletion is best accomplished with parenteral fluids designed for this purpose (see Chap. 11). Also, the only use for albumin in wound healing may be to reduce peripheral edema in a hypoproteinemic patient.

Albumin costs about 30 times more than crystalloid solutions; therefore, unless specifically needed, albumin is less likely to be used. The ability of albumin to remain in the vascular space is also a consideration. For example, colloid use during capillary leak (as occurs in burns, intestinal obstruction, sepsis, or adult respiratory distress syndrome [ARDS]) should be minimized until the capillary leak has been resolved.[19] In patients with burns and intestinal obstruction, the capillary integrity is restored in about 24 hours; however, in sepsis or ARDS, the "leak" may persist for longer periods.

Reported side effects of albumin include urticaria, flushing, chills, fever, headache, and circulatory overload with pulmonary edema (with rapid infusion).[20] Albumin should be used with caution in patients likely to develop fluid overload.

HETASTARCH AND DEXTRAN

Other colloid substitutes used for volume expansion include hetastarch (Hespan) and dextran. These substances are not derived from donor plasma and, therefore, are free of the risk of transfusion-related diseases.

Hetastarch

Hetastarch is a synthetic colloid made from starch and is available as 6% hetastarch in 0.9% NaCl. Its ability to expand the plasma volume is similar to that of a 5% albumin solution; yet, it is less expensive than albumin, making it an appealing colloid preparation.[21] Like albumin, it is not a substitute for blood or plasma.

Hetastarch can be used to expand the plasma volume in patients with shock from hemorrhage, trauma, burns, and sepsis. For the treatment of hemorrhagic shock, hetastarch solution may be given at a rate of 20 mL/kg/hr; slower rates are generally used for patients with burns or septic shock.[22] The typical dose in an adult to expand the plasma volume is 500 to 1,000 mL; however, the required dose and rate of infusion depend on the amount of blood or plasma lost as well as other clinical factors. Doses of more than 1,500 mL/day for a typical 70-kg adult are usually not required.[23]

The IV administration of hetastarch results in plasma volume expansion that decreases over the succeeding 24 to 36 hours.[24] Elimination of hetastarch is hepatic and renal. Therefore, caution should be observed before administering hetastarch to patients with a history of liver disease; also, hetastarch should not be used in patients with renal disease with oliguria or anuria that is not related to hypovolemia.[25] It is sometimes used to initially expand the plasma volume of patients with severe renal impairment; however, these patients are observed especially carefully for volume overload.

Because hetastarch causes osmotic diuresis, urinary volume should not be used as a gauge for the adequacy of intravascular volume replacement. The increased urine volume must not be misinterpreted as a sign of adequate tissue perfusion in this situation.[26]

Mild and transient coagulopathies have been observed after resuscitation with hetastarch.[27] Also, anaphylactoid reactions have been reported with the use of hetastarch.[28] Because serum amylase levels will rise after hetastarch infusion, blood for serum amylase testing should be drawn before initiation of the infusion. The elevated serum amylase does not indicate pancreatitis.

Dextran

Dextrans are polysaccharides that approximate the colloidal activity of albumin when given IV; they are available as low molecular weight dextran (dextran 40) and high molecular weight dextran (dextran 70). Besides its indications for expanding plasma volume, it is used for prevention of thromboembolism and promotion of peripheral perfusion.[29] Dextran is associated with greater risk of anaphylaxis than is hetastarch or albumin.[30]

Dextran can impair blood coagulation and interfere with blood crossmatching.[31] For these reasons, use of dextran 70 for fluid resuscitation has gradually been declining over recent years.[32,33] If it is necessary to draw blood for typing and crossmatching, it should be done before dextran is started.

CRYSTALLOID VERSUS COLLOID RESUSCITATION

For a variety of conditions, both crystalloids and colloids are widely used in clinical practice. The debate regarding which is superior in a given situation is likely to continue because clinical evidence supports the use of both types of fluids. A recently published study that analyzed 37 randomized controlled trials of the use of colloids compared with crystalloids for volume replacement in critically ill patients found no evidence of differences in mortality between the two groups.[34] However, other similar studies have indicated that significant differences do occur; for example, one concluded that crystalloid is superior to colloid for resuscitation after trauma in human beings (causing a 12% reduction in mortality after crystalloid infusion).[35] No consensus has been reached as to which type of resuscitation is superior in a given situation.

Proponents of crystalloids (primarily lactated Ringer's solution and isotonic saline) point to their quick availability and low cost and the fact that they are reaction free. These investigators also point out that clinical trials have shown these fluids are effective plasma volume expanders in a wide range of conditions. Because only a fraction of the volume of isotonic crystalloid solutions administered IV remains in the intravascular space by the end of 1 hour, it is customary to administer at least three times the amount of crystalloid solution as the estimated blood volume lost. A rough guideline for the total amount of crystalloid volume acutely required is 3 mL crystalloid solution for each 1 mL of blood loss.[36] The major part of the administered crystalloid solution shifts into the interstitial space, causing interstitial fluid expansion. Some clinicians worry that expansion of lung ECF can lead

to pulmonary edema; however, several clinical studies do not support this concern.[37] For example, one group found no differences in extravascular lung water either immediately after operation or 1 to 2 days later in 19 aortic surgical patients randomized to either balanced salt solution or colloid resuscitation.[38]

Proponents of colloids argue that a good clinical response can be accomplished with less fluid volume, resulting in less accumulation of edema fluid. This is because colloids remain in the bloodstream longer and pull fluid in from the interstitial space to expand the intravascular volume. A study reported by Hankeln et al.[39] confirmed that substantially more fluid was required to achieve hemodynamic stability when crystalloids (versus colloids) were used in critically ill patients; however, there did not appear to be any measurable difference in the development of pulmonary edema or other complications between the two groups. Potential problems cited as being associated with colloids include their greater expense and their possibilities for binding with ionized fraction of serum calcium and decreasing the circulating levels of immunoglobulins.[40]

Because advantages and disadvantages are associated with both types of resuscitation, the question becomes one of which type is best in a given situation. Generally, the choice of fluids should be guided by considering the urgency and pathophysiology of the condition requiring fluid resuscitation.[41] It is helpful to review some common clinical conditions to compare the efficacy of both crystalloids and colloids.

HEMORRHAGIC SHOCK

In general, it is common practice to initiate the replacement of blood loss with crystalloid fluids (either lactated Ringer's solution or isotonic saline). If hemodynamic stability returns and the hematocrit remains above 30%, further aggressive therapy may not be needed.[42] If stability does not return, consideration is given to adding a colloid (such as 5% serum albumin or an equivalent colloid solution) to the regimen.[43] Of course, blood replacement is needed if the oxygen-carrying capacity of the patient's blood is severely diminished.

For the treatment of hemorrhage, resuscitation with crystalloids (isotonic saline and lactated Ringer's solution) is prudent and of proved efficacy.[44] It is important to note that there is no place for salt-free crystalloid solutions (plain dextrose in water) in resuscitation of acutely hypovolemic patients.[45] Lactated Ringer's solution and normal saline are readily available and are commonly administered while blood is being crossmatched. These solutions can limit the total amount of blood eventually needed for patients with major blood loss. As a rule, several liters are administered quickly while the patient's clinical status is further assessed. How much more is needed depends on the patient's response to the fluids as well as the hematocrit level. Large volumes of crystalloids may ultimately be required to maintain peripheral perfusion (as evidenced by a mean arterial pressure between 70 and 80 mm Hg, a heart rate < 100 beats/min, warm extremities with good capillary refill, adequate central nervous system function, a urine output between 0.5 and 1 ml/kg/hr, and the absence of increasing lactic acidosis).[46] The visible edema that will develop as a major portion of the infused fluid shifts into the interstitial space should not be used as an indicator of adequate intravascular volume expansion. Refer to Chapter 15 for a more thorough discussion of fluid resuscitation in hemorrhagic shock.

ADULT RESPIRATORY DISTRESS SYNDROME

The adult respiratory distress syndrome (ARDS) refers to an acute lung injury that can be caused by a variety of insults. Significant risk factors are sepsis, aspiration of gastric contents, major trauma, and drug overdose.[47] Shock is associated with loss of capillary wall integrity, resulting in "capillary leak." This is especially problematic in the lung because of the subsequent development of ARDS. In ARDS, the increased vascular permeability to large molecular weight proteins results in pulmonary edema. Invasive monitoring with a pulmonary artery catheter is helpful in guiding the clinician in maintaining the lowest intravascular volume that is compatible with adequate tissue perfusion.

Considerably differing thoughts exist regarding which fluid is superior in resuscitating patients with ARDS. Those who favor crystalloids believe that the use of colloids is counterproductive because the colloids "leak" through the damaged pulmonary capillaries into the pulmonary interstitium. Those who favor colloids believe that the sometimes massive volumes of crystalloids needed to achieve adequate tissue perfusion add to the pulmonary edema. Although it is known that crystalloids dilute the plasma oncotic pressure, it is debatable whether this decreases lung function. It appears that neither crystalloids nor currently available colloids have any preferential effects to minimize edema in patients with ARDS.[48] It seems that the development of ARDS is more related to the presence of sepsis than to the type of fluid used in shock resuscitation.[49]

OTHER CONDITIONS

Neither colloids nor crystalloids are superior in the treatment of sepsis because the use of both can be supported in the literature.[50] Colloids may have a greater role than crystalloids in managing patients with burns, anaphylaxis, and venom injuries.[15] Patients with burns, peritonitis, and pancreatitis may need colloid replacement early.[52]

● FLUID AND ELECTROLYTE DISTURBANCES ASSOCIATED WITH BLOOD TRANSFUSIONS

Principal indications for blood transfusion are to correct the diminished oxygen-carrying capacity of the blood, to replace hemostatic components, or to replenish or expand the circulating intravascular volume. Although blood transfusion can be lifesaving when indicated, it should not be undertaken lightly because there are a number of inherent risks with the transfusion process. Among these are immune-mediated reactions to the transfused substances, infections (such as malaria, hepatitis, and acquired immunodeficiency syndrome), and fluid/electrolyte/acid–base disturbances. Only the electrolyte/acid–base disturbances are discussed in this chapter.

Chemical and physical changes in blood are caused by preservatives and prolonged storage. These changes in stored blood can cause electrolyte problems and other related complications.

HYPERKALEMIA

Continual destruction of red blood cells occurs when blood is stored, perhaps reaching a concentration as great as 25 mEq/L after 21 days.[53] Potassium is released from the destroyed red blood cells and is also transferred from intact red blood cells into the surrounding plasma. This leakage of potassium is related to loss of cell membrane integrity resulting from hypoxia. When the stored blood is infused into the recipient, the blood cells are reoxygenated and take up the leaked potassium; however, before this occurs, transient hyperkalemia can develop if blood administration is extremely rapid.

Although hyperkalemia associated with even rapid transfusion is rarely a problem, it has the potential to be very serious. Hyperkalemia is accentuated in patients with metabolic acidosis, renal dysfunction, or both. Hypocalcemia, if also present, decreases cardiac tolerance to the hyperkalemia and increases the risk for arrhythmias.[54] Fatal hyperkalemia has been reported with as little as 2 units of blood administered over a 1-hour period.[55] In situations where hyperkalemia may be of concern (as in neonates or in patients with renal failure), fresher units of blood (<10 days old) or washed cells should be used.[56] Twenty-four hours after massive transfusion, hypokalemia can occur as the red blood cells are reoxygenated and take up potassium from the plasma.[57]

HYPOCALCEMIA

Citrate-phosphate-dextrose (CPD)-preserved bank blood contains excessive amounts of citrate ions. In some situations, the excess citrate may combine with ionized calcium in the recipient's blood, producing a deficiency of ionized calcium. (Recall that it is ionized calcium that controls neuromuscular irritability.) However, the excess citrate usually causes no difficulty because the liver rapidly converts it to bicarbonate. Another safeguard to protect the body from hypocalcemia is the rapid mobilization of calcium from bone when needed.

Citrate-induced decreases in calcium ionization are usually transient and cause no hemodynamic effect in most patients receiving blood transfusions.[58] For example, in a study of 100 patients who received blood during a variety of surgical procedures, only 1 patient developed cardiovascular problems related to hypocalcemia, although 10% of the patients had ionized calcium levels below 2 mg/dL.[59] The accumulation of citrate (with resultant decrease in ionized calcium) is most likely in hypothermic and shock patients receiving massive

transfusions; a rapid fall in the ionized calcium level can cause impaired cardiovascular function, muscle tremors, and changes in the electrocardiogram.[60]

Current recommendations suggest administering calcium only to patients in whom symptomatic hypocalcemia develops.[61] Calcium chloride or calcium gluconate may be administered IV as needed. Because infusions of calcium can be associated with ventricular dysrhythmias, it should not be used indiscriminately.[62]

Although the overall incidence of transfusion-related hypocalcemia is thought to be quite small, certain patients are at increased risk. Most liver transplant patients are anhepatic for part of the surgical procedure and thus cannot metabolize the citrate they receive in blood transfusions during this time.[63] In such patients, calcium supplementation may be needed to prevent decreased ventricular function and hypotension.[64]

Hemodynamic parameters remain stable in most patients with transfusion-related hypocalcemia; however, in patients with underlying cardiac problems, there is increased risk for complications such as hypotension or heart failure. This group of patients may require calcium replacement therapy.[65]

ACID–BASE CHANGES

The pH of 2-week-old bank blood decreases to about 6.5 (due to leakage of lactate and pyruvate into the plasma as a result of red cell hypoxia during storage).[66] Because banked blood is acidic, a metabolic acidosis is expected to occur in the massively transfused recipient.[67] Historically, this led to the prophylactic administration of bicarbonate to patients who received massive blood transfusions. However, this practice was detrimental, often leading to a more severe metabolic alkalosis.[68] Now, it is considered prudent to monitor the arterial blood pH and correct metabolic defects as they are discovered. Because it is more likely that the acidosis seen in massively transfused patients is due to hypoxemia and poor tissue perfusion than it is to the blood itself, the key is to provide adequate volume restoration and perfusion (which will correct any transient acidosis).[69,70]

Although an initial metabolic acidosis may occur during rapid transfusion, metabolic alkalosis may eventually result due to metabolism of citrate to bicarbonate. This is because blood is stored in a solution containing citrate (which eventually is converted to bicarbonate by the liver). Although patients with normal renal function can readily excrete the excess bicarbonate load, those who require large volumes of blood usually also have decreased renal perfusion due to decreased intravascular volume. Thus, patients requiring massive transfusions may have impaired ability to excrete bicarbonate through the kidneys.[71] Also, the presence of renal failure reduces the patient's ability to excrete the excess alkali load. In addition to metabolic alkalosis, patients requiring massive transfusions may develop respiratory alkalosis. This is because of a combination of catecholamine release, hypoxemia, and noncardiogenic pulmonary edema.[72]

HYPERAMMONEMIA

Ammonia concentration in stored blood begins to rise after 5 to 7 days and reaches high levels after 2 to 3 weeks of storage.[73] Healthy patients can tolerate the extra ammonia with no difficulty; however, the ammonia content in stored blood may be of concern in patients with liver failure who require large amounts of blood. Washed cells can be considered as an alternative

to stored blood, although there is no documented advantage to giving washed cells.[74]

FLUID VOLUME OVERLOAD

Fluid volume overload and congestive heart failure are frequent complications of blood transfusions. The onset of circulatory overload is usually gradual, with symptoms becoming more severe as the transfusion continues. Symptoms include cough, shortness of breath, neck vein distention, and pulmonary congestion. Many physicians request hemodynamic monitoring during rapid blood administration. (See procedures for hemodynamic monitoring in Chap. 2.) Individuals with compromised cardiovascular status should be monitored especially closely for fluid volume overload. Packed red blood cells are frequently used for such patients to reduce the volume of the infusion (recall that packed cells are obtained by centrifuging whole blood and drawing off 200–225 mL plasma). Although packed red cells have a reduced plasma volume, it is necessary to use a slow infusion rate for high-risk patients.

REFERENCES

1. Carey C, Lee H, Woeltje K. *The Washington Manual of Medical Therapeutics*, 29th ed. Philadelphia: Lippincott-Raven; 1998:39.
2. Ibid.
3. Narins R, ed. *Clinical Disorders of Fluid and Electrolyte Metabolism*, 5th ed. New York: McGraw-Hill; 1994:1466.
4. Smith E. *Fluids and Electrolytes: A Conceptual Approach*, 2nd ed. New York: Churchill Livingstone; 1991:151.
5. Chernow B, ed. *The Pharmacologic Approach to the Critically Ill Patient*, 3rd ed. Baltimore, MD: Williams & Wilkins; 1994:274.
6. Ibid, p 276.
7. Ibid, p 277.
8. Schwartz S, Shires T, Spencer F, et al. *Principles of Surgery*, 7th ed. New York: McGraw-Hill; 1999:108.
9. Ibid.
10. Ibid, p 107.
11. Healey MA et al. Lactated Ringer's is superior to normal saline in a model of massive hemorrhage and resuscitation. *J Trauma* 1998;45:894.
12. Rose B. *Clinical Physiology of Acid-Base and Electrolyte Disorders*, 4th ed. New York: McGraw-Hill; 1994:405.
13. Ibid, p 406.
14. Chernow, p 965.
15. Condon R, Nyhus L. *Manual of Surgical Therapeutics*, 9th ed. Boston: Little, Brown; 1996:191.
16. Doherty G, Baumann D, Creswell L, et al. *The Washington Manual of Surgery*. Boston: Little, Brown; 1997:46.
17. Chernow, p 280.
18. Doherty G et al, p 46.
19. Chernow, p 281.
20. Shannon M et al. *Appleton & Lange's 1999 Drug Guide*. Stamford, CT: Appleton & Lange; 1999:1019.
21. Doherty, p 47.
22. Ibid.
23. *Physician's Desk Reference*, 53rd ed. Montvalek, NJ: Medical Economics; 1999:934.
24. Ibid, p 933.
25. Ibid, p 934.
26. Doherty, p 47.
27. Schwartz et al, p 108.
28. *Physician's Desk Reference*, p 934.
29. Doherty, p 46.
30. Schwartz et al, p 109.
31. Doherty, p 46.
32. Bapat P, Raine G. Fluid resuscitation with colloid or crystalloid solutions: Use of dextran-70 for fluid resuscitation has been dying out (letter). *BMJ* 1998;31(7153):27.
33. Tierney L, McPhee S, Papadakis M. *Current Medical Diagnosis & Treatment*, 38th ed. Stamford, CT: Appleton & Lange, 1999.
34. Schierhout G, Roberts I. Fluid resuscitation with colloid or crystalloid solutions in critically ill patients: A systematic review of randomized trials. *BMJ* 1998;316(7136):961.
35. Velanovich V. Crystalloid versus colloid fluid resuscitation: A meta-analysis of mortality. *Surgery* 1989;105:65.

36. *Advanced Trauma Life Support*[R] *Program for Doctors*, 6th ed. American College of Surgeons Committee on Trauma; 1997.
37. Schwartz et al, p 107.
38. Shires GT III, Peitzman AB, et al. Response of intraoperative lung water to intraoperative fluids. *Ann Surg* 1983;197:515.
39. Hankeln K et al. Comparison of hydroxyethyl starch and lactated Ringer's solution on hemodynamics and oxygen transport of critically ill patients in prospective crossover studies. *Crit Care Med* 1989;17:133.
40. Schwartz et al, p 107.
41. Narins, p 1469.
42. Doherty, p 47.
43. Ibid.
44. Narins, p 1469.
45. Condon, Nyhus, p 6.
46. Chernow, p 275.
47. Chernow, p 281.
48. Narins, p 1469.
49. Chernow, p 274.
50. Narins, p 1469.
51. Ibid, p 1470.
52. Condon, Nyhus, p 6.
53. Ibid, p 264 .
54. Narins, p 708.
55. Ibid.
56. Condon, Nyhus, p 264.
57. Carey et al, p 374.
58. Chernow, p 778.
59. Howland W et al. Factors influencing the ionization of calcium during major surgical procedures. *Surg Gynecol Obstet* 1976; 58:274.
60. Wilson R et al. Electrolyte and acid-base changes with massive blood transfusions. *Am Surg* 1992;58:535.
61. Condon, Nyhus, p 264.
62. Ibid.
63. Chernow, p 335.
64. Ibid.
65. Narins, p 1484.
66. Condon, Nyhus, p 264.
67. Chernow, p 335.
68. Condon, Nyhus, p 264.
69. Chernow, p 335.
70. Condon, Nyhus, p 264.
71. Narins, p 999.
72. Ibid.
73. Condon, Nyhus, p 264.
74. Ibid.

Parenteral Nutrition

This chapter reviews the effects of parenteral nutrition on fluid and electrolyte balance and describes the nurse's role in caring for patients with imbalances and other metabolic abnormalities caused by this treatment.

INDICATIONS FOR PARENTERAL NUTRITION

Clinicians generally agree that "when the gut works, use it."[1] That is, if gastrointestinal function is present, enteral feedings should be favored over parenteral nutrition. Aside from being less expensive, benefits of enteral feedings compared with parenteral nutrition include better preservation of both immune function and intestinal function.[2] Despite the preference for enteral feedings, however, certain patients require parenteral nutrition because they are unable to meet their nutritional needs by the gastrointestinal tract. Candidates for parenteral nutrition include patients with inadequate small bowel surface area to absorb nutrients (as in massive small bowel resection or severe radiation enteritis) and those in need of temporary "bowel rest" during recovery from a primary gastrointestinal disease condition. Others who may benefit from parenteral nutrition include those who are unable to consume or use sufficient enteral calories to meet their total nutritional needs.

PERIPHERAL PARENTERAL NUTRITION

Occasionally patients need parenteral nutrition support for only a relatively short period of time, making it impractical to access a central vein. Some clinicians have reported success in providing nutrients through peripheral parenteral nutrition (PPN) to a number of patients.[3] Others believe that few patients who need nutrition support meet the criteria for PPN (such as good peripheral veins, relatively low energy and protein needs, and tolerance for relatively large volumes of fluid).[4] The typical PPN solution consists of 5% to 10% glucose, 2% to 5% amino acids, and variable quantities of electrolytes (according to individual need). Fat emulsions are sometimes mixed with the other nutrients; other times they are piggybacked simultaneously.

Candidates for PPN should have good peripheral veins. Even then, because of the high osmolality of the PPN solution, phlebitis at the infusion site will eventually occur. The onset of this complication may be slowed by decreasing the nutrient density of the formula or by decreasing its flow rate. Unfortunately, these maneuvers also decrease the caloric intake. PPN usually involves daily resiting of the cannula as a prophylactic measure to avoid phlebitis.[5] Because of this, venous access eventually becomes difficult.[6] A study of the incidence and severity of infusion phlebitis with PPN in 142 surgical patients found that the administration of an "all-in-one" solution (dextrose, amino acids, and fat emulsions) resulted in significantly less phlebitis than when the PPN was administered in separate containers (with the fat emulsion piggybacked into the infusion site of the glucose and amino acid solution).[7]

The large fluid volume needed for PPN as the sole source of calories limits its use to patients requiring only short-term support (such as 5–7 days). Usually, PPN is used to supplement the nutrient intake of patients who are consuming inadequate nutrients orally or by tube feeding.[8]

TOTAL PARENTERAL NUTRITION FOR CENTRAL ADMINISTRATION

SITE AND DETERMINATION OF NUTRIENT NEEDS

When prolonged parenteral nutritional support is needed, a central vein is the necessary delivery site. Delivery of the solution into the superior vena cava can be accomplished by introducing a central venous catheter through a subclavian vein. Most formulations for total parenteral nutrition (TPN) have an osmolality of 1,800 mOsm/L or greater; fortunately, because the vena cava has a high rate of blood flow, the solution is rapidly diluted and is not harmful to the vessel.[9] Before TPN is initiated, the patient's caloric need is calculated and the appropriate percentage of macronutrients (dextrose, protein, and fat) as well as electrolytes and vitamin needs are determined. Caloric intake is based on actual weight unless the patient is more than 120% of ideal body weight; beyond 40 kcal/kg/day, the excess calories may be a stress to the patient and lead to CO_2 retention and fatty infiltration of the liver.[10] Daily weights are measured; weight gain as lean body mass occurs at a maximum rate of ¼ to ½ lb/day; any increase beyond this value is either as fat or water.[11] Modifications in the TPN formulation are made as needed.

TOTAL PARENTERAL NUTRITION SOLUTION

Nutrients available for TPN infusion include amino acids (protein), glucose (carbohydrate), and fat emulsions. The traditional TPN formula contains 25% dextrose, 4.25% to 5.0% amino acids, as well as electrolytes, vitamins, and trace elements.[12] However, for some patients with limited fluid tolerance, there are more concentrated solutions. The most concentrated intravenous (IV) nutrients available commercially are 70% dextrose in water, 15% amino acid solution, and 20% fat emulsion.[13] The desired proportions of these nutrients are prepared by a pharmacist under a laminar-flow hood to maintain strict sterility.

Dextrose

Dextrose (glucose) is the primary carbohydrate used in parenteral nutrition solutions. The dextrose used in parenteral nutrition solutions furnishes 3.4 kcal/g (Table 11-1). Glucose is the carbohydrate of choice for TPN because it is readily metabolized by all tissues, stimulates secretion of the anabolic hormone insulin,

and usually, is well tolerated in large quantities.[14] Generally, dextrose is used to provide 40% to 65% of the caloric requirement.[15] By furnishing nonprotein calories, glucose allows more efficient use of the infused amino acids.

Recall that CO_2 is an end product of carbohydrate metabolism. Thus, when CO_2 retention is a problem, excessive carbohydrate administration can lead to respiratory acidosis. For example, Covelli et al.[16] observed a rise in $PaCO_2$ within 12 hours after TPN was initiated in a patient maintained on a fixed mechanical ventilator setting; the $PaCO_2$ rose from 43 to 93 mm Hg and the serum pH fell from 7.4 to 7.25 within 24 hours after the carbohydrate intake was increased from 1,500 to 2,500 kcal/day. To minimize excessive CO_2 production, an effort is made to avoid administering excessive calories (particularly in the form of glucose) to patients at risk for hypercapnia (excessive $PaCO_2$).[17]

Amino Acids

Crystalline amino acids are the source of proteins for IV administration. In addition to standard amino acid solutions, special amino acid formulations contain higher essential amino acids (for patients with renal failure) and more branched-chain amino acids (for patients with liver failure). However, the diagnosis of a specific disease does not necessitate the use of a specialty product in all instances. For example, patients with chronic stable renal failure without dialysis may benefit from a solution with a higher proportion of essential amino acids to prevent worsening of uremia while promoting positive nitrogen balance. However, when dialysis is initiated, standard amino acid solutions can be used.[18]

Fat

Fat emulsions made from soybean or safflower oil are available as 10% and 20% emulsions providing 1.1 and 2.0 kcal/mL, respectively.[19] The only advantage of a 20% emulsion is its lower fluid volume for a given caloric yield. Fat emulsions can be delivered via piggyback or as part of a "three-in-one" mixture (depending on the TPN formulation). Patients with diabetes may require a higher percentage of fat calories to prevent hyperglycemia and patients with respiratory failure may require more fat (and less glucose) calories to minimize CO_2 production. The latter is particularly important when attempting to wean patients off ventilators.

TABLE 11-1. Caloric Content and Osmolality of Selected Dextrose Solutions*

Dextrose Concentration	Dextrose		
	g/L	Kcal/L	Osmolality/L
5%	50	170	252
10%	100	340	505
15%	150	510	758
20%	200	680	1,010
25%	250	850	1,263
30%	300	1,020	1,515

*Each gram of dextrose provides 3.4 kcal.

Electrolytes

Electrolyte requirements vary greatly among patients, and even for an individual patient during a course of TPN therapy.[20] For example, potassium requirements are affected by the level of cellular flux associated with reversal of the catabolic state, the level of metabolic stress (being higher when stress is high), the amount of potassium lost by abnormal routes (such as diarrhea), as well as various medications that affect potassium balance (see Table 5-1). Because of the numerous factors affecting electrolyte requirements, it is necessary to closely monitor the serum electrolytes until they are stable; daily electrolyte supplementation is guided by these results.

Despite the variations in electrolyte requirements, each institution typically provides a preprinted order sheet for standard TPN formulations and usual additives. This is because most patients can tolerate relatively standard electrolyte solutions. In fact, it has been estimated that standard electrolyte solutions are suitable for 50% to 80% of patients receiving TPN.[21] One suggested range for electrolyte additives includes sodium, 60 to 80 mEq/day; potassium, 30 to 60 mEq/day; magnesium 8.1 to 20 mEq/day; calcium, 4.6 to 9.2 mEq/day; phosphate, 12 to 24 mmol/day; and chloride, 80 to 100 mEq/day.[22] However, daily requirements for these electrolytes can have wide ranges; for example, 50 to 250 mEq for sodium, 30 to 200 mEq for potassium, 50 to 250 mEq for chloride, 10 to 30 mEq for magnesium, 10 to 20 mEq for calcium, and 10 to 40 mEq for phosphorus.[23]

Acid–base balance is controlled by the amount of acetate (a bicarbonate precursor) and chloride included in the formulation. Acetate concentration is increased if metabolic acidosis correctable by acetate is present.[24] Conversely, if metabolic alkalosis is likely because of gastric fluid loss, more chloride may be added to the formulation.[25] Trace elements added include zinc, manganese, chromium, and selenium.[26] The need for zinc supplementation is greater when large zinc losses are occurring (as from diarrhea or ileostomy output).

Continuous Versus Cyclic Method

Continuous infusion is the most common method for delivering the TPN solution. When TPN is initiated, the rate is gradually increased until the caloric goal is achieved; then, the rate is maintained evenly over 24 hours. After it has been established that the patient is metabolically stable, a few select patients (such as those to receive home TPN) are eligible for cyclic infusion of the solution. With the cyclic method, the solution is infused for 8 to 12 hours and then is turned off for the remainder of the 24-hour period. The cyclic method frees the patient from the infusion for a major part of the day and allows for normal activities. In a report of 36 patients receiving home cyclic TPN through Broviac or Hickman catheters, 80% were able to return to work, school, or housekeeping activities, or at least to care for themselves unaided.[27]

⬤ METABOLIC DERANGEMENTS ASSOCIATED WITH TOTAL PARENTERAL NUTRITION

Virtually any metabolic disturbance may occur during TPN; however, the most common are hyperglycemia, hypophosphatemia, and hypokalemia.[28] Specific derangements are largely reflective of the patient's underlying disease state that can interfere with the ability to metabolize or excrete the infused nutrients (Table 11-2). Essentially, expected abnormalities fall into two categories. First, the addition of too little of an essential electrolyte or nutrient can result in a deficiency state; second, an excess of the electrolytes or nutrients in the parenteral solution may lead to toxicity when they exceed the body's normal metabolic and excretory capacity. Electrolyte abnormalities in patients receiving TPN are primarily detected by evaluating daily laboratory results. When detected early, the imbalance(s) can usually be rectified by altering the electrolyte composition of the formula. For this reason, it is customary to monitor serum electrolytes at least daily during early TPN and at less frequent, but regular, intervals thereafter. Of course, baseline electrolyte values should be obtained before the initiation of central TPN and serious abnormalities corrected before TPN is initiated.

Of great importance during TPN therapy are the major intracellular ions (potassium, phosphate, and
(text continues on page 198)

TABLE 11-2.   Summary of Selected Metabolic Disturbances Associated
With Total Parenteral Nutrition

Problem	Causes	Signs/Symptoms	Management
Hyperglycemia	Too rapid flow rate	Elevated blood sugar	Attempt made to maintain serum glucose < 200 mg/dL (preferably < 140 mg/dL) unless blood sugar is so labile that careful control carries high risk for hypoglycemia
	Increased production of stress hormones, as in sepsis or surgical trauma	Glucosuria Polyuria: Acute weight loss and other signs of fluid volume deficit are associated with severe polyuria	If insulin is needed, it is usually directly to the TPN solution. Less often, it is given SQ according to a sliding scale; if the patient is markedly fluid volume depleted, insulin should not be given SQ because of erratic absorption.
	Patients with diabetes mellitus at high risk		Stable patients who suddenly develop a blood sugar > 200 mg/dL, or who require increasing amounts of insulin, should be evaluated for sepsis or other stressors.
			Administration rate of TPN solution should be temporarily reduced if serum glucose is markedly elevated (such as > 350 mg/dL) and not advanced until < 200 mg/dL.
			If hyperglycemia has caused significant osmotic diuresis, fluid volume deficit must be corrected with appropriate electrolyte solutions.
			Management of nonketotic hyperglycemic hyperosmolar syndrome is described in Chapter 18.
			Prevention: • Initiate infusion slowly and increase gradually (*Example:* rate of a 35% dextrose solution might be initiated at 30 mL/hr/day and increased by the rate of 20 mL/hr/day until the desired flow rate is achieved. • Infuse via a volumetric infusion pump. • Monitor flow rate at least hourly. • If infusion rate falls behind, do not attempt to "catch up" by increasing the flow rate.

Continued

TABLE 11-2.   Summary of Selected Metabolic Disturbances Associated
With Total Parenteral Nutrition—*cont'd*

Problem	Causes	Signs/Symptoms	Management
Hypoglycemia	Sudden discontinuance of TPN solution	Diaphoresis Confusion Agitation	Bolus injection of dextrose; further managment determined by serum glucose and clinical response. Prevention: • Discontinue TPN gradually (over hours) when possible. If not possible, infuse a 5% or 10% dextrose solution at same rate as TPN for several hours. • Ensure adequate caloric intake by GI route before stopping TPN, if feasible.
Hypophosphatemia	Anabolism increases demand for intracellular phosphorus (if inadequate amount is provided in TPN solution, phosphorus is pulled from the extracellular fluid) Factors increasing risk are severe malnourishment and alcoholism	Paresthesias Muscle weakness Muscle pain and tenderness Mental changes	Provide adequate phosphorus in TPN solution; required amount is determined by serum phosphorus levels and clinical indicators. (See text for usual requirements.) Significant hypophosphatemia (<1 mg/dL) requires supplemental phosphorus in a separate IV line. Phosphate is supplied as either a sodium or a potassium salt; the most appropriate form is selected based on the patient's serum potassium concentration and state of renal function.
Hypokalemia	Anabolism increases demand for intracellular potassium	Fatigue Muscular weakness	Provide adequate potassium in TPN solution; required amount is determined by serum potassium levels and clinical indicators. (See text for usual requirements.)

⬤ TABLE 11-2.   Summary of Selected Metabolic Disturbances Associated
With Total Parenteral Nutrition—*cont'd*

Problem	Causes	Signs/Symptoms	Management
Hypokalemia —*cont'd*	Factors increasing risk are severe malnutrition, drugs such as amphotericin and furosemide, as well as loss of GI fluids	Decreased bowel motility Cardiac arrhythmias ECG changes	When hypokalemia is present, consider peripheral IV or oral route for immediate potassium replacement and then adjust potassium in TPN solution. Potassium replacement is described in Chapter 5.
Hypomag-nesemia	Anabolism increases demand for intracellular magnesium Factors increasing risk: alcoholism, drugs such as aminoglycosides and cisplatin, and loss of GI fluids	Increased reflexes Disorientation Cardiac arrhythmias	Provide adequate magnesium in TPN solution; required amount is determined by serum magnesium levels and clinical indicators. (See text for usual requirements.) Severe hypomagnesemia requires magnesium replacement via a separate IV line. Magnesium replacement is described in Chapter 7.
Hypercapnia (excessive PaCO$_2$)	Infusion of calories in excess of patient's need Infusion of TPN solution with a concentration (end-product of carbohydrate metabolism is CO$_2$ and water). Patients at increased risk are those with respiratory function.	Respiratory decompensation (increasing PaCO$_2$) Difficulty weaning from ventilator	If patient is being overfed, reduce caloric intake to tolerable level. Provide more calories as fat and reduce glucose concentration in TPN formula

ECG, electrocardiogram; GI, gastrointestinal; SQ, subcutaneous; TPN, total parenteral nutrition.

magnesium). During nutritional repletion, these ions, derived from the serum, are incorporated in newly synthesized cells. Failure to supplement these ions adequately can lead to hypophosphatemia, hypokalemia, and hypomagnesemia. The intracellular shift of these three electrolytes during nutritional support is referred to as the *refeeding syndrome.*[29]

PHOSPHATE IMBALANCES

Hypophosphatemia is probably the most common imbalance in patients receiving TPN. Although its incidence is only 0.5% to 3% in the general hospital population, it is as high as 31% in patients receiving specialized nutritional support.[30] Hypophosphatemia occurs as a result of new tissue synthesis and a shift of phosphate from the extracellular to the intracellular compartment.

The intracellular consumption of phosphate during protein synthesis may produce a striking deficit in the serum phosphate level if adequate phosphate supplements are not given. A report was recently published in which four patients with chronic renal failure developed significant hypophosphatemia 3 to 5 days after starting TPN.[31] Although one would normally expect to see an elevated phosphate level in patients in chronic renal failure, these individuals developed hypophosphatemia because insufficient phosphate supplementation was provided in the nutritional formula. Apparently a contributing factor in two of the patients was the administration of dextrose through continuous ambulatory peritoneal dialysis (CAPD). Another factor in two patients was the administration of insulin. Recall that the administration of glucose and insulin increases the uptake of phosphate by the cells.

To prevent refeeding hypophosphatemia, at-risk patients should be refed slowly, and phosphorus supplementation should be provided as indicated by frequent monitoring of the serum phosphate level.[32] Examples of those at high risk are severely malnourished patients and chronic alcoholics. To avoid precipitation of calcium phosphate, the amount of calcium and phosphate that can be added to a TPN mixture must be controlled. Significant hypophosphatemia (<1 mg/dL) should be corrected with supplemental phosphate in a separate IV. IV preparations containing either sodium phosphate or potassium phosphate are available and selection of

the most appropriate salt is based on the patient's serum potassium concentration and the state of renal function. Refer to Chapter 8 for a review of the severe metabolic abnormalities associated with hypophosphatemia.

Although rare, hyperphosphatemia is possible if excessive phosphate is added to the TPN solution (particularly in patients who have impaired renal ability to excrete phosphate). Hyperphosphatemia occurred in an obese septic patient whose TPN formulation unintentionally contained triple the amount of required phosphate.[33] Her serum phosphate concentration increased as a result to 3.02 mmol/L (normal 0.76–1.46 mmol/L). The hyperphosphatemia contributed to calcification of her subcutaneous arteries and resulted in widespread infarcts of the skin. Fortunately, the skin lesions gradually healed as her metabolic status improved. See Chapter 8 for a more detailed discussion of phosphorus imbalances.

POTASSIUM IMBALANCES

Potassium abnormalities are common in patients receiving TPN. Hypokalemia in patients receiving TPN can occur as a result of new tissue synthesis with shifts of potassium into the intracellular compartment. Likewise, increased catecholamines caused by the stress of illness or trauma will increase the cellular uptake of potassium.[34] If insufficient potassium is contained in the solution, a significant fall in the serum concentration may occur as early as 6 to 12 hours after beginning TPN.[35]

Serum potassium levels must be monitored closely during the initiation of TPN and the amount of potassium added to the TPN formula adjusted as necessary. Patients who receive insulin for hyperglycemia need to be monitored especially closely for hypokalemia because insulin facilitates transport of potassium into cells and further depresses the serum potassium concentration. (Refer to Chap. 5 for a review of the clinical signs of hypokalemia as well as its treatment.)

It has been recommended that patients receiving TPN whose serum potassium concentration and renal function are normal should receive 60 to 90 mEq potassium per day[36]; occasionally up to 200 mEq is needed per day.[37] Even patients with advanced renal failure who receive TPN usually require potassium, although in a reduced amount.[38] The actual amount needed is determined by serial monitoring of serum potassium levels.

Addition of too much potassium to the TPN solution, or large intake from other sources without cutting back the amount added to the solution, can lead to hyperkalemia (particularly in patients with impaired renal ability to excrete potassium). Hyperkalemia is more likely in patients receiving TPN who are not sufficiently anabolic to use the relatively high potassium load administered in the TPN solution. Tissue necrosis and systemic sepsis also predispose to hyperkalemia. See Chapter 5 for a more detailed discussion of potassium imbalances.

MAGNESIUM IMBALANCES

Hypomagnesemia is less common than hypophosphatemia or hypokalemia in patients receiving TPN. When it occurs, it is usually in patients who are chronic alcoholics, severely malnourished, receiving drugs associated with renal magnesium wasting (such as diuretics, amphotericin B, cisplatin, or cyclosporine),[39] or experiencing large losses of intestinal fluid. Other causes of hypomagnesemia as well as clinical signs are described in Chapter 7. Severe hypomagnesemia requires treatment with up to 100 mEq magnesium sulfate administered over 24 hours through a separate IV line.[40] Hypermagnesemia can occur if excessive magnesium is supplied in the parenteral formula of patients with renal failure.

The daily requirement for magnesium in patients receiving TPN has not been established and recommendations vary from 4 to 42 mEq/day.[41] In the absence of renal insufficiency, patients on TPN seem to tolerate 16 to 30 mEq magnesium per day.[42] See Chapter 7 for a more detailed discussion of magnesium imbalances.

SODIUM IMBALANCES

Hyponatremia is frequently noted and is most often due to the excessive administration of hypotonic fluid.[43]

For example, a young adult trauma patient receiving TPN became hyponatremic because of the daily administration of almost 3 liters of D_5W in a peripheral vein as a diluent for antimicrobial agents administered for sepsis.[44] Other possible causes of hyponatremia in TPN patients include the syndrome of inappropriate antidiuretic hormone secretion, congestive heart failure, cirrhosis, and adrenal insufficiency. Although hyponatremia is common, hypernatremia

occurs far less frequently. For example, Weinsier et al.[45] reported that a serum sodium level less than 125 mEq/L was present in 6% of the patients on TPN in their study; in contrast, there was only a 1% incidence of hypernatremia (serum sodium 160 mEq/L) in the same population. When hypernatremia occurs, it is caused by excessive water loss (as in fever or hyperventilation) or inadequate water intake.

Dilutional hyponatremia is usually managed by decreasing the fluid intake; if sodium intake is inadequate, additional sodium may be given. In contrast, when the problem is hypernatremia, the free water intake should be increased (either in the TPN solution or through another route). See Chapter 5 for a more thorough discussion of sodium imbalances.

FLUID VOLUME IMBALANCES

It is important to monitor patients receiving TPN for fluid volume problems. These can best be detected by maintaining good fluid intake and output records as well as body weight records. Some patients have difficulty tolerating the relatively large fluid load required for TPN; when this occurs, it may be necessary to switch to a more concentrated solution to decrease the fluid volume. Other patients may need additional fluids to meet their needs; this can be provided by increasing the water content in the formula.[46]

CALCIUM IMBALANCES

Because most patients receiving TPN are malnourished and thus have low serum albumin levels, it is likely that their total serum calcium levels will also be below normal. However, because ionization of calcium usually remains normal in hypoalbuminemic patients, this "hypocalcemia" is not physiologically significant and will not result in paresthesias or other signs of tetany. Other causes of hypocalcemia, such as hypomagnesemia, are discussed in Chapter 6. The usual TPN solution contains 5 to 10 mEq calcium per liter. A daily calcium supplement in TPN is needed to prevent bone demineralization. See Chapter 6 for a more thorough discussion of calcium imbalances.

Hypercalcemia can occur in patients receiving TPN for extended periods. Possible causes are metabolic bone disease associated with long-term TPN or the excessive infusion of calcium or vitamin A and D supplements. When hypercalcemia occurs, it is necessary to consider other causes, such as neoplasms or primary or secondary hyperparathyroidism.

HYPERGLYCEMIA

Hyperglycemia is one of the most common metabolic derangements caused by TPN. For example, one prospective study of 100 patients receiving TPN found that 47 patients had serum glucose concentrations greater than 300 mg/dL.[47] Hyperglycemia is more likely to occur in patients receiving more than the required number of calories. Of course, patients with diabetes mellitus are at higher risk. Common causes of hyperglycemia include too rapid or uneven administration of the high dextrose solution and increased levels of glucose-elevating stress hormones (associated with a number of illnesses and injury states). The development or worsening of a glucose intolerance may be a harbinger of sepsis or another complicating condition (such as myocardial infarction). Indeed, hyperglycemia may precede other signs of infection by 18 to 24 hours.[48] When hyperglycemia occurs despite careful management, the cause should be investigated carefully.

Uncontrolled hyperglycemia can lead to hyperosmotic hyperglycemic nonketotic syndrome (HHNS). Fortunately, due to frequent monitoring for glucosuria and hyperglycemia, this complication is less frequent than in the past. In a study of 200 patients receiving TPN, 6 patients developed HHNS; all had familial histories of diabetes mellitus and had negative water balance with hyperglycemia for several days preceding the development of the syndrome.[49] See Chapter 18 for a detailed discussion of HHNS and its management.

Prevention

To prevent hyperglycemia, infusion of the TPN solution must begin slowly and gradually be increased as tolerated. For example, for a patient receiving a 25% dextrose solution, on day 1 the rate might be 40 mL/hr for a total of 960 mL (40 mL X 24 hr). On day 2, the rate might be increased to 80 mL/hr (for a total of 1920 mL). On day 3 the rate might be increased to 120 mL/hr. An infusion pump should be used to ensure even flow of the solution at the correct rate. If the patient falls behind in TPN administration, the rate of infusion should not be abruptly increased to compensate for the deficiency. A common cause of transient hyperglycemia in patients on TPN is inadvertent rapid administration of the TPN solution due to equipment malfunction or operator error.

For patients receiving cyclic TPN, it is customary to begin with a reduced flow rate for 2 hours before initiating the full infusion rate and then to taper the rate of flow for 2 hours before discontinuance. This method is usually reserved for patients who are metabolically stable.

When patients receiving TPN are scheduled to have surgery for a major operation, orders should be clear about what to do with the infusion rate. Although physician preferences vary greatly, the rate of glucose infusion is usually decreased because patients often become less glucose tolerant when subjected to the major stress of surgery.

Detection

During TPN administration, the patient should be closely monitored for glucose intolerance, especially during the early days. In acute care settings, glucose tolerance is usually measured by checking capillary blood sugars every 6 to 8 hours. An attempt is made to maintain blood glucose levels at less than 200 mg/dL (preferably <140 mg/dL) unless the blood sugar level is so labile that careful control carries a high risk for hypoglycemia.[50] If the patient's renal threshold is known, it may be possible to monitor for hyperglycemia by checking urinary glucose content every 6 hours. Urinary glucose levels are not reliable for some patients. For example, patients with renal disease may have glucosuria despite normal blood glucose levels, or they may have high blood sugars and little or no glucosuria.[51]

Insulin Therapy

In the presence of hyperglycemia, it is usually necessary to administer insulin. Regimens vary somewhat but many centers favor adding regular insulin to the TPN solution to achieve more even blood sugar control. For example, mild or moderate hyperglycemia may be managed by adding 1 to 2.5 units regular insulin per 25 g glucose in the TPN solution; greater quantities may be needed for patients with more severe glucose intolerance.[52] Although variable levels of insulin adsorption to the parenteral fluid container and tubing have been demonstrated in laboratory settings, clinical experience has indicated that blood glucose concentrations can be controlled effectively by adding insulin to the TPN solution.

The administration rate of the TPN solution should be temporarily reduced if the serum glucose concentration is more than 350 mg/dL; the TPN administration rate should not be increased until the serum glucose level is less than 200 mg/dL.[53] If HHNS occurs, the TPN solution is stopped until the fluid volume deficit is corrected (usually with isotonic saline) and hyperglycemia is treated IV with low-dose insulin. Refer to Chapter 18 for a discussion of the treatment of HHNS.

HYPOGLYCEMIA

Hypoglycemia is always a possibility when exogenous insulin is supplied directly in the TPN solution or subcutaneously by sliding scale. Also, hypoglycemia is a possible complication of abrupt discontinuance of TPN (especially after the infusion rate has recently been increased, resulting in increased endogenous insulin production). Presumably, the high glucose infusion stimulates hyperinsulinism; abrupt discontinuance of the high glucose fluid may temporarily allow the serum glucose level to fall precipitously.

One study indicated that when TPN was stopped abruptly, serum insulin and glucose concentrations returned quickly to normal levels and no reactive hypoglycemia was observed.[54] The researchers reported that hypoglycemia only occurred when the rate of the TPN solution was transiently increased and then was abruptly stopped. Several other small studies have suggested that TPN can be discontinued abruptly without the risk of hypoglycemia.[55,56] In a study of 11 children who had TPN abruptly discontinued, 6 developed hypoglycemia (glucose concentration < 40 mg/dL) after abrupt discontinuation of the formula.[57] Many authorities believe that TPN solutions should be

tapered in all patients who receive 200 to 300 g or more of IV glucose per day.[58]

Clinically, there is rarely a reason to discontinue TPN abruptly. In most instances, an effort is made to ensure that adequate nutrients (ie, 75% of maintenance calories) are consumed by the enteral route before TPN is stopped. Even when quick discontinuance is needed, there is usually time to taper the solution's flow rate over several hours. If this is not possible, there is no risk and little cost involved in providing coverage with a 5% or 10% dextrose solution in a peripheral vein. For example, 10% dextrose in water may be ordered for 4 hours at the same rate the TPN solution was infusing when stopped.[59]

CASE STUDIES

● **11-1.**[60] A 45-year-old man was admitted for an elective resection of a large temporal arteriovenous malformation. Because of severe hemorrhage during the procedure, he required massive blood transfusions. He was mechanically ventilated but self-extubated himself on the first postoperative day; during this time, he suffered aspiration and required reintubation. He soon developed the adult respiratory distress syndrome (ARDS) and required high positive end-expiratory pressure and fraction of inspired oxygen to maintain adequate oxygenation. He also required chemical paralysis and sedation to minimize oxygen consumption and to control airway pressures. On the second postoperative day, TPN was started. The caloric intake was increased gradually and a low volume of enteral formula was started via a nasojejunal feeding tube. The total caloric intake from both routes was 3,370 kcal/day. The patient's ARDS became progressively more difficult to manage. Hypercapnea (PCO_2 ranged between 65 and 70 mm Hg) was present and was assumed to be due, at least in part, to overfeeding. TPN was discontinued and the enteral feeding was adjusted to deliver 1,440 kcal/day. Within 36 hours of these changes, the PCO_2 dropped to 43 mm Hg and other ventilatory parameters improved. Weekly indirect calorimetry was performed to guide adjustments in nutrient delivery. The ARDS gradually resolved and no further ventilatory support was required by the 59th postoperative day. The patient was discharged 5 weeks later.

COMMENTARY: This patient's high total caloric intake generated excess CO_2. This high production of CO_2, coupled with his lung pathology (ARDS), resulted in ineffective clearing of CO_2 and thus hypercapnea. Fortunately, recognition of overfeeding allowed this patient to ultimately recover.

Refer to Case Study 7-1 for an example of hypomagnesemia associated with TPN and to Case Study 8-1 for an example of hypophosphatemia associated with TPN.

REFERENCES

1. Kudsk K, Minard G. Enteral nutrition. In: Zaloga G. *Nutrition in Critical Care.* St. Louis: Mosby; 1994:331.
2. Heizer W, Holcombe B. Approach to the patient requiring nutritional supplementation. In: Yamada T, et al., eds. *Textbook of Gastroenterology,* vol 1, 2nd ed. Philadelphia: JB Lippincott; 1995:1077.
3. Payne-James J, Khawaji H. First choice for total parenteral nutrition: The peripheral route. *JPEN J Parenter Enteral Nutr* 1993;17:468.
4. Heizer, Holcombe, p 1071.
5. Taylor M. Total parenteral nutrition. Part 1. *Nursing Standard* 1994;8(23):25.
6. Andreoli T, Carpenter C, Bennett J, Plum F. *Cecil Essential of Medicine,* 4th ed. Philadelphia: WB Saunders; 1997:451.
7. Nordenstrom J et al. Peripheral parenteral nutrition: Effect of a standardized compounded mixture on infusion phlebitis. *Br J Surg* 1991;78:1391.
8. Nussbaum M, Fischer J. Parenteral nutrition. In: Zaloga G. *Nutrition in Critical Care.* St. Louis: CV Mosby; 1994.
9. Strausburg K. Parenteral nutrition admixture. *The ASPEN Nutrition Support Practice Manual.* Silver Springs, MD: American Society for Parenteral and Enteral Nutrition; 1998: 8-5.
10. Mirtallo J. TPN composition. Postgraduate Course I. Fundamentals I. Total Parenteral Nutrition. American Society for Parenteral and Enteral Nutrition, 19th Clinical Congress; 1995:52.
11. Ibid.
12. Nussbaum, Fischer, p 386.
13. Heizer, Holcombe, p 1072.
14. Inadomi D, Kopple J. Fluid and electrolyte disorders in total parenteral nutrition. In: Narins R, ed. *Clinical Disorders of Fluid and Electrolyte Metabolism,* 5th ed. New York: McGraw-Hill; 1994:1438.
15. Carey C, Lee H, Woeltje K. *The Washington Manual of Medical Therapeutics,* 29th ed. Philadelphia: Lippincott-Raven; 1998.
16. Covelli H et al. Respiratory failure precipitated by high carbohydrate loads. *Ann Intern Med* 1981;95:579.
17. DeMeo M et al. The hazards of hypercaloric nutritional support in respiratory disease. *Nutr Rev* 1991;49:112.
18. Alpers D, Stenson W, Bier D. *Manual of Nutritional Therapeutics,* 3rd ed. Boston: Little, Brown; 1995:328.
19. Shannon M, Wilson B, Stang C. *Appleton & Lange's 1999 Drug Guide.* Stamford, CT: Appleton & Lange, 1999:579.
20. Alpers et al, p 325.
21. Heizer, Holcombe, p 1072.
22. Doherty G, Baumann D, Creswell L, et al. *The Washington Manual of Surgery.* Boston: Little, Brown; 1997:16.
23. Alpers et al, p 326.
24. Doherty et al, p 16.
25. Heizer, Holcombe, p 1073.
26. Ibid.
27. Freund H et al. A decade of experience with home total parenteral nutrition. *Harefuah* 1991;12:294.
28. Weinsier R, Bacon J, Butterworth C. Central venous alimentation: A prospective study of the frequency of metabolic abnormalities among medical and surgical patients. *J Parenter Enteral Nutr* 1982;6:421.
29. Brooks M, Melnik G. The refeeding syndrome: An approach to understanding its complications and preventing its occurrence. *Pharmacotherapy* 1995;15:713.
30. Clark C, Sacks G, Dickerson R, Kudsk K, Brown R. Treatment of hypophosphatemia in patients receiving specialized nutrition support using a graduated dosing scheme: Results from a prospective clinical trial. *Crit Care Med* 1995;23:1504.
31. Duerksen D, Panineau N. Electrolyte abnormalities in patients with chronic renal failure receiving parenteral nutrition. *JPEN J Parenter Enteral Nutr* 1998;22:102.
32. Marik P, Bedigian M. Refeeding hypophosphatemia in critically ill patients in an intensive care unit. *Arch Surg* 1996;131:1043.
33. Janigan D, Perey B, Marrie T, et al. Skin necrosis: an unusual complication of hyperphosphatemia during total parenteral nutrition therapy. *JPEN J Parenter Enteral Nutr* 1997;21:50.
34. England B, Mitch W. Acid-base, fluid, and electrolyte aspects of parenteral nutrition. In: Kokko J, Tannen R, eds. *Fluids & Electrolytes,* 3nd ed. Philadelphia: WB Saunders; 1996:792.
35. Heizer, Holcombe, p 1072.
36. Inadomi, Kopple, p 1449.
37. Alpers et al, p 326.
38. Inadomi, Kopple, p 1449.
39. Heizer, Holcombe, p 1073.
40. Inadomi, Kopple, p 1475.
41. Ibid.
42. Ibid.
43. Skipper A, Millikan K. Parenteral nutrition implementation and management. *The ASPEN Nutrition Support Manual.* Silver Springs, MD: American Society for Parenteral and Enteral Nutrition; 1998:9-1.
44. Sunyecz L, Mirtallo J. Sodium imbalances in a patient receiving total parenteral nutrition. *Clinical Pharmacy* 1993;12:138.
45. Weinsier et al, p 422.
46. Heizer, Holcombe, p 1077.

47. Weinsier et al, p 422.
48. Inadomi, Kopple, p 1440.
49. Kaminski M. A review of hyperosmolar hyperglycemic nonketotic dehydration: Etiology, pathophysiology and prevention during intravenous hyperalimentation. *JPEN J Parenter Enteral Nutr* 1978;2:690.
50. Inadomi, Kopple, p 1440.
51. Ibid.
52. Ibid.
53. Heizer, Holcombe, p 1076.
54. Sanderson I, Deitel M. Insulin response in patients receiving concentrated infusions of glucose and casein hydrolysates for complete parenteral nutrition. *Ann Surg* 197;179:387.

55. Krzywda E et al. Glucose response to abrupt initiation and discontinuance of total parenteral nutrition. *JPEN J Parenter Enteral Nutr* 1993;17:64.
56. Wagman LD et al. The effect of acute discontinuation of TPN. *Ann Surg* 1986;204:524.
57. Bendorf K, Friesen C, Roberts C. Glucose response to discontinuation of parenteral nutrition in patients less than 3 years of age. *JPEN J Parenter Enteral Nutr* 1996;20:120.
58. Inadomi, Kopple, p 1438.
59. Heizer, Holcombe, p 1077.
60. Sullivan D, Marty T, Barton R. A case of overfeeding complicating the management of adult respiratory distress syndrome. *Nutrition* 1995;11:375.

Tube Feedings

Enteral feedings are commonly used to provide nutritional support for patients who, for some reason, cannot consume adequate nutrients although they have functional gastrointestinal (GI) tracts. Indeed, enteral feedings are believed to be more beneficial physiologically and more cost effective than total parenteral nutrition (TPN). More specifically, enteral nutrition is associated with improved gut and liver function, enhanced immune function, reduced infection rates, and better survival rates in critically ill patients.[1] However, there are problems associated with enteral feedings, just as there are with most therapies. Those related to fluid and electrolyte balance are discussed in this chapter.

⬤ CHARACTERISTICS OF FORMULAS

Before discussing specific problems, it is helpful to review briefly some characteristics of tube feeding solutions. Formulas have evolved from the blenderized whole foods used several decades ago to a multitude of commercially available preparations that can provide total nutrient needs. Although commercially available standardized formulas have many advantages, they must be selected carefully to meet the patient's individual needs. Formulas differ in osmolality, protein and carbohydrate sources, fat content, caloric density, and electrolyte content.

OSMOLALITY

An important characteristic of a tube feeding formula is its osmolality (concentration). Osmolality is primarily a function of the number and size of molecular and ionic particles in a given volume. Most enteral products range in osmolality from 270 mOsm/kg to about 700 mOsm/kg.[2] Commercially prepared feedings usually have this value printed on the product label. If this information is not on the product label, as well as the information on the renal solute load, it is usually available in product brochures. Major determinants of a formula's osmolality include simple carbohydrates, amino acids, electrolytes, and small peptides.[3] Table 12-1 shows the wide variance in osmolalities of some commercially available tube feeding formulas. Whereas some formulas approximate the osmolality of plasma (and therefore are deemed isotonic), others have considerably higher osmolalities (hypertonic). (Recall that plasma osmolality is about 300 mOsm/kg.)

A formula's osmolality affects the renal solute load and thus the water requirements. (The primary determinants of renal solute load are protein and the electrolytes sodium, potassium, and chloride.[4]) A high renal solute load (formed during nutrient use) requires a large water volume for excretion. If the water is not provided, the patient will become dehydrated.[5] Therefore, the renal solute load imposed by a formula should be considered in patients with impaired renal function or those with increased fluid losses (such as from fever or diarrhea).

Hypertonic formulas can cause slowed gastric emptying with nausea, vomiting, and distention; when hypertonic formulas are administered in the small bowel, they cause increased secretion of intestinal fluids. If this fluid is not reabsorbed adequately, diarrhea will result.[6]

ELECTROLYTES

Standard enteral formulas have fixed electrolyte contents, based on usual requirements. This can be a source of fluid and electrolyte problems in tube-fed patients as some patients require additional electrolytes, whereas other patients cannot tolerate the preestablished amounts.

As with TPN, either deficiencies or excesses of electrolytes can occur, varying with the patient's underlying disease condition, general clinical status, and the electrolyte content of the formula being used. For example, starving patients beginning vigorous refeeding may suffer extracellular deficits of potassium, phosphorus, and magnesium as these electrolytes are pulled into the cells during anabolism. Such patients need more of these electrolytes than those who are not undergoing this process. Conversely, patients with renal failure often need limitations on potassium, phosphorus, and magnesium intake. (The electrolyte content of selected enteral formulas is listed in Table 12-1.)

SPECIALIZED FORMULAS

Commercial sources supply specialized products targeted to patients with specific problems, such as renal, hepatic, and respiratory failure. Because numerous products are available, it is important to study the literature supplied by the manufacturer. Widespread use of

TABLE 12-1.   Selected Characteristics of Some Commercially Available Enteral Formulas

Formula	mOsm/ kg	Cal/ mL	% Water	Na (mg/L)	K (mg/L)	Ca (mg/L)	P (mg/L)	Mg (mg/L)
Ensure (R)	470	1.06	85.0	846 (37 mEq/L)	1,564 (40 mEq/L)	530	530	212
Ensure Plus (R)	690	1.50	77.0	1,055 (46 mEq/L)	1,943 (50 mEq/L)	704	704	282
Glucerna (R)	375	1.00	87.3	928 (40 mEq/L)	1,561 (40 mEq/L)	704	704	282
Hepatic Aid II (M)	560	1.10	87.3	288 (13 mEq/L)	196 (5 mEq/L)	—	—	—
Isocal (M)	270	1.06	84.0	530 (23 mEq/L)	1,320 (34 mEq/L)	630	530	210
Isocal HN (M)	270	1.06	84.0	930 (40 mEq/L)	1,610 (41 mEq/L)	850	850	340
Jevity (R)	310	1.06	83.3	933 (40 mEq/L)	1,567 (40 mEq/L)	912	759	303
Nepro (R)	635	2.00	70.0	829 (36 mEq/L)	1,057 (27 mEq/L)	1,373	686	211
Magnacal (SM)	590	2.00	83.0	1,000 (44 mEq/L)	1,250 (32 mEq/L)	1,000	1,000	400
Osmolite (R)	300	1.06	84.0	636 (28 mEq/L)	1,018 (26 mEq/L)	530	530	212
Pulmocare (R)	520	1.50	78.6	1,311 (57 mEq/L)	1,733 (44 mEq/L)	1,056	1,056	423
Sustacal (MJ)	650	1.06	85.0	930 (40 mEq/L)	2,100 (54 mEq/L)	1,010	930	380
Travasorb Hepatic (C)	600	1.10	82.0	235 (10 mEq/L)	892 (23 mEq/L)	491	491	197
Travasorb Renal (C)	590	1.35	77.0	—	—	—	—	—
Two Cal HN (R)	690	2.00	71.2	1,306 (57 mEq/L)	2,422 (62 mEq/L)	1,052	1,052	422
Vivonex TEN (S)	630	1.00	85.0	460 (20 mEq/L)	782 (20 mEq/L)	500	500	200

C, Clintec Nutrition Company; M, McGaw; MJ, Mead Johnson; R, Ross Laboratories; S, Sandoz Pharmaceutical; SM, Sherwood Medical. Information adapted from Zaloga G, ed. *Nutrition in Critical Care.* St. Louis: CV Mosby; 1994:450, with permission.

these formulas is limited somewhat by their expense and controversy about their effectiveness.

Renal Failure

Patients with renal failure tend to be malnourished because of poor dietary intake, particularly when coupled with nutrient losses from dialysis treatments. Although GI problems (such as nausea, vomiting, diarrhea, and GI bleeding) may preclude enteral feedings in some patients, others may benefit from enteral nutrition. When enteral feedings are tolerated, the content of the formula is partly dependent on whether dialysis is used. For patients with acute renal failure, specialized enteral formulas may be necessary; however, once dialysis is instituted, standard enteral formulas may be used to provide a full complement of amino acids.[7] Characteristically, renal enteral formulas are calorically dense and have low to absent electrolyte content as well as moderate protein content (perhaps containing increased amounts of essential amino acids).[8]

Although patients with acute renal failure require less sodium than patients with normal renal function, they still require sodium replacement as a result of obligatory losses from the GI tract and skin. Sodium intake should be matched to output. Potassium, phosphorus, and magnesium are restricted in patients with acute renal failure because these minerals are normally excreted in the urine.[9] When patients are highly catabolic, intracellular electrolytes escape from the cells and cause significant elevations in serum levels. However, when these individuals become anabolic, the opposite occurs (perhaps rendering the patient hypokalemic, hypophosphatemic, and hypomagnesemic).[10] In patients with acute renal failure, it is obvious that nutritional requirements must be evaluated on a daily basis and modifications made as needed.

Hepatic Failure

Some patients with hepatic insufficiency can tolerate the protein contained in standard enteral formulas without developing hepatic encephalopathy. For those who cannot, specialized products with a high branched-chain amino acid content are available. These formulas are calorically dense; also, they are low in protein (to minimize ammonia production).[11] Because they are very expensive, their use can only be justified in patients whose hepatic failure is associated with encephalopathy that worsens with the use of a standard enteral formula.[12,13] Examples of hepatic formulas include Hepatic-Aid II and Travasorb Hepatic.

Respiratory Failure

Patients with compromised respiratory function are frequently malnourished. Although these patients often need nutritional support, they may be unable to tolerate high caloric intake if ventilator weaning is in progress. This is because high caloric intake (especially from carbohydrates) causes increased carbon dioxide production (a problem in patients who are already hypercapneic). It is thus important to not overload pulmonary patients with calories.[14] To meet the needs of patients with compromised respiratory function, special formulas have been developed that are lower in carbohydrate content and higher in fat than standard enteral products. (Examples of such formulas include Pulmocare and Nutrivent.) These diets modestly decrease the production of carbon dioxide and thereby the partial pressure of carbon dioxide in arterial blood ($PaCO_2$).

Glucose Intolerance

The carbohydrate content in standard enteral formulas may not be tolerated by patients with diabetes or stress-induced glucose intolerance. Therefore, low-carbohydrate, high-fat, high-fiber formulas have been designed for such individuals.[15] An example of such a formula is Glucerna.

⬤ FLUID AND ELECTROLYTE DISTURBANCES ASSOCIATED WITH TUBE FEEDINGS

Tube-fed patients tend to have the fluid and electrolyte disturbances associated with their underlying disease and treatment conditions. Therefore, theoretically, it is possible to observe all types of electrolyte disturbances in tube-fed patients. As indicated in the previous discussion, factors related to the enteral formula and its delivery can cause additional disturbances. Understandably, fluid and electrolyte disturbances are more common in patients with severe illness than in relatively healthy persons requiring tube feedings for only short periods. The discussion of imbalances in this chapter is limited to the more commonly encountered disturbances.

SODIUM IMBALANCES

Hyponatremia

Hyponatremia was present in almost one-fourth of the tube-fed patients in two studies.[16,17] Partly the hyponatremia was due to the patients' underlying illnesses, and partly it was due to the concomitant use of intravenous (IV) dextrose and water solutions for parenteral drug administration.

Factors contributing to hyponatremia in tube-fed patients include water-retaining states, such as occurs with the syndrome of inappropriate antidiuretic hormone (SIADH) and abnormal routes of sodium loss, such as diarrhea or diuretic use. Note in Table 4-2 that a number of conditions predispose to this condition. In the presence of excessive antidiuretic hormone activity, large water supplements (by any route) can cause dilution of the serum sodium level, particularly when hypotonic or isotonic feedings are used. Although water added to the formula is usually charted, it is often difficult to determine the amount of fluid used as flushes to maintain tube patency and to administer medications by the tube.[18] The administration of medications by tube requires dilution of the medication as well as numerous water flushes and thus can be a significant source of fluid intake; this is an important consideration in patients with a water-retaining state (such as SIADH).

Hypernatremia

Hypernatremia is a possible electrolyte abnormality in tube-fed patients.[19] However, it is less common today than in the past when high-protein, high-osmolality formulas (about 1,000 mOsm/kg) were often used. Ingestion of large solute loads without a sufficient amount of water can result in dehydration (hypernatremia) and azotemia.[20] Although formulas in use today typically have lower osmolalities, hypernatremia can still develop in patients given inadequate water supplements. This problem is most prevalent in patients unable to make their thirst known (such as those who are unconscious, very young, aphasic, elderly, or debilitated). Elderly patients are more prone to develop hypernatremia with hyperosmolar feedings because of their decreased renal ability to conserve needed water.[21] The very young may also have difficulty in concentrating urine because of immature renal function. With decreased ability to concentrate urine, patients need more fluid to eliminate body wastes. If not provided through the feeding tube or the IV route, it is taken from internal fluid reserves.

Clinical studies have reported variable rates of hypernatremia in tube-fed patients. In one study it occurred in 10% of the tube-fed population (primarily in neurosurgical patients who were unable to conserve free water because of transient diabetes insipidus).[22] In another study, a higher incidence (18%) was reported in an acutely ill tube-fed population, being greatest in patients older than 60 years of age who were receiving feedings with osmolalities greater than 400 mOsm/kg.[23]

FLUID VOLUME IMBALANCES

Fluid Volume Overload

It is possible to cause fluid volume overload when attempting to provide sufficient calories to a patient with renal, cardiac, or hepatic disease. For such patients, a formula supplying 2 kcal/mL is often selected (as opposed to one supplying only 1 kcal/mL). In addition, special low-sodium formulas are available for such patients. As noted in Table 12-1, some formulas have considerably more sodium than others. However, in most situations, the volume of formula needed to provide 2,000 kcal will deliver 40 to 80 mEq sodium.[24]

Edema can also occur when a high-carbohydrate formula is fed to a previously fasting patient. Weight gains of 20 lb in a single week have been reported, accompanied by massive pedal edema.[25] Refeeding with carbohydrate causes an abrupt decrease in urinary sodium excretion in patients who have fasted for as little as 3 days.[26] Fluid retention is most pronounced during the first few days of refeeding.[27] Contributing to edema in tube-fed patients may be the presence of hypoalbuminemia, which favors shifting of fluid from

the vascular to the interstitial space. One study of tube-fed patients found the incidence of edema to be 20% to 25%.[28]

Fluid Volume Deficit Associated With Hyperglycemia

Tube-fed patients are at risk for hyperglycemia because of the high carbohydrate content of some formulas and because of the relative insulin resistance commonly present in acute illness. Patients with mild to moderate hyperglycemia need extra fluid to replace increased urinary fluid losses until the disorder can be controlled by hypoglycemic agents. (When insulin is administered, it is important to remember its contributory effect on the shifting of potassium, phosphorus, and magnesium from the extracellular fluid into the cells.) Occasionally, tube feedings will cause severe hyperglycemia that may progress to a hyperosmolar reaction.[29] In this situation, vigorous hydration is warranted (see Chap. 18).

REFEEDING SYNDROME

When starving (catabolic) patients are started on vigorous enteral feedings, potassium, phosphorus, and magnesium shift from the extracellular space into the cells. This shift occurs as protein synthesis (anabolism) is initiated. Insulin administration further favors intracellular shifting of these electrolytes. Failure to detect developing hypokalemia, hypophosphatemia, and hypomagnesemia, and to furnish replacements as needed, can result in serious consequences because these electrolytes have vital functions.

Although parenteral nutrition has received more attention as a precipitator of the refeeding syndrome, enteral feedings are not without risk.[30] For example, the sudden death of four malnourished children within 6 to 9 days of starting high caloric enteral feedings has been reported.[31] Interventions for dealing with the refeeding syndrome are discussed later in this chapter. Other causes for hypokalemia, hypophosphatemia, and hypomagnesemia exist and are discussed below.

POTASSIUM IMBALANCES

Hypokalemia

Hypokalemia is a common complication of enteral feeding; partly this is related to the refeeding syndrome. However, there are also other causes (such as diarrhea and use of potassium-losing diuretics). Note in Table 12-1 that there is variability in the potassium content in tube-feeding formulas. Hypokalemia can result if the potassium intake is chronically less than body requirements. Clinical indicators of hypokalemia are described in Chapter 5.

Hyperkalemia

If excessive supplements are given in addition to the enteral formula, hyperkalemia could result, particularly in high-risk patients (such as those with renal failure). Even standard formulas may contain more potassium than some patients can tolerate. Clinical indicators of hyperkalemia are described in Chapter 5.

PHOSPHORUS IMBALANCES

Hypophosphatemia

Hypophosphatemia is less common in enterally fed patients than in those fed IV. This is because enteral nutrition solutions usually contain adequate phosphate for patients with normal phosphate stores. However, there is danger of hypophosphatemia during aggressive enteral feeding of starving patients because refeeding causes phosphates to shift into the cells during tissue synthesis. When this happens, the plasma phosphate level may drop precipitously. A recent report described data on two patients with protein-energy malnutrition who developed severe hypophosphatemia during enteral feeding with phosphorus-containing formulas.[32] Additional risk factors in these two patients were present (one had chronic alcoholism and the other had malabsorption because of Crohn's disease). The researchers pointed out that patients with depleted phosphate stores and high metabolic demand have a higher daily requirement for phosphorus than is available in routine isotonic enteral formulas.[33] These case reports emphasize the importance of monitoring daily serum phosphate concentration for at least 1 week after commencement of feeding.[34]

   In another study of tube-fed patients, a 30% incidence of hypophosphatemia was observed, even when phosphate-containing solutions were used.[35] This occurred primarily in patients who received insulin for treatment of hyperglycemia; thus, the hypophosphatemia was probably secondary to a shift of phosphorus into the cells. Other investigators reported

hypophosphatemia in malnourished patients receiving glucose infusions (again, related to a cellular shift).[36] Clinical indicators of hypophosphatemia are described in Chapter 8.

Hyperphosphatemia

Although hypophosphatemia is far more common, hyperphosphatemia has also been observed in tube-fed patients.[37,38] A 14% incidence of hyperphosphatemia was reported by Vanlandingham et al.[39]; the elevated phosphate levels correlated with renal failure (a common cause of this imbalance). This is reflective of the close parallel between electrolyte abnormalities and underlying disease states in tube-fed patients.

MAGNESIUM IMBALANCES

Hypomagnesemia

During anabolism, magnesium requirements increase as the intracellular mass expands. As with the other primary cellular electrolytes (potassium and phosphorus), extracellular magnesium deficiency may result if inadequate amounts are present in the formula or added as supplements (either enterally or parenterally). In a study by Holcombe and Adams,[40] 46% of the patients had lower than normal serum magnesium levels (11 had the problem before the initiation of tube feedings and 9 patients became hypomagnesemic during the course of tube feedings). Clinical indicators of hypomagnesemia are described in Chapter 7.

Hypermagnesemia

Patients with renal failure are at risk for hypermagnesemia if the amount of magnesium contained in the formula exceeds the ability of the kidneys to excrete magnesium. Use of magnesium-containing medications adds to the risk.

ZINC DEFICIENCY

Although several trace element deficiencies may occur in patients receiving long-term enteral feedings as their only nutritional source, zinc deficiency has probably received the most attention. Zinc deficiency has been described in two patients who received tube feedings for 4 and 7 months.[41] Both patients developed skin rashes around the groin and under the breasts and axilla; after supplementation with zinc sulfate, the rashes disappeared and the serum zinc levels returned to normal. Below-normal serum zinc levels occurred in 11% of the tube-fed patients in the study by Vanlandingham et al.[42]

ASSESSMENT FOR FLUID AND ELECTROLYTE DISTURBANCES IN TUBE-FED PATIENTS

ROUTINE LABORATORY AND CLINICAL MONITORING

Although clinical assessment is important, electrolyte disturbances are usually detected by laboratory analyses.

Recommendations vary regarding the frequency of metabolic monitoring in tube-fed patients; however, it seems reasonable to measure serum sodium, potassium, glucose, blood urea nitrogen (BUN), and creatinine daily for the first week and once a week thereafter; and serum phosphorus, magnesium, and calcium at least twice weekly during the first week and once a week subsequently. As evidence of stabilization is gathered, the testing frequency can be gradually decreased. In many situations, the severity of illness dictates how frequently laboratory values are obtained. For example, it may be necessary to check all electrolytes daily in critically ill patients.

Fluid intake and output (I&O) should be monitored and recorded every 8 hours (or hourly in acute situations such as an hyperosmolar reaction). Body weight should be measured and recorded daily. Vital signs should be monitored at least once per shift. Urine glucose and acetone should be checked every 6 hours for the first 48 hours and then once daily if normal. If the renal threshold is in question (as it frequently is in elderly and very ill patients), capillary blood glucose should be measured.

RISK FACTORS FROM UNDERLYING DISEASE AND TREATMENT CONDITIONS

Virtually any electrolyte imbalance can occur in tube-fed patients, usually reflecting abnormalities associated with their primary disease condition(s). Factors related to enteral nutrition (such as the formula itself) can add to the patient's chance of developing fluid and electrolyte problems. Some risk factors for specific imbalances are summarized in Table 12-2.

HYDRATION STATUS

Because tube-fed patients may develop either fluid volume deficit or fluid volume excess, with or without sodium imbalances, it is necessary to monitor the hydration status closely (Table 12-3).

NURSING INTERVENTIONS

PREVENTING THE REFEEDING SYNDROME

Some recommendations suggested by Solomon and Kirby[45] to avoid the refeeding syndrome include:

1. Recognize "at-risk" patients (such as those with chronic cachexia due to prolonged starvation or any patient who has been chronically deprived of adequate nutrition).
2. Test for and correct electrolyte abnormalities before initiating nutritional support in at-risk patients, either orally, enterally, or IV.
3. Begin nutritional repletion slowly and keep increases in calories modest during the first week.
4. Monitor serum sodium, potassium, magnesium, and phosphorus levels and administer supplements as indicated (especially during the first week of refeeding when most of the serious electrolyte problems are likely to occur).

It may be helpful to monitor the pulse rate as a noninvasive method to assess fluid replacement. Most severely malnourished patients have bradycardia; if during nutritional repletion the intravascular volume is increased too rapidly, the heart rate may increase markedly. For example, a heart rate of 80 to 100 beats/min in a previously malnourished, bradycardic patient may be a sign of cardiac stress and warrants close observation.[46]

MANAGING ELECTROLYTE IMBALANCES

A brief summary of interventions for specific electrolyte imbalances associated with tube feedings is presented in Table 12-2. See Chapters 3 through 9 for more detailed information regarding assessment

TABLE 12-2.   Summary of Fluid and Electrolyte Imbalances in Tube-Fed Patients:
Risk Factors and Interventions

Fluid/Electrolyte Imbalance	Examples of Risk Factors	Possible Interventions
Hyponatremia	Excessive water retention associated with increased antidiuretic hormone activity: • Disease conditions such as oat-cell lung tumor and head injury • Medications such as Cytoxan, Oncovin, Diabinese, and Mellaril	Adjust water intake according to serum sodium levels Avoid hypotonic formulas or large water intake in patients at risk for hyponatremia Use calorie-dense formula to limit water intake, as indicated
	Excessive water administration in form of hypotonic enteral formula, water flushes of the feeding tube, or D_5W to administer IV medications	Administer IV medications in isotonic saline (instead of D_5W) if compatible
	Abnormal routes of sodium loss, as in diarrhea or diuretic use	Administer sodium supplements via enteral route, if indicated (If NaCl supplements are prescribed, it is safer to obtain predetermined quantities of NaCl in capsule form from a pharmacist than it is to measure table salt in a teaspoon at the bedside.) Sodium may also be supplemented by IV route, if indicated.
Hypernatremia	Excessive water loss, as in: • Diabetes insipidus • Fever • Hyperventilation	Adjust water intake according to serum sodium levels Change to isotonic formula (if problem is a hyperosmolar formula)
	Use of hyperosmolar enteral formulas with insufficient water supplements	Administer water supplements as boluses via feeding tube, as indicated
	Decreased renal concentrating ability (as in very old and very young patients)	Administer IV medications in D_5W (instead of normal saline), if compatible
	Decreased level of consciousness, inability to recognize or respond to thirst	Rehydrate gradually over a period of several days if severe hypernatremia is present; too rapid correction can cause brain edema

Continued

TABLE 12-2. Summary of Fluid and Electrolyte Imbalances in Tube-Fed Patients: Risk Factors and Interventions—*cont'd*

Fluid/Electrolyte Imbalance	Examples of Risk Factors	Possible Interventions
Hypokalemia	Aggressive refeeding of starving patients	Initiate feedings cautiously in starving patient
	Use of potassium-losing medications: • Furosemide, thiazide diuretics • Aminoglycosides • Amphotericin	Monitor serum potassium levels and administer potassium supplements as indicated (IV route may be necessary)
	Insulin administration	
	Severe diarrhea	
Hypomagnesemia	Aggressive refeeding of starving patients	Initiate feedings cautiously in starving patients
	Use of magnesium-losing medications such as aminoglycosides, cisplatin, and mannitol	Monitor serum magnesium levels and provide magnesium supplements as indicated (IV route may be necessary)
	Insulin administration	
	Chronic alcoholism	
	Diarrhea	
Hypophosphatemia	Aggressive refeeding of starving patients	Initiate feedings cautiously in starving patients
	Insulin administration	Monitor serum phosphorus levels and provide supplements as indicated:
	Chronic alcoholism	Fleet Phospho-Soda is sometimes added to the enteral formula to treat mild to moderate hypophosphatemia; parenteral phosphorus should be used to treat patients with serum phosphorus concentrations < 1.5 mg/dL[43]
	Malabsorption	
	Respiratory alkalosis	
	Diarrhea	

Continued

TABLE 12-2. Summary of Fluid and Electrolyte Imbalances in Tube-Fed Patients: Risk Factors and Interventions—*cont'd*

Fluid/Electrolyte Imbalance	Examples of Risk Factors	Possible Interventions
Hyperkalemia	Use of potassium-conserving diuretics Renal failure	Monitor serum potassium levels; if elevated, consider potassium content of enteral formula, IV fluids, and medications Reduce potassium intake
Hypermagnesemia	Use of magnesium-containing antacids Renal failure	Monitor serum magnesium levels; if elevated, consider magnesium content of enteral formula, IV fluids, and medications Reduce magnesium intake
Hyperphosphatemia	Use of phosphate-containing antacids Renal failure	Monitor serum phosphorus levels; if elevated, consider phosphorus content of enteral formula, IV fluids, and medications Reduce phosphorus intake
Fluid volume deficit	Osmotic diuresis from hyperglycemia	Monitor serum glucose level every 6 hr after feedings are initiated (until stable) Control hyperglycemia by adjusting formula or administering hypoglycemic agent (as indicated)
Fluid volume excess	Use of standard formula with relatively high sodium content in patients with renal, cardiac, or hepatic failure Early period (especially first few days) of refeeding of patients with chronic malnutrition	Assess for fluid excess by daily body weights, intake and output measurement, looking for edema, listening to breath sounds Consider use of low-sodium or calorie-dense formula Initiate refeeding cautiously in chronically malnourished patients; assess fluid volume carefully, monitor for signs of cardiac stress

TABLE 12-3. Summary of Assessment of Hydration Status of Tube-Fed Patients

Assessment	Description
Fluid intake and output	Record volume and type of all fluids given by mouth, tube, and IV (include water used to flush tube to maintain patency and to administer medications) Record all fluid losses, including: • Urine • Liquid feces • Vomitus • Drainage from fistulas, wounds, etc. Consider fluid losses associated with fever, perspiration, hyperventilation, and dry environmental conditions.
Urine concentration	In addition to volume of urine, record its color (ranging from dark amber to pale or colorless). If necessary, measure urinary specific gravity with urinometer or refractometer. (If glucosuria is present, specific gravity will be abnormally high; urinary osmolality is a more accurate measure in this instance.)
Urinary glucose	Monitor for glucosuria at least 3 times daily throughout initial feeding period, particularly in middle-aged and elderly patients. If present, check capillary blood sugar. If renal threshold is in question, omit urinary tests and check capillary blood sugars.
Body weight	Measure body weight daily (using same scales and same clothing). A slight increase in weight is anticipated in the anabolic patient. This gain should not exceed 0.7 kg/day, roughly 1.5 lb/day.[44] A gain greater than this amount probably indicates fluid volume overload.
Edema	Look for dependent edema in feet and ankles of ambulatory patients and in the backs of bedfast patients. Assess breath sounds for pulmonary edema.
Sensorium	Assess for changes in sensorium (from baseline) after feedings are initiated. Severe sodium derangements (either high or low) can affect the patient's level of alertness and responsiveness.
Blood chemistries	Examine blood urea nitrogen/creatinine ratio; if elevated, possibility of fluid volume deficit exists. Examine serum sodium level (if high, indicates need for free water; if low, indicates need for restriction of free water). Look for elevated blood sugar level; if present, patient is at increased risk for osmotic diuresis and fluid volume deficit.

for these imbalances and treatment recommendations.

WATER SUPPLEMENTATION

A perplexing problem for the nurse is determining how much free water is needed for each tube-fed patient. The previous discussion identified several variables affecting this decision. Some key questions to consider include the following. Is there a need for fluid restriction due to SIADH or renal or cardiac disease? Is extra fluid required due to delivery of high-osmolality, high-protein feedings, or increased loss from other routes, such as diarrhea, fistula or wound drainage, hyperventilation, or fever? Is the patient receiving sizable amounts of fluid through the IV route? How does the I&O record look? What is the serum sodium concentration? All of these factors must be considered individually (see Table 12-3).

Given these qualifiers, some rough guidelines exist to help calculate the free water requirements of normal afebrile adults receiving tube feedings. For example, the amount of water needed to replace urine and insensible fluid losses is 30 to 35 mL/kg body weight per day, or 1 mL water per calorie fed.[47] Another consideration in determining the amount of extra water to provide is the amount of water provided in the formula itself. For example, most formulas that provide 1 calorie/mL contain 800 to 850 mL water/L formula; more calorically dense formulas may contain only 600 mL/L.[48] After determining how much water is provided by the enteral formula, it is necessary to calculate how much IV fluid is infused as well as how much water is given through the feeding tube with medications or as flushes to maintain tube patency. Subtracting what is given from what is needed provides the amount of extra water that is needed.

MANAGING DIARRHEA

Incidence and Causes

Severe diarrhea leads to fluid, electrolyte, and nutrient depletion and should be prevented whenever possible.[49] Although the true prevalence of diarrhea in tube-fed patients is difficult to pinpoint (largely because clinicians define diarrhea differently), it is generally agreed that diarrhea is a potential problem in tube-fed patients that must be reckoned with to avoid serious fluid and electrolyte problems.

Reported incidences range from as low as 2% in some populations to as high as 68% in others.[50–52] When GI function is normal, the incidence of diarrhea in tube-fed patients is reported to be 12% to 25%.[53,54] In contrast, about half the patients in intensive care units (ICUs) develop diarrhea.[55] Several factors may account for this higher incidence, such as increased rates of malnutrition (causing decreased ability of the intestinal mucosa to absorb nutrients), multisystem organ disease, multiple medications, and infectious processes. Apparently, critically ill patients who are mechanically ventilated are at even greater risk for diarrhea. A study of 73 critically ill, mechanically ventilated patients reported a 63% incidence of diarrhea.[56] Another study of tube-fed patients found that 26% had documented diarrhea (defined as stools >500 mL/day for at least 2 consecutive days).[57] A single cause was specified in 29 of the 32 episodes of diarrhea. Medications were directly responsible in 61%; other less fre-

quent causes were *Clostridium difficile* and characteristics of the enteral formula. Antibiotics are generally associated with an increased rate of diarrhea; however, they are especially problematic in tube-fed patients. This is because there appears to be a synergistic relationship between enteral feedings and antibiotic treatment that increases the risk for diarrhea.[58] Sorbitol-based elixirs are also problematic in terms of causing diarrhea.

A recent study found that hospitalized, tube-fed patients, especially those fed in the small bowel, are at greater risk for acquiring *C. difficile*-associated diarrhea than are similarly ill non–tube-fed patients.[59] Therefore, the researchers recommended that clinicians test for *C. difficile* in tube-fed patients with diarrhea.

Treatment

Because multiple factors can cause diarrhea, a variety of methods are traditionally tried to alleviate it; among these are medications such as adsorbents (eg, kaolin or pectin) and antimotility agents (eg, Lomotil, loperamide, or paregoric). An old treatment that was recently tested in a group of critically ill tube-fed patients was the administration of banana flakes; when compared to a group that received medical treatments, the incidence of diarrhea was similar.[60] The investigators concluded that banana flakes can be used as a safe, cost-effective treatment for diarrhea in critically ill tube-fed patients. Another group of investigators recently concluded that diarrhea induced by enteral feeding is, at least in part, due to the malabsorption of bile acids and that a bile acid resin-binding agent improves diarrhea induced by enteral feeding in some patients.[61]

Adjustment of Medications

Antibiotics are required for many patients even though it is known they are associated with an increased incidence of diarrhea; as soon as is possible, antibiotics are discontinued. If sorbitol-based or other hyperosmolar medications are suspected of causing the diarrhea, it may be necessary to consult with the pharmacist and physician to find a more suitable method for administering the needed medications. Options for avoiding problems with sorbitol-containing medications include changing to another manufacturer's product or changing the route of administration.[62] The adjustment of liquid medications is an important consideration because numerous patients are switched to liquid medications as soon as they receive a feeding tube; in some situations, enough sorbitol is administered this way to cause diarrhea.[63] Unfortunately, many commonly used liquid medications are sorbitol-based or otherwise hyperosmolar. Agents that most commonly cause problems are those with a high sorbitol content, especially if numerous doses are required over a 24-hour period (such as acetaminophen elixir for fever or discomfort).

A number of medications are hyperosmolar and can cause osmotic diarrhea if given undiluted, especially into the small intestine. Examples of osmolalities of such medications include 10% potassium chloride solution (Adria), 3,000 mOsm/kg; acetaminophen elixir, 65 mg/mL (Roxanne), 5,400 mOsm/kg; and sodium phosphate liquid, 0.5 g/mL (Fleet), 7,250 mOsm/kg.[64] Hyperosmolar medications should be diluted before administration and water flushes given through the tube before and after delivery.[65] This not only dilutes the medication but enhances its absorption. (This should be done with the patient's fluid requirements in mind.) Hyperosmolar preparations should only be administered in the stomach to minimize GI intolerance.[66] At times, the parenteral route may be necessary for electrolyte supplements when they are not tolerated well by the GI tract.

Use of magnesium-containing antacids may also cause diarrhea. When antacids are necessary, it may be helpful to alternate magnesium-containing antacids with magnesium-free antacids[67] or to change to calcium or aluminum antacids.[68] Other medications frequently implicated in diarrhea are penicillin-like antibiotics.

Another possible cause of diarrhea is the administration of metoclopramide, an agent often prescribed to stimulate gastric emptying. It is possible that stopping treatment with this drug will cause the diarrhea to resolve.[69]

Formula Selection

High-Fiber Formulas

Because the colon is the final site of water and electrolyte absorption and ultimately determines fecal composition, diarrhea associated with enteral feedings may result from altered colonic function.[70] In patients who can tolerate high-residue formulas, use of a high-fiber formula is thought to increase the sodium and water absorptive ability of the colon and thus, minimize fecal fluid loss. Commercially available fiber-supplemented formulas are often prescribed to either prevent or treat diarrhea.

Elemental and Chemically Defined Formulas

In certain disease states, there is impaired absorption of nutrients. Among these are intestinal atrophy or loss of absorptive surface associated with profound malnutrition, critical illness, and acquired immunodeficiency syndrome. Several studies have indicated that peptide-based formulas are helpful in avoiding diarrhea in hypoalbuminemic, critically ill patients.[71,72] However, a larger prospective study did not demonstrate any advantage in a peptide-based formula over a standard, polymeric formula.[73] One group of investigators recommended that the use of elemental formulas should be limited to specific conditions in which absorption has been definitely shown to be impaired.[74] There are indications that enteral feeding with elemental diets for patients with human immunodeficiency virus can lessen diarrhea.[75]

Lactose-Free Formulas

Although few formulas contain lactose, it is important to be aware that the presence of intestinal mucosal damage reduces the surface area available for absorption and produces secondary lactose deficiency. Therefore, formulas with little or no lactose are indicated for very ill patients with small bowel conditions that predispose to lactose intolerance (such as intestinal resection, radiation enteritis, and malnutrition).

Formula Dilution and Rate of Delivery

Formulas that are isotonic (approach the osmolality of plasma, 280–300 mOsm/kg) are usually administered at full strength. Even those that are moderately hyperosmotic are usually administered at full strength. When hyperosmolar feedings are thought to be the cause of diarrhea, the rate of flow is usually decreased rather than diluting the formula. Formula dilution may result in greater GI complications and poor nutritional outcomes. If formula dilution is necessary, it should be performed as aseptically as possible to avoid contamination of the formula. Hyperosmolar solutions are less well tolerated in the small intestine than in the stomach.

If the cause of diarrhea is too rapid administration of the formula, it is customary to decrease the rate of flow to the point where no diarrhea occurs.[76] Then, the rate is gradually increased until the desired rate is achieved. Feedings may be administered either intermittently or continuously in the stomach, but only continuously in the intestine.

Temperature of Solution

Recently refrigerated formulas should be started at a slow rate to permit them time to warm to room temperature. Research findings by Kagawa-Busby et al.[77] suggest that cold feedings can predispose to cramping and diarrhea in some patients.

Preventing Contamination of Formula/Feeding System

Enteral nutritional solutions may be an important source of nosocomial infection.[78] This can be particularly dangerous in severely ill, immunocompromised patients.[79] Thus, enteral formulas should be handled with clean technique to prevent microbial contamination. It has been suggested that the complete delivery set (except the feeding tube itself) be changed every 24 hours for patients in a hospital setting to reduce the incidence of contamination.[80,81] When powdered formulas are used, all of the preparation equipment needs to be cleaned meticulously. Some researchers recommend the use of sterile water (versus tap water) when it is necessary to reconstitute or dilute enteral nutrition solutions.[82] Dilution of liquid formulas should be avoided whenever possible because of the risk for contamination. The recommended hang time for prefilled formulas should be provided by their manufacturers. Canned, ready-to-use formulas can generally be kept at room temperature for 8 to 12 hours; however, manufacturers' guidelines should be followed.[83] Clean technique is required while adding formula to the feeding reservoir. The less the reservoir is handled, the less likely the chance for contamination.

CASE STUDIES

● **12-1.**[84] A 75-year-old woman was admitted to the ICU with shortness of breath progressively worsened over a period of 1 week. Her medical history included hypertension, interstitial lung disease, and alcohol abuse. She showed no clinical evidence of liver disease nor of drinking in the week preceding her admission to the ICU. On physical examination, she was alert and fully oriented but moderately malnourished. A chest x-ray showed pulmonary congestion and rales were present. A diagnosis of congestive heart failure was made and she responded to diuresis. Serum electrolytes were found to be within normal range.

After she was stabilized, enteral feedings were started and progressively advanced to 42 kcal/kg/day. On the third day of feedings, her serum phosphorus level began to drop and she became drowsy. On the fourth day of feeding, she developed coma and respiratory failure and required intubation and mechanical ventilation. Her serum phosphorus level on day 5 was 0.5 mg/dL. Despite subsequent correction of the hypophosphatemia, the patient did not regain consciousness and died on the 11th hospital day. It was surmised that hypophosphatemia initiated the chain of events that ultimately led to her death.

COMMENTARY: As pointed out by the authors of this case report, central to the pathophysiology of the refeeding syndrome is a block in the synthesis of adenosine triphosphate and 2,3-diphosphoglycerate, which ultimately leads to neurological and muscular dysfunction.[85] Metabolic encephalopathy associated with hypophosphatemia can cause lethargy and coma; further, respiratory failure can be a consequence of severe hypophosphatemia. Like most malnourished patients, this patient had a normal serum phosphorus concentration on admission. Yet, her total body phosphorus content was diminished by chronic malnutrition. This deficit was unmasked by the initiation of enteral feedings when her body was called on to metabolize the nutrients (especially carbohydrates). It has been recommended that patients at risk for the refeeding syndrome be fed slowly (such as 15–20 kcal/kg/day with about 50% of the administered calories given as fat).[87,88] Further, vigorous replacement of potassium, phosphorus, magnesium, and thiamine may be needed for the first 3 to 5 days until the serum values of these substrates are stable.[89]

● **12-2.**[90] A 22-year-old woman with a history of anorexia nervosa was admitted to the hospital for enteral feedings because she had sustained a weight loss of 55 lb over the previous few months. She was easily tired on exertion and complained of generalized weakness. Her admission body weight was 59 lb and she was 5 ft, 1 in. tall. Lying flat, her blood pressure was 90/50; it dropped to 70/50 when she sat upright. Her pulse rate was 50 beats/min. Because her serum phosphorus level was low (0.47 mmol/L, normal = 0.81–1.45 mmol/L), she was given oral phosphate, 500 mg, twice daily. Tube feedings were started and advanced over several days to full strength at a rate of 100 mL/hr. Although she felt stronger, she became tachycardic on the fourth day. At that time, her serum phosphorus concentration was 0.18 mmol/L (roughly equivalent to 0.5 mg/dL). Because of this, she was started on potassium phosphate supplements IV. On the sixth day, her serum phosphorus level had dropped to 0.16 mmol/L and she developed symptoms of heart failure. Oxygen was started and she was given furosemide IV; her tube feedings were discontinued. In addition, her phosphate supplement was increased orally and IV. By the seventh day, her electrocardiogram was essentially normal and she no longer required oxygen. As she improved, she was restarted on enteral feedings and continued on oral phosphate supplements only. No further complications were noted.

COMMENTARY: The cardiac decompensation noted in this patient during refeeding was likely caused by hypophosphatemia in the presence of cardiac changes due to severe malnutrition.[91,92] Fortunately, the changes were reversible. The authors of this case study emphasized the need to monitor serum electrolyte levels closely in anorectic patients during refeeding, especially during the first week. Further, they indicate a need to start feedings gradually with graded increases in the caloric content of the feeds.[93]

Related case studies are also presented in Chapters 7, 8, 11, and 18.

REFERENCES

1. Zaloga G. *Nutrition in Critical Care,*. St. Louis: CV Mosby; 1994:675.
2. Ibid, p 446.
3. Gottschlich M, Shronts E, Hutchins H. Defined formula diets. In: Rombeau J, Caldwell M, eds. *Clinical Nutrition: Enteral and Tube Feeding*, 3rd ed. Philadelphia: WB Saunders; 1997:225.
4. Ibid.
5. Ibid.
6. Alpers D, Stenson W, Bier D. *Manual of Nutritional Therapeutics*, 3rd ed. Boston: Little, Brown; 1995:297.
7. Matarese L. Rationale and efficacy of specialized enteral nutrition. *Nutr Clin Pract* 1992;9:58.
8. Olree K, Vitello J, Sullivan J, Kohn-Keeth C. Enteral formulations. *ASPEN Nutrition Support Practice Manual*, Chapter 4. Silver Spring, MD: American Society for Parenteral and Enteral Nutrition; 1998:4-6.
9. Zaloga, p 673.
10. Ibid.
11. Olree et al, p 4-6.
12. Ibid.
13. Alpers et al, p 300.
14. Ibid.
15. Olree et al, p 4-5.
16. Vanlandingham S et al. Metabolic abnormalities in patients supported with enteral tube feeding. *JPEN J Parenter Enteral Nutr* 1981;5:322.
17. Bowman ME et al. Sodium imbalances in tube-fed patients. *Crit Care Nurs* 1989;9:22.
18. Ibid.
19. Gault et al. Hypernatremia, azotemia, and dehydration due to high-protein feeding. *Ann Intern Med* 68:778,1968.
20. Pemberton L, Pemberton D. *Treatment of Water, Electrolyte and Acid-Base Disorders in the Surgical Patient*. New York: McGraw-Hill; 1994:99.
21. Walike J. Tube feeding syndrome in head and neck surgery. *Arch Otolaryngol* 1969;89:117.
22. Vanlandingham et al, p 322.
23. Bowman et al, p 24.
24. Alpers et al, p 312.
25. Havala T, Shronts E. Managing the complications associated with refeeding. *Nutr Clin Pract* 1990;5:27.
26. Zaloga, p 770.
27. Ibid, p 771.
28. Heymsfield S et al. Enteral hyperalimentation: An alternative to central venous hyperalimentation. *Ann Intern Med* 1979;90:63.
29. Condon R, Nyhus L. *Manual of Surgical Therapeutics*, 9th ed. Boston: Little, Brown; 1996:205.
30. Zaloga, p 776.
31. Patrick J. Death during recovery from severe malnutrition and its possible relationship to sodium pump activity in the leukocyte. *Br Med J* 1977;1:1051.
32. Maier-Dobersberger T, Lochs H. Enteral supplementation of phosphate does not prevent hypophosphatemia during refeeding of cachectic patients. *JPEN J Parenter Enteral Nutr* 1994;18:182.
33. Ibid.
34. Ibid.
35. Vanlandingham et al, p 324.
36. Hayek M, Eisenberg P. Severe hypophosphatemia following the institution of enteral feedings. *Arch Surg* 1989;124:1325.
37. Holcombe B, Adams M. Metabolic complications associated with enteral nutritional support. *Nutritional Support Services* 1985;5:26.
38. Primrose JN et al: Hyperkalemia in patients on enteral feedings. *JPEN J Parenter Enteral Nutr* 1981;5:130.
39. Vanlandingham et al, p 324.
40. Holcombe, Adams, p 27.
41. Jhangiana et al. Clinical zinc deficiency during long-term total enteral nutrition. *J Am Geriatr Soc* 1986;34:385.

42. Vanlandingham et al, p 324.
43. Zaloga, p 490.
44. Heymsfield et al, p 69.
45. Solomon S, Kirby D. The refeeding syndrome: A review. *JPEN J Parenter Enteral Nutr* 1990;14:90.
46. Ibid.
47. Lord L, Trumbore L, Zaloga G. Enteral nutrition implementation and management. *ASPEN Nutrition Support Practice Manual*. Chapter 5. Silver Spring, MD: American Society for Parenteral and Enteral Nutrition. 1998:5-7.
48. Ibid.
49. Guenter P, Settle G, Perlmutter S, et al. Tube feeding-related diarrhea in acute ill patients. *JPEN J Parenter Enteral Nutr* 1991;15:277.
50. Kelly T, et al. Study of diarrhea in critically ill patients. *Crit Care Med* 1983;11:7.
51. Bliss D, et al. Defining and reporting diarrhea in tube-fed patients—What a mess! *Am J Clin Nutr* 1992;55:753.
52. Heimburger D. Diarrhea with enteral feeding: Will the real cause please stand up? *Am J Med* 1990;88:89.
53. Cataldi-Betcher EL et al. Complications occurring during enteral nutrition support: A prospective study. *JPEN J Parenter Enteral Nutr* 1983;7:546.
54. Jones et al. Comparison of an elemental and polymeric enteral diet in patients with normal gastrointestinal function. *Gut* 1983;24:78.
55. Brinson R, Anderson W, Singh M. Hypoalbuminemia-associated diarrhea in critically ill patients. *J Crit Illness* 1987;2:72.
56. Smith CE et al. Diarrhea associated with tube-feeding in mechanically ventilated critically ill patients. *Nurs Res* 1990;39:148.
57. Edes T, Walk B, Austin J. Diarrhea in tube-fed patients: Feeding formula not necessarily the cause. *Am J Med* 1990;88:91.
58. Bowling T, Silk D. Diarrhea and enteral nutrition. In: Rombeau J, Caldwell M, eds. *Clinical Nutrition: Enteral and Tube Feeding*, 3rd ed. Philadelphia: WB Saunders; 1997:541.
59. Bliss D et al. Acquisition of *Clostridium difficile* and *Clostridium difficile*-associated diarrhea in hospitalized patients receiving tube feeding. *Ann Intern Med* 1998;129:1012.
60. Emery E et al. Banana flakes control diarrhea in enterally fed patients. *Nutr Clin Pract* 1997;12:72.
61. DeMeo M et al. Beneficial effect of a bile acid resin binder on enteral feeding induced diarrhea. *Am J Gastroenterol* 1998;93:967.
62. Johnson D, Nyffelen M. Drug-nutrition considerations for enteral nutrition. *ASPEN Nutrition Support Practice Manual*. Chapter 6. Silver Spring, MD: American Society for Parenteral and Enteral Nutrition. 1998:6-5.
63. Henley E. Sorbitol-based elixirs, diarrhea and enteral tube feeding. (Letter). *Am Fam Physician* 1997;55:2084.
64. Thomas C, Rollins C. Nutrient-drug interaction. In: Rombeau J, Caldwell M, eds. *Clinical Nutrition: Enteral and Tube Feeding*, 3rd ed. Philadelphia: WB Saunders; 1997:533.
65. Edes et al, p 91.
66. Seshadri V, Meyer-Tettambel O. Electrolyte and drug management in nutritional support. *Crit Care Nurs Clin North Am* 1993;5:31.
67. Zaloga, p 572.
68. Eisenberg P. Causes of diarrhea in tube-fed patients: A comprehensive approach to diagnosis and management. *Nutr Clin Pract* 1993;8:119.
69. Zaloga, p 342.
70. Palacio J, Rombeau J. Dietary fiber: A brief review and potential application to enteral nutrition. *Nutr Clin Pract* 1990;5:99.
71. Brinson R, et al. Diarrhea in the intensive care unit: the role of hypoalbuminemia and the response to a chemically defined diet. *J Am Coll Nutr* 1987;6:517.
72. Brinson R, Kolts B. Diarrhea associated with severe hypoalbuminemia: A comparison of a peptide-based chemically defined diet and standard enteral alimentation. *Crit Care Med* 1988;16:130.
73. Mowatt-Larssen C, et al. Comparison of tolerance and nutritional outcome between a peptide and a standard enteral formula in critically ill, hypoalbuminemic patients. *JPEN J Parenter Enteral Nutr* 1992;16:20.
74. Dietscher E et al. Nutritional response of patients in intensive care unit to an elemental formula vs a standard enteral formula. *J Am Diet Assoc* 1998;98:335.
75. Salamone S et al. An elemental diet containing medium-chain triglycerides and enzymatically hydrolyzed protein can improve gastrointestinal tolerance in people infected with HIV. *J Am Diet Assoc* 1998;98:4
76. Eisenberg, p 121.
77. Kagawa-Busby K, Heitkemper M, Hansen B. Effects of diet temperature on tolerance of enteral feedings. *Nurs Res* 1980;29:276.
78. Thurn J et al. Enteral hyperalimentation as a source of nosocomial infection. *J Hosp Infect* 1990;15:203.
79. Moe G. Enteral feeding and infection in the immunocompromised patient. *Nutr Clin Pract* 1991;6:55.
80. Perez S, Brandt K. Enteral feeding contamination: Comparison of diluents and feeding bag usage. *JPEN J Parenter Enteral Nutr* 1989;13:306.
81. Kohn C. The relationship between enteral formula contamination and length of enteral delivery set usage. *JPEN J Parenter Enteral Nutr* 1991;15:567.
82. Fagerman K. Microbiological monitoring of enteral nutrition solutions needed (Letter). *JPEN J Parenter Enteral Nutr* 1989;13:670.
83. Lord et al, p 4-7.
84. Vaszar L, Culpepper-Morgan J, Winter S. Refeeding syndrome induced by cautious enteral alimentation of a moderately malnourished patient. *Gastroenterologist* 1998;6:79.
85. Ibid.
86. Ibid.
87. Ibid.
88. Heymsfield S, Casper K, Funfar J. Physiologic response and clinical implications of nutrition support. *Am J Cardiol* 1987;60:75G.
89. Vaszar et al, p 81.
90. Birmingham C, Alothman A, Goldner E. Anorexia nervosa: Refeeding and hypophosphatemia. *Int J Eat Disord* 1996;20:211.
91. Ibid.
92. Simone G, Scalfi L, Galderisi M, et al. Cardiac abnormalities in young women with anorexia nervosa. *Br Heart J* 1994;871:287.
93. Birmingham et al, p 213.

Clinical Situations Associated With Fluid and Electrolyte Problems

CHAPTER 13

Gastrointestinal Problems

Gastrointestinal (GI) fluid loss is a common cause of water and electrolyte disturbances. This is because of the large fluid volumes in the GI tract and the many ways in which these fluids can be lost, such as vomiting, diarrhea, suction drainage, fistulas, and sequestration into an obstructed bowel. Along with the possibility of fluid volume deficit (FVD), there is the potential for various electrolyte imbalances. Nursing considerations related to these GI fluid and electrolyte losses are discussed in this chapter.

CHARACTER OF GASTROINTESTINAL FLUIDS

In healthy individuals, about 3 to 6 liters of gastric, pancreatic, biliary, and intestinal secretions are secreted into the GI lumen each day.[1] Counting normal fluid intake and endogenous GI secretions, about 9 L/day enters the upper intestinal tract. Most of these fluids are then reabsorbed in the ileum and proximal colon,

resulting in daily loss of only 100 to 200 mL water in feces.

With the exception of saliva, the GI secretions are isotonic with the extracellular fluid (ECF). In addition, material entering the GI tract tends to become isotonic during the course of its absorption. Because many liters of ECF pass into the GI tract and back again, as part of the normal digestive process, this movement is sometimes referred to as the "gastrointestinal circulation." The electrolyte content of GI secretions is summarized in Table 13-1. The usual pH of GI secretions is listed in Table 13-2.

VOMITING AND GASTRIC SUCTION

FLUID AND ELECTROLYTE DISTURBANCES

Major electrolytes in gastric juice are hydrogen (H^+), chloride (Cl^-), potassium (K^+), and, to a lesser extent, sodium (Na^+). Gastric juice is the most acidic of the GI

TABLE 13-1.   Approximate Electrolyte Composition of Gastrointestinal Secretions

Secretion	Usual Maximum Volume/Day	Sodium (mEq/L in Adults)	Chloride (mEq/L in Adults)	Potassium (mEq/L in Adults)
Normal				
Saliva	1,000	100	75	5
Gastric juice (pH < 4.0)	2,500*	60	100	10
Gastric juice (pH > 4.0)	2,000*	100	100	10
Bile	1,500	140	100	10
Pancreatic juice	1,000	140	75	10
Succus entericus (mixed small-bowel fluid)	3,500	100	100	20
Abnormal				
New ileostomy	500–2,000	130	110	20
Adapted ileostomy	400	50	60	10
New cecostomy	400	80	50	20
Colostomy (transverse loop)	300	50	40	10
Diarrhea	1,000–4,000	60	45	30

*Nasogastric suction volume is usually much less than this unless pyloric obstruction exists.
From Condon R, Nyhus L. *Manual of Surgical Therapeutics*, 9th ed. Boston: Little, Brown; 1996, with permission.

TABLE 13-2. Gastrointestinal Secretions and Their Usual pH

Secretion	pH
Saliva	6.0–7.0
Gastric juice	1.0–3.5*
Pancreatic juice	8.0–8.3
Bile	7.8
Small intestine	7.5–8.0
Large intestine	7.5–8.0

*Gastric pH will probably be higher than 3.5 in patients receiving H$_2$-receptor antagonists.

---

secretions with a pH of 1.0 to 3.5 in the fasting state in most individuals not receiving H$_2$-receptor antagonists. Imbalances most often associated with the loss of gastric juice include:

• FVD
• Metabolic alkalosis
• Hypokalemia
• Sodium imbalances
• Hypomagnesemia

Fluid Volume Deficit

If vomiting is prolonged and fluid replacement therapy is inadequate, severe FVD may result, manifested by decreased urinary output, postural hypotension, tachycardia, elevated hematocrit, and elevated blood urea nitrogen (BUN)/creatinine ratio. It is not uncommon to see a 10-point drop in the hematocrit level during the first 12 to 24 hours after fluid replacement.[2] Also, because many liters can be removed daily by gastric suction (depending on the underlying disease process), FVD can easily occur in this situation if fluids are not replaced parenterally.

Metabolic Alkalosis

Excessive loss of gastric juice by vomiting or suction causes metabolic alkalosis (base bicarbonate excess) for several reasons. First, secretions from the stomach contain high concentrations of H$^+$ and Cl$^-$ ions. With loss of Cl$^-$, there is a compensatory increase in bicarbonate ions. (Each milliequivalent of hydrochloric acid lost

from the stomach represents 1 mEq bicarbonate added to the ECF.[3]) The kidneys add to the metabolic alkalosis by failing to excrete all the excess circulating bicarbonate (HCO$_3^-$).[4] Symptoms are generally those of decreased calcium ionization related to the alkaline plasma. (Recall that calcium ionization is decreased in alkalosis.) Because it is the ionized fraction of calcium that controls neuromuscular excitability, symptoms of tetany can occur.

Hypokalemia

As noted in Table 13-1, gastric fluid contains about 10 mEq potassium per liter. With the loss of several liters of gastric fluid, it is clear that hypokalemia could easily develop. In addition to the direct loss of potassium with vomiting and gastric suction, there is a transient renal wasting of potassium early in the period of gastric fluid loss. The metabolic alkalosis described previously accompanies hypokalemia.

Recall that an adult, not eating, requires the daily addition of about 40 to 60 mEq potassium to intravenous (IV) fluids. A patient with large gastric fluid losses may require substantially more.

Sodium Imbalances

The plasma sodium level varies in patients losing gastric fluid by vomiting and gastric suction. Gastric fluid is usually isotonic or mildly hypotonic; therefore, the plasma sodium level will remain essentially normal unless other factors are present. For example, in the hospital setting, if excessive amounts of free water (such as 5% dextrose in water) are given, the plasma sodium concentration may drop below normal. This is particularly likely to occur because vomiting is a potent stimulus for the release of antidiuretic hormone, thus causing water retention. Hyponatremia is less likely to occur in the homebound patient because vomiting usually precludes oral fluid intake until the problem is resolved. Of course, in the presence of other factors that increase free water loss (eg, fever and hyperventilation), the plasma sodium level could be elevated.

Hypomagnesemia

Prolonged vomiting or gastric suction can contribute to magnesium depletion, an imbalance not as likely as those listed previously because the magnesium concentration in gastric juice is relatively low (about 1 mEq/L).[5] However, it can be a problem if losses are prolonged (lasting several weeks) and no magnesium is supplied in the IV fluids. Unfortunately, most routine electrolyte replacement solutions do not contain magnesium (eg, lactated Ringer's solution and isotonic saline have none).

MANAGEMENT OF GASTRIC FLUID LOSS

Treatment of gastric fluid loss requires correction of both the hypokalemia and the hypochloremic alkalosis with adequate amounts of fluid, potassium, and sodium chloride.[6] One author recommends replacing gastric fluid losses with 5% dextrose in 0.45% NaCl with 20 mEq KCl, given milliliter for milliliter of gastric fluid lost in the previous 24 hours.[7] For gastric

fluid losses more than 1500 mL in 24 hours, it has been recommended that the electrolyte content of the lost fluid be analyzed and treatment planned accordingly.[8]

Examples of nursing diagnoses related to loss of gastric fluid loss in vomiting or nasogastric suction include:

- Fluid volume deficit related to loss of isotonic gastric fluid
- Alteration in acid–base balance (metabolic alkalosis) related to loss of hydrogen and chloride ions

Examples of nursing interventions for patients with vomiting are listed in Table 13-3, and those for nasogastric suction are in Clinical Tip: Nursing Interventions for Patients With Gastric Suction.

 TABLE 13-3.   Nursing Interventions for Patients With Vomiting

1. Discourage the intake of plain water if vomiting is prolonged. Instead, encourage the frequent intake of small volumes of fluids containing electrolytes. (See Table 3-1 for a summary of the electrolyte content of commonly available oral fluids.)
2. Report vomiting early so that appropriate treatment can be started before fluid and electrolyte disturbances become severe. The physician will likely prescribe a medication to relieve nausea. If vomiting is prolonged and oral fluids are not retained, parenteral fluids are indicated.
3. Alter physical environment as much as possible to lessen stimuli for nausea (eg, remove sources of unpleasant odors).
4. Promote bedrest when vomiting is severe; avoid quick movements because they often make nausea more severe.
5. Measure, or estimate as accurately as possible, the amount of vomitus so that lost water and electrolytes can be replaced by the parenteral route. In fact, all fluids lost and gained from the body should be measured.
6. Measure body weight daily to detect significant changes in fluid balance. Daily weights are helpful in detecting FVD, particularly if vomitus has not been measured. A patient on a starvation diet should lose about ½ lb/day; a loss in excess of this amount probably implies FVD. A weight gain in this situation implies FVE. Routine IV fluids are low in calories; for example, a liter of 5% dextrose solutions contains only 170 calories.
7. Monitor for imbalances associated with loss of gastric fluid (see preceding discussion).
8. Be familiar with parenteral fluids commonly used to replace gastric fluid. Solutions that may be prescribed include routine solutions (such as isotonic or half-strength saline) with added potassium and magnesium, or special gastric replacement solutions (see Chap. 10).

FVD, fluid volume deficit; FVE, fluid volume excess.

● DIARRHEA

FLUID AND ELECTROLYTE DISTURBANCES

Diarrhea is characterized by increased frequency of stools with excessive water content. It can have many causes, such as infectious agents (viral, bacterial, and parasitic), toxins, and certain drugs. Viral enteritis and bacterial infections with organisms such as enterotoxigenic *Escherichia coli*, *Shigella*, and *Salmonella* are the most common causes of diarrhea in the United States.[9] Common causes in hospitalized patients who develop diarrhea are antibiotics and fecal impactions. Diarrhea is classified into several categories, including osmotic, secretory, structural, and primary motility disorders. Examples of causes of osmotic diarrhea are ingestion of poorly absorbable solutes (eg, lactulose, sorbitol, mannitol, magnesium sulfate, magnesium hydroxide, and sodium phosphate), generalized malabsorption or maldigestion, and certain infections. Secretory diarrhea is caused by abnormal secretion of water and electrolytes into the bowel lumen. Examples of causes of secretory diarrhea include enterotoxigenic bacteria (eg, *E. coli* and *Vibrio cholerae*) and partial or recently relieved intestinal obstruction.[10] Diarrhea secondary to structural changes occur in inflammatory bowel disease, collagen vascular disease, and sprue. Imbalances likely to be associated with diarrhea include:

- FVD
- Metabolic acidosis
- Hypokalemia
- Hypomagnesemia
- Sodium imbalances

FLUID VOLUME DEFICIT

Volume depletion is secondary to sodium and water loss in the diarrheal fluid. Severe diarrhea can lead to a daily loss of 2 to 10 liters of fluid, together with large quantities of electrolytes.[11] Obviously, prolonged diarrhea is a serious threat to water and electrolyte balance.

Metabolic Acidosis

The incidence of acid–base disorders in patients with severe diarrhea is about 70%, and the entire spectrum of disturbances may be seen.[12] However, metabolic acidosis is by far the most common disorder and is especially likely to occur in pediatric patients and in those with secretory or infectious diarrhea. Intestinal fluids are relatively alkaline because of their bicarbonate content; as a result, loss of intestinal fluid is likely to lead to metabolic (hyperchloremic) acidosis. (The plasma chloride level increases as the bicarbonate level decreases.)

Hypokalemia

Diarrhea, due to a multitude of causes, can be associated with excessive stool losses of potassium and result in hypokalemia. The typical electrolyte disorder in patients with diarrhea is hypokalemia with hyperchloremic metabolic acidosis.[13] A clinically significant depletion of total body potassium is likely only when severe chronic diarrhea is present.[14] A profound potassium depletion can occur in patients with colonic villous adenomas that secrete a profuse amount of potassium-rich, watery mucus.

Hypomagnesemia

Magnesium deficit can occur with prolonged diarrhea, particularly if magnesium is not adequately replaced. Most routine electrolyte solutions do not contain magnesium (eg, lactated Ringer's solution and isotonic saline have none).

Sodium Imbalances

The plasma sodium concentration varies in patients with diarrhea, depending on the cause of the problem and related clinical events. As discussed below, the diarrheal fluid may have a sodium content that is similar to, higher than, or lower than that of plasma. Extraneous factors also affect the plasma sodium concentration; among these are the amount of water intake (orally or IV) and the presence of fever or hyperventilation. Fever increases water loss in perspiration, and the compensatory hyperventilation associated with metabolic acidosis increases water loss from the lungs.

When the sodium content of the diarrheal fluid is similar to that of plasma, its loss causes an isotonic FVD (with no change in the plasma sodium level). This is often the case with diarrheal conditions classified as secretory diarrhea.[15] In contrast, diarrhea caused by osmotic conditions tends to be associated with relatively greater losses of water than sodium, resulting in a tendency toward an elevated plasma sodium concentration.[16] Hypernatremic dehydration

---

CLINICAL TIP

Nursing Interventions for Patients With Diarrhea

1. Measure, or estimate as accurately as possible, the amount of liquid feces so that lost water and electrolytes can be replaced (either by oral electrolyte solutions or via the parenteral route). All fluids gained and lost from the body should be measured and recorded on the I&O record. (See discussion of I&O measurement in Chap. 2.)

2. Measure body weight daily to detect significant changes in fluid balance. Daily weights are helpful in detecting fluid volume deficit, particularly if liquid stools have not been measured.

3. Monitor for clinical and laboratory indicators of imbalances commonly associated with the loss of intestinal fluid (see text). Specific imbalances are described in Chapters 3 to 9.

4. Offer oral electrolyte-containing liquids if allowed by the type of diarrhea present. (Some types of diarrhea respond better to temporary fasting and parenteral fluid replacement.) (See Table 24-1.)

5. Monitor response to parenteral fluids (if they are indicated) to replace fluid losses. Commonly used fluids for this purpose are lactated Ringer's solution and half strength saline (0.45% NaCl) with added potassium. Other electrolytes (such as magnesium) are replaced as indicated. Nursing responsibilities in fluid replacement therapy are described in Chapter 10.

I&O, intake and output.

---

due to watery diarrhea is most often seen in children less than 2 years of age.[17] In some types of diarrhea, sodium is lost in excess of water, causing a tendency toward hyponatremia. See Chapter 24 for a discussion of diarrhea in children.

MANAGEMENT OF DIARRHEAL FLUID LOSS

Most acute diarrheal episodes of viral or bacterial origin are self-limited and do not require specific therapy. If diarrhea is due to accumulation of poorly absorbed solutes in the intestine (osmotic diarrhea), it usually subsides with fasting. However, the diarrhea will usually persist despite fasting if it is a form of secretory diarrhea.[18]

Oral rehydration with glucose and electrolytes in infantile diarrhea is described in Chapter 24. For adults with mild dehydration who are not vomiting, rehydration can usually be accomplished by avoiding solid foods for at least 12 hours and taking only clear liquids.[19] Commercially prepared oral rehydration solutions are available, which contain potassium citrate, sodium chloride, sodium citrate, and dextrose (facilitates transport of electrolytes across the intestinal mucosa).[20]

If oral fluids are not tolerated, parenteral fluids are indicated. For moderate increases in stool fluid

(500–1000 mL/24 hr), a replacement fluid of 0.45% NaCl plus 20 mEq potassium acetate (which the liver converts to bicarbonate) might be used.[21] If the stool volume increases to more than 1 L/day, the replacement fluid might be changed to lactated Ringer's solution plus 20 mEq KCl.[22]

Examples of nursing diagnoses for patients with diarrhea include:

- Fluid volume deficit related to loss of isotonic diarrheal fluid
- Alteration in potassium balance (hypokalemia) related to loss of potassium-rich diarrheal fluid

See Clinical Tip: Nursing Interventions for Patients With Diarrhea.

IMBALANCES ASSOCIATED WITH LAXATIVES AND ENEMAS

Laxatives and enemas are frequently used to treat constipation and to cleanse the colon before diagnostic radiological studies and abdominal surgical procedures. Whenever possible, constipation should be treated by nonpharmacological means (Table 13-4). When these

TABLE 13-4. Nursing Interventions Related to Laxative and Enema Abuse

1. Encourage patients to avoid the repeated use of cathartics and enemas and rely on other methods to achieve bowel evacuation regularity.
2. Encourage maximum level of tolerated physical activity. Regular exercise stimulates gut motility and is an important part of a bowel management program. Walking 20–30 minutes a day is a good form of exercise. For immobilized patients, even small increases in activity may be helpful. For example, modest activities such as sitting up in bed or turning and twisting in a chair cause changes in colonic motility.[23]
3. Encourage ingestion of a glass of warm fluid first thing in the morning to stimulate the evacuation reflex.
4. Encourage regular fluid intake to act as a stool softener. For example, a glass or two of water on rising, between meals, and before bedtime should be consumed if tolerated.[24]
5. Encourage adequate bulk in the diet. Wheat bran is an excellent source that is available in many cereals and breads. Most fruits and vegetables are good sources of fiber.[25] Dietary fiber holds water, causing stools to be softer, bulkier, and heavier. The increased bowel bulk causes quicker movement of stool through the colon.
6. Encourage patients to attempt to develop a regular bowel routine. The best time to attempt a bowel elimination is probably after breakfast, because this is the time when the strongest propulsive contractions occur.

measures are not feasible or are ineffective, occasional use of laxatives or enemas may be indicated. However, the fluid and electrolyte problems that may accompany the injudicious use of laxatives and enemas must be considered. These fluid and electrolyte problems vary according to the nature of the laxative or enema solution used.

LAXATIVES

Patients with impaired renal function are at risk for hypermagnesemia and hyperphosphatemia when magnesium salts (such as magnesium citrate, magnesium sulfate, and milk of magnesia) or sodium phosphate solutions are administered because their kidneys are unable to excrete these substances adequately.[26] This can be a problem because magnesium-containing laxatives are frequently administered in quantities sufficient to cause toxic serum levels of magnesium when renal function is impaired.[27] Of interest, several instances have been described in which hypermagnesemia developed in patients with *normal* renal function (after administration of large doses of magnesium sulfate to facilitate poison removal from the GI tract).[28] Magnesium and phosphate cathartics are further contraindicated in patients with poor bowel motility (as occurs in adynamic ileus) because slowed motility increases the likelihood of absorption. A fatal case of

hyperphosphatemia secondary to the administration of Fleet Phospho-Soda as a cathartic to a 64-year-old man with colonic ileus was recently reported.[29]

ENEMAS

Tap Water Enemas

Repeated tap water enemas can result in excessive water absorption by the colon and thus dilutional hyponatremia. Excessive water absorption from the colon has been observed in states of chronic constipation and megacolon. Especially at risk are young children. Also thought to be at increased risk are adults with congestive heart failure (CHF), acquired immunodeficiency syndrome, and malignancy.[30] A case of severe hyponatremia and irreversible brain damage associated with tap water enemas in a patient with spinal cord injury was reported by Chertow and Brady.[31] Before receiving five tap water enemas of 1.5 to 3 liters each over a 10-day period, the patient (a 65-year-old man with C6 quadriplegia) had mild symptomless hyponatremia and a baseline glomerular filtration rate (GFR) of 82 mL/min. During the fifth enema, the patient became confused and developed seizures. Despite treatment with hypertonic saline, the patient remained comatose. The authors emphasized that the colonic mucosa can absorb life-threatening amounts of water in patients with ineffective renal water clearance ability.

Sodium Phosphate Enemas

Sodium phosphate enemas are available over the counter in pediatric (2.25 oz) and adult (4.5 oz) sizes (Fleet, C.B. Fleet Co., Lynchburg, VA). Because these enemas are composed of a hypertonic sodium phosphate solution, they act as an osmotic laxative by causing an increase in fluid volume of the colon, thus distending the colon and causing peristalsis to become more vigorous; ultimately, defecation occurs. However, if defecation does not occur before the hypertonic enema solution is absorbed by the colon, these enemas may produce a series of fluid and electrolyte problems (primarily hyperphosphatemia, hypernatremia, and hypocalcemia). The hyperphosphatemia and hypernatremia are a result of direct absorption of these electrolytes from the enema solution; hypocalcemia is a reciprocal response to hyperphosphatemia.

Imbalances occur primarily in patients unable to eliminate the enema solution adequately before significant absorption occurs. There have been reports of hyperphosphatemia, hypernatremia, and hypocalcemia after the use of sodium phosphate enemas in patients with GI disorders that interfere with prompt elimination of the enema solution (such as megacolon or fecal impaction).[32,33] Because of this finding, the manufacturer warns that sodium phosphate (Fleet) enemas should not be used in patients with conditions predisposing to retention of the enema solution (eg, congenital megacolon, imperforate anus, or colostomy). The manufacturer of sodium phosphate enemas warns that if after the enema solution is administered there is no return of the liquid, a physician should be contacted immediately because dehydration could occur.[34] The manufacturer warns that the enema should not be used in patients with megacolon, bowel obstruction, imperforate anus, or CHF.[35] Further, the manufacturer advises to use caution in patients with impaired renal function or a colostomy, preexisting electrolyte disturbances, or in patients taking diuretics or other medications that may affect electrolyte levels.[36]

Risks in Children

Most published reports of adverse effects from sodium phosphate enemas involve small children; usually the children had GI or renal problems, but sometimes they did not. It is helpful to review some of these cases to fully grasp the potential seriousness of the use of sodium phosphate enemas in young children.

Use of adult-sized sodium phosphate enemas for constipation or bowel cleansing before surgery or diagnostic procedures in children can produce disastrous results. Hypocalcemia and severe hyperphosphatemia occurred in a 4-year-old boy who received adult-sized sodium phosphate enemas for the treatment of constipation.[37] Due to tetany from the hypocalcemia, the child's extremities were stiff and could not be actively or passively moved. After treatment with IV calcium gluconate and oral calcium supplements, and hydration to promote diuresis, the child's condition improved. A similar case was described in which a previously healthy 5-month-old child suffered severe hyperphosphatemia, hypocalcemia, acidosis, and shock after administration of an adult-sized sodium phosphate enema for the treatment of constipation.[38] Still another tragic occurrence involved the administration of four adult-sized sodium phosphate (Fleet) enemas to an 11-month-old boy admitted for surgical correction of an imperforate anus.[39] The child had a sigmoid colostomy constructed shortly after birth. Two enemas were given in each barrel of the colostomy. About 2.5 hours after the enemas were administered, cardiac arrest occurred. Despite extensive resuscitative efforts with IV calcium, phosphate-binding resins per ostomy, and peritoneal dialysis, the child died. The manufacturer of sodium phosphate (Fleet) enemas warns that adult-sized enemas should not be used in children under 12 years of age and that the children's size should not be administered to children less than 2 years of age.[40]

Not all cases of serious electrolyte disturbances in children after sodium phosphate enemas involve the use of adult-sized enemas. A situation was reported in which two sodium phosphate *pediatric* enemas were administered to a girl aged 2 years, 6 months in preparation for a radiographic procedure.[41] She developed coma, tetany, dehydration, hypotension, tachycardia, and hyperpyrexia. Laboratory results indicated severe hyperphosphatemia, hypocalcemia, hypernatremia, and acidosis. Apparently about one-third of the administered enema solution was absorbed systemically.

Although more likely in high-risk patients, electrolyte disturbances from sodium phosphate enemas have also been reported in patients with no obvious underlying disease process.[42–44] Because most of the adverse effects with these enemas involve small children, some investigators reiterate that sodium phosphate enemas should be avoided in children under 2 years of age and that they should be used only with caution in those 2 to 5 years of age, especially if underlying bowel or renal dysfunction exists.[45] Still other researchers recommend against the use of sodium phosphate enemas entirely in small children and infants, indicating that it is incorrect to assume that sodium phosphate solutions are not absorbed by the colon.[46] Because sodium phosphate enemas are available over the counter, it has been recommended that parents be made aware that these enemas can be dangerous to infants and that prominent labeling be provided on the enema containers to indicate the potential dangers associated with their administration to infants.[47] Nurses should take an active part in educating parents about the dangers of nonjudicious use of enemas. Many clinicians favor the use of isotonic saline (0.9% NaCl) as an enema solution for patients of all ages to minimize fluid and electrolyte changes associated with absorption of the enema solution.

Risks in the Elderly

The elderly are also at increased risk for electrolyte disturbances associated with sodium phosphate enemas, particularly if they have atonic colons or renal failure. A recent case report of a 77-year-old woman who developed severe hyperphosphatemia and hypocalcemia after the administration of multiple sodium phosphate (Fleet) enemas to relieve fecal impaction indicates the potential problem in elderly patients.[48] (See Case Study 8-2.) The investigators cautioned against the overaggressive use of sodium phosphate enemas in elderly patients with fecal impactions because of the potential for prolonged retention of the enema solution; they further recommended that isotonic enemas be used instead whenever possible.[49]

A study of 14 elderly subjects (mean age, 78.5 years) indicated that sodium phosphate (Fleet) enemas carry a potential risk for acutely ill elderly patients.[50] To avoid untoward effects due to hyperphosphatemia and hypocalcemia, these researchers recommended that the phosphate load be adjusted to the patient's level of renal function. In that way, the amount of phosphate

that could conceivably be retained by the colon could ultimately be safely excreted by the kidneys.

● STANDARD BOWEL PREPARATIONS VERSUS POLYETHYLENE GLYCOL LAVAGE FOR DIAGNOSTIC STUDIES AND SURGERY

Two commonly used regimens to cleanse the colon before colonoscopy or colon surgery consist of (1) the rapid ingestion (either orally or by nasogastric tube) of a balanced electrolyte-polyethylene glycol (PEG) solution, and (2) a clear liquid or low-residue diet for 1 to 3 days plus a cathartic (such as sodium phosphate or magnesium citrate). In general, use of oral GI electrolyte-PEG lavage solutions has become the standard method for preparing the lower GI tract for colonoscopy.[51] Among the commercially available PEG lavage solutions are GoLYTELY (Braintree Laboratories, Inc., Braintree, MA) and Colyte (Schwarz Pharma, Inc., Milwaukee, WI). When reconstituted with water, COLYTE contains 125 mEq/L sodium, 10 mEq/L potassium, 20 mEq/L bicarbonate, 80 mEq/L sulfate, 35 mEq/L chloride, and 18 mEq/L PEG 3350.[52] About 1.5 liters of a PEG lavage solution is ingested per hour in adults until the rectal effluent is clear or up to 4 liters is consumed. According to the manufacturers, large volumes may be administered without significant changes in fluid and electrolyte balance because the osmotic activity of the PEG lavage results in virtually no net absorption or excretion of ions or water. Although these solutions are advantageous in terms of electrolyte balance, patients often have difficulty consuming the required fluid volume.

The kind of electrolyte imbalance likely to be associated with cathartic use depends on the cathartic itself. Oral sodium phosphate is commonly used for colon preparation before colonoscopy and could conceivably cause hypernatremia, hyperphosphatemia, and hypocalcemia. Although two studies have shown it to be safe for patients with normal renal function,[53,54] it is not recommended for patients with electrolyte imbalance, renal failure, poorly controlled CHF, or advanced liver disease.[55] Some authors have suggested that it may be prudent to evaluate serum electrolytes before the administration of sodium phosphate even in patients with normal renal function.[56] In a clinical study, serum magnesium levels were increased in patients receiving magnesium citrate as a cathartic as opposed to those receiving a PEG lavage solution.[57] Although the serum magnesium concentrations remained within a normal range, the potential for hypermagnesemia could be an important consideration in patients with renal insufficiency because they lack the ability to excrete magnesium normally.

Compared with the traditional method, the major advantage of PEG lavage is the considerably shorter time needed for preparation. Because the food restriction period is shortened considerably, hunger and associated weakness are less problematic. A disadvantage is nausea, abdominal fullness, and bloating (occurring in up to 50% of patients) associated with ingestion of the PEG lavage; abdominal cramps and vomiting occur less frequently.[58] Some patients complain that the PEG lavage solution has a disagreeable mildly salty taste and refuse to drink it. Chilling the solution makes it more palatable. The manufacturers recommend that patients fast for about 3 or 4 hours before ingesting the solution. They emphasize that solid food should not be allowed for at least 2 hours before the solution is given. Only clear liquids are allowed during the interval between PEG lavage solution ingestion and examination.

A disadvantage of the traditional method is the 1- to 3-day period of reduced food intake, resulting in hunger and weakness. Although many patients prefer cathartics over drinking 4 liters of an electrolyte-PEG solution, the use of cathartics after several days of dietary restrictions can present problems for elderly patients. Thus, the elderly patient undergoing rigorous bowel preparation should be observed closely for adverse reactions. The reduced GFR in the elderly potentiates the hazards of any further decrease in ECF volume (as occurs in vigorous catharsis). The aged patient having GI roentgenograms should probably receive IV fluids during the preparation period of reduced oral intake and increased fluid loss (caused by catharsis and enema). Note also that use of radiocontrast agents in diagnostic radiology (particularly in large doses) has been incriminated as predisposing to acute renal failure, especially when the patient has a

severe FVD. See Chapter 25 for further discussion of the effect of standard bowel preparations on elderly patients.

● LOSS OF FLUID THROUGH FISTULAS

Fistulas are abnormal communications between the intestine and the skin (external fistula) or another hollow viscus (internal fistula). They can result from trauma or occur spontaneously as a complication of pancreatitis, inflammatory bowel disease, neoplasia, or other GI disorders. The majority of external GI fistulas that develop postoperatively are the result of technical complications.[59] Fistulas can develop at any level in the GI tract.

The major complications associated with small bowel fistulas include fluid and electrolyte disturbances, sepsis, and malnutrition.[60] Loss of fluids from fistulas can produce serious fluid and electrolyte disturbances. In general, the more proximal the fistula, the greater is the fluid loss. Any fistula that drains 500 mL or more in 24 hours is considered to be a high-output fistula.[61] Failure to adequately replace large fistulous losses can lead to FVD, hypoperfusion, and eventually multiorgan failure.[62]

The electrolytes lost in fistulous drainage depend on the exact site of the fistula. An educated guess regarding imbalances likely to accompany a specific fluid's loss can be made by reviewing the usual electrolyte content of fluid in the region of the fistula (see Table 13-1). When doubt about the fistula's origin exists, sending a sample of the drainage fluid to the laboratory for analysis of pH and electrolyte composition can aid in determining replacement therapy.

Intestinal fluids, including pancreatic and biliary secretions, are relatively alkaline because of their bicarbonate content. Thus, loss of these fluids would likely lead to metabolic acidosis. In contrast, loss of chloride-rich gastric fluid predisposes to metabolic alkalosis.

Although fluid and electrolyte problems are possible with any fistula, they are most likely to be substantial in patients with pancreatic, duodenal stump, and gastrojejunal anastomotic fistulas.[63] Biliary and pancreatic fistulous drainage contains sizable amounts of sodium and bicarbonate, predisposing to FVD and metabolic acidosis. Hyponatremia can easily occur if fluid replacement contains more free water than needed.

Drainage from external fistulas can often be collected with a well fixed stoma appliance. The volume of drainage collected in this device should be measured and recorded on the intake and output record. If the drainage cannot be obtained and directly measured, an estimate should be made of the volume absorbed by dressings and bed linens. Of course, skin care is essential to guard against the effects of autodigestion by GI enzymes. Various skin barrier films and other preparations are available for this purpose.

It seems prudent to provide aggressive nutritional support for patients with fistulas.[64] Nutritional support can be in the form of total parenteral nutrition or enteral feedings. When tolerated, enteral feedings are preferred because they are more effective in maintaining intestinal integrity and therefore in decreasing bacterial translocation and infection. When enteral feedings are used, the feeding tube is inserted about 30 to 40 cm past the fistula.[65]

Several studies have reported increased spontaneous closure rates of fistulas as well as decreased mortality rates when IV hyperalimentation was used.[66,67] Data exist to suggest that somatostatin used in conjunction with nutritional support allows spontaneous closure of fistulas to occur earlier.[68,60]

⬤ IMBALANCES ASSOCIATED WITH ANOREXIA NERVOSA

Anorexia nervosa can be subdivided into the "restricting" form in which the patient loses weight by self-induced starvation and perhaps compulsive exercising, and the "bulimic" form, in which there is a combination of marked dietary restriction and episodes of binge eating, vomiting, and diuretic/laxative abuse.[70] Serious, even life-threatening, fluid and electrolyte problems are understandably possible in patients with eating disorders. The prognosis for severe bulimia nervosa is less favorable than for uncomplicated anorexia nervosa.[71] One study of 168 patients with bulimia or related eating disorders found about 50% had some sort of electrolyte abnormality.[72]

The type of electrolyte abnormalities in anorectic patients depends on whether or not self-induced vom-

iting is the predominant behavior or whether laxative or diuretic abuse is dominant.[71] A careful history is needed to determine which methods are used by the patient to lose weight. Among the more frequent fluid and electrolyte problems observed in patients with eating disorders are FVD, hypokalemia, hypomagnesemia, hypophosphatemia, hyponatremia, hypocalcemia, and either metabolic alkalosis or metabolic acidosis.

FLUID VOLUME DEFICIT

This condition is most likely in patients who take large doses of diuretics and laxatives. Clinically, hypotension (< 90/60 mm Hg) and postural dizziness or syncope may be present. Also, the BUN is elevated out of proportion to the serum creatinine level. Skin turgor may appear normal despite FVD in adolescents or young adults who characteristically have good skin elasticity.

HYPOKALEMIA

Hypokalemia is possible due to excessive losses from vomiting and laxative abuse, coupled with poor dietary intake. If the patient has access to potassium-losing diuretics, such as the thiazides, the likelihood of hypokalemia is even greater. (Chlorothiazide and hydrochlorothiazides are commonly abused diuretic agents.[74]) Hypokalemia is a particularly dangerous imbalance because of the possibility of cardiac arrhythmias. One researcher recommends that patients with serum potassium concentrations less than 2.5 mEq/L be hospitalized for bedrest and treatment.[75] Hypokalemic nephropathy can follow prolonged potassium depletion in anorectics and be associated with the development of polyuria, polydipsia, and elevated serum creatinine levels.[76]

HYPOMAGNESEMIA

Like hypokalemia, hypomagnesemia is possible because of excessive losses from vomiting and diuretic or laxative abuse, coupled with poor dietary intake. Hypomagnesemia has been reported in up to 25% of patients with anorexia nervosa, and is often associated with refractory hypokalemia and hypocalcemia that may not resolve unless the hypomagnesemia is corrected simultaneously.[77]

HYPOPHOSPHATEMIA

Hypophosphatemia is an ominous sign in patients with eating disorders.[78] The etiology of hypophosphatemia is not clear, but it is most likely the result of inadequate oral intake and absorption of phosphorus. It is most problematic during aggressive refeeding when rapid glucose-rich hyperalimentation causes extracellular phosphorus to shift into the cells, thus further lowering the serum phosphorus levels. This may result in myocardial dysfunction and neurological complications, such as convulsions.[79] Thus, plasma phosphorus levels should be monitored for several days in any malnourished patient during refeeding and supplements administered as indicated.

HYPONATREMIA

Hyponatremia may result from excessive sodium losses from diuretic and laxative abuse, as well as from self-induced vomiting. However, it may also result from excessive water intake. Several cases have recently been reported in which patients affected by anorexia nervosa presented with seizures secondary to self-induced water intoxication. One of these was a 17-year-old girl who ingested an average water intake of 7 to 8 L/day.[80] Her history did not include abuse of laxatives or diuretics. On admission to the hospital with a generalized tonic-clonic seizure, her serum sodium level was 116 mEq/L.

HYPOCALCEMIA

Hypocalcemia can result from poor dietary intake and diminished bone stores of calcium after prolonged malnutrition. Ionized levels of calcium are decreased in patients with metabolic alkalosis, a common imbalance in those with vomiting and potassium-losing diuretic abuse.

ACID–BASE IMBALANCES

In a study of 168 bulimic patients, metabolic alkalosis was the most frequent acid–base imbalance.[81] It is commonly associated with loss of gastric fluid from vomiting and with the abuse of potassium-losing diuretics.

Metabolic acidosis (due to the loss of alkaline intestinal fluid) may be the predominant acid–base disturbance if the patient is a heavy abuser of laxatives.

Some patients have been reported to take as many as 100 laxative doses daily.[82] Most commonly taken are stimulant-type laxatives that are available over the counter (such as Correctol, Ex-Lax, and Senokot).[83] The most common diuretic agent used by adolescents and young adults is ammonium chloride (available without a prescription); abuse of this drug compounds the metabolic acidosis caused by laxative abuse.[84]

Patients with eating disorders must be observed closely for life-threatening electrolyte abnormalities. As pointed out by Hofland and Dardia,[85] bulimia is a psychiatric disorder, but morbidity and mortality can occur because of the physical problems. For example, sudden death with unexplained cardiovascular collapse may occur secondary to electrolyte-induced arrhythmias. These arrhythmias may result from imbalances such as hypokalemia, hypomagnesemia, and altered pH disturbances, all of which are commonly present in patients with eating disorders. Although these risks are present in the purely "restrictive" forms of the disease, they are even greater in those who abuse laxatives and diuretics. Refeeding the starving patient also carries increased risks for cardiac dysfunction, especially if performed too aggressively. In general, a cautious and gradual approach with regular blood electrolyte analyses is indicated in the initial period of refeeding.[86]

IMBALANCES ASSOCIATED WITH INTESTINAL OBSTRUCTION

Intestinal obstruction causes interference with the normal progression of intestinal contents and may be termed either complete or incomplete. A mechanical obstruction is defined as an actual physical barrier (eg, adhesions, hernia, tumor, or diverticula) blocking normal passage of intestinal contents. A mechanical obstruction is termed *simple* when the vascular supply is not compromised; it is termed *strangulated* when the vascular supply is inhibited. A functional obstruction is sometimes referred to as *paralytic ileus*, or an *adynamic* or *neurogenic ileus*. As the name implies, the obstruction is caused by ineffective or nonpropulsive peristalsis. Although motor activity is slowed, it is not completely absent. Causes of paralytic ileus can include intra-abdominal conditions such as peritonitis, appendicitis, cholecystitis, and pancreatitis. Other causes involve trauma and systemic conditions such as hypokalemia, uremia, and septicemia.

Simple mechanical obstruction results in a striking accumulation of intestinal fluid and gas above the obstruction. Most of the gas is due to swallowed air, although some results from bacterial fermentation within the gut. Because of distention, large quantities of water and electrolytes are secreted into the bowel lumen, even in the absence of oral intake. Fluid also accumulates within the bowel wall. The edematous bowel wall is not able to absorb the large volume of intestinal secretions; therefore, distention becomes progressively greater, leading to isotonic contraction of the ECF compartment as fluid is sequestered in the bowel (third-space effect). Ten liters or more of fluid can collect in this third-space site and lead to hypovolemic shock. Vomiting or nasogastric suctioning adds to the fluid losses. (Nursing assessment for third-space fluid shift is described in Chap. 3.)

In adynamic ileus, decreased propulsive motility can affect the small intestine and colon, separately or together. As in mechanical obstruction, gas accumulates in the involved intestine, producing marked distention. Fluid also accumulates in the intestine because of decreased absorption. Although third-space fluid loss may be significant, it is not likely to be as great as in mechanical obstruction.

Plasma concentrations of electrolytes are initially preserved because the fluid lost is primarily isotonic; however, the patient usually becomes thirsty and drinks water, thereby developing hyponatremia.[87] Contributing to hyponatremia is the endogenous release of water produced by oxidation. Sodium and other electrolytes (such as potassium and magnesium) are also lost by vomiting or as a result of GI suction after treatment is initiated. If the lost electrolytes are not replaced, deficits will eventually result.

The type of acid–base imbalance likely to be encountered is largely determined by the site of the obstruction. Metabolic alkalosis is common with pyloric or high small intestinal obstruction in which copious vomiting produces loss of acidic gastric juice. Sometimes in upper small intestinal obstruction, the patient will vomit about equal volumes of gastric and intestinal juice, thus preventing serious disturbances in pH levels. If the obstruction is in a distal segment of the small intestine, the patient may vomit larger quantities of alkaline fluids than of acid fluids. (Recall that secretions below the pylorus are mainly alkaline.) Thus, metabolic acidosis can result from a low intestinal obstruction. If the obstruction is below the proximal colon, most of the GI fluids will be absorbed before reaching the point of obstruction, and thus acid–base balance may remain intact. In this situation, solid fecal matter accumulates until symptoms of discomfort develop. Respiratory acidosis can develop in patients with abdominal distention because respirations are compromised by upward pressure on the diaphragm, resulting in carbon dioxide retention. Impairment of renal function due to severe hypovolemia can lead to metabolic acidosis, as can starvation with subsequent ketoacidosis.[88]

CASE STUDIES

● **13-1.** A 16-year-old high school student was brought to the emergency room after experiencing a seizure within a few minutes of complaints of dizziness and faintness. According to her parents, she had a history of restrictive dietary intake (interspersed with brief periods of binge eating) and self-induced vomiting, as well as heavy abuse of laxatives. At the time of admission, her body weight was 79 lb (height, 63 in.). Lying flat, her blood pressure (BP) was 88/54 mm Hg and her pulse rate was 98/min; on standing, her BP dropped to 64/46 mm Hg and her pulse rate increased to 130/min. Blood chemistries revealed:

Sodium = 128 mEq/L
Chloride = 90 mEq/L
Potassium = 2.5 mEq/L
CO_2 content = 29 mEq/L
Magnesium = 1.8 mEq/L
BUN = 30 mg/dL
Calcium = 8.5 mg/dL
Creatinine = 1.2 mg/dL
Phosphorus = 2.6 mg/dL

The patient was treated with IV 0.9% NaCl with added KCl. After stabilization, she was cautiously started on TPN. Several days after treatment was initiated, the patient experienced fluid retention (as evidenced by mild puffiness and bloating).

COMMENTARY: Probably the seizure was caused by FVD, which was associated with cerebral hypoperfusion, and hyponatremia (which predisposed to a reduced seizure threshold because of mild brain swelling). Note that several typical indicators of FVD were present in this patient (eg, postural hypotension, tachycardia, and a BUN elevated out of proportion to the serum creatinine level).

Isotonic saline was not only effective in expanding her ECF volume, it helped correct the lower than normal serum sodium and chloride levels. Both the FVD and hyponatremia were probably due to self-induced vomiting, laxative abuse, and poor dietary intake.

The low serum potassium level (2.5 mEq/L) was quite serious and required admission to an intensive care unit for cardiac monitoring until corrected.

It is not uncommon for anorectics who have chronic FVD to develop a compensatory increased production of aldosterone, which causes the kidneys to conserve sodium and water. This compensatory renal mechanism begins slowly but once initiated persists after FVD is corrected, resulting in temporary fluid retention during purge-free periods.[88] Patients with eating disorders usually find this phenomenon highly distressing and often renew their pattern of vomiting and laxative/diuretic abuse to relieve bloating.

● **13-2.** An 80-year-old woman was admitted to the hospital with a history of diarrhea (average of six watery stools per day) over a period of several weeks. The following laboratory data were obtained:

  Sodium = 135 mEq/L
  Arterial pH = 7.25
  Potassium = 3.0 mEq/L
  $PaCO_2$ = 28 mm Hg
  Chloride = 111 mEq/L
  HCO_3 = 12 mEq/L

COMMENTARY: Note the presence of metabolic acidosis, as indicated by the low pH and bicarbonate concentration. This is a normal anion gap acidosis: Na - (HCO_3 + Cl) = 12 mEq/L (135 - [12 + 111] = 12). The $PaCO_2$ is appropriately reduced as a compensatory change.

● **13-3.** A 40-year-old woman was admitted with a 5-day history of nausea and episodic vomiting. She complained of feeling lightheaded on standing. Lying flat, her BP was 102/68 mm Hg and her pulse rate was 92/min; standing up, her BP fell to

92/60 mm Hg and her pulse rate rose to 110/min. The following laboratory data were observed:

  Sodium = 143 mEq/L
  Arterial pH = 7.53
  Potassium = 2.9 mEq/L
  $PaCO_2$ = 47 mm Hg
  Chloride = 85 mEq/L
  HCO_3 = 36 mEq/L

COMMENTARY: This patient had FVD, as evidenced by the postural changes in BP and pulse rate. She also had metabolic alkalosis (secondary to loss of chloride and hydrogen ions from vomiting), as evidenced by the greater than normal arterial pH and elevated HCO_3 level. The $PaCO_2$ was elevated as a compensatory mechanism. The low serum potassium was related to loss of potassium in vomitus and in the urine (see text for further explanation).

● **13-4.**[90] A 68-year-old woman with a prior history of jejunoileal bypass surgery was admitted to the emergency department with complaints of difficulty walking as well as numbness and tingling in all four extremities. She had ingested 45 mL of Fleet's Phospho-Soda in preparation for a routine colonoscopy. Although she was scheduled to take an additional dose on the day of the procedure, her symptoms prevented her from doing so.

On physical examination, she was found to have tetany in her toes and fingers and a positive Trousseau's sign (elicited in the right arm on inflation of a blood pressure cuff). Laboratory blood work revealed:

  Total calcium = 6.5 mg/dL (normal = 8.4–10.2 mg/dL)
  Phosphorus = 8.8 mg/dL (normal = 2.4–4.4 mg/dL)
  Magnesium = 1.1 mg/dL (normal = 1.7–2.2 mg/dL)
  Albumin = 3.9 g/dL (normal 3.5–5.5 g/dL)

All other laboratory values were within the normal range. Following treatment over the next 24 hours, her symptoms improved dramatically. A review of her medical history revealed that she had had a similar episode almost a year earlier. In that situation, she also had ingested 45 mL of Fleet's Phospho-Soda in preparation for colonoscopy. She subsequently developed numbness in her arms and face and was evaluated in the emergency department and discharged with no diagnosis. Laboratory work at that time revealed a low serum calcium (7.3 mg/dL), a normal serum albumin level, and a high serum phosphorus (8.7 mg/dL). In retrospect, it was recognized that these abnormal values were related to the ingestion of the Fleet's Phospho-Soda.

COMMENTARY: Recall that the ingestion of a high phosphorus load causes a reciprocal drop in the serum calcium level. The low serum calcium level was accentuated by the patient's poor intestinal absorption of calcium due to her jejunoileal bypass. The chronic hypomagnesemia secondary to malabsorption may have also contributed to the development of hypocalcemia because magnesium deficiency can block parathyroid hormone secretion. (Recall that in normal situations when the serum calcium level drops below normal, secretion of parathyroid hormone is increased to cause release of calcium from the bone into the bloodstream.) The fact that the patient had a normal serum albumin level means that the low total serum calcium level reflected a true hypocalcemia. In summary, Ehrenpreis et al.[90] warned against the use of Fleet's Phospho-Soda for bowel preparation in any patient suspected of having small intestinal malabsorption of calcium to avoid the development of severe hypocalcemia.

● **13-5.**[91] An 88-year-old woman was admitted to a hospital after a sudden onset of acute confusion.

Her husband reported that she had been her usual self before going to the bathroom to irrigate her colostomy. Two hours later, she emerged talking "gibberish" and was unable to identify her family members. It was later learned that she had used 4 liters of tap water (instead of the usual 1 liter) to irrigate her colostomy because of difficulty with bowel elimination. On physical examination her vital signs were essentially within their usual range; her body weight was 90 lb. A mental state examination confirmed her disorientation to time, place, and person and inappropriate noncontextual responses. Laboratory data revealed:

Serum sodium = 118 mEq/L
Serum potassium = 3.9 mEq/L
Serum chloride = 87 mEq/L
Serum glucose = 94 mEq/L
Serum creatinine = 1.0 mg/dL

COMMENTARY: Her acute confusional state was secondary to hyponatremia. After treatment with hypertonic saline infusion her sodium level improved; as this occurred, she became more alert and responsive. Two days after her emergency admission her score on the Mini-Mental State Examination was 26 (maximum score, 30). Shiwach[91] emphasized that this case demonstrates that hyponatremia can result from overenthusiastic lavage of a colostomy with water and can present as an acute confusional state, especially in an elderly person who already has mild cerebral changes.

REFERENCES

1. Rose B. *Clinical Physiology of Acid–Base and Electrolyte Disorders*, 4th ed. New York: McGraw-Hill; 1994:389.
2. Kokko J, Tannen R. *Fluids and Electrolytes*, 3rd ed. Philadelphia: WB Saunders; 1996:678.
3. Narins R. *Clinical Disorders of Fluid and Electrolyte Metabolism*, 5th ed. New York: McGraw-Hill; 1994:947.
4. Kokko, Tannen, p 677.
5. Ibid, p 432.
6. Narins, p 680.
7. Pemberton L, Pemberton D. *Treatment of Water, Electrolyte and Acid-Base Disorders in the Surgical Patient.* New York: McGraw-Hill; 1994:54.
8. Ibid.
9. Carey C, Lee H, Woeltje K, eds. *Manual of Medical Therapeutics*, 29th ed. Philadelphia: Lippincott-Raven; 1998:326.
10. Narins, p 1143.
11. Ibid.
12. Ibid, p 1145.
13. Szerlip, Goldfarb, p 92.
14. Narins, p 1143.
15. Rose, p 644.
16. Ibid.
17. Narins, p 1143.
18. Carey et al, p 327.
19. Kroser J, Metz D. Evaluation of the adult patient with diarrhea. *Gastroenterology* 1996;23:629.
20. Ibid.
21. Pemberton, Pemberton, p 55.
22. Ibid.
23. Ellickson E. Bowel management plan for the homebound elderly. *J Gerontol Nurs* 1988;14:16.
24. Yakabowich M. Prescribe with care: The role of laxatives in the treatment of constipation. *J Gerontol Nurs* 1990;16:4.
25. Preece G, Judd C. Constipation in the elderly: Are drugs the only alternative to irregularity? *Canadian Pharmaceutical Journal* 1982;115:136.

26. Yakabowich, p 4.
27. Schwartz S et al. *Principles of Surgery*, 7th ed. New York: McGraw-Hill; 1999.
28. Jones J et al. Cathartic-induced magnesium toxicity during overdose management. *Ann Emerg Med* 1986;15:1214.
29. Fass R et al. Fatal hyperphosphatemia following Fleet Phospho-Soda in a patient with colonic ileus. *Am J Gastroenterol* 1993;88:929.
30. Chertow G, Brady H. Hyponatremia from tap-water enema. *Lancet* 1994;344(8924):748.
31. Ibid.
32. Moseley P, Segar W. Fluid and serum electrolyte disturbances as a complication of enemas in Hirchsprung's disease. *Am J Dis Child* 1968;115:714.
33. Korzets A et al. Life-threatening hyperphosphatemia and hypocalcemic tetany following the use of fleet enemas. *J Am Geriatr Soc* 1992;40:6210.
34. *Physician's Desk Reference*, 53rd ed. Oradell, NJ: Medical Economics Company, 1999:1012.
35. Ibid.
36. Ibid.
37. Edmondson S, Almquist T. Iatrogenic hypocalcemic tetany. *Ann Emerg Med* 1990;19:938.
38. Wason S et al. Severe hyperphosphatemia, hypocalcemia, acidosis, and shock in a 5-month old child following the administration of an adult Fleet enema. *Ann Emerg Med* 1989;18:696.
39. Martin R et al. Fatal poisoning from sodium phosphate enema: Case report and experimental study. *JAMA* 1987;257:2190.
40. *PDR*, p 1012.
41. Sotos J et al. Hypocalcemic coma following two pediatric phosphate enemas. *Pediatrics* 1977;60:305.
42. Swerdlow D et al. Tetany and enemas: report of a case. *Dis Colon Rectum* 1974;17:786.
43. Davis et al. Hypocalcemia, hyperphosphatemia, and dehydration following a single hypertonic phosphate enema. *J Pediatr* 1977;90:484.
44. Levitt M et al. Inorganic phosphate (laxative) poisoning resulting in tetany in an infant. *J Pediatr* 1973;82:479.
45. Craig J et al. Phosphate enema poisoning in children. *Med J Austr* 1994;160:347.
46. Martin, p 2192.
47. Wason et al, p 696.
48. Korzets et al, p 620.
49. Ibid.
50. Grosskopf L et al. Hyperphosphatemia and hypocalcemia induced by hypertonic phosphate enema—an experimental study and review of the literature. *Hum Exp Toxicol* 1991;10:351.
51. Keeffe E. Colonoscopy preps: What's best? *Gastrointest Endosc* 1996;43:524.
52. *PDR*, p 2897.
53. Cohen S, Wexner S, Binderow S, et al. Prospective, randomized endoscopic-blinded trial comparing precolonoscopy bowel cleansing methods. *Dis Colon Rectum* 1994;37:689.
54. Huynh T, Vanner S, Paterson W. Safety profile of 5-h oral sodium phosphate regimen for colonoscopy cleansing: Lack of clinically significant hypocalcemia or hypovolemia. *Am J Gastroenterol* 1995;90:104.
55. Tooson J, Gates L. Bowel preparation before colonoscopy. *Postgrad Med* 1996;100:203.
56. Lieberman D et al. Effect of oral sodium phosphate colon preparation on serum electrolytes in patients with normal serum creatinine. *Gastrointest Endosc* 1996;43:467.
57. DiPalma J et al. Comparison of colon cleansing methods in preparation for colonoscopy. *Gastroenterology* 1984;86:856.
58. *PDR*, p 2898.
59. Schwartz et al, p 1251.
60. Ibid, p 1252.
61. Schwartz, p 1252.
62. Zaloga G, ed. *Nutrition in Critical Care*. St. Louis: CV Mosby; 1994:625.
63. Kokko, Tannen, p 937.
64. Zaloga, p 686.
65. Ibid, p 316.
66. Chapman R et al. Management of intestinal fistulas. *Am J Surg* 1964;108:157.
67. MacPhayden B et al. Management of gastrointestinal fistulas with parenteral hyperalimentation. *Surgery* 1973;74:100.
68. diCostanzo J et al. Treatment of external gastrointestinal fistulas by a combination of total parenteral nutrition and somatostatin. *JPEN J Parenter Enteral Nutr* 1987;11:465.
69. Torres A et al. Somatostatin in the management of gastrointestinal fistulas: A multicenter trial. *Arch Surg* 1992;127:97.
70. Sharp C, Freeman C. The medical complications of anorexia nervosa. *Br J Psychiatry* 1993;162:452.
71. Comerco G. Medical complications of anorexia nervosa and bulimia nervosa. *Med Clin North Am* 1990;74:1293.
72. Mitchell J et al. Electrolyte and other physiological abnormalities in patients with bulimia. *Psychol Med* 1983;13a:273.
73. Comerci, p 1298.
74. Ibid, p 1306.
75. Sharp, Freeman, p 459.
76. Hall R, Beresford T. Medical complications of anorexia and bulimia. *Psychiatric Medicine* 1989;7:165.
77. Sharp, Freeman, p 454.
78. Comerci, p 1301.
79. Sharp, Freeman, p 454.
80. Cuesto M et al. Secondary seizures from water intoxication in anorexia nervosa. *Gen Hosp Psychiatry* 1992;14:212.
81. Mitchell J. Medical complications of anorexia nervosa and bulimia. *Psychiatric Medicine* 1983;1:229.
82. Edelstein C et al. Early clues to anorexia and bulimia. *Patient Care* 1989;23:155.
83. Mitchell J, Boutacoff L. Laxative abuse complicating bulimia: Medical and treatment implications. *Int J Eating Disord* 1986;5:325.
84. Comerci, p 1306.
85. Hofland S, Dardia P. Bulimia nervosa: Associated physical problems. *J Psychosoc Nurs* 1992;30:23.
86. Sharp, Freeman, p 458.
87. Narins, p 1147.
88. Ibid.
89. Comerci, p 1304.
90. Ehrenpreis E et al. Symptomatic hypocalcemia, hypomagnesemia, and hyperphosphatemia secondary to Fleet's phosphosoda colonoscopy preparation in a patient with a jejunoileal bypass. *Dig Dis Sci* 1997;42:858.
91. Shiwach R. Hyponatremia from colonic lavage presenting as an acute confusional state. *Am J Psychiatry* 1996;153:10.

CHAPTER 14

Fluid Balance in the Surgical Patient

Although surgical patients are at great risk for fluid and electrolyte imbalances, these disturbances often can be prevented or minimized by appropriate intervention. Assessment and management of the patient's fluid and electrolyte status begins in the preoperative period and continues into the postoperative recovery period.

● PREOPERATIVE PERIOD

Before surgery, potential perioperative problems should be identified by reviewing the patient's medical, surgical, and anesthesia history, and by looking for specific indicators of potential problems. Preoperative assessment in the ambulatory surgical setting presents a special challenge to the nurse. The health care economy has generated an increase in ambulatory surgery, necessitating creative strategies to perform a preoperative evaluation that is both cost effective and reliable.[1] Various methods (such as telephone interviews and mailed questionnaires) have been used to gain needed information. Some ambulatory surgery centers require previsits for all patients (or at least those who will have general anesthesia); others rely on voluntary previsits.[2] At times, the needed assessment is performed in the surgeon's office or clinic. In any event, the nurse must work with the surgeon and anesthesia department to manage potential problems before or on the day of surgery. Operative blood transfusion requirements and various alternatives such autologous preoperative donation are discussed in the preoperative period. The nurse answers questions and provides information on the process of donation.

FLUID AND ELECTROLYTE DISTURBANCES

Virtually any fluid and electrolyte problem can be seen in surgical patients, depending on the individual history. Because of this, recent studies point to the need to individualize laboratory tests to the patient's medical history, medications, and assessment findings.[3–8] Although thorough tests are still indicated for hospitalized patients scheduled for major procedures, it has been suggested that routine preoperative testing for elective surgical procedures in relatively healthy patients is of questionable value and results of the tests often do not lead to a change in the surgery or anes-

thesia plan. However, any patient (in or out of the hospital) with renal, heart, liver, adrenal, or thyroid disorders, diuretic therapy, and abnormal gastrointestinal losses requires preoperative water and electrolyte evaluation before surgery.[9]

Available laboratory data should be reviewed carefully to detect fluid and electrolyte problems. (See Tables 2-2 and 2-3 for blood and urine tests useful in determining fluid balance status.) Any abnormalities should be called to the attention of the medical staff for early correction. (Specific fluid and electrolyte imbalances are discussed in Chaps. 3 through 9.)

Hypokalemia

Hypokalemia is the most frequent cause for cancellation of elective surgery because this imbalance predisposes to cardiac arrhythmias during the intraoperative period, especially in those with cardiac disease.[10] Patients with hypokalemia caused by use of diuretics should also be screened and treated for hypomagnesemia because of their arrhythmogenic capacity and ability to worsen renal potassium wasting.[11] Correction of potassium deficit should be started only after adequate urine output is established.

Fluid Volume Deficit

Surgical patients are at risk for fluid volume deficit (FVD) for a number of reasons. Prolonged periods of "nothing per os" (NPO) are common in patients who have undergone numerous diagnostic tests before surgical intervention. This is particularly problematic because diagnostic tests may require the use of cathartics and enemas (promoting fluid loss through the intestine) or use of contrast agents (producing osmotic diuresis). In addition, the patient may have suffered fluid losses related to the primary illness requiring surgical intervention.

Before surgery, sufficient fluid must be given to stabilize blood pressure and pulse and increase hourly urine volume to an acceptable range (preferably 50 mL/hr in an adult). The rate of fluid administration varies considerably, depending on severity and type of fluid disturbances, presence of continuing losses, and cardiac status.

Preoperative Fluid Restriction

Various methods have been used to reduce the risk of nausea and vomiting in surgical patients; among these are NPO regimens, preanesthesia and postanesthesia suctioning of gastric contents, and ingestion of antacids.[12] It is still common practice to restrict hospitalized patients to NPO status at midnight before the day of surgery; however, this practice is less common in ambulatory care settings. One reason it may be possible to shorten the fasting period is that currently used anesthetic agents cause less nausea and vomiting than those used in the past.[13,14] It has been suggested that prolonged liquid fasts are unnecessary in healthy patients before ambulatory surgery; ingestion of coffee and pulp-free orange juice (250 mL) 2 to 3 hours before surgery apparently does not increase gastric volume.[15] Goresky and Malby[16] have offered the following recommendations for elective surgical patients: (1) permission for unrestricted intake of clear liquids until 3 hours before the scheduled time of surgery, (2) allowing oral medications to be taken with 30 mL water up to 1 hour before surgery, and (3) use of an H_2-blocker preoperatively for patients at increased risk for regurgitation and aspiration of gastric contents.

CHRONIC CONDITIONS

Certain chronic illnesses predispose to fluid, electrolyte, and acid–base disturbances during the stressful perioperative period. For example, patients with renal failure are at risk for hyperkalemia, metabolic acidosis, hypermagnesemia, and hyponatremia and may require emergent hemodialysis before emergency surgery.[17] Patients with end-stage liver disease are at risk for chronic hyponatremia due to impaired renal sodium handling.[18] Those with chronic obstructive pulmonary disease are predisposed to respiratory acidosis and hypoxemia. Patients who have experienced a myocardial infarction in the last 6 months or those with uncompensated congestive heart failure (CHF) are at high risk for perioperative myocardial infarction and death and therefore are not acceptable candidates for elective surgery.[19] Patients with chronic cardiac conditions should be in the best metabolic control possible before surgery and often require preoperative insertion of a pulmonary artery catheter for monitoring during and after surgery.

MEDICATIONS

As discussed in Chapters 3 through 9, a number of medications can cause fluid and electrolyte disturbances. Some of the more problematic are potassium-losing diuretics. Examples of others include antibiotics predisposing to renal potassium wasting (such as carbenicillin and amphotericin B) and renal magnesium wasting (such as gentamicin).

ALTERED ADRENAL RESPONSE

Adrenal crisis is a life-threatening condition that may result when a patient is unable to make the expected adrenal cortical response to stress. To prevent this problem in the perioperative period, it is important to recognize that supplemental steroids may be needed for patients who have taken supraphysiological dosages of steroids (equivalent to prednisone, 7.5 mg/day) for 1 to 3 weeks in the year before the planned surgery.[20] Exogenous steroids can suppress the hypothalamic-pituitary-adrenal axis and prevent the patient submitted to surgical stress from producing sufficient cortisol. (Recall that the usual daily secretion of cortisol ranges from 15 to 30 mg[21]: in contrast, the normal adrenal production of cortisol is 250–300 mg/day under maximal stress conditions.[22]) Adrenal crisis may present as unexplained hypotension and tachycardia that is often unresponsive to fluid resuscitation and vasopressors.[23] Hyponatremia or hyperkalemia (or both) is usually present.[24] When indications for the prophylactic administration of steroids in the perioperative period are unclear, rapid adrenocorticotropic hormone (ACTH) stimulation testing may be performed.

NUTRITIONAL STATUS

The reasonably well nourished and otherwise healthy individual undergoing an uncomplicated major surgical procedure has sufficient body fuel reserves to withstand the catabolic insult and partial starvation for at least 1 week. However, the nutritionally depleted patient undergoes surgery with a serious handicap. Operative morbidity and mortality are increased enormously in malnourished patients.[25] Atrophy of the mucous membrane linings of the respiratory and gastrointestinal (GI) tracts predispose to infection, as does diminished ability to form antibodies. Hypoproteinemia follows prolonged negative nitrogen balance and increases susceptibility to shock. Diminished supplies of protein and vitamin C retard wound healing.

Because malnutrition greatly increases perioperative risk, the malnourished patient should be identified early so that appropriate intervention can be undertaken. The patient's nutritional history must be reviewed. One study identified 38% of patients undergoing abdominal operations for benign disease demonstrated protein-energy malnutrition.[26] When assessing patients for malnutrition, consider whether the weight is 20% above or below normal, 10% of body weight has been recently lost or gained, physical problems are present that interfere with eating, there has been a loss of appetite for more than 5 days, and the patient has been maintained for more than a week on "routine" intravenous (IV) fluids. (One liter of fluid with 5% dextrose contains only 170 calories, all from carbohydrates; electrolyte solutions without dextrose have essentially no calories.)

Early institution of nutritional support provides essential nutrients for maintenance of gut integrity, prevention of bacterial translocation, and preservation of organ function, wound healing, and immune function.[27] However, research findings do not justify routine use of preoperative total parenteral nutrition to decrease surgical complications or to improve outcomes.[28] It is probably more prudent to provide perioperative nutrients for high-risk patients through the enteral route whenever possible.

🔵 INTRAOPERATIVE PERIOD

INTRAOPERATIVE FLUID MANAGEMENT

Hypotension may develop promptly with the induction of anesthesia if preoperative correction of extracellular FVD has been inadequate. Other factors predisposing to hypotension in the operative period are fluid loss due to bleeding, shifting of intravascular fluid into the surgical site (third-space edema), evaporation of fluid from the exposed peritoneum during abdominal surgery, and inhalation of dry gases. Most patients tolerate a 500-mL blood loss without difficulty because albumin synthesis and erythropoiesis will usually compensate for such minor losses. However, when this volume is exceeded, blood replacement must be considered.

Third-space fluid shift (which cannot be measured directly) can be substantial after extensive dissection of tissue; fluid can also sequester into the lumen and wall of the small bowel and accumulate in the peritoneal cavity. Judicious intraoperative correction of third-space fluid losses with an electrolyte solution (such as lactated Ringer's solution) markedly reduces postoperative oliguria. Although no accurate formula for intraoperative fluid administration is known, balanced salt solution needed during surgery is about 0.5 to 1 L/hr (but only to a maximum of 2–3 liters during a 4-hr major abdominal procedure unless there are other measurable losses).[29] Intraoperative assessment of pulmonary capillary wedge and central venous pressures may be needed to optimally guide fluid replacement in high-risk patients. (Debate on the best type of fluid replacement [crystalloids versus colloids] has continued for many years; isotonic crystalloids, colloids, and hypertonic saline solutions have advantages and disadvantages, depending on the setting.) Refer to Chapter 10 for a review of various fluids and to Chapter 15 for further discussion of parenteral fluids used in resuscitation for hypovolemia.

EFFECT OF CARDIOPULMONARY BYPASS ON FLUID AND ELECTROLYTE BALANCE

Cardiopulmonary bypass (CPB), used for patients undergoing cardiac surgery, has unique effects on body fluids and electrolytes. The hypo-oncotic solution used to prime the pump dilutes plasma proteins and increases movement of water from the vascular space to the interstitial space. Intravascular fluid loss is further enhanced by increased capillary permeability associated with kinin and prostaglandin release from the damaged blood cells and platelets.[30] This fluid loss may persist for up to 8 hours postoperatively, requiring close monitoring of the hemodynamic status with fluid replacement.[31] Because massive extracellular fluid (ECF) volume expansion is required for patients undergoing CPB, a 5- to 15-lb weight gain is expected.[32] It has been shown that patients undergoing CPB without weight gain during the procedure develop significant postoperative problems (such as hypovolemia and poor cardiac function).[33] The expanded ECF can persist for up to 10 days postoperatively.[34] Management of this problem in the postoperative period includes use of diuretics and colloids (such as albumin or hetastarch) to help mobilize the accumulated fluid. (See Chap. 10 for a discussion of colloids.)

There is a tendency to hyponatremia because plasma antidiuretic hormone (ADH) levels during CPB are higher than in other types of surgery (causing excessive water retention with sodium dilution).[35] During the postoperative period, free water intake is minimized to avoid hyponatremia. In patients with preoperative CHF, both fluid and sodium restriction may be indicated. The serum sodium level is influenced to some extent by the type of cardiac surgery. For example, hyponatremia has been reported after mitral commissurotomy, whereas hypernatremia has been reported in a subset of patients undergoing tricuspid value replacement.[36]

Hypokalemia commonly occurs during and after CPB and requires treatment.[37,38] This is especially important in patients who were taking digoxin before surgery (because hypokalemia intensifies the action of digoxin on the myocardium). Conditions aggravating the decrease in serum potassium concentration during CPB include the preoperative use of potassium-losing diuretics, urinary potassium losses, and shifting of potassium into the intracellular space. The obvious danger of hypokalemia is increased risk of arrhythmia. Potassium replacement may be delivered by slow infusion into the extracorporeal circulation or intermittently through a central venous catheter.[39] Intraoperative *hyper*kalemia has been associated with the preoperative use of nonselective β-blockers (because of prevention of β_2-mediated uptake of potassium by muscles).[40]

Hypomagnesemia is also common during and after CPB (due to dilution of plasma magnesium by ECF volume expansion and binding of magnesium by chelating agents in administered stored blood products).[41] Indicators of hypomagnesemia in the postoperative period can include hyperreflexia, enhanced digitalis toxicity, and cardiac arrhythmias. Hypomagnesemia is associated with increased risk of dysrhythmias and prolonged need for mechanical ventilatory support.[42]

Lactic acidosis can result from CPB. It is usually mild in uncomplicated cases and resolves within 18 hours.[43]

EFFECT OF IRRIGATING SOLUTIONS ON FLUID AND ELECTROLYTE BALANCE

Irrigation solutions used during transurethral resection of the prostate (TURP), ultrasonic lithotripsy, and uterine endoscopic laser surgery may be absorbed intravascularly and result in fluid and electrolyte disturbances.[44] Because saline is an electrically conductive solution, fluids that contain no electrolytes must be used. Among the solutions that have been used for irri-

gating purposes in these surgical procedures are glycine, sorbitol, and mannitol.

Transurethral Resection of the Prostate Syndrome

The TURP syndrome consists of a variety of symptoms related to absorption of hypo-osmotic irrigating fluid during transurethral prostatectomy. It has been reported to occur in 5% to 10% of TURP cases.[45] Among the risk factors for the TURP syndrome include preoperative hyponatremia, chronic obstructive pulmonary disease, and CHF.[46]

During TURP, the prostatic veins are opened and the irrigant solutions, which are used to distend the urethra and clear fragments and blood from the operative field, can be absorbed. In the United States, 1.5% glycine is the most commonly used irrigating solution during TURP.[47] On average during a TURP procedure, 10 to 30 mL/min[48] is absorbed, with a range of 300 mL to 4 liters reported.[49] The risk of developing symptoms increases with higher volumes of glycine solution absorption.[50] The fundamental pathology in the TURP syndrome is volume overload and dilutional hyponatremia. The severity and rapidity of the hyponatremia is proportional to the volume of the absorbed irrigant.[51]

Symptoms are often first noticed in the operating room or the recovery area when the patient complains of headache or visual changes. Other signs may include agitation or lethargy, vomiting, muscle twitching, bradycardia, diminished pupillary reflexes, hypertension, and respiratory distress.[52] The appropriate treatment consists of supportive care, fluid restriction, and diuretics; when extreme hyponatremia (< 110 mEq/L) is present, hypertonic saline may be needed.[53] Differentiation of isotonic hyponatremia and hypotonic hyponatremia based on plasma osmolality will guide treatment.[54,55] Measures that can be taken to prevent the TURP syndrome include using low-pressure irrigation and limiting the procedure to less than 1 hour to decrease the degree of volume overload.[56] Use of epidural or spinal anesthesia allows earlier symptom recognition. A new surgical technique, transurethral electrovaporization of the prostate, has been associated with fewer complications (particularly bleeding).[57] Therefore, less irrigant absorption occurs and decreases the development of TURP syndrome.

Hysteroscopic Endometrial Ablation

Hysteroscopic endometrial ablation for menorrhagia is gaining popularity over hysterectomy because it is considered safe and cost effective.[58] During this procedure, a hypotonic irrigating solution (such as 1.5% glycine, 3% sorbitol, or mannitol) is infused into the uterine cavity to wash away operative debris.[59] Because uterine veins are opened during this procedure, there is the possibility of IV absorption of substantial quantities of fluid. Hyponatremia may result and is especially problematic in women of childbearing age because this group is most susceptible to hyponatremic encephalopathy[60-64] (see Chap. 4). The endogenous production of ADH that accompanies surgical stress worsens the hyponatremia by causing water retention. Hyponatremia has been reported as one of the serious complications of hysteroscopic endometrial ablation[65] (see Case Study 14-4).

The presence of symptoms suggesting hyponatremia should lead to immediate testing of the plasma sodium level; if below normal, early and appropriate therapy for the hyponatremia should be instituted before respiratory insufficiency occurs. In patients with general anesthesia during endometrial ablation, the possibility of hyponatremia should be suspected if the patient has a drop in body temperature, shows decreased oxygen saturation, or displays tremulousness or dilated pupils.[66]

Arieff and Ayus[67] described four patients with hyponatremia due to endometrial ablation. Hyponatremia in three of the women was detected early and treated (mean sodium levels were corrected from 102 to 123 mEq/L within the first 24 hours); all three recovered completely. Unfortunately, the fourth patient suffered respiratory arrest before therapy could be initiated; she never regained consciousness and died several days later. Autopsy revealed cerebral edema with tonsillar herniation. (See Chap. 4 for a more thorough discussion of the risks of hyponatremia in menstruant women.)

BLOOD ADMINISTRATION

Because of the hazards of infectious diseases, complications of blood transfusions, and personal choices regarding blood transfusions, many surgical centers are now focused on the reduction of perioperative blood transfusions. Options include preoperative autologous donation of 1 to 3 units of packed red blood cells. The units are reinfused as needed in the intraoperative and postoperative period. A second option is autotransfusion of shed blood during the surgery and in the immediate postoperative period. Autotransfusion is used most commonly with cardiovascular, orthopedic, and vascular surgeries. Another option is normovolemic hemodilution.[68-70] In this procedure, blood is removed in the immediate preoperative period (either in the operative holding area or in the operating room) until a desired hematocrit of 28% to 30% is achieved. During blood removal, crystalloids or colloids are infused to maintain normovolemia. The reduced blood viscosity improves microcirculatory perfusion.[71] Retransfusion occurs in the intraoperative or postoperative period. Although not a new procedure, the optimal surgical candidates and timing of retransfusion are still being researched.

POSTOPERATIVE PERIOD

NEUROENDOCRINE RESPONSE

The neuroendocrine response stimulated by many anesthetic agents is further heightened by surgical stress. Secretion of ACTH and cortisol is increased according to the magnitude of surgery or trauma. Cortisol and ACTH levels generally remain elevated for 2 to 4 days after surgery; however, with extensive trauma or the complications of sepsis or shock, the levels may remain elevated for weeks.[72]

Circulatory instability related to fluid losses during surgery and trauma produces decreased renal perfusion, which in turn stimulates production of substances (renin, angiotensin, and aldosterone) that support the blood pressure through vasoconstriction and sodium and water conservation.[73] In humans, isotonic fluid volume reduction (as occurs in simple blood loss) is one of the most potent stimuli to aldosterone and ADH secretion. Surgery and trauma also cause increased release of ADH through vasoconstriction of the renal artery and stimulation of the hypothalamus; these effects may persist for 12 to 24 hours into the postoperative period. Reduced volumes of concentrated urine can be expected in the early postoperative period due to these hormonal changes. Unfortunately, increased aldosterone secretion results in greater urinary loss of potassium, predisposing to hypokalemia if potassium replacement is inadequate. In elderly surgical patients, the neuroendocrine response to the stress of surgery may result in increased morbidity.[74] Patients undergoing cerebrovascular surgery may have either prolonged inappropriate secretion of ADH (resulting in dilutional hyponatremia) or possibly suppression of ADH secretion (resulting in diabetes insipidus with hypernatremia). Therefore, careful monitoring of plasma osmolality and sodium levels is required (see Chap. 19).

METABOLIC CHANGES

During the first hours after surgical trauma, increased blood glucose levels may result from secretion of growth hormone and glucagon and suppression of insulin release. The extent of negative nitrogen balance that occurs postoperatively is largely related to the magnitude of the injury. After a few days, the altered metabolism is associated with a slow but progressive reaccumulation of protein followed by a reaccumulation of body fat.

FLUID AND ELECTROLYTE IMBALANCES

Fluid Volume Deficit

The most common fluid disorder in the postoperative patient is extracellular FVD.[75] Contributing factors to postoperative FVD include loss of GI fluids, continued third-space fluid shifts, fever, overzealous blood sampling for repeated chemical determinations, hyperventilation, injudicious administration of diuretics, and an unhumidified tracheostomy with hyperventilation.

Among the indicators of FVD are decreased urine output, postural hypotension and tachycardia, diminished skin turgor, decreased capillary refill time, and blood urea nitrogen (BUN) elevated out of proportion to the serum creatinine (see Chap. 3). If fluids are directly lost from the body (as from vomiting or diuresis), body weight will decrease acutely. However, if FVD is due to third-spacing, decreased body weight does not occur because the fluid "lost" from the vascular space pools in another part of the body (such as the surgical site or bowel due to adynamic ileus). Actually, as parenteral fluids are administered to correct the vascular volume deficity, the patient will gain weight. Intake and output (I&O) measurements are manda-

tory when FVD is suspected; in general, in the adult an acceptable hourly urine volume is 30 to 50 mL. Decreased urine volume coupled with tachycardia and decreased blood pressure should cause one to suspect a FVD of several liters.

Fluid replacement must be guided by the intravascular volume status (estimated by vital signs, urine output, and filling pressures when available). Remember that third-spacing from surgical trauma is not limited to the operative period; indeed, it may continue slowly for a few hours or more during the first day of injury.[76] Unrecognized deficits of ECF volume during the early postoperative period may be manifested as circulatory instability. Later, as the third-spacing resolves and fluid shifts back into the intravascular space, diuresis and weight loss will occur. In patients with cardiac or renal dysfunction, the shift of fluid back into the vascular bed may result in CHF or pulmonary edema.

Treatment of FVD depends on the composition of lost fluids. Generally, it can be accomplished with either lactated Ringer's solution or isotonic saline (0.9% NaCl). Use of a large volume of isotonic saline can theoretically produce hyperchloremic acidosis because it contains considerably more chloride than is normally present in plasma. In some situations, normal volume can be accomplished with albumin or other blood products. (See Chap. 10 for a discussion if IV replacement fluids and their recommended use.) Because fluid losses are only roughly estimated, careful monitoring of physiological indices must be done to warn of overhydration when large volumes of fluid are given rapidly. For example, a sudden increase in pulmonary artery occlusion pressure to greater than 20 mm Hg may be an indicator of too much fluid given too rapidly.[77]

Urine Output

Preferably, urinary output should be at least 30 to 50 mL/hr in adults; an hourly urinary output of less than 25 mL should be investigated. The decreased urinary output of stress reaction (healthy physiological response to surgery) must be differentiated from pathological developments. Factors associated with decreased urinary volume in the postoperative patient may include:

- Inadequate preoperative fluid replacement
- Hypovolemia resulting from fluid loss incurred during surgery (either direct loss or subtle third-

space accumulation at the surgical site or intestinal ileus)

- Disturbance in myocardial function causing decreased blood flow to the kidneys and thus decreased urine formation
- Renal failure (a serious cause of postoperative oliguria)

Postoperative renal failure is highest in the elderly patient undergoing cardiac surgery or aortic aneurysm repair.[78] Although oliguric renal failure may occur postoperatively in the patient who has suffered poor renal perfusion during surgery, high-output renal failure is actually more frequent. High-output renal failure is characterized by uremia occurring with a daily urine volume greater than 1,000 to 1,500 mL. It probably represents the renal response to a less severe episode of renal injury than is required to cause the classic oliguric renal failure. Although it is generally easier to manage than oliguric renal failure, high-output failure is more difficult to recognize. Typically, the urine volume is normal or greater than normal and the BUN is increased. A real danger for hyperkalemia exists when potassium is administered to a patient with unrecognized high-output failure.

Fluid Volume Excess

In trauma and postoperative patients, large volumes of fluid may seep from the vascular space into a third-space (such as the surgical site or a generalized interstitial space due to decreased plasma oncotic pressure after albumin loss). As fluids are administered to correct these vascular losses, the body takes on an added fluid load. Part of the administered fluid continues to seep into the third-space site; therefore, hypovolemia may persist despite the appearance of edema (if the fluid has shifted to visible portions of the body) and weight gain. Therefore, the adequacy of fluid replacement must be guided by vital signs and urine output. Of course, it is possible to administer so much fluid that the intravascular space is overloaded.

In the surgical patient without renal failure, the most common causes of intravascular volume overload are iatrogenic; these include overcorrection of a previous volume deficit, a poorly guarded IV line, or a positive gain of water in patients receiving constant humidified ventilatory support. Among the earliest

signs is weight gain during the catabolic period when the patient is expected to lose ¼ to ½ lb/day.[79]

Although volume overload can occur at any time in the postoperative period, it is more common soon after surgery. Daily weight measurement is necessary to detect excessive weight gain due to retained fluid. If pulmonary edema is present, diuretics may be indicated. Observation for pulmonary edema is important because eventually any retained third-space fluid will shift back into the vascular space.

Hyponatremia

A frequent imbalance in the postoperative period is hyponatremia related to excessive ADH secretion. In one study, hyponatremia was present in 4.4% of postoperative patients within 1 week of surgery.[80] Predisposing factors include a temporary increase in ADH release after anesthesia and the stress of surgery. Pain enhances the release of ADH by direct stimulation of the hypothalamus. Nausea, which is frequently present in postoperative patients, can increase ADH release as much as 1,000-fold; the nausea does not have to be associated with vomiting.[81] Because of the tendency for hyponatremia in new postoperative patients, the excessive administration of electrolyte-free solutions during the first 2 to 4 postoperative days should be avoided. In fact, because elevated plasma levels of ADH are essentially a universal postoperative occurrence in the first few postoperative days, some investigators state that it may be important to avoid the use of any hypotonic IV solutions in the immediate postoperative period.[82] In the postoperative period, the kidney can also generate electrolyte-free water from a large sodium excretion in the urine; therefore, even isotonic fluids should be given only as needed for hemodynamic stability and based on the patient's size.[83,84] A serum sodium level between 130 to 135 mEq/L should be heeded; the simple act of restricting free water may be sufficient to avoid the full-blown syndrome of water intoxication (severe dilutional hyponatremia).[85] Cases of permanent brain damage related to profound hyponatremia have been reported in postoperative patients receiving excessive free water. Refer to Case Study 4-5 and the section on postoperative hyponatremia in menstruant women, and to the section on endometrial ablation earlier in this chapter. In patients with chronic hyponatremia (such as those with end-stage liver disease undergoing liver transplant), slow correction in the perioperative period is recommended.[86]

Potassium Imbalances

Hypokalemia is the most common potassium imbalance in surgical patients. However, some authorities believe it is unnecessary and probably unwise to administer potassium during the first 24 hours postoperatively unless a definite potassium deficit exists.[87] This is because trauma causes release of potassium from cells at the surgical site into the extracellular space in the early postoperative period. For patients at risk for renal failure due to hypotensive episodes during the surgical procedure, even small potassium supplements can be detrimental. After the first 24 hours, potassium is administered daily as necessary to replace urinary and GI potassium losses.[88] Generally, a daily supplementation of 60 to 100 mEq is required postoperatively.[89] The needed potassium should be distributed evenly in the total daily maintenance fluids. For example, if 2 liters of fluid is prescribed over 24 hours, and 80 mEq KCl is the required daily potassium supplement, 40 mEq KCl should be added to each liter of solution. This makes far more sense than routinely administering "K-runs" to meet maintenance potassium needs. (See the discussion of IV potassium replacement in Chap. 5.) Special considerations for patients undergoing CPB are discussed earlier in this chapter.

Hyperkalemia is rare in the postoperative patient, except when acute renal failure, rhabdomyolysis, massive hemolysis, or tissue necrosis is present. If hyperkalemia occurs at any time in the postoperative period, the possibility of impaired renal function (manifested by rising serum creatinine in the presence of low, normal, or high urine output) should be explored. Release of cellular potassium by crush injuries and electrical injuries, plus acute renal failure, can lead to lethal hyperkalemia within hours.

Hypocalcemia

Postsurgical hypocalcemia may accompany parathyroidectomy, thyroidectomy, or radical neck dissection. Hypocalcemia reportedly occurs in up to 70% of patients undergoing parathyroidectomy, particularly when a severe hyperparathyroid state was present before surgery.[90] Transient hypocalcemia reportedly occurs in 5% to 10% of patients undergoing thyroidectomy.[91] The hypocalcemia may occur immediately or 1 to 2 days postoperatively and usually lasts less than 5 days.[92]

The etiology for the transient hypocalcemia after thyroidectomy is by no means obvious nor it is likely unifactorial.[93] Various causative mechanisms have been proposed. One is thought to be the inadvertent removal of, or injury to, parathyroid tissue at the time of surgery. If permanent parathyroid damage has not occurred, parathyroid insufficiency resolves as edema at the surgical site lessens and revascularization occurs. Others have postulated that the release of calcitonin secondary to the manipulation of the thyroid gland during surgery may be the culprit (recall that calcitonin lowers the serum calcium level).[94] Still others have postulated that a phenomenon known as the "hungry bone syndrome" is responsible; in this condition, it is thought that there is an abrupt postoperative uptake of calcium in patients who have preexisting osteodystrophy.[95] One likely mechanism for hypocalcemia after radical neck dissection is reduced blood flow to the parathyroid glands after dissection and hemostatic maneuvers.

Permanent hypocalcemia associated with thyroid surgery (which may be defined as a hypocalcemia lasting 2 months or longer) is due to accidental removal of the parathyroid glands or to vascular necrosis.[96] Fortunately, permanent postsurgical hypoparathyroidism occurs in only a small percentage of patients; the frequency of this complication is partially dependent on the technical skill of the surgeon.[97] Indeed, surgeons performing thyroidectomies and parathyroidectomies strive to preserve the blood supply to the parathyroid glands.[98] Extensive neck surgeries (as in radical neck dissection for cancer) are more likely to be associated with permanent hypoparathyroidism than are less involved surgical maneuvers.

Most patients who develop hypocalcemia after neck surgery are asymptomatic; however, some may develop paresthesia, laryngeal spasm, or tetany.[99] It has been recommended that the serum ionized calcium level be checked every 12 hours after neck surgery (and more frequently if symptoms of hypocalcemia are present) until the serum ionized concentration begins to elevate, indicating recovery of the parathyroid glands.[100] The critical period for calcium level monitoring has been described by some authors as being the first 24 to 96 hours after surgery.[101] Of course, symptomatic patients should receive supplemental calcium to increase the serum calcium level to the low normal range.

It is possible that postoperative hypoparathyroidism may manifest itself months to years after neck surgery; therefore, serum ionized calcium levels should be serially monitored in patients at risk. It is also possible that stress can induce hypocalcemia in these individuals; therefore, critically ill patients with a history of neck surgery should have a serum calcium test performed.[102]

Acid–Base Disorders

Surgical patients may have normal pH or develop virtually any acid–base abnormality (depending on individual circumstances). Respiratory acidosis may result from shallow respirations related to anesthesia, narcotics, abdominal distention, pain, or large cumbersome dressings. On assessment, decreased respirations and decreased breath sounds in the bases may be noted. Measures to increase gas exchange, such as frequent coughing and deep breathing, frequent suctioning of tracheobronchial secretions, avoidance of oversedation, and turning and ambulating the patient, will decrease the likelihood of respiratory acidosis.

Subclinical respiratory alkalosis is common in surgical patients.[103] Among the causes are hyperventilation due to pain, hypoxia, central nervous system injury, and assisted ventilation. Respiratory alkalosis is disturbing in the presence of metabolic alkalosis (for which hypoventilation with subsequent carbon dioxide retention is needed for compensatory purposes).

The most common causes of metabolic alkalosis in the surgical patient are loss of gastric acid due to nasogastric draining or vomiting and therapy with potassium-losing diuretics. The most common causes of metabolic acidosis in surgical patients include ketoacidosis, renal failure, lactic acidosis associated with shock, and loss of alkali from biliary and pancreatic drainage.

PARENTERAL FLUID RESUSCITATION

Chapter 10 describes commonly prescribed water and electrolyte fluids and colloids (such as albumin and hetastarch) and Chapter 15 discusses fluid resuscitation for patients with hypovolemic shock after surgery or trauma.

AMBULATORY SURGERY CONSIDERATIONS

Patients undergoing ambulatory surgery will usually recover initially in a postanesthesia care unit and then in some type of phase II recovery or discharge unit. Procedures performed in ambulatory surgery seldom result in significant alterations in fluid and electrolyte status; however, because they do elicit the same stress response (to a much lesser extent), these patients require assessment and nursing interventions related to fluid and electrolyte balance.[104] Blood administration, autologous or donor, may be required.[105] Oral intake is encouraged after the patient is sufficiently alert, able to protect the airway, and not nauseated. Nausea and vomiting can have multiple causes and require individual assessment and management. When IV fluids are used, they are generally continued until the patient is able to tolerate oral fluids[106]; however, this practice is currently being questioned. Jin et al.[107] found that postoperative nausea and vomiting were similar between ambulatory surgery patients who drank fluids before discharge and those who did not take oral fluids until they went home. Time to discharge was slightly less in the nondrinking group.

Assessment for the ability to void as well as for bladder distention is also important. Postoperative instructions for home are ideally given during the preadmission contact and reinforced in the discharge unit. Instructions related to fluid balance usually include:[108]

- Increase oral fluids, especially after urologic procedures and spinal anesthesia.
- Do not drink any alcoholic beverages during the first 24 hours.
- Methods for management of nausea and vomiting
- Notify physician if uncomfortable due to inability to void.

A follow-up phone call the day after surgery allows the nurse to assess the patient's status and address any questions or concerns.

NURSING DIAGNOSES

Clinical Tip: Examples of Nursing Diagnoses for a New Postoperative Patient After Abdominal Surgery lists some possible nursing diagnoses related to fluid and electrolyte balance for a patient who has undergone abdominal surgery.

CLINICAL TIP

Examples of Nursing Diagnoses for a New Postoperative Patient After Abdominal Surgery

NURSING DIAGNOSIS	ETIOLOGICAL FACTORS	DEFINING CHARACTERISTICS
FVD related to actual fluid loss and third-space fluid shift during surgical procedure	Vomiting after reaction to anesthesia GI suction Third-space fluid shift at surgical site	Postural tachycardia Postural hypotension initially; later, low BP in all positions Decreased skin turgor Slowed capillary refill time Oliguria ($<$ 30 mL/hr in adult) Weight change depends on cause (decreased if actual fluid loss, as in GI suction; usually increased if fluid loss is due to third-space shift, provided parenteral fluids are given in an attempt to correct hypovolemia)
Altered tissue perfusion (renal) related to hypotension during surgical procedure	Hypotensive effects of anesthesia Hypovolemia due to direct or indirect loss of fluid Hypovolemia due to inadequate parenteral fluid replacement	Oliguria or polyuria in presence of elevated serum creatinine (see discussion of low-output and high-output renal failure in text)
Alteration in sodium balance (hyponatremia) related to excessive ADH activity	Major surgery with its premedication, anesthesia, decreased blood volume, and postoperative pain results in increased ADH release (causing water retention with sodium dilution)	Serum sodium $<$ 135 mEq/L May be asymptomatic if Na $>$ 125 mEq/L Lethargy, confusion, nausea, vomiting, anorexia, abdominal cramps, muscular twitching (see Chap. 5).
Alteration in acid–base balance (metabolic alkalosis) related to vomiting or gastric suction	Vomiting after reaction to anesthesia Gastric suction, particularly if patient is allowed to ingest ice chips freely	Tingling of fingers, toes, and circumoral region, due to decreased calcium ionization pH $>$ 7.45, bicarbonate above normal, chloride below normal
Altered nutrition (less than body requirements) related to negative nitrogen balance after surgical stress and inadequate caloric intake	Catabolic response to stress of surgery Inability to tolerate oral feedings during first few postoperative days due to decreased GI motility, anorexia, nausea, and general discomfort Failure of health care providers to administer sufficient calories via the parenteral route	Weight loss of approximately ¼ to ½ lb/day in adult (provided fluids are not abnormally retained) Perhaps a decrease in serum albumin, transferrin, and retinol binding protein levels.

ADH, antidiuretic hormone; BP, blood pressure; FVD, fluid volume deficit; GI, gastrointestinal.

CASE STUDIES

● **14-1.** A 60-year-old man underwent surgical repair of an abdominal aortic aneurysm and was brought to the surgical intensive care unit for follow-up care. He was mechanically ventilated with an inspired gas mixture containing 40% oxygen; tidal volume was set at 950 mL and breathing rate at 12 breaths/min. A nasogastric tube was connected to suction. He received 2 liters 5% dextrose in 0.11% NaCl solution every 24 hours for the first 2 postoperative days. In addition, he received 20 mg furosemide IV twice daily. On the morning of the third postoperative day the following laboratory results were obtained:

> Serum sodium = 128 mEq/L
> Serum potassium = 3.3 mEq/L
> Arterial pH = 7.62
> $PaCO_2$ = 26 mm Hg
> HCO_3 = 28 mEq/L
> PaO_2 = 74 mm Hg

COMMENTARY: Furosemide, a powerful diuretic, causes sodium loss in the urine. In addition, some sodium was lost in nasogastric suction. However, very little sodium was replaced via the IV route (5% dextrose in 0.11% NaCl solution contains only about 19 mEq sodium per liter). In addition, pain and surgical stress stimulate production of ADH, which causes water retention (thus diluting the serum sodium level, especially when hypotonic fluid are supplied IV).

The arterial pH of 7.62 indicates alkalosis. A higher than normal bicarbonate level indicates metabolic alkalosis. A lower than normal $PaCO_2$ indicates respiratory alkalosis. Therefore, the patient has two primary acid–base problems (metabolic alkalosis and respiratory alkalosis). Possible causes of metabolic alkalosis include loss of acidic gastric fluid via suction and use of a potassium-losing diuretic. Because the patient was mechanically ventilated at a fixed volume and rate, he was unable to make the usual compensatory respiratory change (hypoventilation) seen when metabolic alkalosis exists. In fact, the high minute volume set by mechanical ventilation caused *hyper*ventilation and thus respiratory alkalosis.

● **14-2.** A 32-year-old woman presented with hypercalcemia and was diagnosed with primary hyperparathyroidism. On neck exploration, the surgeon found four enlarged parathyroid glands and removed three. On the first postoperative day, the total serum calcium was 8.6 mg/dL; it decreased to 6.8 mg/dL by the third postoperative day. At that time, she complained of feeling lightheaded and having paresthesias of the mouth, fingers, and toes. On examination, she was found to have a positive Chvostek's sign. Later, she developed twitching of the facial muscles. She was treated with 10 mL 10% calcium gluconate IV over 10 minutes.

COMMENTARY: The hypocalcemia was caused by surgical hypoparathyroidism (after the removal of three of the four parathyroid glands). A potential serious consequence that could have occurred with this degree of hypocalcemia is laryngeal spasm, which compromises the airway. This patient is likely to recover normal calcium balance after the operative injury heals.

● **14-3.** A 66-year-old woman with a history of coronary artery disease and manic-depressive disorder underwent a coronary artery bypass graft. She was started back on her preoperative dose of lithium on the first postoperative day; at that time, her serum sodium level was 142 mEq/L. After the second dose of lithium, her urine output increased to greater than 400 mL/hr for 4 hours. After that time, her urine output ranged from 250 to 300 mL/hr for the next 24 hours. Her only source of fluid intake was by the oral route; her appetite was described as poor. No IV fluids were infused. By the morning of postoperative day 2, her serum sodium level was 153 mEq/L and reached a high of 170 mEq/L on postoperative day 3. At that time, her serum osmolality was 351 mOsm/kg and her urine osmolality was 228 mOsm/kg. A review of her I&O record for the postoperative period revealed that her fluid output exceeded her fluid intake by 11,000 mL. A toxic lithium level was revealed by laboratory analysis. She had mental status changes and required reintubation on the evening of postoperative day 2. IV water replacement therapy with D_5W was initiated on postoperative day 3. Frequent measurements of the serum sodium level were made to ensure that the serum sodium level was not dropped too quickly.

COMMENTARY: A reduced intake of fluid and sodium can accelerate lithium retention with resultant toxicity.[109] Further, a toxic lithium level can lead to a large output of dilute urine.[110] The more common response to CPB is fluid retention and hyponatremia; therefore, the staff should have been alert to such an excessive diuresis with hypernatremia. More attention should have been paid to the far greater fluid output than fluid intake, as well as the elevating serum sodium level. Once the hypernatremia was detected, it was recognized that gradual correction of the imbalance was indicated to avoid causing adverse neurological changes. (Too rapid a correction of hypernatremia can result in cerebral edema, seizures, permanent neurological damage, and death; see Chap. 4 for a more thorough discussion of the treatment of hypernatremia.)

● **14-4.**[111] A 43-year-old woman was admitted for an elective endometrial ablation for menorrhagia. The medical history was unremarkable except for migraine-type headaches and irritable bowel syndrome. Her preoperative serum sodium level was 139 mEq/L. She underwent hysteroscopic endometrial ablation using 3% sorbitol solution for irrigation. Because she had heavy bleeding, a laparoscopy was performed to rule out perforation. Eight liters of 3% sorbitol irrigation fluid was instilled; the measured affluent was 4,100 mL. During the procedure, she also received 3,800 mL lactated Ringer's solution. The blood loss was estimated at around 300 mL. The procedure was well tolerated and the patient was moved to the recovery room. There she complained of headache and was noted to be drowsy but easily arousable. Facial puffiness was noted and her rectal temperature was found to be 92°F. A positive Babinski sign was noted on the right side. Laboratory tests revealed a serum sodium concentration of 112 mEq/L. Once the hyponatremia was recognized, the patient was moved to an intensive care unit and

treated with 3% NaCl solution; her serum sodium was slowly corrected to 129 mEq/L over the next 12 hours. The next day, the patient was substantially improved and was transferred out of the intensive care unit.

COMMENTARY: The condition described above has been labeled the "female TURP syndrome."[112] The fact that this patient's perioperative fluid intake greatly exceeded the recorded output supports excessive absorption of hypotonic fluid as at least one reason for the rapid decline in the serum sodium level.[113] It is likely that the elevated ADH level commonly observed in surgical patients contributed to the hyponatremia. The sudden decline in the serum sodium concentration likely caused brain swelling and accounted for the neurological symptoms. The authors reported it was appropriate to infuse hypertonic sodium chloride because the fatality rate for hyponatremia is quite high once cerebral edema develops.[114] This is especially true in menstruant women; see Chapter 4 for a more thorough discussion of this topic.

Measures to help prevent complications from fluid overload revolve around three principles: (1) avoiding excess fluid absorption during the procedure, (2) recognizing and treating the fluid overload early should it occur, and (3) using the distending medium least likely to cause serious complications should it be absorbed in excess.[115]

An accurate account of fluid intake and output throughout the procedure is important to detect excess fluid absorption. Also, use of regional anesthesia (when possible) would help detect neurological symptoms early.[116] Finally, for diagnostic hysteroscopy or for operative procedures in which mechanical instruments are used, normal saline and lactated Ringer's solution are the distending media of choice.[117] However, when an intrauterine electrosurgical procedure is planned using a conventional resectoscope, the solution used to wash away the debris must be nonconductive.[118]

REFERENCES

1. Cassidy J, Marley R. Preoperative assessment of the ambulatory patient. *J Perianesth Nurs* 1996;11:334.
2. Burden N. *Ambulatory Surgical Nursing*. Philadelphia: WB Saunders; 1993:155.
3. France F, Lefebvre C. Cost-effectiveness of preoperative examinations. *Acta Clin Belg* 1997;52:275.
4. Haug R, Reifeis R. A prospective evaluation of the value of preoperative laboratory testing for office anesthesia and sedation. *J Oral Maxillofac Surg* 1999;57:16.
5. Johnson H et al. Are routine preoperative laboratory screening tests necessary to evaluate ambulatory surgical patients? *Surgery* 1988;104:639.
6. Meneghini L et al. The usefulness of routine preoperative laboratory tests for one-day surgery in healthy children. *Paediatr Anaesth* 1998;8:11.
7. Wattsman T, Davies R. The utility of preoperative laboratory testing in general surgery patients for outpatient procedures. *Am Surg* 1997;63:81.
8. Narr B et al. Outcomes of patients with no laboratory assessment before anesthesia and a surgical procedure. *Mayo Clin Proc* 1997;72:505.
9. Tolksdorf W. Electrolyte disorders relevant to anesthesia. *Acta Anaesthesiol Scand Suppl* 1997;111:328.
10. Narins R, ed. *Clinical Disorders of Fluid and Electrolyte Metabolism*, 5th ed. New York: McGraw-Hill; 1994:1412.
11. Ibid.
12. Epstein B. Preventing postoperative nausea and vomiting. In: Sleisenger M, ed. *The Handbook of Nausea and Vomiting*. New York: Caduceus Medical Publishers by the Parthenon Publishing Group; 1993:93.
13. Summers S, Ebbert D. *Ambulatory Surgical Nursing: A Nursing Diagnosis Approach*. Philadelphia: JB Lippincott; 1992:264.
14. Goodwin A et al. The effect of shortening the pre-operative fluid fast on postoperative morbidity. *Anaesthesia* 1991;46:1066.
15. Epstein, p 94.
16. Goresky G, Maltby J. Fasting guidelines for elective surgical patients (editorial). *Can J Anaesth* 1990;37:493.
17. Narins, p 1409.
18. Abbasoglu O et al. Liver transplantation in hyponatremic patients with emphasis on central pontine myelinolysis. *Clin Transplant* 1998;12:263.
19. Ibid.
20. Doherty G, Baumann D, Creswell L, et al. *The Washington Manual of Surgery*. Boston: Little, Brown; 1997.
21. Condon R, Nyhus L. *Manual of Surgical Therapeutics*, 9th ed. Boston: Little, Brown; 1996.
22. Doherty et al, p 133.
23. Ibid.
24. Tierney L, McPhee S, Papadikis M. *Current Medical Diagnosis & Treatment*, 38th ed. Stamford, CT: Appleton & Lange; 1999.
25. Dannhauser A et al. Preoperative nutritional status and prognostic nutritional index in patients with bening disease undergoing abdominal operations—part I. *J Am Coll Nutr* 1995;14:80.
26. Ibid.
27. Zaloga G. *Nutrition in Critical Care*. St. Louis: CV Mosby; 1994:298.
28. The Veterans Affairs Total Parenteral Nutrition Cooperative Study Group. Perioperative total parenteral nutrition in surgical patients. *N Engl J Med* 1991;325:525.
29. Schwartz S et al, eds. *Principles of Surgery*, 7th ed. New York: McGraw-Hill; 1999:69.
30. Vaska P. Fluid and electrolyte imbalances after cardiac surgery. *AACN Clin Issues* 1992;3:664.
31. Ibid.
32. Kokko J, Tannen R. *Fluids and Electrolytes*, 3rd ed. Philadelphia: WB Saunders; 1996:749.
33. Ibid.
34. Ibid.
35. Ibid, p 750.
36. Narins, p 1419.
37. Kokko, Tannen, p 750.
38. Nally B et al. Supraventricular tachycardia after coronary artery bypass grafting surgery and fluid and electrolyte variables. *Heart Lung* 1996;25:31.
39. Narins, p 1422.
40. Ibid.
41. Kokko, Tannen, p 750.
42. Narins, p 1422.
43. Ibid, p 1423.
44. Ibid, p 1419.
45. Rhymer J. Hyponatremia following transurethral resection of the prostate. *Br J Urol* 1985;57:450.
46. Ellis R, Carmichael J. Hyponatremia and volume overload as a complication of transurethral resection of the prostate. *J Fam Pract* 1991;33:89.
47. Ibid.
48. Gold M. Perioperative fluid management. *Crit Care Clin* 1992;8:409.
49. Narins, p 1414.
50. Hahn R. Irrigating fluids in endoscopic surgery. *Br J Urol* 1997;79:669.
51. Narins, p 1419.
52. Ellis, Carmichael, p 90.
53. Ayus C, Arieff A. Glycine-induced hypo-osmolar hyponatremia. *Arch Intern Med* 1997;157:223.
54. Dixon B, Ernest D. Hyponatremia in the transurethral resection of prostate syndrome. *Anaesth Intensive Care* 1996;24:102.
55. Ellis, Carmichael, p 90.
56. Grundy P et al. Randomized controlled trial evaluating the use of sterile water as an irrigation fluid during transurethral electrovaporization of the prostate. *Br J Urol* 1997;80:894.
57. Kupeli B et al. Efficacy of transurethral electrovaporization of the prostate with respect to standard transurethral resection. *Journal of Endourology* 1998;12:591.
58. Agraharkar M, Agraharkar A. Posthysteroscopic hyponatremia: Evidence for a multifactorial cause. *Am J Kidney Dis* 1997;30:717.
59. Arieff A, Ayus C. Endometrial ablation complicated by fatal hyponatremic encephalopathy. *JAMA* 1993;279:1230.
60. Ayus C, Wheeler J, Arieff A. Postoperative hyponatremic encephalopathy in menstruant women. *Ann Intern Med* 1992;117:891.
61. Ayus C, Arieff A. Brain damage and postoperative hyponatremia: The role of gender. *Neurology* 1996;46:323.
62. Metheny N. Focusing on the dangers of D_5W. *Nursing97* 1997;October:55.
63. Steele A et al. Postoperative hyponatremia despite near-isotonic saline infusion: A phenomenon of desalination. *Ann Intern Med* 1997;126:20.
64. Agraharkar, Agraharkar, p 719.
65. Arieff, Ayus, p 1230.
66. Ibid.
67. Goodnough L et al. Acute preoperative hemodilution in patients undergoing radical prostatectomy: A case study analysis of efficacy. *Anesth Analg* 1994;78:932.
68. Lisander B. Preoperative haemodilution. *Acta Anaesthesiol Scand* 1988;89S:63.

69. Messmer K. Hemodilution—possibilities and safety aspects. *Acta Anaesthesiol Scand* 1988;32AS:49.
70. Olsfanger D et al. Acute normovolaemic haemodilution decreases postoperative allogeneic blood transfusion after total knee replacement. *Br J Anaesth* 1997;79:317.
71. Schwartz et al, p 97.
72. Kokko, Tannen, p 731.
73. Ibid.
74. Beck L. Perioperative renal, fluid, and electrolyte management. *Clin Geriatr Med* 1990;6:557.
75. Schwartz et al, p 57.
76. Ibid, p 69.
77. Shoemaker W et al. *Textbook of Critical Care*, 3rd ed. Philadelphia: WB Saunders; 1995:261.
78. Beck, p 56.
79. Schwartz et al, p 70.
80. Chung H et al. Postoperative hyponatremia. *Arch Intern Med* 1986;146:333.
81. Narins, p 599.
82. Ayus et al, p 891.
83. Gowrishankar M et al. Acute hyponatremia in the perioperative period: Insights into its pathophysiology and recommendations for management. *Clin Nephrol* 1998;50:352.
84. Steele et al, p 24.
85. Kokko, Tannen, p 742.
86. Abbasoglu et al, p 268.
87. Schwartz et al, p 69.
88. Ibid.
89. Kokko, Tannen, p 744.
90. Condon, Nyhus, p 274.
91. Ibid.
92. Chernow B, ed. *The Pharmacologic Approach to the Critically Ill Patient*, 3rd ed. Baltimore, MD: Williams & Wilkins, 1994:777.
93. Szubin L et al. The management of post-thyroidectomy hypocalcemia. *Ear Nose Throat J* 1996;75:612.
94. Narins, p 1025.
95. See A, Soo K. Hypocalcemia following thyroidectomy for thyrotoxicosis. *Br J Surg* 1997;84:95.
96. Bourrel C et al. Transient hypocalcemia after thyroidectomy. *Ann Otol Laryngol* 1993;102:496.
97. Narins, p 1025.
98. Pemberton L, Pemberton D. *Treatment of Water, Electrolyte, and Acid-Base Disorders in the Surgical patient.* New York: McGraw-Hill; 1994:216.
99. Chernow, p 780.
100. Ibid.
101. Szubin et al.
102. Chernow, p 780.
103. Shires G. *Fluids, Electrolytes and Acid-Bases.* New York: Churchill Livingstone; 1988:8.
104. Burden, p 287.
105. Ibid.
106. Ibid.
107. Jin F et al. Should adult patients drink fluids before discharge from ambulatory surgery? *Anesth Analg* 1998;87:306.
108. Burden, p 358.
109. Shannon M, Wilson B, Stang C. *Appleton & Lange's 1999 Drug Guide.* Stamford, CT: Appleton & Lange; 1999:812.
110. Ibid, p 813.
111. Agraharkar, Agraharkar, p 717.
112. Marino J et al. Hyponatremia during endoscopic curettage: female TURP syndrome? *Anesth Analg* 1994;78:1180.
113. Agraharkar, Agraharkar, p 718.
114. Ibid.
115. Indman P, Brooks P, Cooper J et al. Complications of fluid overload from resectoscopic surgery. *J Am Assoc Gynecol Laparosc* 1998;5:63.
116. Scott S. Pulmonary edema and hyponatremia during hysteroscopic resection of uterine fibroids: Case report. *CRNA: The Clinical Forum for Nurse Anesthetists* 1998;9:113.
117. Indman et al.
118. Ibid.

CHAPTER 15

Hypovolemic Shock in Trauma and Postoperative Patients

Trauma is a leading cause of death in the first four decades of life in the United States. Death in trauma patients has a trimodal pattern. The first peak of death occurs within seconds to minutes of injury and is usually due to blood loss from lacerations of the heart, aorta, or other large vessels or trauma to the brain, brain stem, or high spinal cord. The second peak occurs within minutes to a few hours after injury and is usually due to epidural and subdural hematomas, hemopneumothorax, ruptured spleen, liver lacerations, pelvic fractures, or any injuries associated with significant blood loss. The third peak of death occurs several days or weeks after the initial injury and is primarily due to complications of shock including sepsis, adult respiratory distress syndrome (ARDS), and multiple system organ failure (MSOF). Every attempt should be made to prevent prolonged shock because it can lead to MSOF and late death. Care of a patient in shock requires accurate assessment and timely interventions and continuous evaluation by the nurse. Management of the patient experiencing hypovolemic shock as a result of traumatic injury or after surgical procedures is the focus of this chapter.

🌑 DEFINITION OF SHOCK

Generally, shock has been defined as an abnormality of the circulatory system that results in inadequate organ perfusion and tissue oxygenation.[1] Shock starts when oxygen delivery to the cells is inadequate to meet metabolic demands.[2] Most common in the injured patient is *hypovolemic shock* after acute blood loss, either externally or internally. External blood loss can result from lacerations, amputations, open fractures, or stab or gunshot wounds. Blood is also frequently lost at the injury site, especially after major closed fractures. For example, a fractured tibia or humerus may be associated with a blood loss of 750 mL, whereas a fractured femur may result in a 1.5-liter blood loss.[3] Pelvic fractures may result in even greater blood losses. Depending on the injury site, a significant volume of blood may be sequestered into body cavities such as the thorax, intraperitoneal space, and retroperitoneal space. Fluid losses other than blood also occur as a result of tissue injury; this obligatory edema adds to the deficit in the intravascular volume.[4]

In *cardiogenic shock*, failure of the heart as a pump causes a decrease in tissue perfusion. In the trauma patient, cardiogenic shock may occur if compensatory mechanisms have failed or if cardiac tamponade, tension pneumothorax, air embolus, or cardiac contusion is present.

Neurogenic shock results from the loss of vasomotor tone, which causes vasodilation in much of the peripheral vascular system. Because of this, there is abnormal distribution of the blood volume in the peripheral vessels. Direct injury to the medullary vasomotor center or interruption of sympathetic innervation due to cervical or high thoracic spinal cord injury causes such a loss of vasomotor control.[5] The classic picture of neurogenic shock is hypotension without tachycardia or cutaneous vasoconstriction. Patients with known or suspected neurogenic shock should be treated initially for hypovolemia; vasoactive drugs should not be administered until volume is restored. This directly inhibits compensatory vasoconstriction in response to intravascular fluid loss and thereby exacerbates the hypovolemic shock state. Intracranial injuries alone do not produce circulatory inadequacy until the brain stem and its reticular activating system are profoundly involved.[6] Therefore, the presence of shock in a patient with a head injury indicates a search for another cause, such as internal bleeding from an abdominal injury.

For trauma patients surviving the first 3 days after injury, sepsis is the principal cause of death.[7] *Septic shock* is uncommon immediately after a traumatic insult.[8] How the patient presents with septic shock depends partly on the volume status. For example, septic patients who are also hypovolemic are difficult to distinguish clinically from those in hypovolemic shock. In contrast, in the normovolemic septic patient, an elevated cardiac output, tachycardia, low systemic vascular resistance, and warm, flushed extremities may be evidence of septic shock.[9]

🌑 CLASSES OF SHOCK

The initial assessment and resuscitation of trauma patients is categorized into four classes of hypovolemic shock based on the amount of blood lost (Table 15-1).[10] The classes are related to physiological responses and can be helpful in understanding the clinical manifestations.

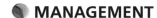

TABLE 15-1. Estimated Fluid and Blood Losses* Based on Patient's Initial Presentation

	Class I	Class II	Class III	Class IV
Blood loss (mL)	Up to 750	750–1,500	1,500–2,000	> 2,000
Blood loss (% BV)	Up to 15%	15–30%	30–40%	> 40%
Pulse rate	< 100	> 100	> 120	> 140
Blood pressure	Normal	Normal	Decreased	Decreased
Pulse pressure (mm Hg)	Normal or increased	Decreased	Decreased	Decreased
Respiratory rate	14–20	20–30	30–40	> 35
Urine output (mL/hr)	> 30	20–30	5–15	Negligible
CNS/mental status	Slightly anxious	Mildly anxious	Anxious and confused	Confused and lethargic
Fluid replacement (3:1 rule)	Crystalloid	Crystalloid	Crystalloid and blood	Crystalloid and blood

*For a 70-kg man.
BV, blood volume; CNS, central nervous system.
From *Advanced Trauma Life Support Course for Doctors,* 6th ed. Chicago: American College of Surgeons; 1997.

COMPENSATORY MECHANISMS

Circulatory reflexes and fluid shifts occur to compensate for the diminished blood volume. Circulatory reflexes trigger a response from the sympathetic nervous system when there is a blood loss greater than 10% of the total blood volume. This causes increased heart rate as well as constriction of arterioles and veins in the peripheral circulation. Fortunately, sympathetic stimulation does not cause significant constriction of either the cerebral or cardiac vessels, although blood flow in many areas of the body is markedly diminished. Thus, blood flow through the heart and brain is maintained at essentially normal levels until the arterial pressure falls below 70 mm Hg.[11] Another compensatory mechanism that occurs over a number of hours involves a fluid shift from the interstitial space to the vascular space, thus increasing blood volume. Still another mechanism triggered by hypovolemia is increased release of the hormones aldosterone and antidiuretic hormone (ADH). Aldosterone increases renal sodium reabsorption and conserves intravascular water.[12] ADH functions to increase water reabsorption in the kidney.

MANAGEMENT

Treatment should be initiated early because prolonged shock leads to cellular swelling and damage, compounding the overall impact of blood loss and hypoperfusion. The overall goal of therapy is to reestablish adequate tissue perfusion and thus oxygen delivery to metabolically active cells. Nursing care is focused on restoring cellular perfusion rather than simply restoring the patient's blood pressure and pulse rate. Of course, active bleeding must be controlled by whatever means necessary.

INITIAL MEASURES

Securing Airway

To restore tissue oxygen delivery, first the airway must be secured. For some patients, a simple jaw thrust may suffice; for others (such as those in class III or class IV shock), endotracheal intubation is required. Once the airway is secured, assessment of respiratory rate and rhythm is performed. Spontaneous hyperventilation is initially noted in major shock, followed by a deterioration in ventilatory efforts. Supplemental high-flow oxygen should be administered to improve oxygen availability for transport to hypoxic tissues. This may be all that is necessary in the spontaneously breathing patient who maintains adequate arterial blood gases. Injury to the thorax or need for surgical intervention in the patient with significant traumatic shock usually necessitates mechanical ventilatory support. Other considerations are the insertion of a urethral catheter to allow for assessment of renal function and to assess urine output, as well as the insertion of a nasogastric tube (unless contraindicated by local fractures) for decompression of the stomach.[13]

Initiating Intravenous Lines

Peripheral Sites

In the presence of severe hypovolemia, the aim of fluid resuscitation is to quickly infuse large volumes of fluid. Flow of intravenous (IV) fluids is directly dependent on the internal diameter of the administration device and inversely dependent on its length; other factors also greatly influence flow rates (Table 15-2). It is possible to achieve high flow rates with a peripheral line. Large peripheral catheters have been developed that can deliver maximal fluid flow to hypovolemic patients. A peripheral access is preferred over a central site; if there is a 20-gauge or larger peripheral IV device already in place, a 7-Fr or 8.5-Fr catheter can be inserted over the existing catheter. Figure 15-1 shows a

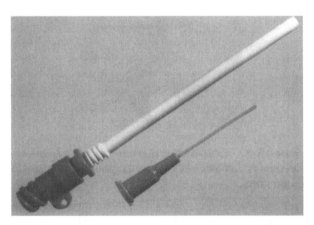

FIGURE 15-1. Arrow RIC 8.5 Fr (Rapid Infusion Catheter) compared with an ordinary 22-gauge device. Both are designed for the peripheral infusion of intravenous fluids; however, markedly higher infusion rates are possible with the wide-diameter device.

photograph of a 8.5-Fr Arrow RIC (Rapid Infusion Catheter) suitable for rapid peripheral fluid administration. Percutaneous access in the upper extremities is preferred, primarily in the antecubital fossae or secondarily at the wrist.[14] If these veins cannot be accessed immediately, it is vital that another route be obtained. For example, cannulation of the saphenous vein in the leg or of the common femoral vein may be considered. Sites are needed both above and below the diaphragm if the patient has thoracic or abdominal injuries. Extremities that show evidence of proximal injury should not be used because of the potential for venous extravasation and fluid loss.[15] When a peripheral site is not available, cannulation of the subclavian vein with a central line introducer (usually 8 Fr) may also be considered.

Central Sites

Recommended central sites for rapid fluid resuscitation include the subclavian,[16] femoral, or internal jugular veins.[17] These sites, cannulated with large-diameter devices, can accept rapid flow rates. A standard 8.5-Fr short introducer sheath is commonly used. Later, this same device can be used as an introducer for a hemodynamic monitoring catheter. It should be noted that typical central venous catheters are not suited for rapid fluid replacement because of their relatively small diameter and long length (causing resistance to rapid flow rate).[18] A wide variety of central venous catheters are in use, varying in length from 6 to 12 inches. Some have single lumens, but most have two or more lumens (Fig. 15-2). The gauge of the lumen and length of the catheter influence the maximal flow rate through that particular IV line. For example, some catheters have triple lumens (two 18-gauge and one 16-gauge lumen; in that event, the 16-gauge lumen would facilitate flow rate more quickly than either of the 18-gauge ports).

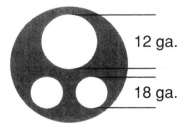

12 ga.

18 ga.

FIGURE 15-2. Cross-section diagram of triple-lumen central venous catheter having one 12-gauge and two 18-gauge ports.

TABLE 15-2.   Factors Affecting Flow Rate and Strategies to Increase Flow Rate in Emergency Situations

Factors Affecting Flow Rate	Strategies to Increase Flow Rate
Catheter diameter	Use largest diameter device available: • Dutky et al.[42] demonstrated in a laboratory study* that the rate of flow increased as the diameter of the device increased (using crystalloid fluids administered by gravity drip). 18 ga: 87 mL/min 16 ga: 125 mL/min 14 ga: 147 mL/min 8.5 Fr: 160 mL/min • See Figure 15-3 to compare the diameters of a rapid-flow infusion catheter and a typical small-diameter catheter. • When a multilumen central venous catheter is available, use the largest port to deliver fluids quickly (eg, fluid can be delivered close to twice as fast through the brown port of a typical Arrow multilumen central venous catheter [CVC] as through the blue or white port).
Catheter length	Use shortest IV device available: • Landow et al.[43] demonstrated in a laboratory study* that flow rate slows as the length of the IV device increases (eg, the flow rate was faster in a 1.25-inch catheter than in a 2-inch catheter) • Note how approximate flow rates (mL/hr) are faster in shorter Arrow multilumen CVCs (7 Fr × 20 cm versus 7 Fr × 30 cm) when normal saline is infused at room temperature through standard tubing under gravity (40-inch head height); under the same conditions, flow rates of up to 11,400 mL/hr can be achieved through the proximal (12 gauge) lumen of a two-lumen 12 Fr × 16 cm Arrow catheter.[44]

Distal Lumen (16 ga) (Brown Port)		Middle Lumen (18 ga) (Blue Port)		Proximal Lumen (18 ga) (White Port)	
7 Fr × 20 cm (3,107 mL/hr)	7 Fr × 30 cm (2,321 mL/hr)	7 Fr × 20 cm (1,506 mL/hr)	7 Fr × 30 cm (993 mL/hr)	7 Fr × 20 cm (1,593 mL/hr)	7 Fr × 30 cm (1,086 mL/hr)

Factors Affecting Flow Rate	Strategies to Increase Flow Rate
IV administration tubing diameter	Use largest diameter IV tubing set available: • Dutky et al.[45] demonstrated in a laboratory study that flow rate was faster with large-diameter tubing (as compared to regular tubing), using crystalloid fluid with gravity drip: Regular tubing with 14-ga catheter: 268 mL/min Large tubing with 14-ga catheter: 417 mL/min Regular tubing with 8.5 Fr catheter: 316 mL/min Large tubing with 8.5 Fr catheter: 805 mL/min

Continued

TABLE 15-2. Factors Affecting Flow Rate and Strategies to Increase Flow Rate in Emergency Situations—*cont'd*

Factors Affecting Flow Rate	Strategies to Increase Flow Rate
Pressure under which fluid is administered	Administer fluid under pressure when possible: • Most facilities have pressure infusion cuffs readily available. • Pumps for rapid fluid infusion are also available. • Landow et al.[46] demonstrated in a laboratory setting that flow rate of a crystalloid solution through a 14-ga catheter under gravity drip was 233 mL/min; in contrast, the flow rate increased to 594 mL/min when 300 mm Hg pressure was applied.
Temperature of fluid to be administered	Warm fluids, as indicated: • Rapidly infused fluids are usually warmed to prevent hypothermia; this also increases flow rate by one-half to one-third.[47] • A suggestion to speed the flow rate of viscous packed red blood cells is to mix them with warmed isotonic saline.
Filters	If a filter is used in the administration set (as for blood), change it as frequently as indicated to avoid clogging and thus slowed fluid flow rate.
Kinking of IV tubing	Use of a large-diameter IV infusion set minimizes the risk for kinking.

*Note that these findings were obtained from studies conducted in a laboratory setting (not in actual patients); thus, the findings were not influenced by factors encountered during actual practice (such as the patient's IV pressure or catheter obstruction from venous valves, venous tortuosity, or occlusion of the catheter's orifice by the patient's venous wall).

Figure 15-3 offers an explanation of the diameters of IV devices according to gauge and French sizes.

FLUID ADMINISTRATION

Selection of Fluids

Crystalloids

To some extent, volume replacement is essential in hypovolemic shock to restore intravascular volume and adequate tissue perfusion. Crystalloids are the primary treatment for a hemorrhaging patient who has adequate red blood cell mass. Crystalloids are defined as isotonic sodium-containing fluids (usually lactated Ringer's solution or 0.9% sodium chloride, also referred to as "normal saline"). The American College of Surgeons' Committee on Trauma recommends isotonic electrolyte solutions for initial replacement of fluid losses; Ringer's lactate solution is the initial fluid of choice, whereas normal saline is the second choice.[19] Although normal saline is a satisfactory fluid, it has the potential to cause hyperchloremic acidosis (especially if renal function is impaired).[20] Recall that isotonic saline

contains 154 mEq chloride per liter (while the plasma chloride concentration is close to 100 mEq/L). In a recently published animal study that compared normal saline to lactated Ringer's as resuscitation fluids following moderate and massive hemorrhage, researchers

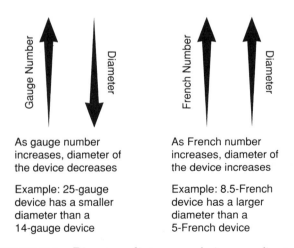

FIGURE 15-3. Diameters of intravenous devices according to gauge and French sizes.

concluded that, with moderate hemorrhage, the two fluids are equivalent; however, in the setting of massive hemorrhage and resuscitation, lactated Ringer's is superior to normal saline.[21]

For trauma victims, fluid resuscitation with isotonic electrolyte solutions is usually initiated in the field by medics. An initial fluid bolus of 1 to 2 liters is given as rapidly as possible for an adult; a dose of 20 mL/kg is used for a pediatric patient.[22] For children, the dose of 20 mL/kg can be repeated once; if there is no response to these two fluid boluses, blood transfusion as well as ongoing crystalloid infusion is required. The patient's response to initial fluid administration must be observed and further action determined accordingly. If the shock state fails to show signs of resolution after aggressive fluid replacement, one should suspect continued blood loss, inadequate fluid delivery, or onset of complications.

Crystalloids Versus Colloids

After administration of the first few liters of a crystalloid, the question of when and if colloids should be added to the regimen frequently arises. The main factors considered when deciding between crystalloids and colloids are the hemodynamic and pulmonary effects of the fluids. The volume of isotonic crystalloids required to attain adequate volume repletion varies from three to seven times the volume of colloids required to reach the same hemodynamic end point.[23] Studies regarding pulmonary status in the "colloid-crystalloid debate" have produced conflicting results. That is, some studies report that pulmonary injury is less likely with crystalloid resuscitation, whereas others state the reverse. Theoretically, based on Starling's law of fluid movement across a semipermeable membrane, excessive volumes of crystalloids might accumulate in the pulmonary interstitium because of a reduction in the colloid oncotic pressure-pulmonary capillary wedge pressure (PCWP) gradient. However, authorities disagree as to the clinical significance of this phenomenon. Some researchers point out that colloids may also extravasate into the interstitial space if there are damaged capillaries (endothelial leakiness). Protein-rich interstitial fluid can accumulate in the lungs and other tissues, causing ARDS and organ failure. However, it appears that the overall volume used and the presence or absence of sepsis affect pulmonary function to a far greater extent than does the type of resuscitation fluid used.[24] Despite continuing theoretical discussions, the avail-

able clinical data do not indicate that colloids have any advantage over crystalloids in initial fluid resuscitation; however, colloids are significantly more expensive and more complex to administer.[25] In a meta-analysis of eight published clinical studies in which patients were randomly assigned to receive either a colloid or a crystalloid regimen, Velanovich[26] found that mortality rates in trauma patients were about 12% less when crystalloid resuscitation was used. In contrast, mortality rates in nontrauma patients were found to be about 8% less when resuscitated with colloid regimens. The meta-analysis further indicated that colloid resuscitation was deleterious in septic trauma patients with capillary leak syndrome (leading to ARDS). Roberts and Bratton agree that despite some theoretical advantages of colloids compared to crystalloid therapy, no decrease in the risk of acute lung injury has been demonstrated.[27]

Hypertonic Saline

Hypertonic sodium chloride solutions contain large concentrations of sodium, ranging from 250 to 1,200 mEq/L. Because of their high sodium content, these solutions are capable of expanding the plasma volume by pulling fluid from the intracellular space into the extravascular space. Therefore, much smaller volumes of hypertonic saline (as compared to isotonic sodium solutions) are needed to increase the intravascular fluid volume. However, some authors point out that although blood pressure may be elevated more rapidly in the first few minutes after resuscitation with hypertonic saline, survival rates do not change.[28] Another consideration is that resuscitation with hypertonic saline can lead to hypernatremia and hyperosmolarity.[29] Proponents of hypertonic saline cite studies that have indicated good clinical response to hypertonic saline administration in trauma patients.[30,31] A recent animal study suggested that hypertonic saline resuscitation after hemorrhagic shock may help protect against the development of lung injury (presumably by suppressing neutrophil activation).[32] Proponents of hypertonic saline also believe that it is effective for volume resuscitation in cases of combined hemorrhagic shock and head injury.[33] Others point out that cerebral dehydration could develop rapidly with subsequent bleeding, as could central pontine myelinolysis due to rapid variations in serum sodium levels.[34] In summary, there is not good agreement in the United States as to the benefits of hypertonic saline in the treatment of trauma victims; therefore, its efficacy remains under investigation.

Blood Products

Blood replacement therapy is needed in patients with blood loss greater than 20% to 25% of their total blood volume (see Table 15-1). It is difficult to predict the actual percentage of blood loss in early treatment; this is generally accomplished by observing the patient's response to fluid resuscitation.

Early in the treatment of hemorrhagic shock, use of hematocrit to guide blood replacement therapy is unreliable (even massive blood loss produces a minimal acute decrease in hematocrit). Later on, after fluid shifts from the extravascular space into the bloodstream have occurred, a hematocrit of less than 30% is usually viewed as need for blood replacement. Theoretically, it is at this point that red blood cell mass should be supplemented to provide adequate oxygen-carrying capacity to the tissues.[35] Although traditionally a hematocrit of 30% has been used as a marker of blood need, more recent clinical data have suggested that the hematocrit be maintained at 33% to 35% in critically ill patients.[36] If the hematocrit is greater than 30% (or the designated level) and hemodynamic stability remains, further aggressive fluid resuscitation may be unnecessary. If the hematocrit falls below the designated level, packed red blood cells (PRBCs) should be transfused. It is important to remember, however, that hemoglobin and hematocrit values alone are unreliable in initially gauging the degree of blood loss because up to 4 hours may elapse before any significant changes are evident.[37] By 2 hours in experimental blood loss, 14% to 36% of the ultimate drop in hematocrit occurs; a 36% to 50% change occurs in 8 hours, and a 63% to 77% change occurs in 24 hours.[38] Although a very low hematocrit suggests significant blood loss or preexisting anemia, an early near normal hematocrit does not rule out significant blood loss (see Case Study 15-1).

PRBCs are obtained by centrifuging whole blood and drawing off about 200 to 225 mL plasma. Although whole blood is preferred, it is not available because of blood bank policies. PRBCs have a hematocrit level of about 70% and can be infused with little difficulty. In a 70-kg person, a unit of red blood cells will increase the hematocrit 3% to 4% (1 g/dL).[39] Full typing and crossmatching before transfusion are desirable when time permits; when not, typing alone may be sufficient. Typing of blood is relatively fast (5–7 minutes); when typing is not

feasible, use of type O, Rh-negative blood may be considered.[40] Unstable patients with more than 40% blood loss (class IV) may require uncrossmatched blood.

Methods to Increase Flow Rates

Strategies to increase flow rates during emergency fluid resuscitation are summarized in Table 15-2. It is important to remember that the rapid infusion of cold fluids can predispose to hypothermia and cardiac dysrhythmias. To prevent hypothermia in patients receiving massive volumes of crystalloids, the fluid may be heated to 39°(102.2°) before use.[41] Specialized blood warmers are used during the rapid administration of blood.

EVALUATING RESPONSE TO RESUSCITATION

Some patients (usually those who have lost < 20% of their blood volume) respond rapidly to the initial fluid bolus and remain stable when the infusion is slowed. No further fluid bolus or immediate blood administration is indicated for this group of patients, although crossmatched blood should be made available. Other patients respond to the initial fluid bolus but show signs of deterioration when the fluids are slowed; most of these patients have lost 20% to 40% of their blood volume, or are still bleeding and require continued crystalloid administration as well as blood transfusion and surgical intervention. Little or no response to fluid resuscitation is seen in a small but significant percentage of injured patients. For most of these, failure to respond to adequate crystalloid and blood administration indicates the need for unlimited blood and fluid resuscitation and immediate surgical intervention to control hemorrhage.

Noninvasive Clinical Signs

Traditionally, a patient's response to resuscitation therapy has been determined by noninvasive clinical indicators such as:

- Systolic blood pressure
- Heart rate
- Level of consciousness
- Urine output
- Pulse pressure

Although urine output is one of the primary indicators of response to fluid resuscitation, it should be recognized that it can be affected by variables other than adequate fluid replacement. For example, diuretics or vasopressors can increase urinary flow rate despite underlying tissue perfusion problems. Within certain limits, adequate volume replacement should produce a urinary output of about 0.5 ml/kg/hr in an adult and 1 mL/kg/hr in the pediatric patient; for children younger than 1 year of age, 2 mL/kg/hr should be maintained.[48]

It is recognized that hypoperfusion and thus poor cellular oxygen delivery can persist although the conventional signs are returned to a normal range. Because of this, current practice reflects an evolving view of how to monitor patients for an appropriate response to fluid resuscitation.[49] Recall that the hypoperfusion of shock creates a cellular oxygen debt and that the overall goal of volume resuscitation is to increase oxygen delivery to the cells. To determine whether this has occurred, it may be necessary to insert a pulmonary artery catheter. Other parameters to assess include hematocrit, blood pH, and lactate levels, which are discussed in the following sections.

During massive fluid resuscitation, it is possible to give too little or too much fluid. Inadequate fluid administration must be guarded against because prolonged hypovolemia predisposes to decreased perfusion of major organs.[50] Conversely, it is possible to administer too much fluid and thereby overwhelm the circulation and perhaps cause pulmonary edema. Volume overload to some extent is common in shock patients during aggressive fluid resuscitation. Because of compensatory increased secretion of aldosterone and ADH, injured patients have an impaired ability to excrete excessive fluid loads. Even when the intravascular volume is not excessive, it is common for skin, muscles, and subcutaneous tissue to become edematous after massive volume resuscitation. This is because about 75% of every liter of balanced salt solution shifts into the interstitial space within 1 hour after administration. Problems associated with the resulting soft tissue edema include a decreased rate of wound healing and an increased propensity to develop pressure sores.

Hemodynamic Parameters

Central Venous Pressure

The response of the central venous pressure (CVP) to fluid administration (when properly interpreted) helps evaluate the adequacy of volume replacement.[51]

Some points to remember about CVP measurements include:

1. CVP is an indirect measure of volume.
2. Normal CVP is 0 to 7 mm Hg when a transducer system is used; it is about 1 to 10 cm water when a water manometer is used.
3. CVP is often low in hypovolemic shock because of inadequate filling of the right heart.
4. The initial CVP and actual blood volume are not necessarily related.
5. A high CVP may be observed even with a volume deficit; for example, patients with generalized vasoconstriction and fluid replacement may show a high pressure related to the application of pneumatic antishock garment or inappropriate use of vasopressors.
6. A minimal rise in the initial, low CVP with fluid therapy suggests the need for further volume expansion.
7. A decrease in CVP suggests an ongoing fluid loss.
8. An abrupt or persistent elevation in CVP suggests volume replacement has been adequate or is too rapid, or that cardiac function has been compromised.
9. A malpositioned catheter or increased intrathoracic pressure from a pneumothorax may cause pronounced elevations of CVP.
10. CVP is best monitored in trends, especially in response to fluid therapy.

Pulmonary Capillary Wedge Pressure

The PCWP is a measure of preload, which reflects left ventricular end-diastolic volume; this measure is easily obtained at the bedside from the pulmonary artery catheter. Although CVP and PCWP do not reflect blood volume accurately in all patients, they are useful in preventing acute volume overload during rapid fluid restoration and fluid challenges. In critically ill patients, a PCWP of 15 to 18 mm Hg is the goal to increase cardiac output.[52]

Lactate Levels

Lactate determinations have been used to assess the adequacy of tissue oxygenation in the critically ill. The most common cause of an elevated blood lactate concentration is hypoperfusion or circulatory shock.[53] When intracellular oxygen is not available, energy is produced by anaerobic metabolic pathways, resulting in increased lactate production. A normal serum lactate level is less than 2.5 mmol/L. A moderate increase to 5.0 to 9.9 mmol/L has an associated mortality of 60% to 75%; a level greater than 10 mmol/L is considered severe and has a mortality rate greater than 95%.[54] Arterial or mixed venous blood specimens are favored for lactate analysis because peripherally obtained venous samples can yield falsely elevated values, depending on the techniques used.[55] If before obtaining the specimen the patient remains at complete rest, venous and arterial levels are virtually alike; however, if even minor movements such as hand clenching are performed, the lactate level in the sample can rise significantly.[56] (Venous stasis from applying a tourniquet has little effect.[57]) Measurement of lactate levels from arterial lines (when present) allows for monitoring of subtle but important serial changes that reflect the patient's response to therapy and provides the clinician with valuable feedback. If an arterial line is not present, a properly drawn specimen from a peripheral venous site is acceptable.

Acid–Base and Electrolyte Changes

The majority of acid–base abnormalities that develop in shock improve spontaneously once adequate ventilation and perfusion are achieved. Early in hypovolemic shock, respiratory alkalosis occurs due to tachypnea; this is followed by a mild metabolic acidosis.[58] Patients with severe traumatic injury and hemorrhagic shock become acidotic as a result of loss of oxygen-carrying capacity and decreased cardiac output.[59] As lactate and hydrogen ions accumulate in shock, a high anion gap metabolic acidosis develops. Respiratory acidosis will also develop as the number of functional pulmonary capillaries decrease, causing carbon dioxide (CO_2) retention. In the final stages of shock, there will be a combined metabolic and respiratory acidosis with an increase in the arterial carbon dioxide tension ($PaCO_2$), a low bicarbonate level, and a very low pH. Metabolic acidosis or metabolic alkalosis may occur after massive blood transfusion (see Chap. 10).

Tissue injury or hemorrhage may cause catecholamine release, which in turn may cause an intracellular shift of potassium and cause hypokalemia.[60] Electrolyte disorders associated with massive transfusions are discussed in Chapter 10. In addition to treatment-related causes of electrolyte imbalances, underlying clinical problems can contribute to the development of specific imbalances.

CASE STUDIES

● **15-1.** After undergoing a sigmoid colectomy and splenectomy, a 47-year-old man was returned to the postoperative recovery room at noon in good condition. At that time, he was receiving lactated Ringer's solution through an 18-gauge port of a triple-lumen central venous catheter (CVC). His vital signs were normal, as was perfusion of the kidneys and brain (as evidenced by an adequate level of consciousness and urinary output). About 4 hours later, he developed seizure-type activity and became unresponsive; the following vital signs were obtained:

Blood pressure = 44/20 mm Hg
Heart rate = 136 beats/min
CVP = 0 cm water
Rapid gasping respirations

Blood work was drawn and showed a hemoglobin of 11 g/dL and a hematocrit of 36%. No bleeding was noted from the abdominal incision. The physician was notified and the IV line was immediately turned to a "wide open" rate (under the influence of gravity). Over the next 5 hours, the patient received lactated Ringer's "wide open" through the 18-gauge port of the CVC, and 2 units of PRBCs was given through the 16-gauge port of the CVC (with the assistance of a pressure cuff). Despite this, the patient's vital signs remained extremely poor, urine output was almost nil, and full consciousness was never regained. The hemoglobin dropped to 6 g/dL and the hematocrit to 19%. The patient was returned to surgery where a short 14-gauge catheter was inserted in the external jugular vein; warmed blood and crystalloids were pumped in through this device. An exploratory laparotomy revealed that a ligature had slipped from the splenic artery and the patient's abdomen was filled with blood. Despite aggressive fluid resuscitation in the operating room and control of bleeding, the patient did not survive.

COMMENTARY: Because a major compensatory shift of fluid from the extravascular extracellular space into the vascular space (to help replace the diminished blood supply) had not had time to occur, the patient's hemoglobin and hematocrit values were close to normal at the time of the hemorrhagic event. Later, hemodilution from this process became more obvious (hemoglobin 6 g/dL and hematocrit 19%).

The patient's clinical status did not improve despite IV fluid given "wide open" because the fluids were administered via gravity with the flow control clamp wide open; because a small port (18-gauge) of a long, narrow CVC was used, the fluid met resistance as it attempted to flow through the catheter. (One could equate this to using a long, narrow ordinary garden hose to apply water to a major fire; instead, of course, one would want to use a wide short hose for this purpose, preferably with the water delivered under pressure.) See Table 15-2 for strategies to administer fluids rapidly when severe hypovolemia is present. Failure of the patient to respond to the inadequate fluid regime described above was an indication that more aggressive fluid resuscitation (along with more rapid surgical intervention) was urgently needed.

A lack of visible incisional bleeding is insufficient to "rule out" hemorrhagic shock after abdominal surgery. In this instance, the patient was bleeding internally. All other clinical signs pointed to hemorrhagic shock; unfortunately, however, they were not recognized.

Although a pulmonary catheter is often helpful in the early diagnosis of hypovolemic shock and to allow titration of fluids during resuscitation to achieve a satisfactory outcome, this patient could have been managed without a pulmonary artery catheter. The blood pressure, heart rate, and CVP should have guided treatment to more aggressive fluid resuscitation along with more rapid surgical intervention. Clinical indicators of hypovolemic shock were obvious, as was the inadequate clinical response to too little fluid resuscitation.

● **15-2.** A 56-year-old man was trapped between two railroad cars in a mining accident. He was hypotensive at the scene of the accident and resuscitated with 3,000 mL lactated Ringer's solution before being transported to a trauma center. On arrival, he was anxious and confused and his vital signs were:

  Blood pressure = 98/60 mm Hg
  Pulse rate = 120 /min
  Respiratory rate = 40/min
  Estimated blood loss at this time = 2,000 mL

He was given an additional 3,000 mL lactated Ringer's before being rushed to surgery. During surgery, he was found to have the following injuries: right diaphragmatic hernia, herniation of kidney and liver into the thoracic cavity, liver laceration, avulsion of the right ureter from the renal pelvis, injury to the lumbar vessels, crush injury to head of pancreas, and serosal tears of the duodenum. The surgical procedure consisted of an exploratory laparotomy with ligation of bleeding lumbar vessels, a repair of the right renal vein, a right nephrectomy, repair of the diaphragm, drainage of the pancreatic injury, and repair of the duodenal serosal tears. During surgery he received the following fluids:

  5% albumin = 500 mL
  Fresh frozen plasma = 785 mL
  Hetastarch = 500 mL
  Platelets = 200 mL
  PRBCs = 12 units
  0.9% NaCl = 1,000 mL

Urinary output from the time of admission through the end of the surgical procedure was 2,000 mL. The total estimated blood loss from the time of injury was 5,000 mL. Because of the need for rapid fluid resuscitation, fluids were warmed and administered under pressure with a fluid infusion warming system (Level 1 H500, Level One Technologies, Rockland, MA).

Vital signs and other data available from the time of admission through the first 24 hours were as shown in Table 15-3. Arterial blood gas, lactate levels, and hematocrit levels were as shown in Table 15-4.

Total intake from the time of injury through the first 24 hours was 20,035 mL; urine output during this time was 6,900 mL. During this same period, he sustained an estimated blood loss of 5,000 mL.

COMMENTARY: The patient experienced class III shock at the time of admission to the trauma center based on estimated blood loss, vital signs, and mental status; see Table 15-1, which worsened during the surgical procedure. (Note the increased heart rate and lowered blood pressure at the third surgical hour.)

On admission, the patient had a combination of metabolic acidosis and respiratory acidosis. For example, the bicarbonate level was below normal

TABLE 15-3.

	Hour 1 (ER)	Hour 3 (OR)	Hour 5 (OR)	Hour 10 (ICU)	Hour 16 (ICU)	Hour 22 (ICU)	Hour 24 (ICU)
Heart rate	120	130	118	98	110	118	113
Blood pressure	98/60	< 60	110/70	166/90	138/78	136/76	140/80
CVP (mm Hg)	—	—	—	6	2	5	13
PCWP (mm Hg)	—	—	—	3	2	6	12

TABLE 15-4.

	Hour 1 (ER)	Hour 2 (OR)	Hour 4 (OR)	Hour 5 (OR)	Hour 6 (OR)	Hour 10 (OR)	Hour 12 (ICU)	Hour 18 (ICU)	Hour 24 (ICU)
pH	7.26	7.23	7.15	7.18	7.3	7.26	7.25	7.35	7.36
$PaCO_2$ (mm Hg)	46	44	40	45	47	43	43	37	43
HCO_3 (mEq/L)	20.2	18	20	18	13	16	23	20	24
Lactate (mmol/L)	—	—	—	—	—	—	5.8	3.6	1.8
Hematocrit	26%	—	—	—	—	—	—	—	33%

(18 mEq/L). The expected $PaCO_2$ in this situation would be as follows (using Winter's formula, see Chap. 9): $1.5(18) + 8 \pm 2 = 33\text{-}37$ mm Hg (instead, it was 44 mm Hg, indicating an excess of $PaCO_2$).

Adding the urinary output to the estimated blood loss, the patient lost a total of about 12 liters fluid; during the same period, he gained about 20 liters by the IV route. The discrepancy of about 8 liters can partially be explained by third-spacing caused by the initial trauma as well as trauma sustained during the surgical procedures. The third-spacing resulted in hypovolemia as fluid shifted from the vascular space into the injured tissues. Fluid was administered in sufficient quantities to keep the vital signs and other parameters within normal limits.

The serum lactate level may be used to assess adequacy of fluid resuscitation. Note how these readings improved from hour 14 to hour 24. Other parameters that improved with resuscitation were vital signs (blood pressure and pulse), hemodynamic readings (CVP and PCWP), hematocrit values, and arterial blood gas values.

REFERENCES

1. American College of Surgeons, Committee on Trauma. *Advanced Trauma Life Support [ATLS] Course for Doctors*, 6th ed. Chicago: American College of Surgeons; 1997:99.
2. Chernow B, ed. *The Pharmacologic Approach to the Critically Ill Patient*, 3rd ed. Baltimore, MD: Williams & Wilkins, 1994: 1110.
3. ATLS, p 105.
4. Ibid.
5. Rice V. Shock, a clinical syndrome: An update. Part I. An overview of shock. *Crit Care Nurse* 1991;11:20.
6. Moore EE, ed. *Early Care of the Injured Patient*, 4th ed. Philadelphia: BC Decker; 1990:77.
7. Cardona V, Hurn P, Mason P, Scanlon A, Veise-Berry S. *Trauma Nursing*, 2nd ed. Philadelphia: WB Saunders; 1994:152.
8. Ibid.
9. Ibid.
10. ATLS, p 108.
11. Guyton A, Hall J. *Textbook of Medical Physiology*, 9th ed. Philadelphia: WB Saunders; 1996:287.
12. Sabiston DC, Lyerly HK, eds. *Sabiston Essentials of Surgery*, 2nd ed. Philadelphia; WB Saunders; 1994:11.
13. Kinney M, Dunbar S, Brooks-Brunn J, Molter N, Vitello-Cicciu J, eds. *AACN's Clinical Reference for Critical-Care Nursing*, 4th ed. St. Louis: CV Mosby; 1998:1099.
14. Moore, p 65.
15. Ibid.
16. Ibid.
17. Dutky P et al. Factors affecting rapid fluid resuscitation with large-bore introducer catheters. *J Trauma* 1989;29:856.
18. Moore, p 64.
19. ATLS, p 107
20. Ibid.
21. Healey M, Davis R, Liu F et al. Lactated Ringer's is superior to normal saline in a model of massive hemorrhage and resuscitation. *J Trauma* 1998;45:894.
22. ATLS, p 107.
23. Chernow, p 275.
24. Ibid, p 280.
25. Moore, p 76.
26. Velanovich V. Crystalloid versus colloid fluid resuscitation: A meta-analysis of mortality. *Surgery* 1989;105:65.
27. Roberts J, Bratton S. Colloid volume expanders. *Drugs* 1998; 55:621.
28. Schwartz S et al, eds. *Principles of Surgery*, 7th ed. New York: McGraw-Hill; 1999:108.
29. Mattox K et al. Prehospital hypertonic saline/dextran infusion for post-traumatic hypotension. *Ann Surg* 1991;213:482.
30. Vassar M et al. Analysis of potential risks associated with 7.5% sodium chloride resuscitation of traumatic shock. *Arch Surg* 1990;125:1309.
31. Angle N, Hoyt D, Coimbra R et al. Hypertonic saline resuscitation diminishes lung injury by suppressing neutrophil activation after hemorrhagic shock. *Shock* 1998;9:164.
32. Soliman M et al. Survival after hypertonic saline resuscitation from hemorrhage. *Am Surg* 1990;56:749.
33. Wisner K et al. Hypertonic saline resuscitation of head-injury: Effects on cerebral water content. *J Trauma* 1990;30:75.
34. Griffel M, Kaufman B. Pharmacology of colloids and crystalloids. *Crit Care Clin* 1992;8:235.
35. Clochesy J, ed. *Critical Care Nursing*. Philadelphia: WB Saunders; 1993:1237.
36. Moore FA et al. Incommensurate oxygen consumption in response to maximal oxygen availability predicts postinjury multiple organ failure. *J Trauma* 1992;33:58.
37. Clochesy, p 1237.
38. Chernow, p 274.
39. Rossi E, Simon T, Moss G, Gould S, eds. *Principles of Transfusion Medicine*, 2nd ed. Baltimore, MD: Williams & Wilkins, 1996:99,
40. Shoemaker W, Ayres S, Grenvik A et al, *Textbook of Critical Care*, 3rd ed. Philadelphia: WB Saunders; 1995:1421.
41. ATLS, p 111.
42. Dutky et al, p 856.
43. Landow L, Shahnarian A. Efficacy of large bore intravenous fluid administration sets designed for rapid volume resuscitation. *Crit Care Med* 1990;18:540.
44. *Arrow Multi-Lumen Central Venous Catheter. Nursing Care Guidelines*. Reading, PA: Arrow International Inc; December, 1994:13.
45. Dutky et al, p 856.
46. Landow, Shahnarian, p 540.
47. Dula D et al. Flow rate variance of commonly used intravenous infusion techniques. *J Trauma* 1981;21:480.
48. ATLS, p 108.
49. Annas C. Changing technology and research shape critical care trauma nursing. *Int J Trauma Nurs* 1994;Fall:20.
50. Ibid.
51. ATLS, p 114.
52. Packman M, Rachow C. Optimum left heart filling pressure during fluid resuscitation of patients with hypovolemic and septic shock. *Crit Care Med* 1983;11:165.
53. Kruse JA, Carlson RW. Lactate metabolism. *Crit Care Med* 1987;5:725.
54. Shapiro B, Peruzzi W, Templin R. *Clinical Application of Blood Gases*, 5th ed. St. Louis: CV Mosby; 1994:173.
55. Narins R, ed. *Maxwell & Kleeman's Clinical Disorders of Fluid and Electrolyte Metabolism*, 5th ed. New York: McGraw-Hill; 1994:1473.
56. Henry J. *Clinical Diagnosis and Management by Laboratory Methods*, 19th ed. Philadelphia: WB Saunders; 1996:206.
57. Ibid, p 207.
58. ATLS, p 109.
59. Ferrera A et al. Hypothermia and acidosis worsen coagulopathies in the patient requiring massive transfusion. *Am J Surg* 1990;160:515.
60. Dunham CM, Cowley RA. *Shock Trauma/Critical Care Manual*. Rockville, MD: Aspen; 1991.

CHAPTER 16

Heart Failure

DEFINITION

Heart failure refers to an inability of the heart to pump enough blood to meet the metabolic needs of tissues throughout the body. Common causes of heart failure (often referred to as congestive heart failure [CHF]) include hypertension, myocardial infarction, cardiomyopathies, and valvular disease.

Left ventricular failure, as seen in hypertensive heart disease or mitral stenosis, typically presents with pulmonary but not peripheral edema. In contrast, pure right ventricular failure initially seen in patients with cor pulmonale, typically presents with edema in the lower extremities and perhaps ascites. Failure of one ventricle often leads to failure of the other; therefore, both types of failure are present. Patients with cardiomyopathies tend to have simultaneous failure of both ventricles, presenting with both pulmonary and peripheral edema. CHF can be chronic or become acutely manifested in the form of pulmonary edema or cardiogenic shock.

MAJOR FLUID AND ELECTROLYTE IMBALANCES

The pathophysiology of CHF includes conditions that, when combined with CHF therapies, predispose patients to a number of potentially serious electrolyte disturbances.[1] For example, decreased cardiac output leads to impaired renal excretion of water and electrolytes (resulting in fluid volume excess) and causes the activation of neurohormonal responses that directly affect electrolyte balance. Further, many medications used to treat CHF affect sodium, potassium, and magnesium balance. The most common serum electrolyte abnormalities in patients with chronic CHF are hypomagnesemia, hypokalemia, and hyponatremia.[2]

Optimal care of the patient with CHF includes the early recognition and management of fluid and electrolyte disturbances. Table 16-1 summarizes the imbalances associated with CHF.

FLUID VOLUME EXCESS

The patient with CHF presents with the classic picture of an expanded extracellular fluid (ECF) volume, that is, swollen legs, engorged neck veins, congested liver,

and pulmonary crackles. Although the ECF is increased, the kidneys respond as if a reduced blood volume is present. The decrease in cardiac output and increase in ventricular end-diastolic pressure set the stage for sodium retention. Decreased cardiac output and increased systemic resistance produce decreased organ flow, especially to the kidney.

Shunting of blood away from the kidneys stimulates secretion of renin, which acts on angiotensinogen to produce angiotensin I, which is subsequently converted to angiotensin II. Angiotensin II is a strong arterial vasoconstrictor that helps to support arterial blood pressure when cardiac output decreases. This arterial vasoconstriction increases the work of the left ventricle as it pumps against the increased pressure (increased afterload). Angiotensin II also stimulates the secretion of aldosterone, which strongly promotes the reabsorption of sodium in the distal tubules and collecting ducts of the kidney. Another effect is venous vasoconstriction, which tends to increase venous return to the heart (increased preload). The result of excessive aldosterone secretion is fluid volume overload due to excessive sodium retention.

Treatment

Refer to the section on methods to decrease preload, presented later in this chapter.

HYPONATREMIA

The pathogenesis of CHF-associated hyponatremia is not well understood. However, it is apparently related to several factors. First, an increase in plasma angiotensin II promotes thirst and results in greater water intake.[3] In addition to activation of the renin-angiotensin-aldosterone mechanism, responses to circulatory failure include stimulation of hormones such as arginine vasopressin (antidiuretic hormone [ADH]), and stimulation of the sympathetic nervous system. ADH acts on the distal tubules to cause water retention; thus, hyponatremia in patients with CHF is primarily due to a limited ability of the kidneys to adequately excrete a water load.[4] The lowered serum sodium concentration does not represent a real decrease of total body sodium; instead, it is a dilution of the actual excessive amount of total body sodium (see Fig. 4-2A).

Contributing to hyponatremia in some patients is the tendency of sodium to shift from the ECF into the cells to replace the potassium loss associated with

TABLE 16-1. Fluid and Electrolyte Disturbances Associated With Congestive Heart Failure

Fluid and Electrolyte Disturbance	Etiology
Fluid volume excess	Secondary hyperaldosteronism (result of decreased renal blood flow associated with decreased cardiac output)
	Excessive aldosterone causes sodium and water retention
Hyponatremia	Although total body sodium content is above normal, excessive secretion of ADH causes relatively greater retention of water, diluting the serum level (see Fig. 4-2A)
	Contributing to the hyponatremia is loss of sodium in, for example, vomiting, diarrhea, and paracentesis; most hazardous if patient is on severely restricted sodium diet and large doses of diuretics
	Contributing to hyponatremia can be the movement of extracellular sodium into the cells to replace the potassium so frequently lost in treatment of heart failure
Hypokalemia	Excessive aldosterone levels predispose to potassium excretion
	Excessive use of potassium-losing diuretics and prolonged loss of potassium by vomiting or diarrhea represent typical causes of potassium deficit
Hypomagnesemia	Similar mechanisms to those described for hypokalemia
	Most likely to be problematic in patients with moderately severe to severe CHF receiving chronic or aggressive thiazide or loop-diuretic therapy
	Frequently contributes to the development of hypokalemia that is resistant to correction by potassium replacement alone
Hyperkalemia	Excessive use of potassium supplements, potassium-sparing diuretics, or angiotensin-converting enzyme inhibitors, in patients with renal dysfunction
Metabolic alkalosis if potassium-losing diuretics are used	Potassium-losing diuretics cause loss of chloride ions and compensatory increase in bicarbonate ions (hence metabolic alkalosis)
Metabolic (lactic) acidosis	Increased liberation of lactic acid from anoxic tissues and failure of body to metabolize it rapidly
	Slowing of circulation interferes with the excretion of metabolic acids
Respiratory acidosis	Pulmonary congestion interferes with elimination of CO_2 from lungs

hyperaldosteronism and use of potassium-losing diuretics.

Hyponatremia commonly complicates the course of CHF and is apparently an ominous prognostic factor.[5] With the exception of patients with hyponatremia due to overdiuresis (combined with hypotonic fluid replacement), hyponatremia in CHF usually indicates a severe clinical stage.[6] Most patients with CHF who have hyponatremia are clinically compromised, have disease of New York Heart Association functional class IV, and are volume overloaded.[7] Consequences of severe hyponatremia are primarily neurological in nature (see Chap. 4). A serum sodium level below 125 mEq/L may lead to arrhythmias.[8]

Treatment

Most patients who present with significant hyponatremia and fluid volume overload are clinically compromised and usually require hospitalization. For inpatients, fluid restriction may be necessary to deal with these problems. Total hypotonic fluid intake may be restricted to less than 1,000 mL in 24 hours.[9] Water intake is usually not restricted in the long-term management of CHF unless there is dilution of the serum sodium to less than 130 mEq/L by excessive water retention.

Diuretics may also be needed and are usually given orally. In some patients with marked edema, however, oral diuretics may be ineffective because of poor absorption by the edematous gastrointestinal (GI) tract; thus, a loop diuretic may need to be given intravenously (IV). If necessary, cardiovascular drug support (eg, dobutamine) may be used to improve the clinical state and increase the renal response to the loop diuretic.[10] The mainstay of chronic management of hyponatremia is use of an angiotensin-converting enzyme (ACE) inhibitor; for mild hyponatremia (serum sodium concentration, 131–136 mEq/L), simply adding or increasing the dose of the ACE inhibitor is often sufficient.[11] Apparently ACE inhibitors can improve hyponatremia in patients with CHF by increasing urinary water excretion.[12]

HYPOKALEMIA

In the patient with CHF numerous conditions predispose to hypokalemia. Among these are increased aldosterone levels, which cause increased loss of potassium in the urine, and frequent use of potassium-losing diuretics. The metabolic alkalosis associated with diuretic use decreases the serum potassium level by driving potassium into the cells and by increasing renal potassium excretion. In volume-overloaded patients, the hypokalemia is in part "dilutional."

Hypokalemia is generally most pronounced in patients with advanced CHF receiving aggressive diuretic therapy and is thought to be associated with a poor prognosis.[13]

Treatment

Regardless of the serum potassium level, patients with CHF (who have good renal function) tend to have reduced total body potassium levels. Therefore, almost all patients with CHF should receive potassium supplementation, a potassium-sparing diuretic (such as spironolactone, amiloride, or triamterene), or an ACE inhibitor; this is especially true if the patient is receiving a potassium-losing diuretic.[14] Hypokalemia is a serious threat because it increases the risk for arrhythmias and sudden death, especially in patients with CHF (because of diseased myocardium and use of arrhythmogenic drugs).[15] A serum potassium concentration of 4.5 to 5.0 mEq/L is favored by most clinicians.[16] In the presence of serious dysrhythmias, IV administration of potassium chloride is best. When hypokalemia does not respond to potassium replacement, it may be necessary to administer magnesium concomitantly.

As is always the case, it is possible to overcorrect an imbalance. Patients with renal dysfunction should be monitored closely for hyperkalemia, especially when receiving potassium supplementation or potassium-sparing agents. Also, the effects of potassium supplementation or potassium-sparing diuretics on patients chronically receiving ACE inhibitors should be followed closely; when the serum potassium levels reach the upper end of the optimal maintenance range, potassium supplements and potassium-sparing diuretics should be discontinued.[17]

HYPOMAGNESEMIA

Hypomagnesemia occurs infrequently in well compensated ambulatory patients with CHF; however, it is prevalent in more severely ill patients.[18] Magnesium deficiency is most likely to occur in patients with severe CHF who are receiving chronic or aggressive therapy with loop or thiazide diuretics. Most of the causes of magnesium deficiency parallel those described above for the development of hypokalemia.

Serum magnesium levels do not correlate strongly with tissue magnesium concentrations; that is, serum magnesium levels may be normal despite the presence of a tissue magnesium deficit. Therefore, supplemental magnesium or other magnesium-retaining agents (eg, potassium-sparing diuretics or ACE inhibitors) should be considered for patients with moderately severe to severe CHF.[19] Hypomagnesemia and whole body magnesium depletion in CHF patients are thought to be arrhythmogenic and probably increase the risk of morbidity and mortality, especially in the presence of digitalis toxicity or acute myocardial infarction and after surgery. Strong evidence implicates magnesium deficiency as an important cause of digitalis-toxic associated arrhythmias; also current evidence suggests that magnesium deficiency has an effect on the development of coronary artery disease and cardiomyopathy.[20] (See Chap. 7 for a discussion of magnesium therapy in cardiac conditions.)

Treatment

Routine magnesium supplementation is probably unnecessary for patients with mild to moderate CHF who are normokalemic and who are receiving an ACE inhibitor or a potassium-sparing diuretic. However, patients with advanced CHF who require aggressive thiazide or loop diuretic therapy and those with uncomplicated hypomagnesemia should be considered as candidates for long-term orally administered magnesium.[21] According to Leier et al.,[22] magnesium is a safe and potentially effective agent in the treatment of CHF, provided the patient has no significant renal dysfunction and reasonable clinical follow-up is performed. When magnesium is needed as an acute intervention, 10 to 20 mL of 10% magnesium sulfate may be prescribed IV over 5 to 10 minutes, usually followed by a 250- to 500-mL infusion of 2% solution during the subsequent 4 to 8 hours.[23]

Magnesium administration is important in the management of hypokalemia that does not respond to simple potassium replacement. Presumably magnesium provides the necessary cofactor required for normal potassium utilization.[24]

METABOLIC ACIDOSIS

Stimulation of the sympathetic nervous system increases heart rate and contractility, which, in turn, increases cardiac output (Fig. 16-1). Blood is preferentially shunted to the brain and heart (away from the skin, skeletal muscles, abdominal organs, and kidneys). This shunting increases arteriovenous oxygen extraction, which can become so severe that the cells shift to anaerobic metabolism, leading to metabolic (lactic) acidosis.

⬤ ASSESSMENT

Knowledge of the pathophysiological mechanisms associated with the usual signs and symptoms of CHF, especially those affecting fluid and electrolyte balance,

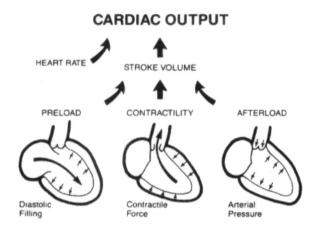

FIGURE 16-1. Factors determining cardiac output.

contributes to effective management of this complex situation (Tables 16-1 and 16-2). The following discussion of assessment of patients with CHF includes both noninvasive and invasive measures.

NONINVASIVE MONITORING

Heart Rate and Blood Pressure

Left ventricular failure is associated with decreased cardiac output. It remains a challenge for clinicians to assess for a decrease in cardiac output without the benefit of invasive hemodynamic monitoring. It is, however, not impossible. *Cardiac output* is defined as the amount of blood pumped by the heart in 1 minute. Normal cardiac output is 4 to 8 L/min. The two components of cardiac output are heart rate and stroke volume. Therefore, an indirect or noninvasive assessment of cardiac output would consist of analyzing these two components. For example, a heart rate that is too fast may indicate a decrease in cardiac output. The heart rate may be increased to make up for a loss of stroke volume in a failing heart.

Assessment of a decrease in stroke volume is also challenging. *Stroke volume* is the amount of blood ejected with each beat. Therefore, stroke volume is one of the three components of systolic blood pressure; the other components are aortic distensibility and left ventricular ejection rate. If there is a drop in systolic blood pressure and you can assume that there has been no change in aortic distensibility or ejection rate, then the drop is most likely due to a decrease in stroke volume. This is particularly true at lower systolic pressures.

TABLE 16-2.   Signs and Symptoms of Congestive Heart Failure and Their Causes

Symptom or Sign	Cause
Fatigue with little exertion or at rest, confusion, headache	Tissue anoxia due to decreased cardiac output
Dyspnea on exertion, later at rest	Cardiac output inadequate to provide for increased oxygen required by exertion (results in increased breathing effort)
Paroxysmal nocturnal dyspnea in left-sided heart failure	When recumbent, edema fluid from the dependent parts returns to the bloodstream, increasing preload and causing decompensation
Cough; sputum may at times be brownish or blood-tinged Adventitious lung sounds (especially crackles)	Pulmonary capillary pressure > 30 mm Hg causes transudation of serum with hemosiderin-filled macrophages into the alveoli, which causes pulmonary congestion and diminished oxygen–carbon dioxide exchange
Tachycardia, various dysrhythmias	Effort to compensate for decreased cardiac output; arrhythmias may be stimulated by hypoxia, digitalis toxicity, hypokalemia, or hypomagnesemia
Presence of third/fourth heart sounds	Associated with rapid ventricular/atrial filling in noncompliant ventricles/atria
Cardiomegaly	Hypertrophy of myocardium helps to maintain stroke volume
Decreased urinary output	Decreased cardiac output and renal blood flow Sodium and water retention caused by excess aldosterone level Increased water retention caused by excess antidiuretic hormone secretion
Nocturia	While resting at night, deficit in cardiac output in relation to oxygen demands is reduced, leading to decreased renal vasoconstriction and increased glomerular filtration rate
Elevated pulmonary capillary wedge pressure or left ventricular end-diastolic pressure	Left ventricle cannot maintain stroke volume in face of increased venous return
Edema (initially in dependent parts, later generalized)	Hydrostatic pressure is greatest in dependent parts of body Progressive cardiac failure causes substantial increase in hydrostatic pressure in all parts of body
Distention of peripheral veins, most noticeable on face, neck, and hands	Elevated venous pressure secondary to cardiac failure
Elevated central venous pressure (> 11 cm H_2O in vena cava)	
Palpable liver, positive hepatojugular reflex	Decreased cardiac output causes damming of venous blood Increase in total blood volume and interstitial fluid volume
Nausea and vomiting	Edema of liver and intestines Impulses arising from the dilated myocardium in acute heart failure Digitalis toxicity
Anorexia	Potassium deficit Digitalis toxicity

Continued

TABLE 16-2. Signs and Symptoms of Congestive Heart Failure and Their Causes—*cont'd*

Symptom or Sign	Cause
Constipation	Poor nourishment and inadequate bulk in diet Lack of activity Depression of motor activity by hypoxia
Orthopnea	Increased interstitial edema decreasing lung compliance and increasing work of breathing; upright position fosters air exchange in upper lungs
Pulmonary edema with severe dyspnea, profound anxiety, coughing of pink frothy fluid, cyanosis, shock, and death	Increased pulmonary venous pressure, which cause serum and blood cells to transudate into the alveoli

PND, paroxysmal nocturnal dyspnea; CVP, central venous pressure.

Therefore, a noninvasive assessment of cardiac output would consist of a close observation for changes in heart rate and systolic blood pressure.

Oxygenation

A decrease in cardiac output leads to symptoms of weakness and fatigue because tissue oxygenation is impaired. Dyspnea is also always present, at first experienced only with exercise. As CHF worsens, dyspnea occurs with progressively less exercise and finally even at rest. Other pulmonary symptoms associated with left ventricular failure include orthopnea, paroxysmal nocturnal dyspnea, dry cough, and fine moist crackles in the lungs. Typically, crackles in the lungs that are induced by cardiac failure are described as dependent on gravity. For example, if the patient is sitting up, the crackles will be heard in the bases of the lungs, but if the patient is lying on the left side, they are heard throughout the left lung. Crackles induced by cardiac failure are due to fluid accumulation in the lungs. Clinicians must be able to distinguish these from pulmonary crackles. Crackles that are pulmonary in origin are due to weak airway walls. Typically, they are heard in all the lung fields. Pulmonary crackles are not dependent on gravity. Patients with left ventricular failure may also demonstrate expiratory wheezing and Cheyne-Stokes respirations. Severe left ventricular failure results in acute pulmonary edema, a potentially life-threatening condition characterized by severe dyspnea and profound anxiety.

Peripheral Edema

Dependent pitting edema (see Fig. 2-3) reflects excessive fluid in the interstitial space and is a major indication in right-sided heart failure. The degree of peripheral edema should be assessed at regular intervals. This can be accomplished by measuring the extremities with a millimeter tape. The patient should be taught to monitor for fluid retention by noting, for example, tight shoes or tight clothing as the day progresses. Right-sided heart failure is associated with jugular vein distention and hepatojugular reflux, which reflect increased venous pressure. The degree of jugular vein distention provides important data regarding fluid volume status and cardiac function; of importance, it can be performed noninvasively (see Fig. 2-1).

Body Weight

Weight gain usually occurs with CHF because of abnormal retention of sodium and water. A simple yet effective method for monitoring fluid volume status is to measure daily body weights.[25] For accuracy, it is best to use the same scale and perform the procedure at the same time each day. Any change in daily weight of more than 0.25 kg (0.5 lb) can be assumed to have resulted from alterations in total body fluid and these measures can be used to monitor therapy with diuretics and other medications. Early in the therapeutic period, a baseline body weight should be obtained to compare with subsequent weight measurements to monitor response to treatment. Daily weight measurements are not only effective in monitoring fluid losses in hospitalized patients, they are also helpful for patients cared for at home. For example, home patients can be taught to chart their weight and to consult a health care provider if a rapid gain or loss of more than 1 kg (2.2 lb) occurs.[26]

Fluid Intake and Output

An important measurement during hospitalization is daily fluid intake and output (I&O). With diuretic administration, urinary output is expected to increase significantly. This increase should parallel the decrease in body weight. Discrepancies in these findings are an indication to check for errors in measurement.

INVASIVE HEMODYNAMIC MONITORING

Hemodynamic monitoring by means of multilumen flow-directed catheters has made it possible to assess pressures directly within the heart chambers and great vessels and to monitor cardiac output. Arterial pressure, central venous pressure (CVP), pulmonary artery pressure (PAP), pulmonary capillary wedge pressure (PCWP), and cardiac output can be measured. The obtained pressure measurements provide information concerning the fluid volume status of both sides of the heart. Several other hemodynamic indices can be derived from these measurements (eg, stroke volume, stroke volume index, and systemic and pulmonary vascular resistance). All these findings are used to monitor the patient's initial status and response to therapy.

In the patient experiencing CHF, CVP is used to monitor the intravascular volume status. The CVP will decrease during periods of hypovolemia (which may occur with overdiuresis) and will increase with hypervolemia, increased venous return, and when right-sided failure worsens.

As indicators of the left ventricle's status in the absence of mitral valve disease, chronic obstructive pulmonary disease, or pulmonary hypertension, PAP and PCWP are more sensitive than is the CVP. The pulmonary artery end-diastolic pressure (PAEDP) and the PCWP reflect the left ventricular end-diastolic pressure (LVEDP). The LVEDP represents the left ventricular filling pressure (preload), which is one of the determinants of stroke volume. An increase in PAEDP or PCWP is the result of the diminished ability of the left ventricle to empty its contents. Symptoms of pulmonary congestion occur when the PAEDP or PCWP exceeds 18 mm Hg. This is the usual situation in pulmonary edema. Cardiac output is another hemodynamic measurement that can be obtained with flow-directed catheters. Decrease in cardiac output can indicate the degree of failure and help determine needed therapy to increase the heart's contractility.

NURSING DIAGNOSES

Clinical Tip: Examples of Nursing Process in Care of Patients With Heart Failure presents three nursing diagnoses that occur at a high frequency in patients experiencing acute or chronic CHF. Also included is information needed for assessment, intervention, and evaluation.

INTERVENTIONS/TREATMENTS

Because the nurse works closely with physicians in the management of fluid balance problems in patients with CHF, the principles of treatment are presented with collaborative actions as a focus.

When possible, therapy is directed at eliminating the disease condition producing CHF (eg, surgical correction of a valvular disorder). When this is not possible, therapy must focus on making the most efficient use of the remaining cardiac function. Unfortunately, most persons with CHF have irreversible cardiac damage. Some evidence, however, suggests that relief of pressure or volume overload (preload and afterload) may lessen or even reverse the decline in contractility; thus, this is an important therapeutic objective.[27] It is now well recognized that a variety of neurohormonal responses, which are initially activated to support the gradually failing heart, may eventually contribute to the progressive nature of the disease and further reduce cardiac function.[28]

DECREASING MYOCARDIAL WORKLOAD

Rest causes a reduction in oxygen need and therefore decreases cardiac workload. It also produces a physiological diuresis. Sometimes rest alone is sufficient to

CLINICAL TIP

Examples of Nursing Process in Care of Patients With Heart Failure

NURSING DIAGNOSIS	ASSESSMENT	INTERVENTIONS	EXPECTED OUTCOMES
Fluid volume excess related to compromised regulatory mechanisms (cardiac failure) *Pathophysiology:* Decreased GFR; kidneys respond by retaining sodium and water (under the influence of aldosterone and ADH)	Weight gain Peripheral edema Intake > output Decreased urinary volume, increased urinary specific gravity Peripheral venous distention Paroxysmal nocturnal dyspnea Increased CVP, PCWP, LVEDP Abnormal breath sounds (crackles) Orthopnea and dyspnea Tachypnea Frothy sputum Hepatomegaly	Assess for fluid volume excess: • Measure I&O; look for I > O • Weigh daily (same scale, same amount of clothing, and same time each day) • Assess lung fields for crackles (compare to baseline) • Monitor changes in vital signs (compare to baseline) Instruct in dietary restrictions (sodium restriction favors diuresis) Restrict fluids as prescribed (may be necessary in patients with severe heart disease to decrease ECF volume) Monitor response to diuretics: • Weight should decline no faster than 1 kg/day (2.2 lb) with diuretic administration • Look for inadequate response to diuretics • Look for excessive response to diuretics (such as weight loss exceeding 2.2 lb/day and BUN elevated out of proportion to serum creatinine) Instruct patient to weigh self daily and report significant weight variations to health care provider Encourage rest periods in which patient lies down (rest, particularly in supine position, favors diuresis) Promote calm environment to decrease sympathetic nervous system stimulation (again, rest favors diuresis) Place in Fowler's position (reduced upward pressure on diaphragm, facilitating ease of breathing) Measures for management of acute pulmonary edema are described in text	Urine output will increase. Weight will decrease to baseline as diuresis occurs. Peripheral edema will lessen. Peripheral venous distention will lessen. Crackles will be absent or diminished. Sputum production will diminish. Dyspnea and tachypnea will diminish. Liver size will diminish. Patient and significant other will verbalize understanding of sodium-restricted diet. Patient will demonstrate ability to weigh self and will verbalize significant variations requiring reporting to health care provider.

CLINICAL TIP

Examples of Nursing Process in Care of Patients With Heart Failure—*cont'd*

NURSING DIAGNOSIS	ASSESSMENT	INTERVENTIONS	EXPECTED OUTCOMES
Activity intolerance related to decreased cardiac reserve *Pathophysiology:* Decreased contractility and increased preload lead to decreased cardiac output and tissue hypoxia	Heart rate increased more than 10% over baseline with activity Heart rate remains increased 2 minutes after exercise Increased LVEDP	Provide bedrest during acute phase of failure (reduces metabolic requirements and thus myocardial workload) Encourage patient to sit in chair when tolerated (pooling of blood in legs decreases venous return and thus preload) Encourage rest 1 hour after meals (since digestion increases metabolic requirements, tolerance to activity is diminished at this time) Monitor response to increases in activity; encourage rest when heart rate increases significantly over baseline and when heart rate remains elevated for longer than 2 minutes after exercise Promote emotional rest (decreases workload of heart by decreasing sympathetic nervous system stimulation) Instruct patient and significant other in prescribed activity regimen Institute measures to maintain normal body temperature, such as avoiding extremes in environmental temperature and prevention of fever (decrease tissue metabolic needs and thus the myocardial workload)	Heart rate will not increase more than 10% above baseline with allowed activity. Heart rate will return to baseline within 2 minutes after allowed activity. Patient or significant other will verbalize understanding of balance between rest and activity.
Impaired gas exchange related to pulmonary congestion *Pathophysiology:* Decreased cardiac output, increased preload, transudation of fluid into alveoli	Dyspnea, orthopnea, PND Crackles (dependent) Cough $PaO_2 < 80$ mm Hg $PaCO_2 > 45$ mm Hg pH < 7.35 ↑ LVEDP ↑ PCWP Alveolar congestion (radiograph)	Elevate head of bed (facilitates ventilation by allowing full chest expansion, draining uppermost alveoli) Tracheal suctioning (removes secretions and thus increases alveolar surface area for gas exchange) Lower feet (decreases venous return and thus preload) Implement medical regimen as appropriate: • Bronchodilators (increases airway diameter) • Oxygen (maintains $PaO_2 > 80$ mm Hg to reduce hypoxia and work of breathing)	Absence or diminishing of dyspnea, crackles $PaO_2 > 80$ mm Hg $PaCO_2 < 45$ mm Hg pH ≥ 7.35 (important to correct acidemia because it predisposes to decreased myocardial contractility) Hemodynamic parameters within normal limits

ADH, antidiuretic hormone; CVP, central venous pressure; BUN, blood urea nitrogen; ECF, extracellular fluid; GFR, glomerular filtration rate; LVEDP, left ventricular end-diastolic pressure; I&O, intake and output; PCWP, pulmonary capillary wedge pressure; PND, paroxysmal nocturnal dyspnea.

alleviate the symptoms of CHF because it diminishes the discrepancy between the heart's ability to pump blood and the oxygenation needs of the tissues. The amount of rest required varies with the person and may range from complete bedrest to only slight restriction of activity.

There is no convincing evidence that prolonged bedrest changes the natural history of CHF.[29] In fact, a gradual exercise program may result in fewer symptoms and a substantial increase in exercise capacity.[30] The patient should be helped to identify an appropriate level of activity that is as nondisruptive to the usual lifestyle as possible. Even somewhat strenuous activities may be tolerated if they are done slowly and are accompanied with frequent rest periods.

Another important nursing responsibility involves monitoring the patient's response to exercise, including changes in pulse and respiratory rate. An increase in heart rate more than 10% over the baseline indicates that an activity may exceed the capacity of the failing heart to respond. Careful reporting of these observations helps to determine the desired amount of activity and aids in the evaluation of the therapeutic regime.

Other interventions to ensure decreased myocardial workload include relief of pain and reduction of fever, if present. Also, patients with CHF often receive oxygen therapy to maintain a partial pressure of oxygen in arterial blood (PaO_2) of at least 80 mm Hg. This reduces hypoxia and the work of breathing. Positioning the patient in a semi-Fowler's position facilitates ventilation by allowing full chest expansion and diaphragmatic excursion. The upright position may also decrease venous return by sequestering blood in the dependent areas.

DECREASING PRELOAD

Venous return is one of the most important determinants of ventricular preload. As preload is increased, so are peripheral edema and pulmonary congestion.

Dietary Sodium/Fluid Restriction

Restriction of dietary sodium is a valuable aid in the management of CHF (see Chap. 3). In general, the fewer sodium ions are in the body, the less water is retained. The degree of sodium restriction necessary to control edema varies with the severity of CHF. Often the dietary sodium intake can be cut in half by not adding salt at the table and in cooking and avoiding foods with a high salt content (see Chap. 3). Limiting sodium intake to less than 2 g daily will facilitate control of symptoms of CHF and minimize diuretic requirements.[31] A stricter diet limited to only 0.5 to 1 g sodium may be required; if so, the patient will need help to achieve the knowledge and motivation necessary to adhere to the recommended diet.

The degree of sodium restriction necessary to control edema also varies with the degree of rest, dosage, and type of diuretic. For example, an ambulatory patient requires more sodium restriction than a patient at bedrest because rest in itself encourages diuresis. A patient receiving potent diuretics has less need for severe sodium restriction than one not receiving diuretics. Indeed, a drastic reduction of sodium intake can be dangerous to the patient receiving a potent diuretic, particularly during bouts of abnormal sodium loss, such as occurs with vomiting or diarrhea.

At times it may be necessary to reduce fluid intake in patients with CHF. Primarily this is done to deal with fluid volume overloaded patients who also have hyponatremia. (See discussion of treatment of hyponatremia earlier in this chapter.)

Diuretics

Diuretics are a valuable aid in the symptomatic treatment of CHF. Their primary purpose is to promote the excretion of sodium and water by the kidneys, thus lowering intravascular volume. Priority nursing responsibilities in the care of patients with CHF include keeping an accurate account of fluid I&O and daily weight measurements. Data obtained from the measurements, in addition to revealing changes in edema accumulation, are invaluable in regulating diuretic dosage and dietary sodium restriction. When diuretics are given to treat an acute exacerbation of CHF, the goal is a net loss of about 0.5 to 1.0 liters of fluid daily.[32]

If hemodynamic monitoring is being used, it may be noted that diuretics produce a decrease in LVEDP (preload) and move the heart's function to a more favorable portion of the Starling curve (Fig. 16-2). This effect decreases pulmonary and systemic congestion and also decreases the degree of backward failure. These effects, in turn, will tend to decrease myocardial need for oxygen. Another advantage of certain diuretics (eg, furosemide) is an increase in venous capacitance with decreased venous return.

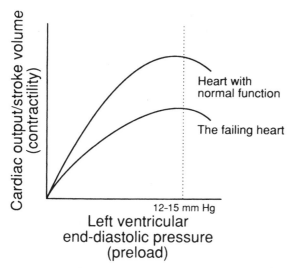

FIGURE 16-2. The Starling mechanism in normal heart function and heart failure.

Because orally administered diuretics (such as furosemide) may be poorly absorbed by the GI tract when right-sided heart failure causes congested abdominal organs, it is sometimes necessary to administer them by the IV route to achieve positive therapeutic results. A recent study in a small group of patients with CHF indicated that oral furosemide solution provided a more potent 24-hour diuretic and natriuretic effect than did an identical dosage in tablet form.[33] The oral form of torsemide, a recently available loop diuretic, may be better absorbed in edematous patients than is orally administered furosemide.[34] Oral and IV doses of torsemide are therapeutically equivalent; therefore, patients may be switched between the two forms with no dosage change.[35] Regardless of the diuretic used, it is important to avoid overdiuresis, which can limit stroke volume and worsen renal function.

Because thiazides (eg, hydrochlorothiazide) and loop diuretics (furosemide, bumetanide, and ethacrynic acid) predispose to hypokalemia, potassium supplementation is often needed. A potassium-sparing diuretic (eg, spironolactone) may also be indicated, particularly because secondary hyperaldosteronism often plays a significant role in advanced CHF. (Recall that spironolactone is an aldosterone-blocking agent.) It should be remembered that ACE inhibitors (such as captopril) cause potassium retention and should not be given simultaneously with potassium-retaining diuretics or with potassium supplements.

Possible side effects of diuretics are disturbances in potassium balance. For example, thiazides and loop diuretics promote renal potassium loss, whereas spironolactone, amiloride, and triamterene promote potassium retention. Acid–base disturbances usually accompany disruptions in potassium balance (metabolic alkalosis with hypokalemia and metabolic acidosis with hyperkalemia). Excessive reduction in the intravascular volume caused by too vigorous diuresis may actually worsen CHF by diminishing the preload stimulus to cardiac contractility. As cardiac output decreases, so do renal blood flow and glomerular filtration rate (GFR), resulting in prerenal azotemia and increased blood urea nitrogen (BUN).

In intractable CHF, the kidney is unable to respond to the usual diuretics. At that point, treatment may consist of a combination of measures involving more severe sodium restriction, more potent diuretics in higher dosage, and fluid restriction to 1,000 mL/day.

Although fluid restriction may be indicated at times, the patient should not be allowed to become volume depleted because volume depletion further impairs cardiac output by decreasing the preload's stimulus on cardiac contractility. It is desirable to use hemodynamic monitoring to guide fluid replacement therapy in seriously ill patients with CHF. Frequent checks of venous pressure and PCWP during fluid administration can give an early warning of circulatory overload or underload and guide the safe administration of needed water and electrolytes. Administration of fluids to patients with CHF requires individualized and cautious attention. Generally, fluid may be given until the LVEDP rises no higher than 15 mm Hg. This level ensures maximum cardiac output while preventing pulmonary edema caused by increased preload. This level is meant to be a guideline for administration of fluids. Individuals with long-standing CHF may have baseline pressures that are much higher than normal due to overstretching of the left ventricle. In these cases the LVEDP may already exceed 15 mm Hg. Therefore, treatment goals should be individualized. Patient at home must understand the precise fluid regimen best suited for their condition and situations that can complicate this regimen (such as increased fluid loss in vomiting and diarrhea).

Monitoring volume, speed, and composition of IV fluids given to patients with CHF is important. Oral fluids should also be monitored carefully in those requiring fluid restriction; the patient's cooperation in this endeavor should be sought. An ongoing assessment of response to fluid intake must occur and alterations made in the treatment plan as indicated.

Vasodilators

Vasodilator drugs are used to inhibit vascular tone in the veins and arteries. Venous vasodilators act on vascular smooth muscle to increase venous pooling. This effect reduces venous return and preload. This would be noted by a decrease in CVP and PCWP and a subsequent improvement in stroke volume. As a result, there is decreased pulmonary congestion and dyspnea. Nitrates are the most common venous vasodilators used to treat CHF. Drugs in this classification include IV nitroglycerin, sustained-release nitroglycerin preparations, topical nitroglycerin ointment and patches, and isosorbide dinitrate. Vasodilators are now considered one of the first-line medications to treat CHF because clinical studies have shown that isosorbide in combination with hydralazine (an arterial vasodilator) can decrease mortality.[36]

Other vasodilators used in the treatment of CHF include ACE inhibitors and hydralazine. These drugs also have an effect on afterload reduction and are discussed later in this chapter. Several vasodilators that are not generally recommended for the treatment of CHF include minoxidil, prazosin, and calcium channel blocking agents.[37]

DECREASING AFTERLOAD

Afterload refers to the pressure against which the ventricle must work to achieve blood flow during systole. In CHF, even in the presence of normal arterial blood pressure, there is a relative worsening of the relationship between contractility and afterload that causes an even greater workload and oxygen need. To reduce the resistance against which the heart must work and to increase cardiac output, arterial vasodilators are one of the first-line medications used in the treatment of CHF.

Hydralazine is one of the most effective arterial vasodilators. It works by reducing systemic vascular resistance (SVR). The drug, by decreasing the SVR, leads to an increase in cardiac output. When used in combination with nitrates, mortality is decreased.

The ACE inhibitors are indirect vasodilators that are also used in treatment of CHF. ACE inhibitors interfere with the conversion of angiotensin I to angiotensin II and thereby decrease the vasoconstrict-

ing action of angiotensin II. Another effect of ACE inhibitors includes a reduction in aldosterone. The overall effect is a decrease in filling pressures and SVR. Drugs in this class include captopril, enalapril, and lisinopril. ACE inhibitors improve cardiac function and decrease mortality.[38] Because aldosterone is inhibited, potassium and magnesium are retained; therefore, supplements of these electrolytes should not be given. Blood pressure must be monitored when therapy is initiated because the patient may experience hypotension due to the effect of the drug. This hypotensive effect is heightened by the concurrent presence of a low intravascular volume (as occurs with too vigorous use of diuretics). An additional consideration before initiating ACE inhibitor therapy is to check serum sodium levels. Patients with serum sodium levels less than 130 mmol/L may be predisposed to an acute drop in blood pressure.[39]

The calcium channel blockers (nifedipine, verapamil, and diltiazem) are not indicated for the routine treatment of systolic heart failure because they demonstrate a negative inotropic effect. These agents may be helpful in the less frequent diastolic failure (eg, dilated cardiomyopathy). These agents inhibit the influx of extracellular calcium during muscular contraction, producing arterial vasodilation and decreased afterload. They may also improve myocardial relaxation during diastole, thus allowing more complete filling when diastolic compliance is impaired.[40]

INCREASING MYOCARDIAL CONTRACTILITY

Administration of positive inotropic agents (medications that increase the strength of cardiac contractility) affects one factor contributing to stroke volume and, therefore, to cardiac output.

Digitalis

The most commonly used inotropic agent is digitalis. This medication increases the force and velocity of myocardial contraction. As the heart contracts more forcefully, tissue perfusion increases and the compensatory responses caused by hypoxia decrease, allowing a corresponding improvement in renal function with diuresis. Digitalis increases the intracellular calcium concentration by inhibiting the sodium-potassium-adenosine triphosphatase (Na-K-ATPase) pump, resulting in increased intracellular sodium, which then exchanges with calcium. The role of digitalis in CHF has been evaluated.[41] It was found that digitalis is effective in treating patients with CHF complicated by atrial fibrillation with a rapid ventricular response. It is now recommended that patients with CHF be treated selectively based on the severity of ventricular dysfunction, symptoms, degree of neuroendocrine activation, and risk of toxicity.[42]

When digitalis preparations are used, be alert for toxic symptoms, such as aversion to food, nausea and vomiting, blurred or distorted vision, confusion, and dysrhythmias. Increased myocardial automaticity may reflect alterations in transmembrane concentrations of sodium, potassium, and calcium. Conduction disturbances can occur secondary to changes in the refractory period.

Remember that symptoms of digitalis toxicity may be induced by hypokalemia, hypomagnesemia, hyponatremia, or hypercalcemia because these imbalances sensitize the heart to digitalis. Hypokalemia occurs frequently in patients with CHF because of the simultaneous administration of potassium-losing diuretics. Often, a potassium supplement (see Chap. 5) or potassium-sparing diuretics will be used to prevent hypokalemia in a digitalized patient. Potassium replacement is often the initial therapy of choice for ectopic rhythms associated with digitalis toxicity. The serum potassium level should be maintained in the high normal range.[43] If potassium administration does not correct the arrhythmia, hypomagnesemia should be suspected.

Other Positive Inotropic Agents

Efforts to find another oral positive inotropic agent have been underway for years. Unfortunately, the digitalis derivatives are the only available oral inotropic agents in the United States at this time.[44]

🔵 DYSRHYTHMIAS IN HEART FAILURE

All types of dysrhythmias can occur in patients with CHF. The relationship between dysrhythmias and CHF is complex. CHF can cause dysrhythmia development. Pathological dysrhythmias can cause CHF, or dysrhythmias may be a consequence of treatment

strategies. At any rate, patients with advanced CHF are prone to dysrhythmias that further alter their hemodynamic status. Alterations in heart rate can cause a decrease in cardiac output and systemic blood pressure. Left untreated, some dysrhythmias are considered life-threatening and may predispose individuals to thromboembolic events or sudden cardiac death.

Dysrhythmias in CHF can be due to the disease process itself. Ischemic heart disease, hypertension, and valvular heart disease all have dysrhythmic complications. Unfortunately, dysrhythmias are poorly tolerated in patients with CHF.

Dysrhythmias can also be due to electrolyte disturbances. Hypokalemia, hyperkalemia, and hypomagnesemia are electrolyte disturbances that may cause dysrhythmias. Hyperkalemia is not a common problem, but it may occur if renal insufficiency is present. Hyperkalemia may also occur secondary to the reduction in aldosterone seen with the use of ACE inhibitors.[45] Hypokalemia and hypomagnesemia are more frequent and are often side effects of diuretic therapy used to treat CHF.

Treatment

Antidysrhythmic therapy in patients with CHF requires an awareness of the effects that the CHF may have on drug metabolism. Patients with renal or hepatic insufficiency secondary to CHF are often at risk for altered metabolism and clearance. Drugs with the potential for negative inotropic effects should be used cautiously or avoided because they can lead to the worsening of CHF.

Atrial fibrillation is one of the most common dysrhythmias seen in patients with CHF. It is particularly dangerous for those who already have some degree of ventricular dysfunction. Management of atrial fibrillation concentrates on the restoration of sinus rhythm and rate control. Restoration of sinus rhythm is difficult in this population because drugs such as quinidine possess negative inotropic properties and, therefore, may not be tolerated. Rate control is best achieved with digoxin. Small, frequent doses of a cardioselective β-blocker, such as metoprolol, may also be appropriate.[46] When pharmacological therapy is ineffective, cardioversion may be considered. Patients with CHF and atrial fibrillation are also at risk for embolic events. Therefore, warfarin is recommended for patients with atrial fibrillation.

Ventricular dysrhythmias are also common in CHF. Treatment of ventricular ectopic beats begins with finding a precipitating cause, such as hypokalemia, intake of caffeinated beverages, or alcohol. Antidysrhythmic agents used to treat ventricular ectopy may include mexiletine or metoprolol.

Ventricular tachycardia seen in patients with CHF is of relatively brief duration, polymorphic, and irregular.[47] Amiodarone is an effective agent used to suppress ventricular dysrhythmias.

Heart block is also common in patients with CHF. This may be due to the disease process itself, the effect of agents used to treat CHF, or electrolyte disturbances. First- and second-degree heart block do not require treatment, other than perhaps an adjustment of therapy. Complete heart block is treated with pacing or isoproterenol. Long-term treatment may involve placement of a permanent pacemaker.

Patients with CHF who are prone to dysrhythmias may also benefit from insertion of an implantable cardioverter defibrillator. The use of these devices for prophylactic therapy in CHF is currently being investigated. Other nonpharmacologic approaches to treatment of dysrhythmias include surgical correction of atrial fibrillation or ventricular tachycardia. Ablation therapy and cardiac transplantation are also alternatives available to some individuals.

Potassium and Magnesium Replacement

There are several recommendations for electrolyte supplementation in patients with CHF. Diuretic-induced hypokalemia is commonly associated with a metabolic alkalosis and a coexisting chloride deficit. Therefore, potassium chloride is the preferred supplementation. The dosage of potassium chloride is individualized, and depends on the use of other medications, such as ACE inhibitors or concomitant diuretics.[48] (See Chap. 5 for specifics on treatment of hypokalemia.)

Hypomagnesemia is most often caused by chronic diuretic therapy, digitalis, or malnutrition in patients with severe chronic CHF. There is a relationship between hypokalemia and hypomagnesemia; magnesium is a cofactor that ensures appropriate function of the Na-K-ATPase pump. Therefore, hypokalemia may persist until the magnesium deficiency is corrected.[49] Another potential problem of magnesium deficiency in patients with CHF is the susceptibility to lethal dysrhythmias and sudden death. Patients with hypomagnesemia have more frequent premature ventricular contractions and episodes of ventricular tachycardia. When patients with hypomagnesemia were compared to patients with normal magnesium levels, patients with a low serum magnesium concentration had a poorer prognosis during follow-up, with 45% and 71% surviving for 1 year, respectively.[50]

In addition to increasing the incidence of dysrhythmias, hypomagnesemia increases peripheral resistance and decreases myocardial oxygenation.[51] Therefore, treatment should be aimed at prevention when applicable. Magnesium supplementation reduces the frequency of asymptomatic ventricular dysrhythmias (possibly due to secondary changes in potassium homeostasis) and produces a minor degree of vasodilation.[52] (See Chap. 7 for specifics on treatment of hypomagnesemia.)

● PULMONARY EDEMA

Cardiogenic pulmonary edema is a result of excessive accumulation of lung water due to left ventricular failure or excessive administration of IV fluid. Pulmonary edema is an emergency situation. To deal with it, the patient should be quickly placed in a high Fowler's position to reduce venous pressure and preload. This position facilitates fluid gravitation to the pleural bases so that less dependent areas of the lung are better ventilated and the work of breathing is decreased. Humidified oxygen is best delivered by a face mask. In extreme cases, endotracheal intubation and mechanical ventilation may be needed. Positive end-expiratory pressure (PEEP) may be used but should be done with caution because an excessive increase in intrathoracic pressure compromises cardiac output.

The IV administration of morphine sulfate may be used to achieve multiple effects:

1. Reducing preload through peripheral venous dilation and thereby decreasing venous return to the heart
2. Reducing afterload by decreasing arterial blood pressure
3. Reducing anxiety (and thereby decreasing sympathetic nervous system stimulation)

Diuretics may be given by IV push to promote a rapid diuresis and thus decrease preload and pulmonary congestion. A vasodilator, such as nitroglyc-

erin, may be given IV or sublingually to decrease preload. However, remember that an excessive drop in
preload may abolish the stimulus for contractility
caused by myocardial stretching. To monitor the
patient's response and allow early detection of complications, measure arterial pressure, cardiac output, and
LVEDP at regular intervals. An inotropic agent, such
as digitalis, may be given IV. Digitalis is most effective if the patient is experiencing a supraventricular
tachycardia.

Patients with acute pulmonary edema may develop
severe acid–base problems (respiratory acidosis and
metabolic [lactic] acidosis). Reversal of the pulmonary
edema is usually effective in restoring acid–base balance by improving gas exchange and allowing metabolism of excess lactate into bicarbonate. Alkali therapy
should be used only for refractory and severe metabolic
acidosis (pH < 7.00–7.10).[53]

CARDIOGENIC SHOCK

Cardiogenic shock develops when the cardiac output is
insufficient to meet the metabolic demands of the body
due to either an absolute decrease in cardiac output or
a severe increase in metabolic demands. Acute myocardial infarction is the most common cause. Cardiogenic
shock is characterized by left ventricular failure, low
cardiac output, arterial hypotension, and peripheral
vasoconstriction. Most often the patient will have a
systolic blood pressure less than 90 mm Hg. When the
mean arterial pressure falls below 75 to 85 mm Hg,
there is danger that coronary blood flow will be inadequate, leading to further damage to the myocardium. A
urinary output of less than 20 mL/hr is also common,
reflecting a decreased GFR. Mental status is impaired
due to cerebral hypoxia. Poor skin perfusion secondary
to peripheral vasoconstriction can cause cold, clammy
skin.

Treatment of cardiogenic shock depends on the
underlying cause. One basic problem that many
patients will encounter is cellular hypoxia related to
decreased cardiac output. Oxygen may be given by a
high-flow system such as a Venturi mask or endotracheal intubation. Atelectasis and retention of carbon
dioxide must be prevented by initiating measures to
mobilize secretions and then suctioning the patient as
often as necessary. The goal of these interventions is to

prevent or minimize acidosis and to maintain a PaO_2
greater than 80 mm Hg. When acidosis is pronounced
(pH < 7.2), myocardial contractility is reduced.
Inotropic agents, such as dopamine, dobutamine, norepinephrine, or amrinone, may be given to strengthen
contractility, maintain adequate blood pressure, and
redistribute blood flow to the vital organs. Arterial
vasodilators, such as nitroprusside, may be given to
decrease afterload in the presence of severe, persistent
vasoconstriction.

Intravenous fluids should be given to correct hypovolemia, if present. However, fluids must be given cautiously to prevent overload and pulmonary congestion.
Maintaining PCWP at 15 mm Hg ensures adequate
left ventricular filling.

An intra-aortic balloon pump may be used in the
presence of severe cardiac injury when recovery is still
possible. In this procedure, a catheter with a balloon
is placed into the aorta. The pump is set so that the
balloon inflates during ventricular diastole and
deflates during systole. This cycle provides better
coronary artery and systemic perfusion with no
increase in peripheral resistance to left ventricular
output.

ELECTROLYTES IN CARDIAC ARREST/RESUSCITATION

Cardiac arrest in patients with CHF may be the result
of pulmonary edema, drug toxicity, electrolyte abnormalities, or dysrhythmias. Pathophysiologic changes in
acid–base metabolism have been a subject of interest in
recent studies.

SODIUM BICARBONATE

Acidosis during cardiac arrest results from inadequate
ventilation and poor oxygen delivery to the tissues.
When cardiac arrest is of short duration, sodium
bicarbonate is generally unnecessary because the provision of cardiopulmonary resuscitation (CPR) limits
the accumulation of carbon dioxide. Use of sodium
bicarbonate after brief arrest apparently does not
improve defibrillation success or increase survival.[54]
Thus, adequate ventilation and perfusion are advocated as the best ways to prevent or treat acidosis
early in cardiac arrest. Sodium bicarbonate is still rec-

ommended as appropriate therapy when CPR is prolonged.[55] When bicarbonate is deemed necessary, 1 mEq/kg is given as an IV bolus; half this dose is given every 10 minutes thereafter as necessary.[56] Possible problems associated with the use of sodium bicarbonate are hyperosmolarity, hypernatremia, or metabolic alkalosis with resultant hypokalemia and hypocalcemia. Also, the oxyhemoglobin curve may be shifted to the left so that there is a decreased release of oxygen to already hypoxic tissues.

POTASSIUM

Extracellular potassium levels are often elevated during CPR. The energy-dependent sodium–potassium pump is impaired by cellular ischemia. This allows potassium to leak out of the cells and extracellular levels to rise. One result of this can be myocardial electromechanical dissociation; when hyperkalemia is the cause, calcium chloride may be useful.[57]

MAGNESIUM

Magnesium infusions can be given to correct selected life-threatening arrhythmias, especially torsade de pointes or dysrhythmias refractive to other agents. It can also be given prophylactically to patients with a myocardial infarction and hypomagnesemia (see Chap. 7). Magnesium ions are involved in keeping intracellular potassium, calcium, and phosphorus levels constant (which may explain the effectiveness of magnesium in reversing dysrhythmias).

CALCIUM

Hypocalcemia during cardiac arrest is due to the movement of calcium from the extracellular to the intracellular compartment. This is a sign of breakdown of basic cellular control mechanisms due to extreme cellular stress.[58] Although calcium is important in myocardial contraction and impulse formation, studies have not demonstrated benefit from calcium administration in cardiac arrest.[59] Calcium is probably helpful when hyperkalemia, hypocalcemia, or calcium channel blocker toxicity is present.[60] Calcium must be used with caution in patients receiving digitalis because it may precipitate digitalis toxicity.[61]

CASE STUDIES

● **16-1.** Mrs. C, a 60-year-old woman with a history of hypertension and myocardial infarction, was admitted to the hospital with complaints of dyspnea and increased pitting edema of the lower extremities. She reported that she had not adhered to her sodium-restricted diet for several weeks and that she had recently increased in weight from her usual 55 to 68 kg. At the time of her last physician visit, her serum sodium level was 135 mEq/L and her serum creatinine was 1.3 mg/dL. Blood work revealed:

Na = 128 mEq/L
K = 4.0 mEq/L
Creatinine = 2.0 mg/dL
BUN = 75 mg/dL

COMMENTARY: Hyponatremia and fluid volume overload were due to the patient's worsening CHF. The high BUN and creatinine levels reflected a reduced GFR secondary to a decreased cardiac output. The symptoms that caused her to seek medical attention were dyspnea and edema, both associated with increasing cardiac failure. No symptoms related to hyponatremia were present. She was treated with furosemide, an ACE inhibitor, and a low-sodium diet. Water intake was restricted until the serum sodium level normalized. Following treatment in the hospital, the serum sodium level returned to the lower limit of normal, the excess body fluid was eliminated, and her renal function returned to the baseline level. Discharge instructions included information about her new medications (furosemide and an ACE-inhibitor) and the need to adhere to her sodium-restricted diet.

● **16-2.** Mr. H has chronic CHF and receives regular visits from a home health nurse. On a recent visit, the nurse notices that he is not quite his usual talkative self. In fact, he has trouble getting up from his chair to open the door and tells the nurse to let herself in. At the previous visit his blood pressure was 118/68 mm Hg and his pulse was 88 beats/min. Currently his blood pressure is 96/64 mm Hg and his pulse is 110 beats/min.

COMMENTARY: A noninvasive assessment of this patient's cardiac output reveals that his systolic blood pressure is low and his heart rate is fast. This alerts you to the possibility that his cardiac output may be low. Remember that cardiac output is comprised of heart rate and stroke volume. Stroke volume is one of the three components of systolic blood pressure. Therefore, any rise in heart rate or any drop in systolic blood pressure alerts you to the possibility that stroke volume has dropped. If stroke volume has dropped, cardiac output will be lower.

● **16-3.** Mr. D is hospitalized in the cardiac surgical intensive care unit. He has a long-standing history of mitral valve disease and has had his mitral valve replaced with a prosthetic valve. His medications include furosemide and digoxin. Electrocardiographic monitoring reveals that he is in atrial fibrillation with a rapid ventricular response.

COMMENTARY: Electrolyte disturbances that may be present include hypokalemia and hypomagnesemia. These would most likely be due to diuretic therapy and the use of digoxin. Checking both of these electrolyte levels would be warranted. Remember that dysrhythmias may be due to valvular heart disease, electrolyte disturbances, or drugs used to treat CHF. Careful consideration of all these factors is warranted in this case.

REFERENCES

1. Dei Cas L, Metra M, Leier C. Electrolyte disturbances in chronic heart failure: metabolic and clinical aspects. *Clin Cardiol* 1995;18:370.
2. Douban S, Brodsky M, Whang D, Whang R. Significance of magnesium in congestive heart failure. *Am Heart J* 1996;132:664.
3. Oster J, Preston R, Materson B. Fluid and electrolyte disorders in congestive heart failure. *Semin Nephrol* 1994;14:485.
4. Elisaf M, Theodorou J, Pappas C, Siampoulos K. Successful treatment of hyponatremia with angiotensin-converting enzyme inhibitors in patients with congestive heart failure. *Clin Pharmacol* 1995;86:477.
5. Leier C, Dei C, Metra M. Clinical relevance and management of the major electrolyte abnormalities in congestive heart failure. *Am Heart J* 1994;128:564.
6. Ibid, p 567.
7. Ibid.
8. Carey C, Lee H, Woeltje K. *The Washington Manual of Medical Therapeutics*, 29th ed. Philadelphia: Lippincott-Raven; 1998:111.
9. Leier et al, p 567.
10. Ibid.
11. Ibid.
12. Elisaf et al, p 477.
13. Dei Cas et al, p 373.
14. Leier et al, p 568.
15. Ibid.
16. Ibid, p 569.
17. Ibid, p 570.
18. Dei Cas et al, p 568.
19. Leier et al, p 569.
20. Douban et al, p 564.
21. Leier et al, p 572.
22. Ibid.
23. Ibid.
24. Ibid, p 571.
25. Kinney M, Dunbar S, Brooks-Brunn J, Molter N, Vitello-Cicciu J. *AACN's Clinical Reference for Critical Care Nursing*, 4th ed. St. Louis: CV Mosby, 1998:438.
26. Trelawny J. Can we improve diuretic response in heart failure? *Br J Hosp Med* 1996;55:616.
27. Parmley W. Pathophysiology and current therapy of congestive heart failure. *J Am Coll Cardiol* 1989;13:771.
28. Barnet D, Pouleur H, Francis G. The changing face of heart failure. In: Barnet D, Pouleur H, Francis G, eds. *Congestive Cardiac Failure: Pathophysiology and Treatment*. New York: Marcel Dekker; 1993:3.
29. Tierney L, McPhee S, Papadakis M. *Current Medical Diagnosis & Treatment*, 38th ed. Stamford, CT: Appleton & Lange; 1999:406.
30. Ibid.
31. Carey et al, p 117.
32. Ibid.
33. Cohen N, Golik A, Dish V et al. Effect of furosemide oral solution versus furosemide tablets on diuresis and electrolytes in patients with moderate congestive heart failure. *Miner Electrolyte Metab* 1996;22:248.
34. Andreoli T, Carpenter C, Bennett J, Plum F. *Cecil Essentials of Medicine*, 4th ed. Philadelphia: WB Saunders; 1997:36.
35. Shannon M, Wilson B, Stang C. *Appleton & Lange's 1999 Drug Guide*. Stamford, CT: Appleton & Lange, 1999:1383.
36. Cohn J et al. A comparison of enalapril with hydralazine-isosorbide dinitrate in the treatment of heart failure. *N Engl J Med* 1991;325:302.
37. Kayser S. Management of chronic congestive heart failure, part II—selection of treatment. *Prog Cardiovasc Nurs* 1994;9:33.
38. The SOLVD Investigators. Effect of enalapril on survival in patients with reduced left ventricular ejection fractions and congestive heart failure. *N Engl J Med* 1991;325:293.
39. Kayser, p 35.

40. Shub C. Heart failure and abnormal ventricular function: Pathophysiology and clinical correlation (part 2). *Chest* 1989;96:906.

41. Uretsky B et al. Randomized study assessing the effect of digoxin withdrawal in patients with mild to moderate chronic congestive heart failure: Results of the PROVED trial. *J Am Coll Cardiol* 1993;22:955.

42. Weintraub N, Chaitman B. Newer concepts in the medical management of patients with congestive heart failure. *Clin Cardiol* 1993;16:380.

43. Carey et al, p 116.

44. Tierney et al, p 410.

45. Kayser, p 36.

46. Campbell R. Sudden death and arrhythmias. In: Barnet D, Pouleur H, Francis G, eds. *Congestive Cardiac Failure: Pathophysiology and Treatment.* New York: Marcel Dekker; 1993:343.

47. Ibid, p 356.

48. Kayser, p 36.

49. Ibid.

50. Gottlieb S, Baruch L, Kukin ML et al. Prognostic importance of the serum magnesium concentration in patients with congestive heart failure. *J Am Coll Cardiol* 1990;16:827.

51. Hix C. Magnesium in congestive heart failure, acute myocardial infarction and dysrhythmias. *J Cardiovasc Nurs* 1993;8:22.

52. Bashir Y, Sneddon J, Stauton A et al. Effects of long-term oral magnesium chloride replacement in congestive heart failure secondary to coronary artery disease. *Am J Cardiol* 1993;72:1156.

53. Rose B. *Clinical Physiology of Acid-Base and Electrolyte Disorders*, 4th ed. New York: McGraw-Hill; 1994:472.

54. Cummins R, ed. *Advanced Cardiac Life Support.* Dallas, TX: American Heart Association, 1997:7-14.

55. Geheb M, Krus J, Haupt M, Desai T, Carlson R. Fluid and electrolyte abnormalities in critically ill patients. In: Naris R, ed, *Maxwell and Kleeman's Clinical Disorders of Fluid and Electrolyte Metabolism*, 5th ed. New York: McGraw-Hill; 1994:1479.

56. Cummins, p 7-15.

57. Martin G et al. Hyperkalemia during human cardiopulmonary resuscitation: incidence and ramifications *J Emerg Med* 1989;7:109.

58. Geheb et al, p 148.

59. Cummins, p 7-17.

60. Ibid.

61. Ibid.

Renal Failure

Among their numerous cardinal functions, the kidneys excrete water, electrolytes, and organic materials after conserving whatever amounts of these substances the body requires. They act both autonomously and in response to blood-borne messengers, such as the mineralocorticoids and antidiuretic hormone. They excrete the breakdown products of protein metabolism, drugs, and toxins; produce the hormone erythropoietin (which is essential for red blood cell production); and convert an unusable form of vitamin D to one that the body can use. Failure of renal function causes a variety of water and electrolyte disturbances and other metabolic derangements (Fig. 17-1). Topics to be considered in this chapter include fluid and electrolyte disorders associated with acute and chronic renal failure.

Renal failure is classified as either acute or chronic. *Acute renal failure* (ARF) refers to a sudden (hours or days) steep decrease in kidney function. *Chronic renal failure* (CRF) refers to a gradual, progressive decrease over months or years, allowing time for the development of partial adaptation to the condition. To some degree, both types of renal failure are characterized by the accumulation of nitrogenous waste products (urea and creatinine) and the inability to regulate fluid and electrolyte homeostasis. The glomerular filtration rate (GFR) must usually decline by 50% or more before clinically significant increases in the serum creatinine and blood urea nitrogen (BUN) concentrations are observed.[1] Because the clinical presentation and management of ARF and CRF are somewhat different, it is helpful to consider them separately.

ACUTE RENAL FAILURE

Acute renal failure is often classified according to its anatomical site of involvement, such as prerenal, intrarenal, or postrenal.

- *Prerenal* refers to hypoperfusion of the kidney that results in azotemia without actual renal parenchymal damage.
- *Intrarenal* refers to actual parenchymal damage and may be subdivided into primary vascular, glomerular, interstitial, and tubular.[2]
- *Postrenal* refers to an obstruction in urine formation distal to the tubular site of urine formation.

Acute renal failure has many diverse causes (Table 17-1); however, by far the most common is acute tubular necrosis. This condition usually complicates a systemic insult such as shock, trauma (particularly involving skeletal muscle), sepsis, or exposure to nephrotoxic agents. Conditions associated with renal hypoperfusion at first result in decreased urine output and prerenal azotemia; if left untreated, acute tubular necrosis can develop. For this reason, it is important to make an early differentiation between prerenal azotemia and acute tubular necrosis (Table 17-2). Other times, ARF may be due to an obstruction in the urinary tract distal to the site of urine formation (such as in the ureter or bladder neck); this too is correctable if detected and treated early.

Acute renal failure may also be classified as either reversible or irreversible. In *irreversible renal failure*,

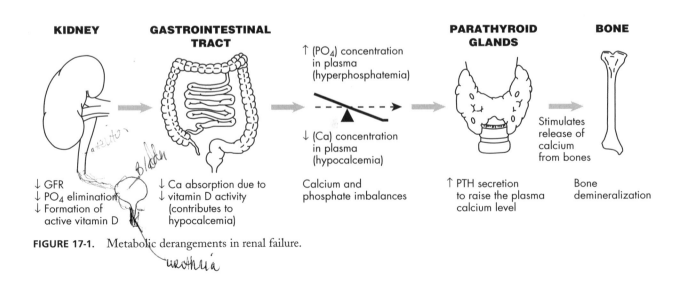

FIGURE 17-1.   Metabolic derangements in renal failure.

🔵 **TABLE 17-1.**   Causes of Acute Renal Failure

Acute tubular necrosis
  Ischemia
  • Prolonged hypovolemia (as in hemorrhage, profound vomiting and diarrhea, diuretic abuse, burns, or osmotic diuresis associated with diabetes)
  • Sepsis
  Nephrotoxic drugs
  • Aminoglycosides (eg, tobramycin, gentamicin, amikacin)
  • Amphotericin B
  • Radiocontrast agents — *Rotten Eggs .*
  • Cisplatin
  • Nonsteroidal anti-inflammatory drugs   *Nsaids*
  Endogenous nephrotoxins
  • Myoglobin (rhabdomyolysis: trauma, muscle disease, seizures, severe exercise)
  • Hemoglobin (as in intravascular hemolysis, transfusin reactions, toxic hemolysis)
  Heavy metals
  • Mercury
  • Arsenic
  Organic solvents
  • Carbon tetrachloride
  • Toluene
  Glycols
  • Ethylene glycol *- ETOH*
  • Oxalic acid
Interstitial nephritis (acute pyelonephritis, allergic nephritis, hypercalcemia, uric acid nephropathy, myeloma of the kidney)
Glomerulonephritis (acute poststreptococcal, systemic lupus erythematosus, Goodpasture's syndrome, bacterial endocarditis)
Renal vascular disease (as in periarteritis or hypersensitivity angiitis)
Urinary tract obstruction (as in ureteral calculi or accidental ligation, bladder neoplasms, or urethral stricture due to prostatic hypertrophy)   *C Section*

---

kidney function does not return and uremia progresses, requiring that the patient undergo lifetime dialysis or receive a kidney transplant. *Reversible renal failure* can be divided into two phases—oliguria and diuresis. The oliguric (maintenance) phase usually lasts 1 to 2 weeks and is followed by the diuresis (recovery) phase after which normal renal function often returns. However, the oliguric phase may be absent or permanent or may last 2 to 6 weeks or longer.

Acute renal failure may occur in the presence of diminished, normal, or even high urine output. Although one most often thinks of oliguria as being present, reports suggest that about 20% to 60% of all cases of ARF may be of the nonoliguric type.[3] Total anuria is defined as zero urine output, anuria as less

Anuria
than 50 to 100 mL/day, oliguria as less than 400 mL/day, nonoliguria as 400 to 1,000 mL/day, and polyuria as greater than 1 to 2 L/day.[4] More important than the volume of urine is the ability of the kidney to excrete solutes. A convenient indicator of ARF is an abrupt twofold increase in the plasma creatinine concentration.[5] Anuria is generally thought to be a poor prognostic indicator and is more likely to require renal replacement therapy. In contrast, nonoliguric ARF (such as caused by nephrotoxic injury from aminoglycosides) represents a less severe injury and usually results in fewer complications and quicker recovery.[6]

Five percent of hospital admissions and 30% of intensive care unit admissions will have ARF; 2% to 5% of hospitalized patients will develop this condi-

TABLE 17-2. Differentiation Between Prerenal Azotemia and Acute Tubular Necrosis

Laboratory Finding	Prerenal Azotemia	Acute Tubular Necrosis
BUN/Cr ratio	> 20:1	10:1
Urine Na (mEq/L)	< 20	> 40
Urine osmolality (mOsm/kg)	> 500	< 350
Urine/plasma osmolality	> 1.5	< 1.1
Urine/plasma creatinine	> 40	< 20

tion.[7] ARF is particularly likely to occur after cardiac surgery.[8] Mortality in patients with ARF depends on the cause of the condition; it is generally higher in surgical and post-traumatic patients than in medical patients. Various studies have reported mortality rates from as low as 8% to as high as 75%.[9,10] Most deaths occur in the first week following the onset of ARF and are primarily related to the underlying cause of failure.

Fluid, electrolyte, acid–base, and other derangements commonly encountered in the patient with ARF are summarized below.

FLUID VOLUME OVERLOAD

It is common for acutely ill patients with diminishing urine output to undergo vigorous intravenous (IV) fluid replacement (usually with a saline solution) to attempt to prevent ARF and rule out prerenal causes for oliguria. If oliguric renal failure ensues despite this action, the patient invariably becomes fluid overloaded. Loop diuretics are sometimes administered to patients with fluid overload in an attempt to convert oliguric failure to polyuric failure; however, a substantial proportion of patients do not respond. In these cases, renal replacement therapy is usually necessary. Untreated fluid overload can ultimately lead to pulmonary edema with infiltrates; if severe enough to cause hypoxemia, the patient may require mechanical ventilation (an ominous sign).[11]

Fluid Replacement

Because fluid balance is precarious in patients with ARF, meticulous attention must be paid to maintaining salt and water intake. To plan appropriate fluid replacement therapy, a reliable assessment of all fluid losses and gains must be maintained. This can be done by keeping accurate intake and output records and weighing the patient daily.

Oliguric Phase

The amount of fluid administered during this phase must be carefully planned while considering the body as a closed system. In patients with oliguric renal failure, fluid replacement must allow for insensible losses from the skin and lungs, the small amount of urine excreted by the kidneys, and fluid losses such as vomitus, gastric suction, diarrhea, or wound drainage. Insensible losses can be estimated as about 0.5 mL/kg body weight per hour (the usual loss in a normal, resting, afebrile adult).[12] For example, a 70-kg person would normally lose about 850 mL of insensible fluid over the course of a day; fever increases the insensible loss by about 13% for each degree of Celsius temperature elevation. Also considered by the physician when planning fluid replacement therapy is the amount of water that results from the endogenous oxidation of proteins, fats, and carbohydrates. This amount of water production (about 500 mL in a typical adult) partially offsets insensible water losses.[13] Therefore, replacement of insensible fluid loss requires about 400 mL/day in an average 70-kg man[14]; the amount of urine produced as well as the amount of other fluid losses (such as diarrhea) are then added to this amount and given to the patient. Accurate daily weights provide a check of the patient's overall fluid balance status and give an indication of the adequacy of fluid therapy; during the oliguric phase of ARF, the patient should lose 0.2 to 0.5 kg body weight per day.[15] To help safeguard against fluid overload, it is important to eliminate all unnecessary infusions (such as "keep vein open" fluids) and to administer IV medications in the smallest possible volume of fluid. To provide nutritional support to the critically ill patient with ARF, it is not unusual to administer 1.5 to 2 liters of total parenteral nutrition (TPN) formulations per day; this may necessitate the use of continuous hemofiltration to prevent fluid overload.[16]

Diuretic Phase

During the diuretic phase of ARF, the kidneys usually excrete a hypotonic urine containing about 50 mEq sodium chloride per liter.[17] The actual amount of urine excreted is largely determined by how well fluid balance was maintained during the oliguric phase; the urine volume is expected to be greater in patients who gained an excess of salt and water than in those who did not. Despite large losses of urine during the diuretic phase, a daily fluid intake in excess of 3,500 mL should seldom be allowed to replace these losses. To achieve appropriate fluid and electrolyte replacement during this phase, it is necessary to carefully measure the urine output and at times to analyze its electrolyte content. Although a weight loss of several pounds is generally expected during this phase, it is not unusual to see a gradual improvement in renal function without a large diuresis in a patient who was well maintained during the oliguric phase.

HYPONATREMIA

Hyponatremia is a relatively common imbalance because patients with renal failure typically receive an excess of free water (as in dextrose solutions) IV and orally as part of their nutritional support; the situation is aggravated because the impaired kidneys are unable to excrete free water normally. To help prevent hyponatremia, it is wise to limit water intake to less than 500 mL/day in oliguric euvolemic patients who are not undergoing ultrafiltration.[18] The usual treatment for hyponatremia in patients with ARF is fluid restriction rather than sodium replacement; however, at times, sodium replacement is indicated. When symptomatic hyponatremia is present, the condition may be corrected by dialysis or by the cautious administration of hypertonic sodium chloride (3% or 5%); dialysis is usually the treatment of choice. A danger of rapidly developing hyponatremia is cerebral edema, which can lead to serious neurological sequelae.[19]

HYPERNATREMIA

In patients with ARF, the ability to retain needed water is impaired; therefore, the possibility for hyper-natremia exists if relatively more sodium than water is administered. Fortunately, this imbalance is uncommon; when it is seen, it is often because excessive amounts of hypertonic sodium bicarbonate or antibiotics rich in sodium (such as carbenicillin) have been administered or excessive sodium has been administered in TPN formulations.[20]

Hypernatremia occurs most often in the diuretic phase of ARF when urine output tends to be excessive and relatively more water than sodium is excreted. Probably the best way to prevent hypernatremia is to measure the volume and electrolyte content of the urine and to replace the losses with oral or IV fluids of similar tonicity. If urinary electrolyte content cannot be measured, it has been suggested that the urine volume be replaced with 0.45% saline (milliliter for milliliter).[21]

HYPERKALEMIA

Hyperkalemia is a major cause of death during the oliguric phase of ARF. Because elimination of potassium occurs almost exclusively through the kidneys, it is not surprising that hyperkalemia is a common imbalance in oliguric patients; however, it does not generally occur unless renal failure is severe (GFR < 10 mL/min).

Although an increase in the serum potassium concentration is primarily due to the inability of the injured kidneys to excrete potassium, another cause is a release of cellular potassium into the bloodstream as a result of hypercatabolism. The cells contain large concentrations of potassium (close to 150 mEq/L) as opposed to relatively low (only about 4 mEq/L) in the bloodstream. Another way to conceptualize this is to consider that about 75% of all the body's potassium is contained in the muscles while only about 2% is contained in the extracellular fluid (ECF; bloodstream and interstitial fluid).[22] Therefore, endogenous release of potassium into the vascular space during even normal tissue breakdown (catabolism) is an important consideration. For example, the serum potassium concentration in a "normally" catabolic patient rises about 0.5 mEq/L/day as a result of protein breakdown; in contrast, the serum potassium concentration may increase as much as 1 to 2 mEq/L within a few hours when the patient is extremely catabolic.[23] Metabolic acidosis aggravates hyperkalemia by driving potassium out of the cells into the ECF.

Because of the danger of hyperkalemia during the oliguric phase of ARF, it is important to minimize the endogenous production of potassium by treating infections, debriding necrotic tissue, draining accumulations of blood, and providing nonprotein calories in the form of glucose and fat. It is also important to avoid administering exogenous potassium in the form of medications (such as potassium penicillin) and in potassium-containing enteral and parenteral products.

Although clinical signs of hyperkalemia include paresthesias, muscle weakness, and paralysis,[24] cardiac abnormalities predominate and are the most life-threatening problems. The untoward effects of hyperkalemia on the heart are made worse by the presence of hyponatremia, hypocalcemia, and acidosis. For example, a serum potassium concentration of 8.5 mEq/L when the serum sodium concentration is 140 mEq/L may be less detrimental than when the serum potassium concentration is 7 mEq/L and the serum sodium concentration is 120 mEq/L.[25] When death occurs from hyperkalemia, it is usually from ventricular fibrillation. Electrocardiographic (ECG) changes associated with hyperkalemia follow definite patterns that are most apparent in the precordial leads. Not only is the extent of the hyperkalemia important, so is its rate of its development; death from hyperkalemia is less likely in patients with CRF because of adaptive changes that occur over time in these individuals. Because nonoliguric ARF is associated with less renal damage than is oliguric renal failure, it tends to pose a lesser problem in regard to the development of hyperkalemia.

If severe hyperkalemia develops, potassium redistribution or removal, or both, must be achieved; methods to accomplish this are described below and summarized in Table 17-3.

Emergent Management

The serum potassium concentration should be measured frequently (such as twice daily) in patients with ARF; when it is 6 mEq/L or greater, frequent ECGs should also be obtained, especially if the concentration is rising.[33] Concomitant factors such as hyponatremia, hypocalcemia, and acidosis make the cardiac effects of hyperkalemia more severe. The ECG is especially helpful because it represents a summation of the influences of potassium as well as various other extracellular electrolytes on cardiac function. The presence of life-threatening cardiac abnormalities is an indication to institute emergency measures to protect the heart and lower the serum concentration.

Calcium

The IV administration of calcium does not change the serum potassium concentration but it does rapidly antagonize the effect of potassium on the myocardium. If needed, 5 to 10 mL of a 10% calcium chloride solution can be given IV by syringe at a rate of 2 mL/min (during continuous ECG monitoring).[34]

Insulin and Glucose

The administration of hypertonic dextrose and regular insulin (usually in a ratio of 1 unit insulin to 5 g dextrose) promotes the temporary transfer of extracellular potassium into the cells. This requires 30 to 60 minutes to achieve but usually lasts for several hours. Once started, dextrose–insulin therapy should not be stopped until the total body potassium has been reduced by other means (this is because of the danger of a rapid shift of potassium back from the cells into the ECF and return of the dangerous levels of hyperkalemia).

Sodium Bicarbonate

Correction of acidosis by the administration of sodium bicarbonate promotes a shift of potassium into the cells while at the same time providing sodium to antagonize the cardiac effects of potassium. These effects are short-lived (1–2 hours) and thus must be backed up with methods (such as dialysis or cation exchange resins) to lower actual body potassium levels.

Albuterol

Albuterol, a β_2-adrenergic agent, causes an acute decrease in plasma potassium and thus is sometimes used to treat hyperkalemia. It acts by stimulating the pancreas beta receptors to release insulin with a resultant temporary shift of potassium into the cells.[35] It may be administered by inhalation or IV. A group of hemodialysis patients who received a 10-minute nebulizer treatment using 10 mg albuterol had a 0.6 mEq/L decrease in the plasma potassium concentration; a greater decrease (1.0 mEq/L) was observed in patients who received a 20-mg dose.[36]

The above emergency measures allow time for instituting measures designed to remove potassium from the body, either by the administration of cation exchange resins or the use of dialysis.

TABLE 17-3.   Measures to Treat Hyperkalemia

Approach	Method	Benefits/Potential Complications
Lower total body potassium concentration	Decrease dietary potassium intake according to level of renal function (usually < 40 mEq/day during oliguric phase of ARF)[26]	Contributes to decreased plasma potassium concentration.
	Increase fecal excretion of potassium by administering sodium polystyrene sulfonate (Kayexate) 30–60 g in divided doses (orally or by retention enema)	Reduces serum potassium concentration by about 1 mEq/L in 24 hours in normally catabolic patient with ARF;[27] because the resin adds sodium to the body, there is potential for fluid volume overload.
	Increase renal excretion of potassium by the administration of a loop diuretic (such as furosemide, 40–160 mg IV or orally)[28] Hemodialysis Peritoneal dialysis	Amount of potassium removed depends on level of remaining renal function; potential for hypovolemia and hypotension if diuresis is excessive.
Shift potassium into cells temporarily when life-threatening hyperkalemia is present	Administer 5–10 units regular insulin with 25 g glucose IV; can be repeated every 15 minutes as needed[29]	Onset of action is 15–60 minutes; effect lasts about 4–6 hours;[30] potential for hypoglycemia.
	Administer $NaHCO_3$ (44–88 mEq) IV	Reduces severity of acidosis and also provides sodium to antagonize effect of hyperkalemia on the heart; onset of action is 15–30 minutes; effects last about 1–2 hours; possibility for fluid overload due to sodium infusion—also possibility that symptoms of hypocalcemia will be exacerbated if acidosis is overcorrected.
	Administer nebulized albuterol (10–20 mg in 4 mL normal saline, inhaled over 10 minutes)[31]	Onset of action is 15–30 minutes; effect lasts about 2–4 hours; may cause tachycardia.
Antagonize cardiac conduction abnormalities associated with life-threatening hyperkalemia	Administer 10 mL of 10% calcium gluconate IV (2–3 mL/min)	Onset of action is 1–5 minutes; effect lasts about 30 minutes;[32] may exacerbate digitalis toxicity.

Cation Exchange Resins

The cation exchange resin sodium polystyrene sulfonate (Kayexalate) is effective in removing potassium when given orally or by retention enema. Oral therapy may be started with 40 g Kayexalate plus 20 mL of (70%) sorbitol.[37] Each gram of the resin adds about 1 to 2 mEq sodium while withdrawing 1 mEq potassium. (The addition of sodium ions can pose a problem for patients with diminished cardiac reserve.) Treatment with oral Kayexalate can be repeated every 2 to 4 hours as required until the serum potassium concentration is brought into a normal range. Enema therapy requires 50 to 100 g Kayexalate in 200 mL water; the solution is given rectally and should be retained for 30 to 45 minutes; the enema can be repeated every 1 to 4 hours as needed.[38]

Dialysis

Hemodialysis is the treatment of choice for reducing the serum potassium concentration quickly, but it has the attendant risks of rapid electrolyte shifts and complications associated with obtaining venous access. Because conventional intermittent hemodialysis is not well tolerated by hemodynamically unstable patients with ARF, a variety of alternative therapies may be considered. For example, peritoneal dialysis fulfills the requirement for slow continuous fluid removal with simultaneous dialysis (provided the patient has not undergone recent abdominal surgery). When peritoneal dialysis is not feasible, one of the slow continuous ultrafiltration methods may be used, such as continuous venovenous hemofiltration (CVVH), continuous venovenous hemodialysis (CVVHD), continuous arteriovenous hemofiltration (CAVH), and continuous arteriovenous hemodialysis (CAVHD). Slow continuous therapies allow large volume and solute removal with minimal effect on blood pressure, heart rate, and cardiac output.

HYPOKALEMIA

Hypokalemia is a rare imbalance in patients with ARF. One possible cause is sustained physical exertion in a hot climate; individuals with this type of renal failure often have suffered excessive sweating with resultant hypovolemia and a marked, cumulative negative potassium balance. They are prone to develop rhabdomyolysis (breakdown of striated muscle) and ultimately hyperkalemia. In a hospital setting, the most common causes of hypokalemic ARF are aminoglycoside nephrotoxicity and overzealous use of diuretics.[39]

HYPERPHOSPHATEMIA

Renal phosphate retention is inevitable when the GFR is abruptly reduced to less than 25% of normal. In general, the serum phosphate level rises from 5 to 8 mg/dL during the oliguric phase of ARF; however, it may occasionally be as high as 15 to 18 mg/dL (especially in tumor-lysis syndromes).[40] Serum phosphate levels elevate early in the course of ARF and parallel inversely the development of hypocalcemia.

Although patients in CRF with hyperphosphatemia are often treated with phosphate-binding antacids, those with ARF usually are not. This is because patients with ARF are usually confined to bed and are more prone to constipation or obstipation; the negative effects of severe constipation (such as anorexia and hyperkalemia) outweigh the risk of transient mild to moderate hyperphosphatemia. However, when the serum phosphorus concentration is greater than 8 mg/dL, it may be necessary to administer a phosphate-binding agent.

HYPOCALCEMIA

Hypocalcemia is invariably present during the oliguric phase of ARF. A decrease in the total serum calcium occurs within the first 2 to 4 days and may reach concentrations as low as 7.5 to 5 mg/dL. Symptoms associated with the hypocalcemia are infrequent because there is a concomitant metabolic acidosis. (Recall that acidosis increases the concentration of the ionized fraction of calcium; because it is the ionized portion of total calcium that regulates neuromuscular function, symptoms of the low total calcium are uncommon.) Probably the most significant feature of hypocalcemia is its potential to worsen the adverse cardiac effects of hyperkalemia.

Although the cause of hypocalcemia is not fully understood, it is related to the inability of the kidneys to excrete phosphate normally. Because the serum calcium concentration is usually inversely proportional to the serum phosphate concentration, hyperphosphatemia promotes hypocalcemia. Another cause of hypocalcemia is a deficiency in the amount of active vitamin D available to promote intestinal absorption of dietary calcium. (Recall that the kidneys are the site of conversion of 25-hydroxyvitamin D to its active form, 1,25-dihydroxyvitamin D_3; with decreased functional renal cells, the amount of active vitamin D formed is diminished.) Still another reason for hypocalcemia is the resistance of bone to the attempts of parathyroid hormone (PTH) to stimulate calcium release from bone stores.

HYPERMAGNESEMIA

Because the kidneys are the major site of magnesium excretion, it is understandable why there is a tendency toward hypermagnesemia when the GFR is reduced. Usually the level of hypermagnesemia in patients with ARF is mild to moderate; however, a profound elevation may occur if the patient is erroneously given magnesium-containing antacids or laxatives. When this occurs, magnesium intoxication is possible and is characterized by central nervous system depression, muscular weakness, and, when extreme (8–10 mEq/L), circulatory collapse.[41] Management of magnesium intoxication includes the administration of calcium gluconate to antagonize the effects of magnesium as well as dialysis against a magnesium-free dialysate to reduce the serum magnesium concentration. Magnesium levels usually return to normal during recovery from acute renal failure.

METABOLIC ACIDOSIS

Because the kidneys are the primary route for the elimination of acids normally generated from the body each day, it is not surprising that patients with ARF develop metabolic acidosis. Of course, failure to excrete acids leads to an accumulation of hydrogen ions and acidosis. The acidosis is made worse by the presence of trauma or sepsis because the acid load generated by these conditions is far above normal. The damaged kidneys are unable to excrete the acids, which then must be buffered by bicarbonate (milliequivalent for milliequivalent); thus, the serum bicarbonate concentration falls below normal. The degree of acidosis that develops in the patient with ARF depends on the cause of the failure, the rate of endogenous acid production, and the rate of recovery of residual renal function. In general, the rate of development of metabolic acidosis is greater in patients with oliguric failure than in those with nonoliguric failure.

Patients with ARF typically have a high anion gap (AG) metabolic acidosis due to the retention of strong acids and accompanying anions not routinely measured by the laboratory; these include sulfate, phosphate, and a variety of organic acids. The increased AG associated with the metabolic acidosis of ARF is almost invariably less than 30 mEq/L unless there are superimposed causes of acidosis (such as lactic acidosis).[42] In the absence of hypercatabolic states, the high AG metabolic acidosis of ARF is usually relatively mild and is not progressive. The general rule is a serum bicarbonate concentration of 12 to 18 mEq/L and an arterial pH of 7.25 to 7.30.[43] Mild metabolic acidosis (bicarbonate ≥ 16 mEq/L) generally does not require therapy. A moderate level of acidosis may be corrected with sodium bicarbonate, 650 to 1,300 mg orally three times a day.[44] However, when the serum pH is less than 7.2, parenteral sodium bicarbonate therapy and dialysis against an alkaline bath are indicated.[45] When parenteral sodium bicarbonate is administered, care must be taken to avoid fluid volume overload and too rapid correction of the acidosis (which decreases the ionized calcium level and predisposes to tetany). (Recall that the patient in renal failure is already hypocalcemic; however, symptoms are not common because metabolic acidosis is also present and favors increased calcium ionization). Severely catabolic patients (such as those with sepsis, shock, or major trauma) are prone to develop severe acid accumulation, which in turn causes a rapid fall in the serum bicarbonate and pH to dangerous levels. Systemic acidosis with a pH less than 7.1 to 7.2 has a number of adverse consequences, including depressed myocardial contractility, susceptibility to cardiac dysrhythmias, and hyperkalemia resulting from a shift of cellular potassium into the bloodstream.

ANEMIA

Anemia may develop within 48 hours after the onset of ARF. The red blood cells are normal in color (normochromic) and shape (normocytic) but are decreased in number. The hematocrit usually stabilizes at a level of 20% to 25%. The inadequate production of a renal enzyme that stimulates release of erythropoietin is the probable cause of anemia. (Recall that erythropoietin normally stimulates the bone marrow to produce red blood cells; thus, a deficit of this substance results in anemia.) Other factors that may contribute to the occurrence of anemia include high plasma levels of urea, potassium, and hydrogen ions. The life span of red blood cells is decreased when uremia is present, further contributing to the development of anemia. Mild bleeding, such as bruising or bleeding of gums, may occur early. Severe bleeding may occur into the gastrointestinal tract, lungs, or brain. The cause of the bleeding tendency in uremic patients is thought to be related to platelet defects resulting in impaired conversion of prothrombin to thrombin. A decrease in platelet adhesiveness leads to an increased bleeding time. If blood transfusion should become necessary, blood less than 10 days old or washed cells will be less likely to contribute to hyperkalemia.

INCREASED SUSCEPTIBILITY TO INFECTION

Patients with ARF or CRF are highly susceptible to infection; in fact, infections complicate the course of ARF in 50% to 90% of patients and are responsible for 30% to 70% of the deaths in these individuals.[46,47] Simple measures to prevent pneumonia (such as incentive spirometry) and urinary tract infection (such as the removal of indwelling urinary catheters as soon as feasible) plus the scrupulous care of wounds and IV devices are important to prevent hospital-acquired infections.[48]

CHRONIC RENAL FAILURE

The most frequent causes of CRF include diabetes mellitus (about 30% of the cases) and hypertension (about 25% of the cases).[49] In contrast to ARF, which is often reversible, CRF almost invariably leads to a progressive decline in renal function. If it occurs slowly, the loss of as much as 75% of renal function is ordinarily not associated with serious changes in fluid, electrolyte, or acid–base balance. Even when renal function is reduced to 10% to 25% of normal, compensatory mechanisms are able to maintain a relative degree of balance. Partly this is because as the renal tubular mass decreases in patients with CRF, an increase in the functional capacity of the remaining nephrons (a process referred to as magnification) occurs. When the degree of renal impairment reaches 90%, however, a series of prominent fluid, electrolyte, and acid–base abnormalities occur.[50]

The fluid and electrolyte disturbances observed in patients with ARF are similar to those found in patients with CRF. A major difference is the frequent development of renal osteodystrophy in patients with advanced CRF.[51]

FLUID VOLUME EXCESS

As the GFR decreases in patients with CRF, the kidneys lose their ability to adjust sodium excretion in response to dietary sodium intake and changes in the ECF volume. As a result, fluid retention is common and is manifested by peripheral edema, pulmonary edema, and hypertension. A moderate limitation in sodium intake (ie, 80–100 mEq daily) may be needed.[52] In contrast, euvolemic, normotensive patients need not limit salt intake. Diuretics are sometimes used to produce natruresis; when the GFR is less than 20 mL/min, thiazide diuretics are ineffective and the more potent loop diuretics are needed. The use of potassium-sparing diuretics is strongly discouraged in moderate to severe CRF because of the danger of life-threatening hyperkalemia.

When fluid volume excess and other imbalances become too severe to manage by medical therapies, dialysis becomes necessary. During dialysis therapies, fluid removal is usually achieved by ultrafiltration to achieve a clinically derived value for "dry weight." In most dialysis centers, dry weight usually reflects the lowest weight a patient can tolerate without intradialytic symptoms and hypotension in the absence of overt fluid overload.[53]

Patients on hemodialysis usually gain both sodium and water between the end of one dialysis treatment and the beginning of the next; in a compliant patient, the gain is usually manifested by a weight gain of 1 to 2 kg.[54] However, in a noncompliant patient, it may be 5 kg or greater.[55]

METABOLIC ACIDOSIS

In mild CRF, the metabolic acidosis is often of the normal AG type; however, as the renal failure increases in severity, the AG increases, resulting in a high AG acidosis. Even then, the AG rarely exceeds 20 mEq/L.[56] As a rule, the bicarbonate level stabilizes at 15 to 18 mEq/L and the arterial pH at 7.25 to 7.35 unless another condition is present that disrupts acid–base balance. Most patients require 50 to 100 mEq bicarbonate daily to manage metabolic acidosis; sodium bicarbonate tablets are often the choice to provide this treatment. The need for bicarbonate replacement can be minimized by limiting dietary protein intake (and thereby limiting acid production) and by using bicarbonate dialysates.

Hemodialysis corrects the metabolic acidosis caused by CRF by furnishing bicarbonate or a potential bicarbonate (such as acetate) in the dialysate that is then transferred across the dialyzer into the patient's bloodstream during the treatment.[57] However, after hemodialysis, the pH and plasma bicarbonate level steadily decrease until the next treatment. In the United States, hemodialysis is the predominant method used to treat patients for chronic (and acute) failure.[58] It is usually started when the patient's creatinine clearance decreases below 10 mL/min. This change usually corresponds to a serum creatinine concentration of 8 to 10 mg/dL.[59]

Continuous ambulatory peritoneal dialysis (CAPD) has several advantages over hemodialysis. It provides stable values for urea, creatinine, and electrolytes (including bicarbonate) from day to day and before and after dialysis treatment.[60] Also, it is technically easier to use and is less expensive than conventional hemodialysis. In the United States, more than 40,000 patients use long-term peritoneal dialysis treatments.[61]

HYPERKALEMIA

With the gradual onset of renal failure, there is time for the development of adaptive changes that augment potassium excretion as well as translocation of potassium into the cells; as a result, patients with CRF can tolerate higher serum potassium concentrations better than patients with ARF. Another compensatory change that occurs over time in patients with CRF is a greater ability to excrete potassium in the stool; the fraction of dietary potassium eliminated in feces can rise from 12% in patients with normal renal function to 35% in patients with CRF.[62] For this reason, it is especially desirable to prevent constipation in these patients. Unfortunately, constipation is a common problem because of the use of large doses of phosphate binders to lower the serum phosphate level.

It is important to remember that despite the development of certain protective mechanisms, potentially fatal hyperkalemia remains a threat in patients with CRF and renders the regulation of serum potassium concentration very important. Dietary potassium restriction to less than 60 to 70 mEq/day is indicated after the GFR has fallen below 10 to 20 mL/min.[63]

Medications that tend to elevate the serum concentration of potassium (such as the angiotensin-converting enzyme [ACE] inhibitors, or cyclosporine in renal transplant patients) increase the probability of the development of hyperkalemia. Once mild hyperkalemia develops, it can usually be managed by potassium exchange resins. Moderate potassium elevations (4.5–5.5 mEq/L) are generally monitored monthly; more severe elevations (> 5.5 mEq/L) are checked at least twice monthly.[64] These moderate elevations may also be managed by oral or rectal potassium-exchange resins.

Rapid treatment of severe hyperkalemia is accomplished by the IV administration of insulin and glucose or perhaps by the administration of aerosolized albuterol when an IV access line has not yet been established. Albuterol sulfate (20 mg dissolved in 4 mL saline) inhaled over 10 minutes decreases the plasma potassium level for about 2 to 4 hours by driving potassium temporarily into the cells.[65]

To manage hyperkalemia in patients undergoing hemodialysis, the potassium concentration in the dialysate is lower than the serum potassium content. The typical dialysate potassium concentrations are in the range of 0 to 3 mEq/L (with 1 or 2 mEq/L considered standard).[66] The total removal of potassium during a typical dialysis treatment is about 50 to 80 mmol.[67] Potassium shifts during dialysis predispose to arrhythmias, especially in patients with cardiovascular disease. Because of this, the potassium content in the dialysate is adjusted as needed on an individual basis.

Severe hyperkalemia is less likely to be present in patients undergoing CAPD than in those treated by hemodialysis.[68] This is probably because CAPD continuously removes potassium, whereas hemodialysis treatments are intermittent. Patients on CAPD are far more likely to have *hypo*kalemia than are predialysis hemodialysis patients; probably this is because CAPD patients take in less dietary potassium and have more residual renal excretion of potassium than do hemodialysis patients.

HYPERMAGNESEMIA

Magnesium excretion is diminished in patients with CRF; however, hypermagnesemia is rarely dangerous unless the patient ingests medications high in magnesium or receives it IV. Patients with CRF should be cautioned to avoid all magnesium-containing laxatives and antacids.

HYPERPHOSPHATEMIA

In patients with CRF, the remaining intact nephrons undergo hypertrophy and secrete proportionately more phosphate per unit; this adaptive process can maintain normal serum phosphate concentrations until the nephron mass is reduced to less than 25% of normal. When hyperphosphatemia is a problem, it is managed by dietary phosphate restriction and the administration of phosphate-binding agents. Oral phosphate-binding agents (such as calcium acetate, calcium carbonate, or calcium citrate) may be given with meals to lower the serum phosphate level while also replacing calcium. For example, calcium acetate (Phoslo) when taken with meals combines with dietary phosphate to form insoluble calcium phosphate, which is then excreted in the feces. Because patients with end-stage renal failure may develop hypercalcemia when given calcium with meals, no other calcium supplements should be given concurrently with calcium acetate. The recommended dose of calcium acetate (PhosLo) for the adult dialysis patient is 2 tablets with each meal; the dosage is adjusted to gradually lower the serum phosphate level below 6 mg/dL so long as hypercalcemia does not develop.[69] Although aluminum hydroxide is also an effective phosphate-binding agent, it is associated with osteomalacia and neurological complications.[70] Aluminum salts replace calcium in the skeleton. Excessive deposits of aluminum can lead to skeletal weakness and also decreased red blood cell production. Foods rich in phosphorus that may need to be limited include eggs, dairy products, and meat.

HYPOCALCEMIA

Intestinal calcium absorption begins to fail as renal failure progresses; when the serum creatinine exceeds 2.5 mg/dL, calcium absorption is detectably reduced.[71] Factors that influence calcium absorption adversely include frank uremia, phosphate retention, and acidemia. Although hypocalcemia would normally stimulate mobilization of calcium from bone (under the influence of PTH), there is an altered responsiveness in bone that is apparently mediated by uremic toxicity.

Goals to promote calcium homeostasis include the management of hyperphosphatemia and metabolic acidosis as well as providing calcium and active vitamin D for more normal bone metabolism. Dietary phosphate intake may be limited to 700 mg/day or less. Also, phosphate-binding agents are frequently used; these agents may be calcium-based compounds that also provide extra calcium. Replacement of calcium is important because intestinal calcium absorption is suboptimal; as a rule, 1 to 2 g elemental calcium is sufficient oral replacement in patients with CRF. Vitamin D (administered as 1,25-dihydroxyvitamin D_3) is empirically given at a dosage of 0.25 to 0.5 ug/day (using caution to avoid hypercalcemia).[72]

It is important to undertake measures to control hyperphosphatemia while supplementing calcium because the danger of metastatic calcifications in soft tissues becomes more prominent when concentrations of both calcium and phosphate mutually increase in the blood. (When plasma concentrations of calcium and phosphate are normal, their product [calcium X phosphate] is about 30–40; a value exceeding 60–70 is thought to be dangerous.) Metastatic calcification may occur in the skin (causing pruritus), the eye (causing band keratopathy and conjunctival irritation), the heart (causing conduction abnormality), the lung (causing pleural scarring), and the blood vessels (causing occlusive disease).[73]

Because acidosis has an adverse effect on calcium balance, acidosis must also be treated. A major part of acidosis control in the chronic setting is restriction of dietary protein; this, in turn, minimizes acid production. Protein intake may be limited to 0.6 g/kg body weight.

BONE CHANGES

Chronic negative calcium balance produces renal osteodystrophy in patients with CRF, especially those who must undergo long-term dialysis. Osteitis fibrosa remains the most common form of bone disease and results from overactivity of the parathyroid glands as a result of hypocalcemia and low 1,25-vitamin D_3 levels.[74] The bone disease is characterized by fibrosis of the marrow space; it can be mild to severe, pure or mixed with aluminum bone disease. Dialysis patients acquire aluminum either through oral aluminum-containing phosphate binders or through the water supply. The aluminum accumulates, because of lack of renal excretion, and deposits at the mineralization front of growing or remodeling bone. This impairs bone mineralization and leads to osteomalacia.

ANEMIA

Normocytic, normochromic anemia occurs in almost all patients with CRF. Routine administration of erythropoietin to patients with end-stage renal disease results in improvement of the anemia and decreases the need for blood transfusions.[75] Recombinant erythropoietin (epoetin alfa) is used in patients who have hematocrit values less than 30% to 35%; iron stores must be adequate to ensure a good response.[76] The patient must have adequate amounts of available iron for optimal red blood cell development. Serum ferritin levels need to be 100 mg/dL or greater, and transferrin saturation levels need to be 20% or greater.

CARDIOPULMONARY CHANGES

Hypertension due to salt and water retention becomes increasingly common as CRF progresses in severity.[77] To help control this problem, dietary salt restriction to 2 g/day may be indicated. Medications to control hypertension may include ACE inhibitors or losartan (if the serum potassium and GFR rate permit), diuretics, and β-blocking agents.[78] Pericarditis may occur when the BUN is markedly elevated (such as 100 mg/dL) and is an absolute indication to start hemodialysis.[79] Congestive heart failure is common and is due to fluid volume overload, hypertension, and anemia. Salt intake needs to be curtailed and diuretics may be of benefit. Thiazide diuretics are not effective when the GFR is less than 10 to 15 mL/min; however, loop diuretics may be tried. ACE inhibitors are helpful but are typically not used if the serum creatinine is greater than 3 mg/dL (because of the risk for hyperkalemia and decreased renal function); these risks are less relevant when the patient is on dialysis.[80] Several case reports and a randomized trial suggest that losartan may cause the same negative renal effects as ACE inhibitors; therefore, renal function should be monitored when patients receive either agent.[81]

A summary of the effects of renal failure on the various body systems is presented in Table 17-4 and a summary of fluid, electrolyte, and acid–base imbalances associated with renal failure is presented in Table 17-5.

CASE STUDIES

● **17-1.** A 50-year-old man was admitted with acute pulmonary edema secondary to a myocardial infarction. On admission, he was given furosemide IV and then was continued on an oral dose of 40 mL/day. The pulmonary edema resolved and he was having an uneventful recovery when on the ninth day it was noted that his BUN had risen from 10 mg/dL on admission to 110 mg/dL and his plasma creatinine (Cr) had increased from 1 mg/dL to 4.5 mg/dL. An acute weight loss of 6 kg was also noted. His skin turgor was poor and his neck veins were flat. A review of laboratory data revealed:

Urine Na = 2 mEq/L
Urine osmolality = 550 mOsm/kg
BUN = 110 mg/dL

Serum Cr = 4.5 mg/dL
BUN/Cr ratio 20:1

COMMENTARY: All of the above signs pointed to prerenal failure secondary to fluid volume depletion following the excessive diuresis. The low urine sodium concentration indicated renal conservation of sodium (a normal renal response to fluid volume depletion). The urine osmolality was high as the kidneys attempted to retain needed fluid.

● **17-2.** A 70-year-old woman with congestive heart failure was admitted with distended neck veins and pedal edema. On admission, her BUN was 20 mg/dL and her serum creatinine was 1.2 mg/dL. A 5-kg weight loss occurred after 3 days of diuretic therapy; although a marked improvement was noted in her clinical status, a mild degree of pulmonary edema persisted. The BUN had elevated to 90 mg/dL and the serum creatinine elevated to 3.0 mg/dL.

COMMENTARY: The elevated BUN and serum creatinine levels (BUN/Cr ratio 30:1) were the result of renal hypoperfusion secondary to excessive diuresis. Her heart disease was so severe that she could not be both edema free and have a normal plasma creatinine concentration. Therapy was initiated to improve her cardiac output.

● **17-3.** A 25-year-old woman with a 10-year history of progressive renal failure was admitted with mild hypertension. Laboratory data include:

Serum Na = 139 mEq/L
Serum K = 5.9 mEq/L
Serum Cl = 105 mEq/L
Serum HCO_3 = 14 mEq/L
BUN = 80 mg/dL

COMMENTARY: The low bicarbonate level indicates metabolic acidosis (the expected acid–base imbalance in a patient with CRF). In renal insufficiency, metabolic acidosis is due to the inability of the kidneys to excrete the daily hydrogen load.

The AG is calculated by subtracting the sum of the serum bicarbonate and chloride levels from the serum sodium level.

$AG = Na - (HCO_3 + Cl)$
$AG = 139 - (14 + 105) = 20$ mEq/L

(Note that this is above the normally accepted range for most laboratories; the usual expected range is 12 ± 2 mEq/L.) This high AG acidosis

TABLE 17-4. Summary of Effects of Renal Failure on the Major Body Systems

System	Effects
Integumentary	Itchy, dry, scaly skin; probably due to calcium and phosphate disturbances.
	Excretion of urochrome pigment through sweat glands produces a yellow color in the skin.
	Skin also may appear pale as a result of anemia.
	Purpura and ecchymoses may occur as the result of platelet dysfunction and increased capillary fragility.
	In very late stages, uremic frost (urea crystals excreted through sweat glands, heaviest on nose, forehead, and neck) may be observed.
Gastrointestinal	Anorexia, nausea, vomiting and ileus are common as a result of the effects of uremic toxins on the gastrointestinal mucosa.
	Acute stress of severe illness coupled with platelet dysfunction leads to gastrointestinal bleeding.
	Unpleasant metallic taste in mouth and ammonia odor to the breath are noted.
	Stomatatitis; salivary urea is hydrolyzed by urease into ammonia, causing mucous membrane irritation.
	Constipation associated with decreased fluid intake and bulk in diet as well as decreased activity.
Pulmonary	Pulmonary edema related to fluid volume excess.
	Pneumonia may occur as a result of the patient's poor resistance to infection.
	Metabolic acidosis may produce a compensatory increase in both the rate and depth of respirations.
Cardiac	Congestive heart failure (contributed to by the combination of fluid overload, hypertension, anemia, and acidosis).
	Dysrhythmias may occur as a result of hyperkalemia, hypocalcemia, and severe acidosis.
Neurological	Gradual diminution of mental acuity over a period of time, leading to coma (resulting from uremic toxins and acidosis).
	Transient episodes of agitated psychotic behavior (hallucinations and paranoid delusions) interspersed with periods of lucidity.
	Peripheral neuropathy (numbness, pain, and burning sensations in the legs and arms—may progress to motor weakness and paralysis).
Skeletal	Over a sustained period, hyperphosphatemia and hypocalcemia lead to osteodystrophy.
Hematologic	Anemia occurs and is related to a combination of decreased erythropoietin and decreased red cell survival time; it is also related to blood loss.
	Platelet dysfunction leads to elevated bleeding time and to clinically important bleeding.
	Defects in granulocyte and chemotaxis and phagocytic activity predispose to infection.
Endocrine	Due to increased peripheral insulin resistance, glucose intolerance occurs in patients with CRF when the GFR is < 10–20 mL/min; on the other hand, circulating insulin levels are higher due to decreased renal insulin clearance (therefore, patients might be either hyperglycemic or hypoglycemic, depending on which condition is predominant).
Reproductive	Decreased libido; impotence in men, decreased ovulation in women.

TABLE 17-5.   Summary of Fluid, Electrolyte, and Acid–Base Problems Commonly Associated With Renal Failure

Imbalance	Pathophysiology
Fluid volume excess	As the GFR decreases, the kidneys lose their ability to adjust sodium excretion in response to sodium intake and changes in the ECF volume; therefore, if excessive fluids are administered, fluid volume excess will occur.
Hyperkalemia	Because potassium elimination occurs primarily through the kidneys, potassium retention will occur when renal function is seriously impaired (GFR < 10 mL/min).
	Metabolic acidosis adds to the hyperkalemia by driving cellular potassium into the extracellular space.
	Increased endogenous release of potassium from the cellular breakdown (catabolism) of infected or necrotic tissue raises the serum potassium level—the more catabolic the patient, the higher the rise in the serum potassium concentration.
	High intake of protein causes the serum potassium level to elevate.
	Certain medications (such as ACE inhibitors or cyclosporine following renal transplantation) predispose to hyperkalemia.
Hyperphosphatemia	Renal phosphate retention is inevitable when the GFR is reduced to < 25% of normal.
	The major consequence of hyperphosphatemia is the associated reciprocal decrease in the serum calcium concentration.
Hypocalcemia	Hypocalcemia is invariably present during the oliguric phase of ARF; a decrease occurs within the first 2–4 days and may reach concentrations as low as 5–7.5 mg/dL.
	Besides phosphate excess, other causes of hypocalcemia include a deficiency in active vitamin D, which, in turn, decreases the amount of dietary calcium absorbed through the gut, and resistance of bone to the attempts of PTH to stimulate calcium release from bone stores.
	Prolonged hypocalcemia in CRF leads to bone demineralization.
Hypermagnesemia	Renal magnesium retention occurs when the GFR is reduced to < 30% of normal; in general, magnesium retention does not result in symptoms until the serum magnesium level exceeds 4–5 mg/dL: most patients with CRF do not exceed this range.
	Usually the hypermagnesemia is only mild to moderate unless the patient is inadvertently given medications containing magnesium (such as magnesium-containing antacids or laxatives).
Metabolic acidosis	The damaged kidneys are unable to excrete the acids produced during metabolism; these acids must then be buffered with bicarbonate, causing the serum bicarbonate level to drop below normal.
	Usually the bicarbonate stabilizes at 12–18 mEq/L and the arterial pH at 7.25–7.30; however, hypercatabolic conditions cause the acidosis to become much worse (sometimes with arterial pH values dropping below 7.1).
	The acidosis is typically a high anion gap metabolic acidosis (owing to the accumulation of sulfate, phosphate, and a variety of organic acids); the anion gap in ARF is almost invariably < 30 mEq/L, whereas it is usually < 20 mEq/L in CRF.

Continued

TABLE 17-5.   Summary of Fluid, Electrolyte, and Acid–Base Problems Commonly Associated With Renal Failure—*cont'd*

Imbalance	Pathophysiology
Hyponatremia	Hyponatremia is a relatively common imbalance because patients with renal failure typically receive an excess of free water IV or orally.
	The impaired kidneys are unable to excrete excess free water; therefore, to help prevent this condition, water intake is often reduced to < 500 mL/day in oliguric euvolemic patients who are not undergoing ultrafiltration.
	A danger of rapidly developing hyponatremia is cerebral edema with serious neurological sequelae.
Hypernatremia	Hypernatremia is uncommon in patients with ARF; it may occur during the polyuric phase as relatively dilute urine is excreted; it may also follow the administration of excessive amounts of hypertonic $NaHCO_3$ or sodium-containing antibiotics.

reflects the retention of phosphate, sulfate, and other organic anions.

The patient's serum potassium level is above normal because renal failure causes poor renal excretion of potassium; further, metabolic acidosis favors shifting of cellular potassium into the plasma.

Oral bicarbonate replacement will likely keep the serum bicarbonate level at more than 15 to 18 mEq/L. Attention is given to avoiding overcorrection of the low serum bicarbonate level because alkalosis favors decreased calcium ionization. Of course, because hypocalcemia is a chronic problem in renal patients, it is important to avoid exacerbating symptoms by overcorrection of acidosis.

● **17-4.**[82] A young man with multiple contusions was found unconscious and admitted to the emergency room. His urine was brown and positive for blood. Laboratory data revealed:

Plasma Na = 150 mEq/L
Plasma K = 7.5 mEq/L
Plasma Cl = 113 mEq/L
BUN = 125 mg/dL
Serum Cr = 17 mg/dL
pH = 7.30

HCO_3 = 14 mEq/L
$PaCO_2$ = 30 mm Hg

He was diagnosed as having ARF secondary to rhabdomyolysis (a condition in which myoglobin is released into the bloodstream from injured muscles). The subsequent attempt of the kidneys to excrete the myoglobin resulted in acute tubular necrosis and accounted for the heme-positive urine.

COMMENTARY: The plasma potassium concentration of 7.5 mEq/L was life-threatening and required immediate treatment. It occurred because large amounts of potassium were released from the injured muscle cells into the bloodstream; the presence of metabolic acidosis added to the hyperkalemia by fostering a shift of potassium from the cells into the extracellular space. Using the formula, AG = Na - (Cl + HCO_3), it was noted that a high AG metabolic acidosis was present; this is characteristic in ARF. The BUN/Cr ratio was close to 10:1.

● **17-5.**[83] A 35-year-old woman underwent a kidney transplant. During surgery, she received 1 liter lactated Ringer's, 1 liter 0.9% NaCl, and 20 g mannitol. The surgery was uneventful and urine output appeared promptly. Postoperatively, her urine output averaged about 1,000 mL/hr (due to a temporary acute tubular dysfunction). She then received 0.45% NaCl IV at a rate to match her hourly urine output. Two boluses of 0.9% NaCl were required to keep her blood pressure in the normal range. Fifteen hours postoperatively, the patient suffered a generalized seizure; she was drowsy but arousable. Blood work revealed:

Na = 120 mEq/L
K = 3.4 mEq/L
Total Ca = 7.0 mg/dL

To treat these abnormalities, her IV fluid was changed to 0.9% NaCl at a rate to replace her urine volume; she also received 1 g calcium gluconate and 2 g magnesium sulfate.

COMMENTARY: It was concluded that the most likely basis for her seizure was acute hyponatremia, brought about by the excessive infusion of a hypotonic saline solution. During a period of 14 hours, she had received a total of 1,009 mEq Na (13.1 liters of 0.45% NaCl, which contains 77 mEq Na/L). However, her urinary loss of sodium during the same time was calculated at 1,441 mEq. Therefore, she had a total sodium deficit of 432 mEq during this period. In other words, hyponatremia in this patient represented the administration of large amounts of IV fluid that were hypotonic to her polyuric losses. The patient subsequently recovered following treatment. A lesson to be learned from this case is that plasma and urine electrolytes should be monitored frequently (such as every 2–4 hours) when polyuria occurs after transplantation and the urine should be replaced with IV therapy appropriate for both volume and tonicity.[84]

● **17-6.** A 63-year-old man with diabetes mellitus whose renal function had worsened over the last few years noticed that his urine output had been decreasing (as has the number of voids per day). On a visit to his physician, the following symptoms were noted:

Body weight 88 kg (normal is 83 kg)
Shortness of breath
Wet breath sounds
Muscle weakness (especially in legs)
Low urine output (< 180 mL/24 hr)

Increased thirst
Decreased level of consciousness

Laboratory results included:

Plasma Na = 132 mEq/L
Plasma K = 6.2 mEq/L
Plasma Cl = 106 mEq/L
BUN = 42 mg/dL
Serum Cr = 5.5 mg/dL

It was concluded that his renal disease had progressed to end-stage renal disease and that hemodialysis was indicated. A subclavian double-lumen central venous catheter was inserted the next morning and the patient was scheduled to have an arteriovenous access inserted in his left forearm. A hemodialysis treatment was performed the afternoon after the subclavian catheter was inserted. Following this treatment the patient's dry weight was 84 kg and the following laboratory values were obtained:

Plasma Na = 142 mEq/L
Plasma K = 4.7 mEq/L
Plasma Cl = 116 mEq/L
BUN = 15 mg/dL
Serum Cr = 3.5 mg/dL

Clinically, the patient appeared much improved. His shortness of breath and wet breath sounds disappeared. Although he was still weak, his level of consciousness was significantly improved.

COMMENTARY: The hemodialysis treatment was effective in reducing the patient's fluid volume overload, hyperkalemia, high BUN, and serum creatinine. The patient was scheduled to receive hemodialysis three times per week. Without this treatment, serious fluid volume overload and hyperkalemia, as well as other uremic abnormalities, would develop. It is not unusual for patients to feel exhausted after a hemodialysis treatment. This is largely due to the shifting of fluids and particles from the patient to the dialysate over a short period of time. Note that the patient lost 4 kg of weight during the hemodialysis treatment. It is important to monitor for hypotension and excessive fluid loss during hemodialysis.

● **17-7.** A 48-year-old woman who had been on hemodialysis for 3 years was apparently doing well but wished to switch to peritoneal dialysis so that she could be more independent. She discussed her wishes with her physician who agreed to the change in treatment. A Tenchkhoff peritoneal catheter was instilled and her incision healed without complication. She remained on hemodialysis while she trained for peritoneal dialysis at home. Following her training classes, her vital signs were within normal limits, her lungs were clear, her catheter exit site was clean, and her dry weight was 55 kg. Her laboratory values were:

    Plasma Na = 142 mEq/L
    Plasma K = 4.1 mEq/L
    Plasma Cl = 115 mEq/L
    BUN = 10 mg/dL
    Serum Cr = 2.1 mg/dL

The patient was started on five 2-liter dialysate exchanges daily. After the first month of peritoneal dialysis, her weight had increased to 62 kg and she had dependent edema and wet breath sounds. Her laboratory values were:

    Plasma Na = 138 mEq/L
    Plasma K = 6.2 mEq/L
    Plasma Cl = 105 mEq/L
    BUN = 60 mg/dL
    Serum Cr = 19 mg/dL

It was discovered that the patient had not been leaving her peritoneal dialysate fluid in as long as prescribed; she had used only three exchanges per day (not the prescribed five exchanges). Because of this, fluid and wastes were inadequately removed. The patient indicated she had developed progressively greater difficulty in remembering how many exchanges she had performed. A peritoneal dialysis treatment was administered while the patient was seen at the clinic. She returned home with her peritoneal dialysis prescription reinforced to accomplish five exchanges daily. The patient's in-clinic dialysis laboratory values were:

    Plasma Na = 142 mEq/L
    Plasma K = 5.0 mEq/L
    Plasma Cl = 115 mEq/L
    BUN = 33 mg/dL
    Serum Cr = 9 mg/dL

COMMENTARY: Although patients on peritoneal dialysis have more flexibility than those on hemodialysis, it must be emphasized to them that interruptions in the peritoneal fluid and dialysate exchanges can lead to progressive changes in laboratory values and clinical status.

● **17-8.** A 23-year-old man with acute myelogenous leukemia had a bone marrow transplant; his weight following this procedure was 78 kg. Two weeks later, he developed graft versus host disease (GVHD) and his BUN, creatinine, and bilirubin levels began to progressively elevate. For the next 2 weeks, his urine output remained greater than 30 mL/hr. However, during the third week following his bone marrow transplant, his urine output dropped to less than 10 mL/hr, he gained 5 kg (weight, 83 kg), and his level of consciousness was decreased. Laboratory values were:

    Plasma Na = 123 mEq/L
    Plasma K = 6.5 mEq/L
    Plasma Cl = 108 mEq/L
    BUN = 222 mg/dL
    Serum Cr = 50 mg/dL

His output was only 6 mL/hr and his temperature was 101.4°F. His blood pressure was 86/40 and his pulse rate was 120 beats/min. Because he was fluid volume overloaded, hyperkalemic, and had markedly elevated BUN and serum Cr levels, he was transferred to the intensive care unit and placed on CVVH. After 17 hours, his laboratory values had significantly improved:

    Plasma Na = 142 mEq/L
    Plasma K = 4.1 mEq/L
    Plasma Cl = 118 mEq/L
    BUN = 100 mg/dL
    Serum Cr = 20 mg/dL

His vital signs were also improved (blood pressure, 118/72; pulse, 92; and temperature, 99.6°F). His body weight was 80 kg.

COMMENTARY: With the initiation of CVVH, the critical care team was able to correct the patient's fluid volume overload and hyperkalemia. There were significant improvements in the BUN and serum creatinine levels. The patient remained on CVVH for 5 days, during which time GVHD worsened. This led to the generation of large amounts of BUN and creatinine, causing the patient's condition to progressively degenerate. He ultimately suffered cardiac arrest and died.

● **17-9.** A 50-year-old man with liver failure caused by chronic alcohol abuse developed hepatic-renal failure. Before this, he weighed 90 kg. His serum albumin level remained close to 3.0 g/dL for the previous year; food intake was essentially limited to snack foods and alcohol. Over a period of about a year his abdominal girth progressively increased while he continued to lose weight. On being seen in a clinic, the following laboratory values were obtained:

Plasma Na = 130 mEq/L
Plasma K = 5.1 mEq/L
Plasma Cl = 105 mEq/L
BUN = 200 mg/dL
Serum Cr = 30 mg/dL

He weighed 78 kg and his vital signs included blood pressure of 72/56 and pulse rate of 112/min. Due to his worsening BUN and serum creatinine (as well as liver enzymes), he was admitted to the hospital for hemodialysis treatments and close monitoring. Because he was hypotensive, it was decided that CVVH was more appropriate than hemodialysis. To help correct his malnourished state, TPN was added in the filtration replacement port of the dialyzer. After being on CVVH for 24 hours, his laboratory values were:

Plasma Na = 140 mEq/L
Plasma K = 4.4 mEq/L
Plasma Cl = 115 mEq/L
BUN = 120 mg/dL
Serum Cr = 10 mg/dL

His weight was maintained at 78 kg but his vital signs improved to blood pressure of 112/70 and pulse rate of 96/min.

COMMENTARY: Patients with advancing liver failure often present with signs and symptoms of fluid volume overload, increased abdominal girth, low serum albumin levels, elevated BUN levels, and elevated liver enzyme levels. These patients may be admitted to critical care units and placed on a continuous renal replacement therapy until they are stable enough for a liver transplant. It is likely that TPN will be maintained following release from the critical care unit.

● **17-10.** A 76-year-old woman with type 1 diabetes mellitus and a double above-the-knee amputation had been maintained on hemodialysis for 5 years. She was dialyzed three times per week, on a Monday-Wednesday-Friday schedule. During her years on hemodialysis, she had varying weight gains between dialysis treatments. Her most current set of laboratory values were:

Plasma Na = 139 mEq/L
Plasma K = 6.6 mEq/L

Plasma Cl = 114 mEq/L
BUN = 38 mg/dL
Serum Cr = 12 mg/dL

Her weight was 79.6 kg, her blood pressure was 112/76, and her pulse rate was 88/min.

While attending a family reunion on a Sunday afternoon, she ate large quantities of strawberries and watermelon. (One cup of raw strawberries contains 6.5 mEq potassium; 1 cup of watermelon contains 5 mEq potassium.) When she came to the hemodialysis unit on Monday morning, she was listless, confused, and not her usual self. Although her goal dry weight was 73 kg, her weight at this time was 83 kg. Stat laboratory data included:

Serum Na = 132 mEq/L
Serum K = 10.2 mEq/L
Serum Cl = 108 mEq/L
BUN = 75 mg/dL
Serum Cr = 30 mg/dL

Her pulse rate was 44/min and her blood pressure was 90/40. She was placed on her hemodialysis prescription with a 0-mEq potassium concentration in the dialysate. During the dialysis treatment, her heart rate dropped to 30/min. She also became hypotensive and lost consciousness. A temporary pacemaker was inserted while she was in the dialysis unit. Following the hemodialysis treatment, her weight was 78 kg. She was admitted to the coronary care unit and was found to have a third-degree heart block. While in the coronary unit, a permanent pacemaker was inserted and paced at 72 beats/min. Her laboratory values following the hemodialysis treatment were:

Plasma Na = 140 mEq/L
Plasma K = 6.8 mEq/L
Plasma Cl = 114 mEq/L
BUN = 36 mg/dL
Serum Cr = 10 mg/dL

COMMENTARY: Although changes in fluid and electrolyte levels are common between dialysis treatments, this patient's were intensified by her high consumption of potassium-containing foods. It was necessary to carefully reduce her weight and serum potassium level because her history of cardiovascular disease increased her likelihood of developing complications if rapid shifts were achieved. Dietary counseling was provided to prevent this unfortunate set of circumstances from recurring.

REFERENCES

1. Arieff A, DeFronzo R. *Fluid, Electrolyte, and Acid-Base Disorders*, 2nd ed. New York: Churchill Livingstone; 1995:643.
2. Narins R. *Maxwell & Kleeman's Clinical Disorders of Fluid and Electrolyte Metabolism*, 5th ed. New York: McGraw-Hill;. 1994: 1175.
3. Kokko J, Tannen R. *Fluids and Electrolytes*, 3rd ed. Philadelphia: WB Saunders; 1996:517.
4. Narins, p 1177.
5. Arieff, DeFronzo, p 633.
6. Kokko,& Tannen, p 517.
7. Tierney L, McPhee S, Papadakis M. *Current Medical Diagnosis & Treatment*, 38th ed. Stamford, CT: Appleton & Lange, 1999.
8. Hilberman M, Myers BD, Carrie BJ et al. Acute renal failure following cardiac surgery. *J Thorac Cardiovasc Surg* 1979;77:880.
9. Wing AJ, Broyer M, Brunner FP et al. Acute [reversible] renal failure. In: Combined Report on Regular Dialysis and Transplantation in Europe. XIII 1982. *Proc Soc Eur Dial Transplant Assoc* 1983;20:64.
10. Cameron JS. Acute renal failure in the intensive therapy unit: The nephrologist's view. In: Bihari D, Neild G, eds. *Acute Renal Failure in the Intensive Therapy Unit*. London: Springer-Verlag; 1990:3.
11. Arieff, DeFronzo, p 640.
12. Ibid, p 663.
13. Ibid.
14. Narins, p 1183.
15. Ibid.
16. Kokko, Tannen, p 518.
17. Narins, p 1184.
18. Arieff, DeFronzo, p 663.
19. Ibid.
20. Ibid, p 637.
21. Ibid, p 664.
22. Ibid, p 636.
23. Ibid, p 665.
24. McCarty M, Jagoda A, Fairweather P. Hyperkalemic ascending paralysis. *Ann Emerg Med* 1998;31:104.
25. Narins, p 1185.
26. Kokko, Tannen, p 519.
27. Arieff, DeFronzo, p 666.
28. Tierney et al, p 847.
29. Narins, p 1205.
30. Tierney et al, p 847.
31. Ibid.
32. Narins, p 1205.
33. Arieff, DeFronzo, p 665.
34. Condon R, Nyhus L. *Manual of Surgical Therapeutics*, 9th ed. Boston: Little, Brown; 1996:156.
35. Chmielewski C. Hyperkalemic emergencies. In: Gould K, ed. *Fluid and Electrolyte Emergencies. Crit Care Nurs Clin North Am* 1998;10:456.
36. Allon M. Hyperkalemia in end-stage renal disease: Mechanism and management. *J Am Soc Nephrol* 1995;6:1134.
37. Schrier R. *Manual of Nephrology*, 4th ed. Boston: Little, Brown, 1995.
38. Ibid.
39. Arieff, DeFronzo, p 637.
40. Narins, p 1189.
41. Arieff, DeFronzo, p 667.
42. Narins, p 1188.
43. Arieff, DeFronzo, p 668.
44. Carey C, Lee H, Woeltje K. *The Washington Manual of Medical Therapeutics*, 29th ed. Philadelphia: Lippincott-Raven; 1998:232.

45. Doherty G, Baumann D, Creswell L, Goss J, Lairmore T, eds. *The Washington Manual of Surgery*. Philadelphia: Lippincott-Raven, 1997:111.
46. Rasmussen HH, Pitt EA, Ibels LS et al. Prediction of outcome in acute renal failure by discriminant analysis of clinical variables. *Arch Intern Med* 1985;145:2015.
47. Kennedy AC, Burton J, Luke RG et al. Factors affecting prognosis in acute renal failure. *Q J Med* 1973;42:73.
48. Arieff, DeFronzo, p 662.
49. Tierney et al, p 873.
50. Kokko, Tannen, p 488.
51. Arieff, DeFronzo, p 673.
52. Narins, p 1197.
53. Jaeger J, Mehta R. Assessment of dry weight in hemodialysis: An overview. *J Am Soc Nephrol* 1999;10:392.
54. Arieff, DeFronzo, p 793.
55. Ibid.
56. Kokko, Tannen, p 502.
57. Arieff, DeFronzo, p 796.
58. Kliger A, Haley W. Clinical practice guidelines in end-stage renal disease: A strategy for implementation. *J Am Soc Nephrol* 1999;10:872.
59. Jones C, McQuillan G, Kusek J et al. Serum creatinine levels in the U.S. population: Third national health and nutrition survey. *Am J Kidney Dis* 1998;32:984.
60. Arieff, DeFronzo, p 801.
61. Popovich R, Moncrief J, Nolph K et al. Continuous ambulatory peritoneal dialysis. *J Am Soc Nephrol* 1999;10:901.
62. Narins, p 1204.
63. Tierney et al, p 879.
64. Narins, p 1201.
65. Baer C. Care of the critically ill chronic renal failure patient. In: Gould K, ed. *Fluid and Electrolyte Emergencies. Crit Care Nurs Clin North Am* 1998;10:441.
66. Arieff, DeFronzo, p 805.
67. Ibid, p 806.
68. Ibid, p 807.
69. *Physicians' Desk Reference*, 53rd ed. Montvale, NJ: Medical Economics Company; 1999:767.
70. Ibid, p 3263.
71. Kokko, Tannen, p 516.
72. Brensilver J, Goldberger E. *Water, Electrolyte and Acid-Base Syndromes*, 8th ed. Philadelphia: FA Davis; 1996:209.
73. Ibid, p 507.
74. Schrier, p 165.
75. Andreoli T, Bennett J, Carpenter C, Plum F. *Cecil Essentials of Medicine*, 4th ed. Philadelphia: WB Saunders; 1997.
76. Tierney et al, p 877.
77. Towsend R, Cirigliano M. Hypertension in renal failure. *Dis Mon* 1998;44:243.
78. Tierney et al, p 877.
79. Ibid.
80. Ibid.
81. Esmail Z, Loewen P. Losartan as an alternative to ACE inhibitors in patients with renal dysfunction. *Ann Pharmacother* 1998;32:1096.
82. Szerlip H, Goldfarb S. *Workshops in Fluid and Electrolyte Disorders*. New York: Churchill Livingstone; 1993.
83. Zaltzman J. Post-renal transplantation hyponatremia. *Am J Kidney Dis* 1996;27:599.
84. Ibid.

CHAPTER 18

Diabetic Ketoacidosis and Hyperosmolar Syndrome

A relative or absolute insulin deficiency can result in severe hyperglycemia, which in turn leads either to diabetic ketoacidosis (DKA) or hyperosmolar hyperglycemic nonketotic syndrome (HHNS), depending on which type of diabetes mellitus is present. DKA and HHNS can be viewed as opposite ends on the spectrum of metabolic derangements, and episodes of DKA and HHNS occurring simultaneously, rather than alone, have been reported.[1]

In 1997 the Expert Committee on the Diagnosis and Classification of Diabetes Mellitus updated the classification and diagnostic criteria for diabetes. Diabetes mellitus is diagnosed by one of three methods and the diagnosis must be confirmed on a subsequent day. The three methods are:

1. The acute symptoms of diabetes (polyuria, polydipsia, polyphagia, and weight loss) with a random plasma glucose concentration greater than 200 mg/dL
2. A fasting plasma glucose value greater than 126 mg/dL
3. A 2-hour plasma glucose level greater than 200 mg/dL during an oral glucose tolerance test[2]

Type 1 diabetes (formerly insulin-dependent diabetes mellitus [IDDM], type I diabetes, or juvenile-onset diabetes) can develop at any age, although most cases are diagnosed before age 30.[3] Persons with type 1 diabetes mellitus are insulinopenic and require exogenous insulin to prevent ketoacidosis and sustain life. An absolute deficiency of insulin, resulting from autoimmune destruction of pancreatic beta cells, predisposes persons with type 1 diabetes to ketosis. In 20% to 30% of cases, DKA may be the first manifestation of diabetes and is responsible for 2% to 14% of all hospitalizations attributable to diabetes.[4] DKA is life-threatening and, despite treatment advances, mortality rates remain between 1% and 10%, depending on treatment circumstances and locale.[5]

Type 2 diabetes (formerly known as type II diabetes, noninsulin-dependent diabetes mellitus [NIDDM], or adult-onset diabetes) usually begins in middle or later adulthood, is typically diagnosed after age 30, and accounts for about 90% of the known diabetic cases in the United States.[6] Persons with type 2 diabetes mellitus may have decreased, normal, or even increased serum insulin levels. The metabolic problems associated with type 2 diabetes mellitus are believed to result from peripheral insulin resistance, with decreased tissue sensitivity or responsiveness to exoge-

nous or endogenous insulin.[7] About 80% of type 2 diabetics are obese,[8] and many can be managed by dietary and weight control measures. In some cases, oral medications are required. Table 18-1 lists the oral medications currently used in the management of type 2 diabetes mellitus.

A percentage of persons with type 2 diabetes may require some exogenous insulin for proper blood glucose control, at least initially or during times of stress (such as illness or surgery).[9] Persons with type 2 diabetes are not as prone to ketosis; instead, they are at risk for HHNS when their hyperglycemia is severe, although in very rare cases, decompensated type 2 diabetes can result in DKA.[10]

It is not fully understood why these individuals are resistant to ketosis. Although HHNS occurs less frequently than DKA, it is on the increase because of the rising population of elderly adults who have type 2 diabetes mellitus. It is a serious complication of many types of medical and surgical therapies in the elderly diabetic and has a higher mortality rate than DKA.[11]

Use of the term "coma" for these conditions is somewhat misleading because only a small percentage of patients are actually comatose when treatment is initiated.[12] However, both DKA and HHNS cause severe derangements of fluid and electrolyte balances, affecting almost all systems of the body; these emergency situations require expert and prompt intervention.

● DIABETIC KETOACIDOSIS

HYPERGLYCEMIA AND HYPEROSMOLALITY

Diabetic ketoacidosis results from profound insulin deficiency and the effects of the counterregulatory hormones: glucagon, catecholamines, cortisol, and growth hormone. Underuse of glucose (most cells are relatively impermeable to glucose in the absence of insulin), excessive production of glucose from fats and amino acids by the liver (gluconeogenesis), and excessive production of glucose from glycogen (glycogenolysis) all lead to hyperglycemia. Glucagon appears to be the primary hormone responsible for stimulation of hepatic gluconeogenesis and the direct activation of glycogen breakdown.[13] Because of these processes, the blood glucose concentration rises markedly and increases plasma osmolality.

TABLE 18-1.   Oral Medications Used in Management of Type 2 Diabetes*

Generic Name	Brand Name	Classification
tolbutamide	Orinase	First-generation sulfonylurea
chlorpropamide	Diabinese	First-generation sulfonylurea
acetohexamide	Dymelor	First-generation sulfonylurea
tolazamide	Tolinase	First-generation sulfonylurea
glyburide	Diabeta Micronase Glynase Prestabs	Second-generation sulfonylurea
glipizide	Glucotrol Glucotrol XL	Second-generation sulfonylurea
glimepiride	Amaryl	New sulfonylurea
repaglinide	Prandin	Meglitinide
metformin	Glucophage	Biguanide
acarbose	Precose	α-Glucosidase inhibitor
troglitazone	Rezulin	Thiazolidinedione

*Medical management of type 2 diabetes now encompasses a variety of drugs that may have complementary or additive effects when used in combinations. The sulfonylureas and repaglinide increase the secretion of insulin into the portal circulation. Metformin, troglitazone, and acarbose have principal actions at the liver, muscle and adipose tissue, and intestinal lumen, respectively, all assisting whatever insulin is available in regulating glucose levels.

The following formula is used to calculate plasma osmolality, the normal range of which is 280 to 300 mOsm/L:

$$pOsm = 2(Na + K) + G/18 + BUN/2.8 = 280{-}300 \text{ mOsm/kg}$$

In the following example, it is possible to see how hyperglycemia increases plasma osmolality.

Example: Patient with hyperglycemia:

Na = 139 mEq/L
K = 4 mEq/L
Serum glucose = 1,800 mg/dL
Blood urea nitrogen (BUN) = 30 mg/dL

$$pOsm = 2(139 + 4) + 1800/18 + 30/2.8 = 397 \text{ mOsm/kg}$$

This elevated osmolality of extracellular fluid (ECF) produces cellular dehydration as water shifts from the cells to the ECF.

Other researchers use the following formula (omitting the urea component) to calculate the effective osmolality, because urea diffuses freely across cell membranes and does not create an osmotic gradient between the intracellular and extracellular spaces:

$$\text{Effective } pOsm = 2(Na + K) + \text{Serum glucose}/18$$

These investigators reason that this equation can calculate a more clinically relevant value.[14–16]

OSMOTIC DIURESIS AND FLUID VOLUME DEFICIT

When the blood glucose level exceeds the renal threshold (normal, 180 mg/dL), glucose spills into the urine, taking water and electrolytes with it and increasing urine volume. Specific gravity (SG) of the urine is elevated due to the high glucose content. The polyuria eventually leads to fluid volume deficit (FVD). As the FVD worsens, glomerular filtration rate (GFR) decreases, as does renal blood flow, causing the patient to become oliguric or even anuric despite marked hyperglycemia. This FVD presents a danger of potential renal tubular damage with its resultant acute renal failure.

ELECTROLYTES

Potassium

Probably the most important electrolyte disturbance that occurs in DKA is the marked deficit in total body potassium. Causes of potassium depletion include:

1. Starvation effect with lean tissue breakdown
2. Depletion of tissue glycogen stores (potassium is normally deposited in the cells with glycogen)
3. Loss of intracellular potassium
4. Potassium-losing effect of aldosterone (aldosterone is stimulated by FVD)
5. Loss of potassium with osmotic diuresis
6. Severe anorexia (reducing intake) and vomiting (increasing loss of potassium)

Before treatment, the patient with DKA may have a normal or elevated serum potassium level, although there is a marked deficit of total body potassium. Factors that tend to elevate the serum potassium level in the untreated patient include:

- Plasma volume contraction with oliguria, which interferes with renal excretion of potassium
- Metabolic acidosis (potassium shifts out of the cells into the extracellular compartment as hydrogen is buffered intracellularly)

This hyperkalemia is quickly alleviated by fluid replacement therapy and reestablishment of urine output. After treatment is begun, the serum potassium level decreases rapidly and usually reaches its lowest point within 1 to 4 hours. Reasons for the decreased serum potassium level at this time include:

- Dilution by the intravenous (IV) fluids
- Increased urinary potassium excretion due to plasma volume expansion
- Formation of glycogen within the cells using potassium, glucose, and water from the ECF (a shift of potassium into the cells)
- Correction of acidosis with reentry of potassium into the cells

Because insulin tends to lower serum potassium levels by enhancing its movement back into cells, it is believed that use of low-dose insulin therapy in the management of DKA is less likely to be associated with rapid decreases in serum potassium than is the use of high-dose insulin therapy.

Phosphorus

Hypophosphatemia almost invariably occurs during treatment in the patient with DKA and for many of the same reasons that hypokalemia occurs. (Recall that both imbalances involve primarily cellular electrolytes.) One potentially serious consequence of phosphorus deficiency is decreased erythrocyte 2,3-diphosphoglycerate (2,3-DPG); a low level of 2,3-DPG may result in decreased peripheral oxygen delivery. Decreased myocardial function has also been observed when the serum phosphate concentration is less than 2 mg/dL.[17] When the serum phosphate concentration decreases to less than 0.5 mg/dL, serious disturbances in metabolism and neurological abnormalities (both central and peripheral) may result; seizures, respiratory failure, impaired leukocyte and platelet function, abnormal skeletal muscle function, and gastrointestinal bleeding have been reported.[18]

Sodium

Plasma sodium concentration is usually below normal; this is partly due to hyperosmolality of the ECF. Accumulation of glucose in the ECF creates an osmotic gradient, causing water to be pulled out of the cells into the ECF and resulting in dilution of the plasma sodium level. If vomiting is present, the hyponatremia becomes more severe. Sodium also moves into the cells as they become depleted of potassium, further lowering the plasma sodium level.

KETOSIS

Severe insulin deficiency causes excessive hydrolysis of triglycerides (from peripheral fat stores) yielding a greater release of free fatty acids (FFA) and glycerol and activates ketogenic pathways in the liver. The excess fatty acids are converted by the liver to ketones, resulting in ketosis. The insulin deficiency also interferes with uptake of the ketones by peripheral tissues, further increasing the buildup of ketones in the bloodstream. The ketones (ketoacids) present in DKA are β-hydroxybutyrate and acetoacetate. Because ketones are strong acids, with one hydrogen ion created with each ion of β-hydroxybutyrate and acetoacetate, this overproduction and impaired metabolism soon overload the body's buffers, resulting in metabolic acidosis.[19] The anionic charge of bicarbonate is replaced by the negatively charged ketones.

The type of metabolic acidosis that occurs in DKA is manifested by a decrease in bicarbonate with a reciprocal increase in the anion gap (AG) as large amounts of unmeasured anions are produced. Calculate AG using the following formula:

$$AG = Na - (HCO_3 + Cl) = 12 - 15 \text{ mEq/L}$$

Example: Patient with ketoacidosis:

Na = 131 mEq/L
Cl = 95 mEQ/L
HCO_3 = 5 mEq/L

$$AG = 131 - (5 + 95) = 31 \text{ mEq/L}$$

Calculation of AG is important in the assessment of acid–base disturbances in DKA because other findings may be misleading. For example, the vomiting that frequently accompanies DKA can superimpose a metabolic alkalosis on the preexisting ketoacidosis, making the plasma pH appear nearly normal. Measurement of the AG will reveal the abnormal levels of ketone ions that are disrupting metabolism.

Excessive ketosis leads to ketonuria and even excretion of volatile acetone from the lungs (resulting in the classic "fruity" odor of the breath associated with DKA). It is not unusual for the plasma pH to drop to 7.25 or below and for the bicarbonate level to drop to 12 mEq/L or less. Possibly the greatest risks of prolonged uncorrected acidosis are decreased cardiac function, arrhythmia, and impaired hepatic handling of lactate.[20]

The body attempts to compensate for the metabolic acidosis associated with DKA by means of the kidneys and lungs. The kidneys eliminate hydrogen ions and conserve bicarbonate ions, resulting in decreased urinary pH. The lungs attempt to lighten the acid load by blowing off extra carbon dioxide, resulting in the deep, rapid breathing known as Kussmaul respiration. The expected decrease in arterial carbon dioxide pressure ($PaCO_2$) to compensate for metabolic acidosis can be calculated by the following formula:

$$\text{Expected } PaCO_2 \text{ (mm Hg)} = 1.5 \, (HCO_3) + 8 \pm 2$$

Example: The expected $PaCO_2$ in a patient with a bicarbonate level of 12 mEq/L would be between 24 and 28 mm Hg:

$$PaCO_2 = 1.5 \, (12) + 8 \pm 2 = 24\text{--}28 \text{ mm Hg}$$

A decrease below the calculated amount indicates a superimposed respiratory alkalosis; failure of the $PaCO_2$ to decrease to the expected level indicates a complicating respiratory acidosis (a dangerous combination).

It is usual practice to obtain arterial blood gas values when a patient is suspected of having DKA. When these data are not available, findings from venous blood can be useful in determining the degree of acidosis present. For example, a recent study found a high correlation between results from arterial and venous blood specimens in a group of patients with DKA.[21]

● HYPEROSMOLAR HYPERGLYCEMIC NONKETOTIC SYNDROME

Hyperosmolar hyperglycemic nonketotic syndrome is a disorder that develops in middle-aged or elderly type 2 diabetics (sometimes not yet diagnosed), often as a result of stress caused by physical impairment such as renal or cardiovascular disease, infections, or effects of pharmacological therapy with drugs such as steroids or diuretics. Too rapid introduction of total parenteral nutrition (TPN) may also precipitate HHNS (see Chap. 11). The condition develops more slowly than DKA; it is not uncommon for patients to experience polyuria, polydipsia, weight loss, and weakness for days and even weeks before seeking medical attention. Impaired thirst mechanism or impaired ability to replace fluids will exacerbate the tendency toward HHNS. Hyperglycemia may be extreme (> 600 mg/dL and generally between 1000 and 2000 mg/dL), but without the ketosis of DKA.[22–24] The plasma pH is usually normal or only slightly low. The absence of ketoacidosis was formerly attributed to the higher residual insulin levels in these patients, but this explanation is no longer considered entirely adequate.[25,26]

The FVD is profound in HHNS and may be life-threatening. Some sources report mortality rates as high as 50%, depending on the severity of the hyperosmolality and the occurrence of sequelae such as thromboembolic and respiratory complications.[27] Death from HHNS is associated with factors such as advanced age (> 70 years), nursing home residency, hyperosmolality, and hypernatremia.[28]

Although there is a deficit of total body sodium, the serum sodium level may be normal or elevated because of a relatively greater loss of water. The plasma bicarbonate level is normal or slightly reduced. The BUN is usually more elevated than in DKA (60–90 mg/dL) and reflects the more severe FVD and the catabolic state. The serum creatinine is often elevated in HHNS, reflecting the common association of HHNS with underlying renal impairment. Potassium and phosphate depletion may occur, as they do in DKA.

RULING OUT HYPOGLYCEMIA AND OTHER CAUSES OF COMA

Hypoglycemia can often be seen in the individual treated with oral diabetes medications as well as the person requiring insulin and occurs as a result of a mismatch of nutrient intake, activity level, and medication timing. Characteristically, signs and symptoms of hypoglycemia can be divided into two major categories, neurogenic and neuroglycopenic. The neurogenic symptoms are those associated with triggering of the autonomic nervous system and the release of epinephrine or acetylcholine from autonomic neurons or epinephrine from the adrenal medulla. The neuroglycopenic symptoms are associated with a lack of glucose availability to the brain with resultant cerebral dysfunction.[29]

Clinically, hypoglycemia can be divided into mild and severe. Mild hypoglycemia is recognized and appropriately treated by the individual. Symptoms such as sweating, excessive hunger, palpitations, tachycardia, and nervousness are characteristic of mild hypoglycemia. Severe hypoglycemia is characterized by unresponsiveness, unconsciousness, or convulsions and always requires the assistance of another person for treatment.[30] With the advent of intensive therapy for the treatment of diabetes and prevention of the chronic complications, a two- to threefold increase in severe hypoglycemia has been seen.[31] Thus, the incidence of severe hypoglycemia occurring in the home setting or community may increase as more patients are practicing intensive therapy for glucose management.

In treating an unconscious diabetic patient, it should be determined whether hyperglycemia or hypoglycemia exists. When in doubt, in a hospital setting, an emergency room, or an environment with paramedical assistance, it is best that IV glucose in the dose of 25 g be administered (one ampule of $D_{50}W$).[32] Outside of the hospital setting or when IV access is unavailable, a 1-mg intramuscular injection of glucagon is the treatment of choice, although it has a slightly slower and less predictable recovery rate than IV glucose.[33] With either treatment, if hypoglycemia is the problem, the patient's condition will improve quickly; if DKA or HHNS is the problem, the small amount of dextrose or the mobilization of hepatic glycogen stores by glucagon will do no harm. Of course, a blood glucose determination should be made as quickly as possible.

Serum glucose measurement is an important first step in the evaluation of the diabetic patient with altered consciousness. A finding of hypoglycemia or hyperglycemia, however, may not fully explain the cause of the altered consciousness or coma. A thorough evaluation is needed so that other pathology, such as stroke, uremia, or drug intoxication, does not go untreated. Conversely, the signs and symptoms of hypoglycemia or hyperglycemia may mimic other conditions; for example, abdominal pain in patients with DKA may simulate an abdominal emergency. For this reason, even when there is no history of diabetes, serum glucose should be measured promptly in acutely ill patients. Recall that DKA or HHNS may be the first manifestation of diabetes in some individuals. Patients with alcoholic ketoacidosis may also occasionally have some degree of hyperglycemia, making differential diagnosis problematic.[34]

TREATMENT OF DIABETIC KETOACIDOSIS AND HYPEROSMOLAR HYPERGLYCEMIC NONKETOTIC SYNDROME

FLUID REPLACEMENT

Adequate and prompt rehydration is vital and must consider the patient's cardiovascular and renal status. Fluid replacement is usually begun with the administration of 1 to 3 liters of isotonic saline (0.9% NaCl) infused at the rate of about 1 L/hr. Isotonic (normal) saline will expand the ECF and will begin to correct the hyperosmolality. In some patients with HHNS in whom there is significant hypernatremia, hypertension, or risk for congestive heart failure, half-strength saline (0.45% NaCl) may be used. When there is a concern about the adequacy of the patient's cardiovascular status, central venous pressure or hemodynamic monitoring may be needed to help gauge the best rate of fluid replacement. Total fluid intake in 8 hours should not exceed 5 liters.[35]

After the initial infusion of normal saline, the IV fluid may be changed to half-strength saline to dilute the hyperosmolar plasma and provide free water for renal excretion. As fluid replacement continues, the rate and volume will be determined by the status of the patient. Patients with HHNS may need larger amounts of fluids to correct the FVD. When the plasma glucose levels decrease to the range of 250 to 300 mg/dL, solutions containing 5% dextrose should be used to prevent hypoglycemia and other complications that might occur as a result of a too rapid fall in blood glucose level. As soon as oral intake is adequate, IV fluids can be discontinued.

INSULIN ADMINISTRATION

The aim of insulin therapy is to give enough rapid-acting (Lispro) or short-acting (Regular) insulin to correct the problem without subjecting the patient to the risk of hypoglycemia. Regular insulin and Lispro are the only clear insulin preparations. Regular insulin is the only insulin product routinely used for IV administration although theoretically Lispro may also be given IV. (Lispro is an insulin analog identical to human insulin in structure with the exception of the juxtaposition of lysine and proline in positions 28 and 29 on the beta chain of the insulin molecule. This molecular alteration yields an insulin with a faster rate of absorption than regular human insulin. Lispro tends to peak in one-half the time and double the concentration of a comparable dose of regular insulin and is used immediately before eating to provide better coverage of postprandial glycemic excursions.[36]) Although it can also be given intramuscularly or subcutaneously, the continuous IV route is best for the very ill patient because absorption of insulin from poorly perfused muscle and fat depots may be erratic, especially if the patient is hypotensive.

Studies have demonstrated that large insulin doses are generally no more effective in correcting DKA than small doses. The low-dose regimen lowers blood sugar concentrations smoothly, improves ketosis, and repairs acidosis at rates indistinguishable from those obtained by higher dose regimens. In addition, patients are less likely to develop hypoglycemia and hypokalemia than are patients receiving large doses.[37] Of course, when

low doses do not achieve the desired effect, as in cases of insulin "resistance," larger doses must be given. Patients with HHNS will require somewhat less insulin than those with DKA.

The insulin dose for continuous IV infusion is usually 4 to 10 U/hr or 0.1 U/kg/hr. Sometimes an initial bolus of 5 to 10 units is given when therapy is initiated, although some studies have not documented any benefits from such a bolus.[38,39] The adsorption of insulin to IV containers and tubing has been documented, but there is disagreement about the extent to which it affects insulin delivery, particularly in low-dose therapy. To minimize the effect of adsorption, the infusion set should be flushed with the insulin solution to saturate the binding sites before connecting it to the patient. According to Peterson et al.,[40] the insulin-binding effect will be minimal if the solution contains a concentration of at least 25 units insulin to 500 mL saline and 50 mL of the solution is flushed through the entire apparatus before it is infused into the patient.

Of primary importance is the individualization of the dosage of insulin to the response of the patient and adjustment of that dosage on the basis of ongoing blood glucose determinations. After initiation of IV insulin therapy, if no improvement in blood pH, AG, bicarbonate, or plasma glucose is seen in 2 to 3 hours, the insulin infusion rate can be doubled.[41] A too rapid drop in blood glucose level creates the risk of complications such as hypoglycemia and hypokalemia. There is also a risk that cerebral edema may occur from the osmotic gradient created between brain and serum osmolality by a too rapid decline in blood glucose concentration.[42] Although cerebral edema is an uncommon occurrence in adults, it can be fatal in children or lead to developmental disabilities for years after resolution of the DKA episode.[43] A controlled-rate infusion pump should be used to ensure accurate administration of the insulin. If one is not available, the solutions should be administered through a volume-controlled administration set. When the patient's condition is sufficiently stabilized, the insulin can be administered subcutaneously.

ELECTROLYTE REPLACEMENT

Potassium

Potassium is not added to the IV fluids until the first 2 or 3 liters has been administered and adequate urinary output has been established, unless serum potassium levels have already decreased to normal or below. Potassium replacement is usually accomplished by adding 20 to 40 mEq potassium chloride or potassium phosphate to 1 liter of 0.45% NaCl, infused at a rate appropriate to the status of the patient. Occasionally, larger amounts of potassium are needed if the hypokalemia is severe. Because the IV administration of potassium is always associated with risk of hyperkalemia, it is wise to monitor the serum potassium level at 1- or 2-hour intervals and to use serial electrocardiogram (ECG) tracings. (Rules for safe potassium administration are discussed in Chap. 5, Clinical Tip: Nursing Considerations in Administering Potassium Intravenously.) Oral potassium-containing fluids may be given when the patient is able to tolerate them.

Phosphorus

Because phosphate is lost during the osmotic diuresis of DKA and HHNS, some authorities favor replacing at least a part of the lost potassium with potassium phosphate. This can also reduce the risk of hyperchloremia associated with sole use of potassium chloride salts.[44] It is imperative, however, that significant renal failure be ruled out before phosphate is administered IV; serum phosphate levels should be monitored to prevent possible hyperphosphatemia. Administering too much phosphate can induce hypocalcemia; therefore, calcium levels should also be monitored if phosphate is administered. When oral intake is tolerated, skim milk is a good source of phosphorus. It is thought that phosphate replacement accelerates the recovery of reduced red blood cell 2,3-DPG levels, thereby decreasing hemoglobin–oxygen affinity and improving tissue oxygenation.

Bicarbonate

There has been controversy over the use of bicarbonate in the treatment of DKA. It is used for management of hyperkalemia and is generally considered to be necessary in cases of severe acidosis (pH < 7.1).[45] When bicarbonate is used to correct pH, it is not corrected above a level of 7.1; to normalize the pH could result in paradoxical central nervous system (CNS) acidosis.[46] Too rapid correction of acidosis can also induce hypokalemia (as potassium shifts into the cells). When bicarbonate is given, it should be infused with the IV fluids, not administered by bolus. Some authorities believe that bicarbonate replacement is unnecessary

because insulin therapy reverses the biochemical abnormalities of DKA including the bicarbonate deficit.

Sodium

Isotonic saline that is administered initially supplies enough sodium to correct any sodium loss. Because the patient with DKA or HHNS may lose proportionately more water than sodium, a hypotonic solution (such as 0.45% NaCl) will be ordered after the 2 to 3 liters of isotonic saline. Hypotonic solutions provide free water to correct cellular dehydration.

Other Electrolytes

Losses of calcium and magnesium may occur as a result of the osmotic diuresis. Often they are not considered of clinical consequence, but in some cases, magnesium is replaced if renal function is adequate.[47]

TREATMENT OF PRECIPITATING FACTORS

In addition to the above therapies, treatment will include identification and treatment of concurrent health problems, particularly those that might have been precipitating factors in the development of DKA or HHNS. Table 18-2 lists common precipitating factors for each condition.

● USE OF THE NURSING PROCESS

NURSING ASSESSMENT

Nursing care of the patient with HHNS or DKA involves meticulous, ongoing assessment to detect significant changes. Tables 18-3 and 18-4 outline the clinical manifestations of DKA and HHNS. To achieve ongoing assessment, it is best to use a diabetic flow sheet, which often includes the following data:

1. Vital signs (blood pressure, temperature, pulse, and respirations)
2. Weight
3. Fluid therapy (type, amount, and flow rate)
4. Insulin therapy (number of units per hour IV, intramuscularly, and subcutaneously)
5. Hourly urine volume

TABLE 18-2.   Factors Contributing to Development of DKA or HHNS in Susceptible Patients

Diabetic Ketoacidosis (DKA)	Hyperosmolar Hyperglycemic Nonketotic Syndrome (HHNS)
Infections, illness	Chronic renal disease
Physiological stresses (eg, trauma, surgery, myocardial infarction, dehydration, pregnancy)	Chronic cardiovascular disease
	Acute illness, infection
	Surgery, burns, trauma
Psychological/emotional stress	Hyperalimentation, tube feedings
Omission/reduction of insulin	Peritoneal dialysis
Failure of insulin delivery system (pump)	Mannitol therapy
Excess alcohol intake	Pharmacological agents:
	• Chlorpromazine
	• Cimetidine
	• Diazoxide
	• Diuretics (thiazide, thiazide-related, and loop diuretics)
	• Glucocorticoids and immunosuppressive agents
	• L-asparaginase
	• Phenytoin
	• Propanolol

6. ECG tracings
7. Level of consciousness
8. Deep-tendon reflexes
9. Relevant laboratory data, which may include:
   • Blood glucose (bedside)
   • Blood and urine ketones
   • Arterial blood gases (pH, $PaCO_2$, PaO_2, HCO_3)
   • Potassium
   • Magnesium
   • Bicarbonate
   • Sodium and chloride
   • Calcium and phosphorus
   • BUN and creatinine
   • White blood cell count
   • Hematocrit
10. Calculations
    • AG
    • Serum osmolality

Decisions as to which of the above parameters will be monitored, by whom, and at what intervals will be made based on the patient's status and protocols related to the care setting (such as the emergency room, critical care unit, and nursing unit). Response to therapy must be observed and recorded carefully. This involves constant vigilance over the patient's clinical status so that critical judgments can be made to provide optimal therapy.

NURSING DIAGNOSES

Although many nursing diagnoses are relevant to the diabetic patient, Clinical Tip: Examples of Nursing Diagnoses Related to Patients With Diabetic Ketoacidosis or Hyperosmolar Hyperglycemic Nonketotic Syndrome deals with diagnoses that relate primarily to fluid, electrolyte, and acid–base balance aspects of nursing care of patients with, or at risk for, DKA or HHNS. The listed etiologies and defining characteristics are those most likely to be applicable. In some situations, there may be others. Chapters 3 through 9 provide detailed descriptions of specific imbalances.

NURSING INTERVENTIONS

Nursing care of the patient with DKA or HHNS is complex and involves many traditional nursing actions plus sophisticated monitoring of the responses to medical therapy. The care plan includes many interventions that relate to the fluid and electrolyte status of the patient. Some of those most frequently used are outlined below.

TABLE 18-3.   Clinical Signs of DKA and Their Probable Causes

Clinical Signs	Probable Causes
Hyperglycemia (Normal blood glucose is 80–120 mg/dL. Elevations associated with DKA may be as high as 4000 mg/dL.)	Faulty glucose metabolism causes glucose to accumulate in the bloodstream (lack of insulin decreases glucose uptake by most cells and also increases gluconeogenesis in the liver)
Glucosuria	Blood glucose level exceeds renal threshold (normally 180 mg/dL, higher in the elderly) causing glucose to spill into the urine
Polyuria (initially) with high specific gravity	Osmotic diuretic effect of hyperglycemia, high renal solute load
Polydipsia	Thirst due to cellular dehydration (cells become dehydrated when water is drawn from them by the hypertonic ECF)
Anorexia, nausea, vomiting	Follows onset of DKA; interferes with fluid intake (hastening the development of fluid volume deficit)
Poor skin turgor, dry mucous membranes, poor tongue turgor	FVD
Acute weight loss	FVD (parallels degree of this imbalance)
Ketonemia and ketonuria	Excessive accumulation of ketones in the bloodstream causes them to spill out into the urine
Cherry red skin and mucous membranes	Marked peripheral vasodilatation associated with ketosis
Deep "air hunger" respirations (Kussmaul)	Compensatory mechanism to increase plasma pH by the elimination of large amounts of carbon dioxide
Acetone odor to breath (similar to that of overripe apples)	Acetone, a volatile ketone, is vaporized in the expired air (may be obscured by the odor of vomitus)
Abdominal pain (can simulate acute appendicitis, pancreatitis, or other acute abdominal problems)	Apparently due to the DKA per se (Note: Anorexia, nausea, and vomiting precede the abdominal pain when it is due to DKA; this is in contrast to most surgical emergencies in which the pain usually occurs first.)
Postural hypotension	FVD (eventually may be hypotensive even when supine)
Fatigue, muscular weakness	Lack of carbohydrate utilization, hypokalemia
Hypothermia or normal temperature	Fever is present only when there is a concurrent illness causing it
Blurred vision	Osmotic changes in lenses of eyes
Oliguria, anuria (late)	FVD causes decreased renal blood flow and decreased GFR. (Before assuming that urine formation is scanty, check for a distended, atonic bladder.)
Depressed sensorium (ranging from somnolence to frank coma)	Level of consciousness correlates best with level of hyperglycemia and plasma osmolality

🔵 **TABLE 18-3.** Clinical Signs of DKA and Their Probable Causes—*cont'd*

Clinical Signs	Probable Causes
Laboratory Data	
Hyperglycemia	Related to insulin lack (see above)
Elevated serum osmolality (normal; 280–295 mOsm/kg)	Related primarily to high glucose level; elevated BUN contributes to elevated level
Potassium variations	Serum potassium concentration may be elevated before treatment; later, however, may drop to seriously low levels (see explanation in text)
Hypophosphatemia	Osmotic diuresis
Increased BUN (often increased to 40 mg/dL; normal is 10–20 mg/dL)	Fluid volume deficit, decreased GFR, increased protein metabolism, increased hepatic production of urea (due to insulin lack)
Increased creatinine (normal is 0.7–1.5 mg/dL)	Prerenal azotemia due to FVD
Leukocytosis	FVD, acidosis, adrenocortical stimulation
Decreased serum bicarbonate (usually < 15 mEq/L, may be extremely low; normal is 24 mEq/L)	Excessive ketonic anions in the bloodstream cause a compensatory drop in bicarbonate
Decreased arterial pH (usually < 7.25; may be as low as 6.8 in severe cases; normal is 7.35–7.45)	Associated with the metabolic acidosis caused by ketosis
High anion gap (AG) acidosis (normal AG is < 12–15 mEq/L)	Due to excessive ketones in the bloodstream
Increased hemoglobin, hematocrit, total protein	FVD (causes concentration of formed elements in blood)
Increased liver function tests	Does not necessarily reflect acute or chronic liver damage, as most often values return to normal in several weeks

1. Monitor degree of FVD and response to fluid replacement therapy.
   A. Assess blood pressure (supine and sitting, if possible) and pulse. (A drop in systolic pressure by more than 10 to 15 mm Hg on position change from lying to sitting is indicative of FVD. Remember that a severely volume-depleted patient will be hypotensive even in the supine position. The pulse will be rapid and of a weak volume as the heart pumps faster to compensate for the below-normal plasma volume.
   B. Observe neck veins. (Collapse of the neck veins when the head is raised is a sign of FVD.)
   C. Check skin and tongue turgor and degree of moisture of mucous membranes.
   D. Monitor urinary output.
      i. If patient is too stuporous to void, insert a retention catheter, using meticulous aseptic technique. (Recall that diabetic patients are very prone to urinary infections.) Remove the catheter as soon as the patient is able to empty the bladder by voiding.
      ii. Measure hourly urine volume in a device calibrated for accurate reading of small amounts (see Fig. 2-7). (Output should be at least 30–50 mL/hr. Oliguria related to FVD can lead to renal tubular damage and must be prevented. The hourly urinary output should

TABLE 18-4.   Summary of Hyperosmolar Hyperglycemic Nonketotic Syndrome

The typical patient at risk for HHNS has either undiagnosed diabetes or type 2 diabetes managed with oral diabetes medications, insulin, or diet alone; the typical patient at risk for DKA requires insulin for everyday management and to sustain life.

HHNS tends to occur in middle-aged or elderly type 2 diabetics, often those suffering from underlying renal and cardiovascular impairment. In at-risk patients, the condition is often precipitated by the stress of an acute illness or by treatment with corticosteroids, diuretics, mannitol, phenytoin, and glucose solutions.

Onset of HHNS tends to be more gradual and insidious than that of DKA. (It is not uncommon for patients to experience polyuria, polydipsia, weight loss, and weakness for many days, and even weeks, before seeking medical attention.)

Hyperglycemia and related symptoms of hyperosmolality are often more pronounced in HHNS than in DKA. Abnormal neurological signs may occur, such as focal or generalized seizures. If water loss leads to hypernatremia, fever may occur.

HHNS is not associated with ketoacidosis; it has been postulated that in HHNS there is sufficient insulin to prevent ketosis but not enough to prevent hyperglycemia.

---

increase if parenteral fluid replacement is adequate. Report a urine volume of < 30 mL/hr as well as failure of output to increase with fluid replacement.)

 iii. Measure SG of urine. (Urinary SG is elevated in FVD; if low with a scanty volume, renal damage may be present and should be reported. Heavy glucosuria invalidates SG readings; see Table 2-3.)

 iv. Compare the 8-hr and 24-hr intake and output as well as the total output. (During treatment, intake must exceed output until the FVD is corrected.)

 v. Monitor the BUN and creatinine levels. (An elevated BUN reflects FVD when elevated out of proportion to the serum creatinine level. See Table 2-2 for further discussion of these tests.)

E. Calculate the approximate degree of FVD.

 i. Weigh patient on admission and ascertain, if possible, the preillness weight. (A rapid loss of 1 kg [2.2 lb] of body weight is roughly equivalent to a loss of 1 liter of body fluid. Loss of weight from not eating may amount to 0.5 lb/day. Acute weight loss of 5% body weight constitutes a moderate FVD; 8% or greater is a severe FVD. Many cases have been reported in which as

much as 10% to 20% of body weight has been lost acutely in patients with DKA and HHNS).

 ii. Weigh patient each morning before breakfast. (Monitor for acute changes in body weight; anticipate that weight gain will parallel correction of the FVD.)

 iii. If preillness weight cannot be determined, FVD may be calculated with a formula using the patient's plasma osmolality:

$$\text{FVD (L)} = \frac{(\text{Patient's pOsm} - \text{Normal osmolality})}{\text{Normal osmolality}} \times$$

$$\text{Liters of body fluid (0.6} \times \text{Body wt in kg)}$$

Example: Assume an adult patient has a plasma osmolality of 340 mOsm/kg and weighs 70 kg. (Use 280 mOsm/kg as the normal value.):

$$\text{Liters of body fluid} = 0.6 \times 70 = 42$$
$$\text{FVD (L)} = (340 - 280)/280 \times 42 = 9 \text{ L}$$

F. Monitor neurological status. Look for depressed sensorium and focal neurological signs. A depressed sensorium results most often from hyperosmolality of body fluids and occurs to some degree in most cases of DKA and HHNS. Because of this it is necessary to consider the following points:

CLINICAL TIP

Examples of Nursing Diagnoses Related to Patients With Diabetic Ketoacidosis or Hyperosmolar Hyperglycemic Nonketotic Syndrome

NURSING DIAGNOSIS	ETIOLOGICAL FACTORS	DEFINING CHARACTERISTICS
Fluid volume deficit related to hyperosmotic diuresis	Hyperglycemia Hyperosmolality	Initially: Polyuria Later: Oliguria or anuria Other symptoms of FVD (see Chap. 3)
Alteration in potassium balance (hypokalemia) related to increased potassium loss and insulin therapy (shift into cells)	Osmotic diuresis Dilution by IV fluids Increased excretion Reentry into cells	Drop in serum potassium for 1–4 hours after therapy (symptoms of hypokalemia in Chap. 5)
Alteration in tissue perfusion: Renal, related to FVD	Severe FVD Decreased GFR Decreased renal blood flow	Oliguria or anuria are symptoms of prerenal failure (see Chap. 17)
Alteration in phosphorus balance (hypophosphatemia) and magnesium balance (hypomagnesemia) related to osmotic diuresis and insulin therapy	Osmotic diuresis Rapid fall in levels (especially phosphate) once fluid therapy is begun Reentry into cells	Symptoms of hypophosphatemia (see Chap. 8) Symptoms of hypomagnesemia (see Chap. 7)
Alteration in acid–base balance (metabolic acidosis) related to increased production and decreased use of ketones in DKA	Insulin deficiency in type 1 diabetes Increased activity of counter-regulatory hormones Release of FFA from peripheral fat stores	Ketonemia Decreased plasma pH Ketonuria Decreased plasma HCO_3 Elevated anion gap Kussmaul respirations "Fruity" breath odor Clinical signs of acidosis (see Chap. 9)
Alteration in nutrition: less than body requirements, related to insulin deficiency	Decreased glucose uptake and storage Decreased protein synthesis and fat assimilation Gastric retention Anorexia, nausea, and vomiting	Early: Weight loss and hunger in spite of adequate food intake; abdominal pain Later: Reduction in muscle mass and fat stores
Sensory-perceptual alteration related to effects of DKA and HHNS	Elevated serum osmolality FVD Severe elevated BUN Acidemia in DKA	Changes in level of consciousness Change in usual response to sensory stimuli
Risk for hypoglycemia related to insulin therapy	Insufficient dextrose in IV fluids Erratic absorption of insulin from peripheral sites Excess insulin	Rapid drop in blood glucose Negative urine glucose

Continued

CLINICAL TIP

Examples of Nursing Diagnoses Related to Patients With Diabetic Ketoacidosis or Hyperosmolar Hyperglycemic Nonketotic Syndrome—*cont'd*

NURSING DIAGNOSIS	ETIOLOGICAL FACTORS	DEFINING CHARACTERISTICS
Risk for uncontrolled diabetes related to inadequate management or stress factors	Insulin supply or use not adequate for metabolic needs Food intake excessive for exogenous or endogenous insulin supply Physiological or psychological stressors such as illness, surgery, personal crisis	Lack of adjustment of regimen during illness, infection, or severe emotional stress Decreased insulin dosage when food intake decreases Manipulation of insulin dose related to fear of hypoglycemic reaction Inadequate health care during periods of illness or severe crisis
Potential for HHNS related to pharmacologic or other medical therapy	Type 2 elderly diabetic receiving drugs or therapies that can precipitate HHNS (see Table 18-2)	Hyperglycemia Polyuria Water intake inadequate to compensate for osmotic diuresis
Knowledge deficit of diabetic sick day management related to lack of exposure to diabetic sick day guidelines	No previous history of attending diabetic education program Poor understanding of diabetic sick day management	Does not follow sick day diet; does not monitor blood glucose levels; does not manipulate insulin dosage during illness
Ineffective management of therapeutic regimen related to complexity of diabetes regimen	Lack of understanding of diabetes regimen Patient's denial of the importance of the diabetes regimen	Does not take insulin or oral diabetes agents as prescribed; does not regularly self-monitor blood glucose levels; does not follow appropriate dietary recommendations.

FFA, free fatty acid; FVD, fluid volume deficit; DKA, diabetic ketoacidosis; HHNS, hyperosmolar hyperglycemic nonketotic syndrome; GFR, glomerular filtration rate.

---

i. Maintain an adequate airway (a comatose patient with airway obstruction will require intubation).

ii. Insert nasogastric tube when indicated (gastric retention with regurgitation of contents is not uncommon).

G. Regulate fluid replacement rate and volume according to protocol and patient status. Consider the following facts:

i. After the initial infusion of saline solutions to rehydrate the patient, dextrose solutions are indicated to keep the serum glucose from falling too rapidly.

ii. Central venous pressure or hemodynamic monitoring may be needed in elderly patients and those with compromised cardiovascular or renal status.

iii. The patient with HHNS may need larger amounts of fluid than the patient with DKA because the degree of FVD is often worse in HHNS.

2. Monitor electrolyte status and response to replacement therapy.

A. Monitor potassium levels at frequent intervals (1–2 hours) during the initial period of therapy. (The initial serum potassium level may be normal or elevated because of plasma volume contraction and shift from the intracellular fluid to the ECF; the potassium level drops rapidly with plasma dilution and reentry of potassium into the cells. Replacement therapy after the first 2 to 3 liters of fluid should prevent a precipitous drop in serum potassium. Recall that potassium should not be administered to a patient with oliguria. See Chap. 5 for nursing considerations in the safe administration of potassium solutions.)

B. Use serial ECG tracings and other appropriate assessment parameters to detect effects of hypokalemia and to monitor responses to potassium infusion (see Chap. 5).

C. Promptly report abnormal laboratory levels of other electrolytes, such as a low phosphorus level. (Recall that decreased serum phosphorus levels often parallel those of low potassium. In fact, these electrolytes are often replaced together, in the form of potassium phosphate. See Chap. 8 for a description of hypophosphatemia.)

3. Monitor degree of hyperglycemia and response to insulin therapy.

A. Monitor blood sugar levels closely by use of capillary blood (finger stick) and a blood glucose meter plus regular laboratory determinations. Of course, a decrease in the plasma glucose level is the earliest sign of effective therapy.[48] (Recall that blood sugar determinations are much more accurate than urine glucose tests. Renal threshold varies among individuals, increases with age, and may be affected by renal disease.)

B. Monitor administration of insulin-containing IV infusions to prevent too rapid decrease in blood sugar level and serum osmolality. (Cerebral edema may occur with a too rapid drop in blood sugar levels. Blood glucose should decrease at an optimum rate of 60–120 mg/dL/hr.[49] At a blood glucose level of 250 mg/dL, IV solutions containing dextrose in saline should be used for both fluid replacement and insulin infusion to prevent the development of hypoglycemia.[50–52] Some clinicians recommend maintaining the serum glucose level at about 200 mg/dL for the first 12–24 hours before allowing it to decrease to a normal level.)[53]

C. Observe the patient closely to prevent occurrence of hypoglycemia, and evaluate serum glucose measurements. (Hypoglycemia can be a major complication of therapy. A recent retrospective study indicated that 30% of patients hospitalized with DKA developed hypoglycemia during the first 14 days of treatment.[54] In the study, the risk of hypoglycemia

was increased by the presence of fever, hepatic disease, renal disease, and "nothing by mouth" status.[55] When severe, hypoglycemia may have serious CNS effects and is potentially fatal. Of course, one should report a rapid drop in blood sugar level.)

4. Monitor altered acid–base balance (acidemia) and response to therapy, especially in type 1 diabetic patients with DKA.

A. Monitor serum and urine ketones. (As a result of overproduction and decreased use, ketones build up in the blood and are excreted in the urine.)

B. Observe rate and depth of respirations. (Extra carbon dioxide is blown off by Kussmaul respirations, which are stimulated by the acidemia and help to bring the arterial pH back toward normal. Be alert for a change from deep, rapid respirations to rapid, shallow, gasping breaths. This may indicate a severe drop in blood pH < 7 or impaired flow to the respiratory center because of FVD and circulatory collapse. The patient loses the compensatory action of Kussmaul breathing when this occurs and the acidosis becomes more severe.)

C. Check for "fruity" breath odor. (This occurs as acetone is excreted from the lungs but may be masked by the odor of vomitus.)

D. Observe for cherry-red color of skin and mucous membranes. (This is characteristic of DKA due to marked peripheral vasodilation; improvement of skin color indicates response to therapy.)

E. Observe for signs of decreased cardiac function and arrhythmias. (This constitutes the greatest risk of prolonged, uncontrolled acidosis.)

F. Monitor blood and urine pH and serum bicarbonate levels. (Plasma pH may fall to 7.25 or below and urine pH falls as kidneys eliminate hydrogen ions in an attempt to correct the acidosis. The serum HCO_3 may fall to 12 mEq/L or lower. An increase in serum bicarbonate to 15–20 mEq/L may be expected usually between 12 and 24 hours after treatment has begun.)[56]

G. Assess for presence and characteristics of abdominal pain. (Abdominal pain may occur in DKA and is preceded by nausea and vomiting. Other abdominal emergencies [eg, pancreatitis and surgical abdomen] may coexist with or may have triggered DKA. In these conditions, the pain usually precedes other symptoms.)

5. Use nursing measures to prevent and monitor for other complications that may occur with DKA or HHNS, such as:

    A. Respiratory or urinary tract infections, septic shock, adult respiratory distress syndrome

    B. Thromboembolic complications

    C. CNS deterioration, prolonged coma

    D. Gastrointestinal bleeding

        (These complications have been responsible for deaths in some cases of DKA and HHNS.)

6. Use nursing measures to teach the recovering patient how to prevent recurrences of DKA and HHNS.

    A. Have the patient describe his or her daily routine and demonstrate methods used to carry out the diabetic regimen.[57] This enables one to assess the patient's understanding of the regimen and the degree of accuracy with which procedures such as glucose self-monitoring, meal planning, and insulin administration are being carried out. Some reteaching may be necessary and should be carefully evaluated for effectiveness.

    B. Review with the patient factors that could disrupt control of diabetes, leading to hyperglycemia and DKA or HHNS. (Many persons with diabetes are not aware of the less obvious precipitating factors [see Table 18-2]. The patient should be able to describe the factors and their effect on diabetes control.)

    C. Discuss early symptoms of hyperglycemia with the patient. (Polyuria, polydipsia, polyphagia, fatigue, weakness, blurred vision, and headache should be discussed with the patient as commonly occurring symptoms of poor control.)

    D. Assist the patient to learn a method of testing for elevated serum glucose and ketones. (Self-monitoring of serum glucose with a blood glucose meter is best, but testing with visual strips can also be effective. Ketones can be detected by the urine dipstick method. The patient should demonstrate testing methods in a simulated or real home setting and should interpret the

results accurately.) Instruct the patient to monitor urine ketones anytime the blood glucose level is greater than 240 mg/dL or when illness occurs.

    E. Provide the patient with realistic "sick day instructions" and identify different health care resources for daily routines, in emergencies, and when away from home. (See Clinical Tip: Sick Day Instructions. Stress the importance of keeping regular appointments with the health care provider to prevent loss of control. An after-hours telephone number to be used in serious or emergency situations should be provided when possible. Instruct the patient, when traveling, to seek help at emergency rooms of medical centers or community hospitals.)

    F. Use careful and tactful assessment methods to identify cultural and socioeconomic factors that may interfere with maintaining the diabetes regimen.[58]

        i. Provide services of a social worker or counselor as indicated, especially in cases of recurrent DKA or HHNS.[59]

        ii. Review the meal plan with the client and suggest low-cost substitutes when possible.

        iii. Explore insurance reimbursement policies with the patient and identify less expensive sources of food, equipment, and supplies. (Economic factors such as low income, unemployment, lack of insurance coverage, or pressing family needs may prevent even the most committed patient from maintaining the proper regimen.)

        iv. Make sure the meal plan and exercise and medication schedules have been adjusted to the patient's lifestyle and work schedule. (Shift workers and others who have unusual schedules may experience difficulty maintaining control with a "typical" regimen.)

        v. Tailor instructional materials to the reading and learning level of the patient. (Functional illiteracy and perceptual learning disabilities are more widespread than is commonly recognized.)

        vi. When indicated, include family members or significant others in the education process. (When a family member has diabetes, the whole family must cope with it. Family conflict can interfere with good control. Some patients may need family assistance with certain aspects of the regimen.)

EVALUATION

This important step of the nursing process measures the effectiveness of nursing care for the patient with DKA or HHNS. Evaluation is based on progress made toward short-term and long-term goals.

Short-term goal achievement is demonstrated by:

1. Return of blood sugar to desired levels without any episodes of hypoglycemia
2. Correction of FVD with optimal cardiovascular function and urinary output
3. Electrolyte levels approaching or within normal limits
4. Prevention or correction of complications
5. Prevention of immediate recurrence of DKA or HHNS

Long-term goal achievement is demonstrated by:

1. Control of blood glucose levels within a range appropriate for the individual
2. Prompt intervention when stressors are present that precipitate hyperglycemia
3. Maintenance of general health, growth and development, and activity levels appropriate to the individual

The importance of the nurse's role in the care of the diabetic patient cannot be overemphasized. Skillful use of the nursing process in the care of the patient with DKA or HHNS will contribute greatly to a successful outcome. Equally challenging is the nurse's role as a clinician and health care educator preparing the patient

to maintain control of the diabetes in a way that will prevent recurrences of DKA or HHNS and will enable the best possible level of health.

CASE STUDY

● **18-1.** Mrs. K, a 35-year-old insulin-dependent diabetic, developed viral gastroenteritis with nausea and vomiting. Two days before admission, she omitted her insulin because she was not eating. Her husband brought her to the emergency department because she was becoming increasingly lethargic.

On initial examination, she was found to have tachycardia (pulse rate, 140/min) and deep, rapid (Kussmaul) respirations. Her blood pressure lying flat was 98/70. She was able to void only a few milliliters; the urinary glucose and ketone levels were both 4+. Her skin and mucous membranes were dry and she had a fruity odor to her breath. The following laboratory blood work data were obtained from venous blood:

Glucose = 940 mg/dL
Sodium = 130 mEq/L
Potassium = 6.8 mEq/L
Bicarbonate = 5 mEq/L
BUN = 45 mg/dL
Creatinine = 2.2 mg/dL
Arterial pH = 7.07
Bicarbonate = 2.6 mEq/L
$PaCO_2$ = 13 mm Hg

On the basis of the examination and the laboratory findings, a diagnosis of DKA was made. Mrs. K then was treated with 0.9% sodium chloride IV to correct the FVD and with low-dose regular insulin (5 U/hr). Over the course of the first 16

TABLE 18-5.

Time	Blood Glucose (mg/dL)	Arterial pH	Sodium (mEq/L)	Potassium (mEq/L)	Bicarbonate (mEq/L)	Chloride (mEq/L)	BUN/ Creatinine
5 PM	940	7.07	130	6.8	5	90	45/2.2
7 PM	520		132	6.6	7	100	43/1.9
9 PM	400	7.26	136	4.3	8	105	44/1.6
2 AM	325		140	4.5	16	115	30/1.4
9 AM	300		142	4.4	23	115	22/1.1

CLINICAL TIP

Sick Day Instructions

1. Contact your physician immediately if you have pain, fever, persistent diarrhea, difficulty breathing (rapid, labored respirations), moderate or large ketones, blood glucose levels greater than or equal to 300 mg/dL unresponsive to increased insulin, mental status changes, or you are vomiting and cannot hold down food or liquid.

2. Always take your usual dose of insulin or oral diabetes medication. Never omit your medication even if you are unable to eat.

3. Test your blood glucose level every 3 to 4 hours around the clock or a minimum of four times a day. It is essential that blood glucose levels be tested at least before each meal and at bedtime.

4. If you do not routinely check your blood glucose levels, buy a vial of 25 visual blood glucose strips, a finger lancet device, and lancets to use when you are ill. Check these supplies every 6 months to be sure they have not expired. Once the vial of strips has been opened, they will expire in 4 months.

5. If you have type 1 diabetes and your blood glucose levels are greater than 240 mg/dL, test your urine for ketones. Ketone testing should be done when you are ill from any cause. Patients with type 2 diabetes rarely have ketosis; however, positive nonfasting urine ketones in a patient with type 2 diabetes is a worrisome finding that requires further evaluation. If ketones are present along with high serum glucose levels, you will need extra insulin. Regular (short-acting) or lispro (rapid-acting) insulins should be used. Consult your physician immediately to obtain guidelines for how much regular or lispro insulin you should use and how often to take it. During most illnesses, 10% of the total daily dose can be given safely as a supplemental dose of rapid- or fast-acting insulin every 1 to 4 hours.

6. Drink 8 ounces of caffeine-free and alcohol-free liquid every hour. Fluids that are acceptable are water, caffeine-free tea, consomme, fruit juices, broth made from bouillon cubes, and regular or diet sodas. If your glucose levels are elevated drink calorie-free liquids. If your glucose levels are low and you are unable to eat, drink fluids with calories such as regular soda or Gatorade so that 15 grams of carbohydrate are taken every 1 to 2 hours. If you are unable to take liquids because of nausea and vomiting, consult your physician immediately. A medication may be prescribed to stop the nausea and vomiting.

7. If you cannot follow the usual meal plan, refer to the food suggestions for sick days.

8. Over-the-counter and prescribed medications may contribute to hyperglycemia or hypoglycemia. Consult with your physician before taking any of these medications.

9. Allow friends and family to care for you. Rest and do not exercise.

FOOD SUGGESTIONS FOR SICK DAYS

Apple sauce (sweetened)	½ cup	Lifesavers	5
Baked custard	½ cup	Milk (lowfat or skim)	1 cup
Cooked cereal	½ cup	Popsicle (twin-pop)	1
Eggnog	½ cup	Pudding (sweetened)	¼ cup
Fruit juices (unsweetened):		Regular ice cream	½ cup
Apple	½ cup	Regular Jello	⅓ cup
Cranberry	⅓ cup	Regular soda	¾ cup (6 oz)
Grape	½ cup	Saltine crackers	6
Orange	½ cup	Sherbet	¼ cup
Fruit yogurt	⅓ cup	Soup	1 cup
Frozen yogurt on a stick	1 bar	(vegetable, noodle, or cream)	
Gatorade	1 cup	Toast	1 slice
Gelatin	⅓ cup	Tomato juice	1½ cups
Honey	3 tsp	Vegetable juice	1½ cups
Hershey's syrup	2 Tbs		

Developed by Mary Kay Macheca, MSN(R), RN, CS, ANP, CDE

hours of treatment, the laboratory data in Table 18-5 were recorded.

COMMENTARY: DKA developed because the patient unwisely omitted her insulin during a time of increased need. The laboratory data indicate a severe high AG metabolic acidosis (pH 7.07). The AG is calculated by subtracting the sum of the bicarbonate and chloride levels from the serum sodium level (130 - [5 + 90] = 35 mEq/L). The calculated AG is 35 mEq/L; the accepted normal range is 12 to 15 mEq/L. This indicates an excess of about 20 mEq/L of ketones (flooding the bloodstream due to insulin lack). The deep rapid (Kussmaul) respirations were the body's attempt to compensate for the extremely low serum pH.

Signs of FVD included hypotension, tachycardia, dry skin and mucous membranes, low urinary output, and a high BUN/creatinine ratio. The serum sodium concentration was low initially because of the high serum glucose concentration (which pulled water out of the cells, thus diluting the serum sodium concentration). The serum potassium level was elevated initially due to the effect of starvation (release of potassium from the cells), acidosis (which also facilitates movement of cellular potassium to the bloodstream), and decreased renal excretion of potassium (due to the poor renal perfusion associated with FVD).

Notice how all of the abnormal parameters gradually corrected to normal (or near normal) during the course of the first 16 hours of treatment. This was accomplished solely by the combination of low-dose insulin and fluid volume replacement with isotonic saline. These treatments allowed the metabolic defects to be corrected. For example, the formation of ketones was stopped by the insulin. The metabolic acidosis corrected itself as this occurred; no bicarbonate was administered. As the blood glucose level decreased, the serum sodium level increased. This correction of the dilutional hyponatremia occurred because water was no longer being pulled out of the cells to the intravascular space. In addition, isotonic saline contains a sizable amount of sodium and helped correct any sodium losses from vomiting. The potentially dangerous serum potassium level (6.8 mEq/L) decreased to normal as the starvation effect (due to insulin lack) and the metabolic acidosis were corrected by treatment with insulin and fluid resuscitation. The gradual drop in the BUN and serum creatinine levels reflected improved renal perfusion secondary to fluid resuscitation.

After stabilization, the patient received education about rules to be followed during sick days (see Clinical Tip: Sick Day Instructions).

REFERENCES

1. Wachtel T, Tetu-Mouradjian L, Goldman D, Ellis S, O'Sullivan P. Hyperosmolarity and acidosis in diabetes mellitus: A three-year experience in Rhode Island. *J Gen Intern Med* 1991;6:501.
2. Expert Committee on the Diagnosis and Classification of Diabetes Mellitus. Report of the Expert Committee on the Diagnosis and Classification of Diabetes Mellitus. *Diabetes Care* 1997;20:1183.
3. Skyler J et al, eds. *Diagnosis and Classification. Medical Management of Type I Diabetes*, 3rd ed. Alexandria, VA: American Diabetes Association, 1998:7.
4. Genuth S. Diabetic ketoacidosis and hyperglycemic hyperosmolar nonketotic coma. *Curr Ther Endocrinol Metab* 1997;6:438.
5. Genuth S. Diabetic ketoacidosis and hyperosmolar hyperglycemic nonketotic syndrome in adults. In: Lebovitz H et al, eds. *Therapy for Diabetes Mellitus and Related Disorders*, 2nd ed. Alexandria, VA: American Diabetes Association, 1994:65.
6. Zimmerman BR, ed. *Diagnosis and Classification. Medical Management of Type 2 Diabetes*, 4th ed. Alexandria, VA: American Diabetes Association, 1998:9.
7. Ibid, p 23.
8. Ibid, p 9.
9. Ratner R. Pathophysiology of the diabetes disease state. In: Funnell M, Hunt C, Kulkarni K, Rubin R, Yarborough P, eds. *A Core Curriculum for Diabetes Education*, 3rd ed. Chicago: American Association of Diabetes Educators, 1998:174.
10. Davidson M, Schwartz S. Hyperglycemia. In: Funnell M, Hunt C, Kulkarni K, Rubin R, Yarborough P, eds. *A Core Curriculum for Diabetes Education*, 3rd ed. Chicago: American Association of Diabetes Educators, 1998:415.
11. Genuth, 1997, p 439.
12. Carroll P, Matz R. Uncontrolled diabetes mellitus in adults: Experience in treating diabetic ketoacidosis and hyperosmolar nonketotic coma with low-dose insulin and a uniform treatment regimen. *Diabetes Care* 1983;6:579.
13. Oster J, Kopyt N, Kleeman C, Dunfee T, Kreisberg R, Narins R. Diabetic acidosis and coma. In: Narins R, ed. *Maxwell and Kleeman's Clinical Disorders of Fluid and Electrolyte Metabolism*, 5th ed. New York: McGraw-Hill; 1994:828.
14. Matz R. Hyperosmolar nonacidotic uncontrolled diabetes: Not a rare event. *Clinical Diabetes* 1988;6:30.

15. Pope D, Dansky D. Hyperosmolar hyperglycemic nonketotic coma. *Emerg Med Clin North Am* 1989;7:854.
16. Siperstein M. Diabetic ketoacidosis and hyperosmolar coma. *Endocrinol Metab Clin North Am* 1992;21:425.
17. O'Connor LR et al. Effect of hypophosphatemia on myocardial performance in man. *N Engl J Med* 1977;297:901.
18. Oster, p 840.
19. Marshall S, Walker M, Alberti K. Diabetic ketoacidosis and hyperglycemic non-ketotic coma. In: Alberti K, Zimmet P, Defronzo R, eds. *International Textbook of Diabetes Mellitus*, 2nd ed. Chichester, UK: Wiley; 1997:1217.
20. Davidson J. Diabetic ketoacidosis and the hyperglycemic hyperosmolar state. In: Davidson J, ed. *Clinical Diabetes: A Problem-Oriented Approach*, 2nd ed. New York: Thieme; 1991:400.
21. Brandenburg M, Dire D. Comparison of arterial and venous blood gas values in the initial emergency department evaluation of patients with diabetic ketoacidosis. *Annals of Emerg Med* 1998;31;459.
22. Wachtel T. The diabetic hyperosmolar state. *Clin Geriatr Med* 1990;6:797.
23. White N, Henry D. Special issues in diabetes management. In: Haire-Joshu D, ed. *Management of Diabetes Mellitus: Perspectives of Care Across the Life Span*, 2nd ed. St. Louis: Mosby–Year Book; 1996:350.
24. Zimmerman BR, ed. *Detection and Treatment of Complications. Medical Management of Type 2 Diabetes*, 4th ed. Alexandria, VA: American Diabetes Association, 1998:123.
25. Wachtel, p 798.
26. Oster, p 853.
27. Wachtel, p 803.
28. Genuth, 1994, p 72.
29. White, Henry, p 351.
30. Macheca M. Diabetic hypoglycemia: How to keep the threat at bay. *Am J Nurs* 1993;93:26.
31. The Diabetes Control and Complications Trial Research Group. The effect of intensive treatment of diabetes on the development and progression of long-term complications in insulin-dependent diabetes mellitus. *N Engl J Med* 1993; 329:982.
32. Cryer P, Fisher J, Shamoon H. Hypoglycemia. *Diabetes Care* 1994;17:739.
33. Patrick A, Collier A, Hepburn D, Steedman D, Clarke B, Robertson C. Comparison of intramuscular glucagon and intravenous dextrose in the treatment of hypoglycemic coma in an accident and emergency department. *Arch Emerg Med* 1990;7:76.
34. Davidson, 1991, p 403.
35. Kitabchi A, Fisher J, Murphy M, Rumbak M. Diabetic ketoacidosis and the hyperglycemic, hyperosmolar, nonketotic state. In:

Kahn C, Weir G, eds. *Joslin's Diabetes Mellitus*, 13th ed. Philadelphia: Lea & Febiger, 1994:760.
36. White J, Campbell RK, Yarborough P. Pharmacologic therapies. In: Funnell M, Hunt C, Kulkarni K, Rubin R, Yarborough P, eds. *A Core Curriculum for Diabetes Education*, 3rd ed. Chicago: American Association of Diabetes Educators, 1998:304.
37. Kitabchi A, Matteri R, Murphy M. Optimal insulin delivery in diabetic ketoacidosis (DKA) and hyperglycemic, hyperosmolar nonketotic coma (HHNK). *Diabetes Care* 1982;5(suppl):78.
38. Carroll, Matz, p 582.
39. Lindsay R, Bolte R. The use of an insulin bolus in low-dose insulin infusion for pediatric diabetic ketoacidosis. *Pediatr Emerg Care* 1989;5:78.
40. Peterson L, Caldwell J, Hoffman J. Insulin adsorbance to polyvinyl chloride surfaces with implications for constant infusion therapy. *Diabetes* 1976;25:72.
41. White, Henry, p 348.
42. Oster, p 858.
43. Rogers B, Sills I, Cohen M, Seidel G. Diabetic ketoacidosis: Neurologic collapse during treatment followed by severe developmental morbidity. *Clin Pediatr* 1990;29:456.
44. Skyler, p 128.
45. White, Henry, p 349.
46. Skyler, p 130.
47. Davidson, 1991, p 410.
48. Ibid, p 405.
49. White, Henry, p 348.
50. Ibid, p 348.
51. Ellis E. Concepts of fluid therapy in diabetic ketoacidosis and hyperosmolar hyperglycemic nonketotic coma. *Pediatr Clin North Am* 1990;37:316.
52. Skyler, p 128.
53. Ibid, p 128.
54. Malone M, Klos S, Gennis V, Goodwin J. Frequent hypoglycemic episodes in the treatment of patients with diabetic ketoacidosis. *Arch Intern Med* 1992;152:2474.
55. Ibid.
56. Davidson, Schwarz, p 428.
57. Redman B. Teaching: Theory and interpersonal techniques. *The Process of Patient Education*, 7th ed. St. Louis: Mosby–Year Book; 1993:136.
58. Redman B. Assessment of motivation to learn and the need for patient education. *The Process of Patient Education*, 7th ed. St. Louis: Mosby-Year Book; 1993:24.
59. Henderson G. The psychosocial treatment of recurrent diabetic ketoacidosis: An interdisciplinary team approach. *Diabetes Educator* 1991;17:122.

Fluid Balance in the Patient With Brain Injury

About 500,000 cases of head injury occur each year in the United States; of these, about 10% of the injured die before reaching the hospital.[1] Despite these somewhat grim statistics, research is leading to an increased understanding of the mechanisms responsible for brain cell dysfunction following traumatic brain injury (TBI). Current emphasis is on the prevention of secondary brain injury associated with decreased oxygen delivery. This chapter discusses these concepts in relation to the management of fluid and electrolyte imbalances associated with TBI.

CEREBRAL EDEMA

CLASSIFICATION

The pathophysiology of brain injury varies according to etiology and severity, but the threat from cerebral edema is common. By definition, *cerebral edema* is an increase in brain water content with resultant increased brain tissue volume.[2] Untreated cerebral edema, despite the etiology, leads to elevated intracranial pressure (ICP).[3]

Cerebral edema can be classified into three different forms: (1) vasogenic, (2) cytotoxic (or cellular), and (3) hydrostatic (or interstitial). It is helpful to review briefly the features of these types of brain edema because therapeutic interventions for them can vary.

Vasogenic Edema

The most common form of brain edema, vasogenic edema, occurs in conditions such as trauma, brain tumor growths, abscess, hemorrhage, infarction, encephalitis, and lead encephalopathy, and after brain radiation.[4] In this type of edema, the volume of extracellular fluid (ECF) is increased due to an elevation in plasma protein and greater capillary permeability.[5]

Cytotoxic (Cellular) Edema

This type of edema may be viewed as a secondary form of injury resulting from alteration in cell membrane function and ion transport.[6] All the cellular elements of the brain (neurons, glia, and endothelial cells) may swell, with a consequent reduction in the ECF space in the brain.[7] Most commonly associated with this form of edema are acute hypo-osmolality (hyponatremia) and cerebral hypoxia (such as occurs after cardiac arrest or asphyxia). Cellular swelling is related to failure of the adenosine triphosphate (ATP)-dependent sodium pump within the cells, which causes sodium to accumulate rapidly within the cell and water to follow to maintain osmotic equilibrium.[8] However, patients with chronic hyponatremia do not suffer cerebral swelling (because the brain cells have had time to adapt by losing intracellular osmoles, mainly potassium).

Advances in research are clarifying the biochemical cascade that underlie secondary injury to the brain tissue. Biochemical changes, loss of calcium homeostasis and release of free radicals (polyunsaturated fatty acids), and excitatory amino acids are believed to induce brain cellular edema associated with ischemia and hyperosmolar states by inhibiting $(Na^+\text{-}K^+)$-ATPase activity.[9,10] As a result, new pharmacotherapies are being developed to block or inhibit these destructive responses.[11]

Hydrostatic Edema

Hydrostatic (or interstitial) edema is characterized by an increase in the interstitial fluid surrounding the cells. It is related to blockage of cerebrospinal fluid (CSF) absorption, most commonly by obstructive hydrocephalus.[12]

DISRUPTION IN PRESSURE AND VOLUME EQUILIBRIUM

Cerebral edema represents a disruption in the pressure and volume equilibrium within the intracranial compartments. These compartments, encased in the inelastic cranial vault, contain brain tissue, blood, and CSF. In adults, the pressure is maintained by an intracranial volume of about 1,900 mL, of which about 80% represents brain volume, 10% blood volume, and 10% CSF volume.[13] When one compartment increases in volume, there must be a reciprocal compensatory change in one or both of the other components to maintain a constant total pressure. This is known as the Monro-Kellie doctrine. Because the brain is relatively incompressible, compensation occurs through shunting of CSF into the spinal dural sac, an increased CSF absorption, or a decreased cerebral blood volume. When the total volume of brain mass, blood, or CSF exceeds the compensatory capacity, any additional increase in brain mass causes an exponential increase in ICP. Once ICP is raised to the stage of decompensation, intracranial hypertension results and the risk of brain displacement with herniation through the foramen magnum occurs.

CEREBRAL PERFUSION PRESSURE AND CEREBRAL BLOOD FLOW

Cerebral perfusion pressure (CPP) is defined as the difference between the mean arterial blood pressure (MAP) and ICP (MAP - ICP = CPP). In noninjured individuals, with mean blood pressures between 50 and 160 mm Hg, cerebral blood flow (CBF) remains relatively constant through a process known as autoregulation.[14]

Unfortunately, after severe TBI, pressure autoregulation may be lost. Thus, an elevated ICP can cause the CPP to drop and lead to profound reductions in CBF. Of course, reduced CBF can result in either global or regional ischemia and increase the severity of brain injury.[15] Similarly, a low MAP can lead to reduced CBF. In the past, the treatment of patients with head injuries mainly focused on controlling ICP. However, it is now recognized that maintaining the CPP is equally important. Not only must ICP be controlled, the systemic blood pressure must be maintained at a sufficiently high level to maintain an adequate cerebral perfusion. Efforts are made to keep the CPP at 70 mm Hg or more in patients with TBI because pressures less than 70 mm Hg are generally associated with a poor outcome.

Brain injury is adversely affected by hypotension and hypoxia; therefore, rapid cardiopulmonary stabilization is of primary importance in patients with new brain trauma. Mortality is significantly higher in severely injured patients who present with hypotension on admission than in those who are normotensive (60% versus 27%).[16] Hypoxia from an inadequate airway also significantly increases poor outcome, as does inadequate fluid resuscitation. As will be discussed later in the chapter, dehydration is no longer recommended for patients with TBI; further, hypotonic fluids and glucose-containing fluids are not recommended in severely injured patients.[17] Commonly used fluids for resuscitation of those with TBI include 0.9% NaCl (normal saline) and lactated Ringer' solution.[18]

ELEVATED INTRACRANIAL PRESSURE

ASSESSMENT

The most reliable data for assessing ICP are obtained through continuous ICP monitoring. Normal ICP is a mean pressure between 0 and 10 mm Hg with normal fluctuations of up to 12 mm Hg attributable to transient physiological variations. Readings above 15 mm Hg are considered elevated.[19] However, absolute numbers of ICP must be evaluated within the context of the clinical condition being treated, because compliance varies.[20]

Several techniques exist for continuous ICP monitoring. These include intraventricular catheters, subarachnoid screws or bolts, epidural sensors, fiberoptic catheters, and ultrasonic transcranial Doppler.[21] Direct monitoring is highly valuable in assessing changes in ICP because it provides clinicians with visual pressure readings and waveforms. Neurosurgical centers use continuous ICP monitoring in all patients with severe brain injuries to detect deterioration and guide therapeutic interventions.

When direct ICP monitoring is not available, clinical assessment becomes the primary method by which changes in ICP are determined. The symptoms of increased ICP are eventually the result of a reduction in CBF or mass effect or both.[22] The classic signs and symptoms of elevated ICP include papilledema, headache, and vomiting. Unfortunately, these symptoms do not become evident until relatively late; therefore, interventions performed at this point are less helpful than when elevated ICP is in an earlier state of development. Earlier signs of elevated ICP can be detected by assessing for changes in the level of consciousness, motor and sensory function, pupil size and reactivity, vital signs (hypertension with or without bradycardia), and other signs of neurological dysfunction. Baseline assessment should be performed and compared with data obtained from subsequent assessments for early recognition of significant changes.

Deterioration in the Level of Consciousness

This is often the first sign of deterioration in the patient's condition because an increase in the ICP results in decreased cerebral oxygenation. The cells most sensitive to a reduction in oxygen supply are those of the cerebral cortex involved with higher intellectual functions, including thinking processes (such as memory and orientation). Changes in wakefulness should also be noted.[23]

Loss of Motor and Sensory Function

As the ICP rises, motor and sensory functions are compromised and focal changes may be observed. Motor loss progresses from hemiparesis to hemiplegia on the side of the body that is opposite the cerebral lesion. As the increase in ICP continues, the patient becomes progressively less responsive to light and deep touch, as well as to painful sensations.

Pupillary Changes

Change in pupil size usually occurs on the same side as the lesion (or pressure increase). The response to direct light in this pupil progresses from "equal and reactive" to "nonreactive." With continued deterioration, the patient reaches the terminal stage where pupils may become bilaterally nonreactive to light stimuli. The pupillary changes are all related to compression of the third (oculomotor) cranial nerve.

Alterations in Vital Signs

During the compensatory phase of increased ICP, systolic blood pressure increases to a level slightly higher than that of the CSF pressure (this response is known as the Cushing reflex and is due to brain ischemia). Blood pressure drops as the patient's condition continues to deteriorate and the decompensatory phase begins.

During the compensatory phase, the pulse rate drops to less than 60 beats/min. On palpation, the pulse is full and bounding. This change in rate and quality is related to an attempt by the heart to pump blood into vessels with increased resistance as a result of the increased ICP. During the decompensatory phase, the pulse rate becomes rapid and irregular, and the quality becomes thready.

Abnormalities in respiratory patterns vary according to the level of brain dysfunction. Cheyne-Stokes respiration is often the first irregular breathing pattern observed, although as brain dysfunction progresses, other abnormal breathing patterns become apparent.[24] Increased ICP can also result in acute neurogenic pulmonary edema, which further contributes to alterations in the respiratory pattern.[25]

During the compensatory phase of increased ICP, the body temperature usually remains within normal limits. In the decompensatory phase, however, it may rise very high as a result of hypothalamic dysfunction.

Papilledema

Papilledema is commonly seen in patients with chronic increased ICP; however, it is rarely seen in patients with head injury, even in the presence of raised ICP.[26] Usually by the time papilledema occurs, the ICP has reached markedly elevated levels. The aforementioned signs and symptoms, therefore, are more reliable indicators of the beginning stages of increased ICP.

Headache

Although not always present with increased ICP, headache represents pressure against those intracranial structures that are sensitive to pain. These structures include the middle meningeal arteries and branches, the large arteries at the base of the brain, the venous sinuses, and the dura at the base of the skull. When headache is present in the patient with increased ICP, it typically is worse on arising in the morning.

Vomiting

Vomiting is not always present with increased ICP. When it occurs, it is characteristically projectile in nature and indicates pressure against the vomiting center in the medulla.

MANAGEMENT

Management of the patient with elevated ICP is being carefully reviewed. Nursing and medicine are both reviewing research findings in an attempt to develop scientifically based protocols that will improve patient outcomes.

Basic to all interventions is ongoing neurological assessment. Depending on the patient's condition, the neurological and vital signs must be assessed every 15 minutes to every 4 hours. The assessment should include mental status, level of consciousness, motor and sensory function, pupillary size, reaction to light, and eye movements. Results of each examination should be compared with those of previous assessments; significant changes should be promptly reported. Early subtle signs must be identified and acted on immediately because these signs can herald a change from a compensatory neurological status to one of irreversible decompensation.

In addition to continuing assessments, nursing care must be provided to meet the patient's basic needs. Nursing interventions for patients with elevated ICP have been the subject of clinical research.[27,28] It has been found that some necessary interventions (such as suctioning and body positioning) increase ICP. Motor activity may cause a sustained increase in ICP.[29] For patients in whom required nursing interventions can precipitate dangerous levels of increased ICP, sedation may be needed. Potent analgesics (such as fentanyl, midazolam, or lorazepam) are sometimes used to control ICP.[30] In addition, efforts should be directed toward nursing interventions that prevent or minimize increased ICP.

Head elevation of 30 degrees has been considered a routine nursing procedure to foster venous drainage and thus lower or control ICP. Interestingly, clinical studies examining head position and ICP have produced conflicting results. The conclusion from these studies is that the optimal head position is best determined on an individual basis, considering the need to keep the CPP (> 70 mm Hg) while not causing an increased ICP.[31]

Therapeutic interventions used in the management of increased ICP continue to include hyperventilation, osmotic diuretics, fluid restriction, temperature control, and ventricular drainage. Debates continues as to the relative effectiveness of these interventions; also, there is undoubtedly a need for additional research to support or refute them.[32]

Maintenance of Adequate Ventilation

If respiratory insufficiency is present as a result of brain injury, elevated levels of carbon dioxide (hypercapnia) and decreased levels of oxygen (hypoxemia) would be expected. Both hypercapnia and hypoxemia are potent vasodilating factors and thus contribute to increased ICP. Although hypercapnia and hypoxemia often occur together, hypercapnia alone will stimulate vasodilation.[33]

Because the effects of inadequate ventilation on ICP are so harmful, it is important to maintain respiratory function. Rate and quality of respirations should be assessed, and breath sounds should be auscultated at regular intervals. Interference with breathing related to complete or partial obstruction of the airway by mucus can be alleviated by periodic suctioning. For those severely injured patients who are intubated, guidelines have been developed to reduce the consequences of hypoxia and hypercapnia during suctioning. These include preoxygenating patients to prevent suction-induced hypoxia, limiting suctioning to less than 10 seconds, and limiting the suction passes to only one or two. The use of suction at a negative pressure of more than 120 mm Hg and the use of catheters that occlude more than 50% of the endotracheal tube should be avoided.[34] The drainage of secretions pooled in the mouth can be facilitated by turning the patient from side to side at least every 2 hours.

Assessment of respiratory status must ultimately rely on arterial blood gas analyses. Findings from blood gas studies are crucial in planning measures to minimize increases in ICP. Some authorities recommend that the partial pressure of oxygen in arterial blood (PaO_2) be maintained at least at 70 mm Hg (by intubation if necessary).[35] The partial pressure of carbon dioxide in arterial blood ($PaCO_2$) is often purposely lowered below normal as a therapeutic measure for increased ICP.

Hyperventilation

Lowering the arterial carbon dioxide pressure by inducing hyperventilation results in cerebral vasoconstriction; the presumed benefits of this procedure include a decreased cerebral blood volume with subsequent lowering of ICP. (This works only in patients whose cerebrovascular vessels are able to respond by vasoconstricting.) Clinical studies have indicated that an acute reduction in $PaCO_2$ of 5 to 10 mm Hg lowers ICP 25% to 50% in most patients.[36] When hyperventilation is used, reducing the $PaCO_2$ to 30 to 35 mm Hg is thought to be optimal because lower levels may result in focal ischemia due to excessive vasoconstriction.[37]

The use of hyperventilation to control ICP in patients with TBI has become increasingly controversial.[38] Despite the controversy, a recent study indicated that it is still routinely used in the treatment of patients with TBI in many medical centers that specialize in neurotrauma.[39] Current thinking is that hyperventilation should be used in moderation, for as limited a time as possible.[40] Valid concerns about the safety of hyperventilation involve its potential to cause severe vasoconstriction and decreased CBF, resulting in ischemic injury. It is believed that the resulting ischemia causes vasodilatation (which contributes to cerebral edema), offsetting the effects of further hyperventilation.[41] In severely injured patients, evidence suggests that hyperventilation for more than 6 hours may decrease the ability of cerebrovascular vessels to constrict in response to a lowered $PaCO_2$ level.[42] These patients experience an ischemic phase 12 to 24 hours after injury; if hyperventilation is initiated too early (within the first 24 hours), it may contribute to detrimental patient outcomes.[43] Therefore, authorities suggest that the use of prophylactic hyperventilation ($PaCO_2 \leq 35$ mm Hg) be avoided in the first 24 hours after severe TBI.[44] However, brief periods of hyperventilation may be necessary when periods of increased ICP do not respond to other therapies (such as osmotic diuretics, CSF drainage, sedation, and paralysis).[45] Monitoring CBF helps identify when cerebral ischemia develops after the use of hyperventilation.

Measurement of oxygen saturation in the blood in the jugular bulb with a catheter is a useful method for evaluating cerebral oxygenation. This measurement is known as the jugular venous oxygen saturation (SjO_2). It represents a ratio of the supply to the demand for cerebral oxygen. A normal value should be between 60% and 80%. If the SjO_2 is between 50% and 55%, cerebral hypoxemia should be suspected. A low SjO_2 indicates rising oxygen demands and may be due to anemia, respiratory insufficiency, or low cardiac output.[46]

Before administering high concentrations of oxygen during the hyperventilation process, the respiratory system should be assessed for lung pathology; if present, specific guidelines for oxygen therapy must be provided by the physician.

Fluid Therapy

Controversy exists over the optimal fluid management for patients with TBI.[47] There is disagreement as to the appropriate type as well as quantity of fluid to use to maintain adequate hydration while avoiding an increased ICP.

Type of Fluid

Although there is no single best fluid for patients with TBI, Zornow and Prough point out that isotonic crystalloids (such as 0.9% NaCl and lactated Ringer's solution) are widely used and can be justified on a scientific basis.[48] Others concur that normal saline (0.9% NaCl) and lactated Ringer's solution are considered suitable fluids.[49] Free water (such as 5% dextrose in water) should be avoided because it predisposes to brain swelling.[50]

Medical center policies differ as to fluid therapy protocols. However, it has been suggested that all dextrose-containing solutions be used cautiously in patients after TBI.[51] An early study by Welsh and Ginzberg demonstrated that hyperglycemia exacerbated ischemic brain injury in laboratory models.[52] Other investigators have reported similar findings.[53] Even though the link to humans is difficult to prove, experimental evidence is compelling to urge avoidance of glucose-containing solutions.[54]

Centers in the United States usually resuscitate hypovolemic, patients with TBI with isotonic crystalloids (such as lactated Ringer's or 0.9% NaCl). In contrast, hypertonic saline solutions are used in the prehospital transport of similar patients in Europe.[55] Animal studies have supported the efficacy of small volumes of hypertonic saline solutions in reversing shock and decreasing ICP (by decreasing brain water content in uninjured portions of the brain).[56–58] When used in humans, these solutions should be given in judicious amounts and with frequent monitoring of the serum sodium concentrations.

Volume of Fluid

In the past, fluid restriction was advocated for patients with TBI; however, evidence indicates that this practice can lead to a worsened neurological outcome.[59,60] Failure to maintain an adequate vascular volume interferes with CPP. After a cerebral insult, the brain's ability to autoregulate may be disrupted. Recall, CPP equals MAP minus ICP. Thus, the low MAP associated with hypovolemia has serious implications for the CPP. The level at which CPP should be maintained is not known; however, evidence indicates that 70 to 80 mm Hg may be the critical threshold.[61] Sustained low CPP readings have been directly associated with morbidity and mortality in neurological patients. Care must be taken not to restrict fluids excessively, especially in patients receiving dehydrating agents (such as osmotic or loop diuretics).

In patients who require osmotic or other diuretic therapy (described below), liberalization of iso-osmotic fluid intake to prevent dehydration is appropriate, based on the following clinical parameters. These factors must be considered in determining fluid needs of patients at risk for cerebral edema:

- It is generally agreed that the desired amount of fluid to be administered should be based on the patient's serum osmolality, blood urea nitrogen (BUN), and electrolyte levels. Remember that the neurological patient is at risk for sodium imbalances in either direction.
- Fluid therapy must also provide for any abnormal losses (such as occur from gastric suction, abdominal bleeding, or third-space fluid shifts related to major fractures). Care of the patient with TBI with chest, abdominal, or orthopedic injuries is complicated. The clinician must judiciously balance fluid intake to maintain adequate circulating volume while not overloading the cerebral circulation.

Osmotic Agents and Other Diuretics

Elevated ICP may also be treated with osmotic diuretics (such as mannitol) or loop diuretics (such as furosemide). Fortunately, despite the presence of TBI, there is usually a significant portion of the brain with an intact blood–brain barrier. Mannitol creates a concentration gradient across the blood–brain barrier and thus pulls water out of brain tissue into the intravascular space where it is subsequently eliminated through the kidneys. Furosemide has a diuretic effect on the renal tubules and possibly reduces CSF formation. Used in combination, mannitol and furosemide seem to have a synergistic effect in controlling elevated ICP.[62] The primary osmotic diuretic, mannitol, reduces ICP consistently and increases CPP within 10 to 20 minutes or less in patients with TBI with increased ICP.[63] The most common dosage is 0.25 g/kg; it can be administered every 4 to 6 hours to maintain the ICP within a normal range or it may be used only as needed to treat peaks of increased ICP. In addition to its osmotic effect, mannitol produces a transient rise in MAP.[64]

Assessment of Hydration

Measurement of fluid intake and output (I&O) is mandatory; frequency should be designated by the physician (such as every 15–30 minutes or hourly). To facilitate accurate measurements, an indwelling urinary catheter is usually used for adults and a pediatric collection device for children. The rate of intravenous

(IV) fluid infusion is usually adjusted to maintain a urine flow of at least 30 to 50 mL/hr.[65] A volume less than this amount (or an amount designated by the physician) should prompt discontinuance of mannitol to prevent fluid overload and fulminant congestive heart failure. (This is because the kidneys must be able to excrete the fluid being pulled into the bloodstream.) Serum creatinine and BUN levels should be monitored to evaluate renal function and hydration status. (Osmotic diuretics are contraindicated in patients with significant renal disease because these individuals cannot effectively eliminate the excess fluid volume.) Variations in body weight should be monitored to detect excessive fluid retention or loss; an accurate in-bed scale is most useful. The serum osmolality should be measured at regular intervals. It should not exceed 320 mOsm/kg; the diuresis resulting from mannitol administration may exacerbate hypovolemia and hypotension.[66]

Assessment of Electrolyte Levels

Measurement of electrolytes, primarily sodium and potassium, is of vital importance in monitoring response to mannitol therapy. With mannitol use, there is initially an expansion of the plasma volume caused by diffusion of water into the bloodstream; therefore, hyponatremia is a possible complication. Later, as the fluid is excreted through the kidneys, hypernatremia may be observed (as relatively more water is excreted than sodium). Mannitol should not be administered if the serum sodium level exceeds 150 mEq/L.[67] Because the serum sodium level can be either decreased or increased with mannitol therapy, measured serum levels should be observed closely and abnormalities reported at once. Similarly, serum potassium levels may be variable. Hyperkalemia can occur when potassium levels build up in the bloodstream during the presence of oliguria; conversely, hypokalemia can result when potassium is eliminated during the osmotic diuresis. Chapters 4 and 5 contain descriptions of sodium and potassium imbalances.

A potential problem associated with mannitol use (and other osmotic diuretics) is a rebound increase in ICP.[68] The rebound may result from retention of mannitol in the brain tissue as the blood mannitol level is dropping; this situation reverses the pressure gradient and allows water to diffuse back into the brain tissue, increasing ICP.

Animal models have shown that hypertonic saline solutions are effective in controlling ICP.[69,70] There have been anecdotal reports of the successful treatment of increased ICP with hypertonic saline in patients who did not respond to large doses of mannitol.[71] Fisher et al.[72] compared the effect of hypertonic saline (3% NaCl) to that of isotonic saline (0.9% NaCl) in 18 pediatric patients with head injuries and found that the hypertonic saline was associated with a drop in ICP of 4 mm Hg as compared to an increase of 0.7 mm Hg with isotonic saline.

Corticosteroids

The efficacy of corticosteroids in the treatment of increased ICP is doubtful; however, they are effective in some forms of cerebral edema.[73] They are believed to be beneficial in vasogenic edema (as seen in brain tumor and abscess) but are not effective in cytotoxic edema (as in acute hyponatremia or hypoxia) and are of uncertain effectiveness in hydrostatic edema.[74] The most common corticosteroid given for control of increased ICP is dexamethasone. When dexamethasone is administered, one should anticipate complications such as hyperglycemia, gastrointestinal bleeding, and increased incidence of infection. It is customary to monitor blood glucose levels during massive steroid therapy. Antacids are usually administered to patients receiving large doses of steroids, and H_2-receptor antagonists may be used to decrease gastric acidity.

High-Dose Barbiturate Therapy

In recent years, barbiturates (most commonly pentobarbital) have been used to manage elevated ICP, primarily in patients who have not responded to more conventional methods. Barbiturates induce a significant decrease in CBF and cerebral metabolism.[75] The subsequent effect is a lowering of cerebral blood volume and ICP. To date, clinical trials have not demonstrated improved patient outcome. It is not known if the effects are sustained or if the eventual outcome is altered.[76] With barbiturate therapy, continuous monitoring of ICP, arterial and preferably pulmonary capillary wedge pressures, and cardiac output is indicated.[77]

A major risk of barbiturate therapy is acute hypotension. This can profoundly affect the patient with a compromised myocardium. Hypothermia may also develop; however, core body temperature should not be allowed to drop below 34°C (93.2°F) because of the risk of cardiac instability.[78]

Certain components of the neurological assessment (such as level of consciousness and ability to follow commands) are, of course, negated by barbiturate therapy. However, pupillary dilatation as a result of brain stem compression will still occur at serum barbiturate levels of up to 3 or 4 mg/mL.[79] After achievement of a satisfactory ICP (< 20 mm Hg for 24–48 hours), gradual reduction of the barbiturate dosage can begin.[80]

Temperature Control

Any elevation in body temperature must be controlled because this will increase the brain's need for oxygen, thereby increasing CBF and, in turn, ICP. Elevated temperature can be treated with antipyretic medications used alone or in conjunction with a cooling blanket.

Ventricular Drainage

In an attempt to control erratic increases in the ICP, a ventriculostomy may be performed in some patients. This involves the insertion of a drainage catheter into a cerebral ventricle for the purpose of draining off excess CSF. Because of the continual threat of infection, these patients are frequently given prophylactic antibiotics.

Nursing responsibilities in caring for a patient with ventricular drainage include:

- Promoting absolute sterility of the equipment
- Maintaining a sterile dry dressing at the catheter and incision site
- Keeping the collection container adjusted to a level indicated by the physician
- Observing the drainage system for kinks to assure patency of the tube
- Observing and recording the amount of drainage in the collection container

⬤ SYNDROME OF INAPPROPRIATE ANTIDIURETIC HORMONE SECRETION

PATHOPHYSIOLOGY

When hyponatremia occurs in the presence of neurological injury, the syndrome of inappropriate antidiuretic hormone secretion (SIADH) is often suspected. (However, other causes of hyponatremia such as cerebral salt wasting also need to be considered.) As discussed in Chapter 4, a variety of central nervous system disorders may produce SIADH. Among these are head injury, encephalitis, meningitis, and brain tumors. The exact mechanisms by which SIADH is produced are unknown; presumably, relatively excessive vasopressin (ADH) is released from the neurohypophysis.[81]

In addition, SIADH can cause cerebral edema due to cellular swelling (cytotoxic edema). For the most part, SIADH is self-limiting and subsides as the brain tissue heals; however, it can last for weeks or even months.

CLINICAL SIGNS

The clinical criteria for SIADH include hyponatremia, a relatively high urine sodium concentration (> 20 mmol/L), and a urine osmolality that exceeds serum osmolality. Refer to Table 4-4 for a detailed summary of clinical manifestations and laboratory findings in SIADH and to Table 4-5 for a summary of nursing assessment for this condition. Table 19-1 compares the clinical presentation of SIADH to other conditions associated with sodium imbalances in patients with neurological injuries.

MANAGEMENT

As is the case with all causes of SIADH, restriction of electrolyte-free water intake is indicated. Adequate free water restriction will eventually increase the serum sodium concentration. In nonedematous patients, extra salt is sometimes given in the diet or in the form of salt tablets in combination with mild fluid restriction.[82] However, if severe symptoms are present, it may be necessary to cautiously infuse a hypertonic saline solu-

---

TABLE 19-1   Comparison of Pathophysiology, Clinical Signs, and Treatment of SIADH, CSW, and CDI

Clinical Problem	Pathophysiology	Typical Clinical Findings	Usual Laboratory Findings	Usual Treatment
SIADH (Syndrome of Inappropriate Antidiuretic Hormone Secretion)	High secretion of ADH, causing the kidneys to retain water	Fluid intake exceeds urine output; Increased body weight; No change in CVP	Hyponatremia, Urine Na > 20 mEq/L; No change in BUN/Cr ratio; Serum osm < Urine osm	Fluid restriction; Demeclocycline, if needed; 3% or 5% NaCl, if needed
CSW (Cerebral Salt Wasting)	Sodium loss into urine, results in extracellular fluid volume deficit	Decreased body weight; Fluid intake less than fluid output; Decreased CVP; Perhaps dry skin and mucous membranes	Hyponatremia Urine Na > 20 mEq/L, BUN/Cr ratio increased; Serum osm < Urine osm	Fluid replacement with sodium-containing fluid (such as 0.9% NaCl) to expand the ECF
CDI (Central Diabetes Insipidus)	Low secretion of ADH, causing increased loss of water by the kidneys	Polyuria; Polydipsia (if alert); Decreased body weight	Hypernatremia; Dilute urine (SG often < 1.010); Serum osm > Urine osm	Fluid replacement; Vasopressin

Adapted from Zafonte R, Watanabe T, Mann N, Ko D. Psychogenic polydipsia after traumatic brain injury: A case report. *Am J Phys Med Rehabil* 1997;75:246, and Harrigan M. Cerebral salt wasting syndrome: A review. Neurosurgery 1996;38:152.

ADH, antidiuretic hormone; BUN, blood urea nitrogen; Cr, creatinine; CVP, central venous pressure; ECF, extracellular fluid; SG, specific gravity.

tion (such as 3% or 5% NaCl). As discussed in Chapter 4, these solutions are extremely dangerous and should be handled with care. Hypertonic saline should be administered only in intensive care units under close observation. They are best administered in 100-mL containers to avoid an inadvertent excessive dosage. The reader is referred to Clinical Tip: Nursing Considerations in Administration of Hypertonic Saline Solutions in Chapter 4 for additional information regarding nursing considerations in administering hypertonic saline and to Table 4-6 for a list of nursing interventions related to SIADH therapy.

CEREBRAL SALT WASTING

PATHOPHYSIOLOGY

Cerebral salt wasting (CSW) is a syndrome characterized by hyponatremia, renal sodium loss, and extracellular volume contraction.[83] It is most often seen in patients with subarachnoid hemorrhage; however, it also occurs in patients with head trauma and brain tumors.[84] The mechanism by which the renal salt wasting associated with CSW occurs is not fully understood; however, there are indications that atrial natriuretic peptide (ANP) is probably involved.[85] It is believed that intracranial disease may decrease the ability of the brain to control ANP secretion.[86] This has led to an assumption that enhanced ANP activity may account, in part, for the observed salt wasting and volume depletion seen in patients with subarachnoid hemorrhage.[87] Other factors are also likely involved (such as direct neural effects on the kidneys).[88] Further research is required to fully understand this clinical syndrome.[89]

CLINICAL INDICATORS

The hyponatremia seen in CSW is attributed to true sodium loss; in contrast, the hyponatremia associated with SIADH is due to the dilutional effect of retained water. Therefore, careful assessment of the patient's fluid volume status is the most helpful feature to distinguish between these two entities. It is necessary to obtain highly accurate daily weights and measurements of fluid I&O, along with daily urinary sodium measurements.[90] As noted in Table 19-1, patients with

CSW who are not adequately hydrated will lose weight and have others signs of ECF deficit, such as decreased CVP. (In contrast, patients with SIADH do not have signs of ECF deficit.) A weight loss of more than 1 kg/day (or other signs of decreased fluid volume) in the presence of worsening hyponatremia favors the diagnosis of CSW.[91]

MANAGEMENT

Although hyponatremia is present in both CSW and SIADH, opposite treatment strategies are recommended (see Table 19-1). Whereas SIADH requires fluid restriction to allow water loss to exceed fluid intake, CSW requires intravascular volume resuscitation and sodium replacement. Isotonic sodium solutions (such as 0.9% NaCl) or colloid (such as 5% albumin or fresh frozen plasma) may be used to expand the intravascular volume to reduce the stimulus for ADH secretion.[92]

When CSW presents in patients with subarachnoid hemorrhage, there is an increased risk of brain infarction due to cerebral vasospasm. Therefore, a protocol referred to as hypervolemic, hypertensive therapy is instituted to reduce this risk. Hypervolemia should be guided by a CVP of more than 10 cm H_2O or a pulmonary artery wedge pressure (PAWP) of more than 12 mm Hg.[93] Hypertensive therapy (a blood pressure of 10 mm Hg more than normal value) is controlled by the administration of calcium entry blocking agents (such as nimodipine). This complex protocol is based on broad experience rather than prospective study.[94]

CENTRAL DIABETES INSIPIDUS

PATHOPHYSIOLOGY

Recall that ADH (also called vasopressin) is synthesized in the supraoptic nucleus of the anterior hypothalamus. It is then stored in the posterior lobe of the pituitary gland and released in response to many stimuli (the most important of which is increased plasma osmolality). Unfortunately, after head trauma, ADH deficiency can occur. When this happens, the condition is called central diabetes insipidus (CDI). Inadequate ADH causes the excretion of a large volume of dilute urine; left untreated, this can lead to dehydration, hypovolemia, and hemoconcentration. Depending on the site of the lesion, CDI can be permanent or transient.[95]

CLINICAL SIGNS

Central diabetes insipidus is manifested by an abrupt onset of polyuria and polydipsia. The usual urine volume is 8 to 10 L/day.[96] Conscious patients usually exhibit extreme thirst and will drink large volumes of fluid, if able. For unknown reasons, there may be a preference for iced drinks. Because of the sustained polyuria, sleep deprivation can be a problem. Failure to consume enough fluids to adequately match the large urine volume will produce profound volume depletion. Because the unconscious patient cannot experience thirst, or respond to it, there is a need to replace fluids by the parenteral route, titrated according to urine output and laboratory results. Classic laboratory findings include hypernatremia and slight serum hyperosmolality. Urine specific gravity is usually less than 1.005 and urine osmolality less than 200 mOsm/kg. Although the fluid deprivation test is sometimes used to establish a diagnosis of CDI, it must be done cautiously while observing the urine output and serum sodium level; regardless of fluid restriction, the patient with CDI will continue to excrete a large urine volume (perhaps leading to profound hypovolemia and hypernatremia).

It should be noted that CDI may be triphasic in critically ill patients. That is, it may occur transiently for a few days after surgery or trauma and then resolve for a few days, only to recur.[97] Therefore, one should closely monitor urine output and laboratory values. Especially important are serum sodium and osmolality, as well as urine specific gravity or osmolality.

Refer to Table 4-9 for a summary of clinical manifestations of diabetes insipidus and to Table 4-10 for a summary of assessments for this condition.

MANAGEMENT

Patients with large urinary losses from CDI need fluid replacement. It may be given by mouth if the patient is conscious. If not, it may be given by the parenteral route in the form of lactated Ringer's solution or half-normal saline, depending on the patient's volume status and degree of water deficit.[98] To avoid producing cerebral edema, only half the water deficit plus insensible water loss should be replaced in the first 24 hours; the rest of the deficit can be replaced over the next 24

to 48 hours.[99] Frequent assessment of neurological status is indicated to look for cerebral edema, a complication that can result from accumulation of intracellular solute during dehydration.[100] In addition to water, magnesium and potassium may be needed to replace losses of these electrolytes in the urine.

Acute diabetes insipidus after surgery or trauma may be treated with short-acting aqueous Pitressin. After a period, the treatment may be temporarily discontinued to determine if the diabetes insipidus is transient or permanent.

With the administration of ADH substances, it is conceivable that the patient may become fluid overloaded if fluid intake (IV and oral) exceeds fluid output. Fluid overload may also result if third-space fluid accumulations from other injuries shift back into the vascular space at the time ADH is being administered. Excessive water retention may cause the serum sodium level to drop below normal. Rapid vacillations in the serum sodium level can cause a worsened neurological status related to shifts in the brain water content. Close assessment of neurological signs and laboratory data are required during treatment.

CASE STUDIES

● **19-1.** A 35-year-old man was injured in a multiple vehicle accident and sustained a basilar skull fracture and multiple facial bruises. On admission to the emergency room, the patient was unconscious, with a Glasgow coma scale score of 7 and no focal neurologic abnormalities. A long bone fracture was discovered, and the patient received fluid resuscitation of large amounts of lactated Ringer's solution. Mannitol (100 mg) was given to treat his head injury. Twelve hours after the injury, the patient's urine output was noted to exceed 1 L/hr and the following laboratory data were available:

Serum sodium = 175 mEq/L
Serum potassium = 4.3 mEq/L
Serum chloride = 134 mEq/L
Serum osmolality = 365 mOsm/L
Urine sodium = 10 mEq/L
Urine osmolality = 80 mOsm/L

COMMENTARY: The laboratory data are consistent with CDI. The serum sodium is markedly elevated, as is the serum osmolality. In contrast, the urine sodium and osmolality are low, reflecting large water loss in the urine. Basilar skull fracture is commonly associated with CDI.

After treatment with vasopressin, the urine volume should diminish and the serum sodium level should decrease. Note that while a conscious patient with CDI would likely experience thirst and therefore drink extra fluids, an unconscious patient cannot make these responses. Thus, continued loss of large volumes of urine without adequate fluid replacement could result in severe hypovolemia.

● **19-2.** A 30-year-old woman presented in the emergency room with complaints of severe headache, vertigo, and stiff neck. She denied chest pain and had a normal electrocardiogram. Previously, she had been in good health and denied a history of hypertension or drug use. A head computed tomogram was done in the emergency room and showed a subarachnoid hemorrhage.

On admission to the intensive care unit (ICU) she was lethargic, but opened her eyes when her name was called and responded appropriately to orientation questions before drifting back to sleep. Her pupils were 4/4 and brisk, her extraocular movements (EOM) were intact, her face was symmetrical, and her tongue was midline. She moved all extremities well; however, her left grasp was slightly weaker than the right.

A cerebral angiogram confirmed a right internal communicating artery aneurysm. the heart rate was 80 to 110 beats/min, mean blood pressure (MBP) was 90 to 118 mm Hg, respirations were 16 to 24 breaths/min, and her oxygen saturation was 94% to 98% on room air. She was started on nimodipine (60 mg PO every 4 hours), Decadron (4 mg PO every 6 hours), Colace (100 mg PO bid), Dilantin (200 mg PO bid), Zantac (150 mg

PO bid), Apresoline (5–20 mg IVP PRN), and morphine (1–2 mg IV push) for pain.

Twenty-four hours after her initial subarachnoid hemorrhage, she underwent a craniotomy for aneurysm clipping. On return to the ICU, she was alert and oriented to her name and could follow simple commands using all four extremities; her speech was clear but occasionally inappropriate. Her pupils were 2/2 brisk, her face was symmetrical, and her EOMs were intact. A left radial arterial line (A-line) was placed in the operating room to monitor her MBP; orders were received to maintain the pressure at more than 100 mm Hg. In addition, a pulmonary artery catheter was placed in her right subclavian vein to monitor PAWP every hour and cardiac output readings every 2 hours. Twenty hours after surgery, the patient's level of consciousness changed; she became lethargic and did not follow commands. No other neurological deficits were apparent. Her MBP was 70 mm Hg, CVP 2 mm Hg, and the pulmonary capillary wedge pressure was 5 mm Hg (all indicative of hypovolemia). At this time, her serum sodium level was 130 mEq/L.

COMMENTARY: This patient was experiencing a cerebral vasospasm, a potential complication from subarachnoid hemorrhage. Because of failure to administer IV fluids in sufficient volume to match her urinary sodium loss, she developed fluid volume deficit with hyponatremia (which in turn contributed to the cerebral vasospasm). Hyponatremia can signal either SIADH or CSW. In this case, because the hyponatremia coexisted with clinical signs of fluid volume deficit, it was more likely a problem of CSW (true sodium loss in the urine). The patient required additional administration of 0.9% NaCl to reduce the adverse effects of the cerebral vasospasm and hyponatremia.

REFERENCES

1. American College of Surgeons, Committee on Trauma. *Advanced Trauma Life Support [ATLS] Course for Doctors*, 6th ed. Chicago: American College of Surgeons; 1997:221.
2. Zink BJ. Traumatic brain injury. *Emerg Med Clin North Am* 1996;14:115.
3. Mcintosh TK, Smith DH, Meaney DF, Kotapka MJ, Gennarelli TA, Graham DI. Neuropathological sequelae of traumatic brain injury: Relationship to neurochemical and biomechanical mechanisms. *Lab Invest* 1996;24:315.
4. Williams MA, Razumovsky AY. Cerebrospinal fluid circulation, cerebral edema, and intracranial pressure. *Curr Sci* 1993;6:847.
5. Ibid, p 847.
6. Richmond TS. Cerebral resuscitation after global brain ischemia: Linking research to practice. *AACN Clinical Issues* 1997;8:171.

7. Zink, p 123.
8. Williams, p 848.
9. Richmond, p 173.
10. Zafonte R. The pathophysiology of brain injury: Understanding innovative drug therapies. *Journal of Head Trauma Rehabilitation* 1998;13:1.
11. Ibid, p 1.
12. Winston KR, Breeze R. Hydraulic regulation of brain parenchymal volume. *Neurol Res* 1992;13:251.
13. Kanter MJ, Narayan RK. Intracranial monitoring. *Neurosurg Clin North Am* 1991;2:258.
14. ATLS, p 226.
15. Liebert MA. Guidelines for cerebral perfusion pressure. *J Neurotrauma* 1996;13:693.
16. ATLS, p 234.
17. ATLS, p 240.
18. ATLS, p 241.
19. Hall CA. Patient management in head injury care: A nursing perspective. *Intensive and Critical Care Nursing* 1997;13:329.
20. Doyle PJ, Mark PW. Analysis of intracranial pressure. *J Clin Monitor* 1993;5:81.
21. Hartman A, Stingele R, Schnitzer M. General treatment strategies for elevated intracranial pressure. In: Hacke W, ed. *Neuro Critical Care*. Berlin: Springer-Verlag; 1994:102.
22. Ibid, p 104.
23. Ibid, p 107.
24. Ibid.
25. Ibid.
26. Ibid, p 104.
27. Mitchell P, Mauss N. Relationship of patient-nurse activity to intracranial pressure variations. *Nurs Res* 1978;27:4.
28. Boortz-Marx R. Factors affecting intracranial pressure: A descriptive study. *J Neurosci Nurs* 1985;4:89.
29. Parsons C, Smith A, Page M. The effects of hygiene interventions on the cerebrovascular status of severe closed head injured patients. *Res Nurs Health* 19985;8:178.
30. Zink, p 135.
31. Simmons BJ. Management of intracranial hemodynamics in the adult: a research analysis of head positioning and recommendations for clinical practice and future research. *Neuroscience Nursing* 1997;29:44.
32. Roberts I, Schierhout G, Alderson P. Absence of evidence for the effectiveness of five interventions routinely used in the intensive care management of severe head injury: A systematic review. *J Neurol Neurosurg Psychiatry* 1998;65:729.
33. Kerr ME, Rudy EB, Brucia J, Stone KS. Head-injured adults: recommendations for endotracheal suctioning. *J Neurosci Nurs* 1993;25:89.
34. Kerr, p 89.
35. Greenberg J, Brawansky A. Cranial trauma. In: Hacke W, ed. *Neuro Critical Care*. Berlin: Springer-Verlag; 1994:696.
36. Ibid, p 152.
37. Geraci EB, Geraci TA. Hyperventilation and head injury: Controversies and concerns. *J Neurosci Nurs* 1996;2:381.
38. Yundt K, Diringer M. The use of hyperventilation and its impact on cerebral ischemia in the treatment of traumatic brain injury. *Crit Care Clin* 1997;13:163.
39. Ghajar J, Harira R, Narayan R et al. Survey of critical care management of comatose, head-injured patients in the United States. *Crit Care Med* 1995;23:560.
40. ATLS, p 241.
41. Geraci, Geraci, p 385.
42. Kerr, p 90.
43. Geraci, Geraci, p 387.
44. Bullock R, Chesnut R, Clifton G et al. The use of hyperventilation in the acute management of severe traumatic brain injury. In: Bullock R, Chesnut R, Clifton G et al, eds. *Guidelines for the Management of Severe Head Injury*. New York: Brain Trauma Foundation; 1995.
45. Yundk, Diringer, p 175.
46. Dearden N. Jugular bulb venous oxygen saturation in the management of severe head injury. *Current Opinion in Anaethesiology* 1991;4:279.
47. Zornow M, Prough D. Fluid management in patients with traumatic brain injury. *New Horizons* 1995;3:488.
48. Ibid, p 488.
49. Marshall RS, Mayer SA. *On Call Neurology*. Philadelphia: WB Saunders; 1997:128.
50. Schwartz S, Shires G, Spencer F et al, eds. *Principles of Surgery*, 7th ed. New York: McGraw-Hill; 1999:1484.
51. Zornow, Prough, p 491.
52. Ginsberg MD, Welsh FA, Budd WW. Deleterious effect of glucose pretreatment in recovery of cerebral ischemia in the cat: local cerebral blood flow and glucose utilization. *Stroke* 1980;11:347.
53. Lanier W, Stangland K, Scheithauer B et al. The effects of dextrose infusion and head position on neurologic outcome after complete cerebral ischemia in primates: examination of a model. *Anesthesiology* 1987;66:39.
54. Marshall SB, Marshall LF, Vos HR, Chestnut R. *Neuroscience Critical Care*. Philadelphia: WB Saunders; 1990:195.
55. Zornow, Prough, p 494.
56. Battistella F, Wisner D. Combined hemorrhagic shock and head injury: effects of hypertonic saline (7.5%) resuscitation. *J Trauma* 1991;31:182.
57. Wisner D, Schuster L, Quinn C. Hypertonic saline resuscitation of head injury: Effects on cerebral water content. *J Trauma* 1990;30:75.
58. Prough D, Whitley J, Taylor C et al. Regional cerebral blood flow following resuscitation from hemorrhagic shock with hypertonic saline: Influence of a subdural mass. *Anesthesiology* 1991;75:319.
59. Rosner M, Daughton S. Cerebral perfusion pressure management in head injury. *J Trauma* 1990;30:933.
60. Chesnut R, Marshall L, Klauber M et al. The role of secondary brain injury in determining outcome from severe head injury. *J Trauma* 1993;34:216.
61. Liebert, p 693.
62. Zink, p 135.
63. American Association of Neurological Surgeons. *Guidelines for the Management of Severe Head Injury*. New York: Brain Trauma Foundation; 1995;10-3.
64. Davis A, Briones T. Intracranial disorders. In: Kinney M, Dunbar S, Brooks-Bruns J et al, eds. *AACN Clinical Reference for Critical Care Nursing*, 4th ed. St. Louis: CV Mosby: 1998:692.
65. AANS, 10-3.
66. Ibid.
67. Grande PO, Asgeirsson B, Nordstrom CH. Physiologic principles for volume regulation of a tissue enclosed in a rigid shell with application to the injured brain. *J Trauma* 1997;42:823.
68. Ibid, p 827.
69. Zornow M, Scheller M, Shackford S. Effect of a hypertonic lactated Ringer's solution on intracranial pressure and cerebral water content in a model of traumatic brain injury. *J Trauma* 1989;29:484.
70. Scheller M, Zornow M, Oh Y. A comparison of the cerebral and hemodynamic effects of mannitol and hypertonic saline in a rabbit model of acute cryogenic brain injury. *J Neurosurg Anesth* 1991;3:291.
71. Worthley L, Cooper D, Jones N. Treatment of resistant intracranial hypertension with hypertonic saline: Report of two cases. *J Neurosurg* 1988;68:748.

72. Fisher B, Thomas D, Peterson B. Hypertonic saline lowers raised intracranial pressure in children after head trauma. *J Neurosurg Anesth* 1992;4:4.
73. Roberts, p 731.
74. Williams, p 848.
75. Marshall, p 199.
76. Ibid.
77. Ibid.
78. Ibid.
79. Ibid, p 200.
80. Ibid.
81. Hund EF, Bohrer H, Martin E, Hanley DF. Disturbances of water and electrolyte balance. In: Hacke, ed. *Neuro Critical Care.* Berlin: Springer-Verlag; 1994:924.
82. Harrigan, p 158.
83. Zafonte R, Mann N. Cerebral salt wasting syndrome in brain injury patients: A potential cause of hyponatremia. *Arch Phys Med Rehabil* 1997;78:540.
84. Hund, p 925.
85. Harrigan, p 155.
86. Harrigan, p 154.
87. Ibid, p 155.
88. Ibid.
89. Ibid.
90. Ibid.
91. Charbel F. Commentary to: Kurokawa Y, Uede T, Ishiguro M et al. Pathogenesis of hyponatremia following subarachnoid hemorrhage due to ruptured cerebral aneurysm. *Surg Neurol* 1996;46:500.
92. Adams HP. Prevention of brain ischemia after aneurysmal subarachnoid hemorrhage. *Neurol Clin* 1992;10:251.
93. Steiner H, Fink M, Kremer P, Diringer M. Subarachnoid hemorrhage. In: Hacke W, ed. *Neuro Critical Care.* Berlin: Springer-Verlag; 1994:648.
94. Alvisi C, Giulioni M, Ursino M. The control mechanism involved in post-subarachnoid hemorrhage vasospasm. *J Neurosurg Sci* 1991;35:1.
95. Shucart W, Jackson I. Management of diabetes insipidus in neurosurgical patients. *J Neurosurg* 1976;44:65.
96. Morrison G, Singer I. Hyperosmolal states. In: Narins R, ed. *Maxwell and Kleemans Clinical Disorders of Fluid and Electrolyte Metabolism,* 5th ed. New York: McGraw-Hill; 1994:630.
97. Ibid, p 637.
98. Robinson AG, Verbalis JG. Diabetes insipidus. *Curr Ther Endocrinol Metab* 1997;6:1.
99. Ibid, p 5.
100. Ibid, p 6.

Acute Pancreatitis

PATHOPHYSIOLOGY

Acute pancreatitis is a nonbacterial inflammation of the pancreas that is thought to be caused by digestion of the gland by its own enzymes.[1] The pancreas becomes edematous and may pull enough fluid into itself to produce hypovolemia; swelling may be severe enough to compress the vascular bed and cause ischemia and necrosis. In addition, severe pancreatitis can produce irritation of the peritoneal surface (measuring 1.0–1.5 m[2]) and cause the transudation of substantial volumes of protein-rich fluid. An analogy can be made between the injury induced by severe pancreatitis and a chemical burn. Tissue changes are characterized by pancreatic and peripancreatic edema and fat necrosis; this form of the disease is sometimes referred to as *edematous pancreatitis*.[2] A more severe form involves extensive pancreatic and peripancreatic fat necrosis and hemorrhage into and around the pancreas (referred to *hemorrhagic* or *necrotizing pancreatitis*.[3] Only about 10% to 15% of the patients with pancreatitis have a severe attack; however, the mortality and serious morbidity in this group may be greater than 50%.[4] Death in most patients with severe acute pancreatitis is related to multiple system organ failure.[5]

ETIOLOGICAL ASSOCIATIONS

The annual incidence of acute pancreatitis is about 10/100,000 in the adult population.[6] Collectively, biliary tract stone disease and alcohol abuse account for about 80% of the cases of pancreatitis.[7] Among other possible causes are trauma and operation and certain drugs. About 2% of the cases of pancreatitis in adults are induced by drugs.[8] Sometimes the cause is unknown and is labeled idiopathic.

FLUID AND ELECTROLYTE DERANGEMENTS

HYPOVOLEMIA

In acute pancreatitis, pancreatic inflammation and autodigestion lead to peripancreatic edema and loss of edema fluid or blood into the retroperitoneal tissue. As a result, profound hypovolemic can occur. The severity of the hypovolemia depends on the extent of fluid and blood lost in the retroperitoneum and peritoneal cavity, the volume of fluid sequestered in the bowel during adynamic ileus, and the volume of vomitus or fluid loss from nasogastric (NG) suction. Acute renal failure (ARF) may follow untreated severe intravascular volume depletion; in this case, both the blood urea nitrogen (BUN) and the serum creatinine levels will increase. The hematocrit may be elevated in edematous pancreatitis because of plasma loss from the vascular space (causing the red blood cells to be suspended in a smaller blood volume) or low in hemorrhagic pancreatitis as a result of blood loss.

Note in Table 20-1 that the estimated amount of fluid sequestered in the abdomen after the onset of pancreatitis is one of the prognostic signs for risk of complications, as is the extent to which the hematocrit is decreased (reflecting the amount of blood loss in hemorrhagic pancreatitis).

HYPOCALCEMIA

Hypocalcemia has been reported to occur in 40% to 75% of patients with acute pancreatitis.[9] In part, the drop in the total serum calcium level (sum of the ionized and bound fractions) is related to the con-

 TABLE 20-1.   Ranson's Criteria: Prognostic Signs Used to Estimate Risk of Major Complications or Death From Acute Pancreatitis

At time of admission or diagnosis:
  Age > 55 yr
  WBC > 16,000/mm[3]
  Blood glucose > 200 mg/dL
  Lactate dehydrogenase level > 350 IU/L
  Glutamic-oxaloacetic transaminase level
    > 250 SFU/dL
During initial 48 hr:
  Hematocrit decrease > 10 percentage points
  BUN increase > 5 mg/dL
  Serum calcium < 8 mg/dL
  PaO_2 < 60 mmHg
  Base deficit > 4 mEq/L
  Estimated fluid sequestration > 6,000 mL

current hypoalbuminemia predictably associated with the leakage of protein-rich fluid into the peritoneal cavity. (Recall that when hypoalbuminemia is present, the total serum calcium appears lower than it actually is.) This probably explains why tetany is only rarely seen in patients with acute pancreatitis, despite the presence of a low total serum calcium level.[10] However, there does also appear to be a true decrease in ionized calcium.[11] A significantly reduced ionized calcium level or the presence of hypocalcemic symptoms warrants calcium replacement. Calcium supplementation may be indicated to prevent cardiac dysrhythmias.

Several hypotheses have been proposed to explain the hypocalcemia of acute pancreatitis. For example, discovery of calcium ions deposited in areas of fat necrosis in the pancreas led to the proposal that calcium soap formation was the main cause of hypocalcemia in pancreatitis.[12,13] However, if this were the only cause, it would be difficult to explain why parathyroid hormone does not quickly stimulate the release of calcium stored in the bones. It is thought that decreased secretion of parathyroid hormone contributes to the hypocalcemia.[14–16] Although the exact etiology of hypocalcemia is not certain, the degree of hypocalcemia is often used as a prognostic sign in the patient with acute pancreatitis (see Table 20-1).

HYPOMAGNESEMIA

Mild hypomagnesemia may occur during acute pancreatitis. As is the case with hypocalcemia, at least in part, hypomagnesemia has been attributed to precipitation of magnesium ions in the inflamed tissues in and around the pancreas as insoluble magnesium soaps.[17] Also, like with hypocalcemia, hypomagnesemia is often at least partially related to hypoalbuminemia (meaning that much of the change may be in bound rather than in ionized magnesium). Of course, contributing to the hypomagnesemia may be a direct loss by means of vomiting, gastric suction, and diarrhea. If the pancreatitis is due to alcoholism, the hypomagnesemia is likely to be more severe (because of the multiple magnesium-lowering effects of alcohol). Patients with acute pancreatitis and hypocalcemia commonly have intracellular magnesium deficiency despite normal serum magnesium concentrations; therefore, magnesium deficiency may play a significant role in the pathogenesis of hypocalcemia.[18]

HYPOPHOSPHATEMIA

Hypophosphatemia may occur in patients with acute pancreatitis and is usually associated with respiratory alkalosis.[19] It has also been reported in patients with acute pancreatitis in the absence of respiratory alkalosis. Possible reasons for the association include increased catecholamine production, alterations in circulating insulin or glucagon, or the intravenous (IV) administration of glucose.[20] Alcoholic patients are more likely to have low serum phosphate levels than are nonalcoholic patients.

ACID–BASE DISTURBANCES

Acid–base disturbances may vary widely, depending on clinical circumstances. For example, hypokalemic, hypochloremic, metabolic alkalosis may result from the frequent vomiting associated with acute pancreatitis, as well as from the gastric suction used during treatment to put the pancreas "at rest" and to alleviate an adynamic ileus. On the other hand, a high anion gap (AG) metabolic acidosis is likely in the presence of poor tissue perfusion; a normal AG metabolic acidosis may be seen with early ARF.

The pulmonary complications to which patients with pancreatitis are predisposed (such as pneumonia, pleural effusions, pulmonary edema, pulmonary emboli, and atelectasis) may cause respiratory acid–base problems (either acidosis or alkalosis). Severe pain may stimulate ventilation and cause respiratory alkalosis.

● DIAGNOSIS/PROGNOSTIC INDICATORS

The patient with acute pancreatitis usually presents with severe epigastric pain that radiates to the back, causing abdominal guarding and inability to find a comfortable position. Other common symptoms include nausea and vomiting, mild fever, tachycardia, and tachypnea. Among conditions to consider in differential diagnosis are perforated peptic ulcer, acute cholecystitis, biliary colic, and small bowel obstruction and infarction.

Heavily relied on in the diagnosis of acute pancreatitis is increased serum amylase activity coupled with abdominal pain. Total serum amylase activity level rises

2 to 12 hours after symptom onset and remains elevated for several days in most cases.[21] Values greater than five times the upper limit of normal are found in about 80% to 90% of the cases.[22] A number of investigators have studied commonly used combinations of clinical and laboratory data that can indicate the severity of pancreatitis within the first 48 hours after hospital admission.[23–25] Those listed by Ranson[26] are summarized in Table 20-1. When fewer than three criteria are present, the mortality is predicted to be 1%; when three or four are present, 15%; when five or six are present, 40%; and when seven criteria or more are present, 100%. The criteria differ slightly according to the cause of pancreatitis (gallstone-related versus nongallstone-related). Ranson's criteria are said to be able to distinguish between patients who have mild or severe pancreatitis 90% of the time; however, they are not as accurate in predicting mortality.[27] Other investigators have applied the APACHE II criteria to patients with pancreatitis; an advantage of this set of criteria is that it can be used at any point in the patient's illness (not just the first 48 hours).[28]

● COMPLICATIONS

Nearly 25% of all attacks of pancreatitis are severe and lead to complications; the mortality rate approaches 9%.[29] Severe disease can be associated with both local and systemic complications. Among the local complications are necrosis, pseudocysts, abscesses, fistulas, and gastrointestinal hemorrhage. The two most common systemic complications of acute pancreatitis are renal and respiratory failure.

In a study of 267 consecutive patients admitted with acute pancreatitis, 63 (24%) developed multiple system organ failure (defined as two or more organ systems).[30] Most common in this patient population were renal, respiratory, and cardiovascular failure. To some extent, the multiple system organ failure may be caused by secondary pancreatic infections.

ACUTE RENAL FAILURE

In the above-mentioned study of 267 consecutive patients with acute pancreatitis, renal failure occurred in 16%; overall mortality from ARF was 81%.[31] For the most part, ARF is explained on the basis of hypo-

volemia and hypotension.[32] In fact, renal failure from inadequate fluid replacement is a frequent finding in patients who die from pancreatitis.[33] The need for adequate fluid resuscitation to prevent this complication is obvious. Sufficient fluid replacement should be given to maintain adequate circulatory blood volume and urine output. (See discussion of fluid replacement on page 7.)

RESPIRATORY FAILURE

Respiratory complications (such as atelectasis, pleural effusions, pneumonia, and adult respiratory distress syndrome [ARDS]) are among the more frequent life-threatening features of patients with acute pancreatitis. Frequently there is evidence of basilar atelectasis resulting from abdominal distention and splinting of the diaphragm. Pleural effusions (a result of inflammation from pancreatic enzymes and extravasation of fluids) are most often found on the left side; however, they may be bilateral.[34] About 30% of patients with acute pancreatitis develop arterial hypoxemia (PaO_2 < 70 mm Hg) and require supplemental oxygen by mask.[35] Because the onset of hypoxemia is often insidious, in most patients it is prudent to determine arterial blood gases every 12 hours for the first several days after admission.[36] Factors contributing to respiratory complications may include:

- Immobility and retained secretions
- Release of pancreatic enzymes into the systemic circulation, which may cause damage to pulmonary tissues
- Pleural effusions and accumulation of ascitic fluid (interfere with respirations)
- Overzealous fluid replacement therapy

In most cases, the respiratory failure usually improves as the acute attack of pancreatitis subsides; however, some patients progress to a more severe form of respiratory failure similar in all respects to ARDS. Marked hypoxemia can occur and mandate mechanical ventilation, an ominous prognostic sign. The mortality rate for acute pancreatitis patients with ARDS who require mechanical ventilation is greater than 50%.[37]

In a laboratory study performed on rats with experimentally induced pancreatitis, the initial manifestations of pancreatitis-associated lung injury revealed a pronounced clustering of polymorphonuclear leukocytes in pulmonary microvessels, followed by severe damage of alveolar endothelial cells.[38] The increase in vascular permeability of the lung resulted in interstitial edema formation. Structural changes were maximal after 12 hours and reversed completely after 84 hours. The structural appearance of pulmonary injury in the laboratory animals was similar to that reported in the early stages of ARDS.

It has also been suggested that pancreatitis-associated ARDS may result from degradation of surfactant by circulating enzymes (such as phospholipase) released from the inflamed pancreas.[39] Others indicate that the pathogenesis of pancreatitis-associated ARDS is unclear.[40]

⬤ TREATMENT

The treatment of acute pancreatitis is primarily supportive and includes vigorous IV fluid replacement, elimination of oral intake, possible use of NG suction, adequate parenteral analgesics for pain relief, correction of electrolyte and glucose abnormalities, and renal and respiratory support as needed. The patient with severe pancreatitis is best cared for in an intensive care unit where close monitoring of fluid and electrolyte status can be maintained. Laboratory data recommended to monitor the course of such patients include serum electrolytes (including serum calcium), serum creatinine and BUN, white blood cell count, hematocrit, arterial blood gases, and serum aspartate transaminase and lactic dehydrogenase.[41] Because hyperglycemia occurs in at least one-fourth of patients with acute pancreatitis,[42] blood glucose levels should also be monitored at regular intervals. Fortunately, the hyperglycemia usually resolves as the pancreatitis improves.

FLUID REPLACEMENT

Maintenance of an adequate circulating blood volume is of paramount importance in the patient with acute pancreatitis. The need for restoring volume cannot be overemphasized because the death rate from this disease in the acute stage is directly correlated with the adequacy of fluid resuscitation. Not only does hypovolemia predispose to ARF, pancreatitis itself may be made worse by the hypovolemic shock state because of impaired pancreatic perfusion.[43]

Fluid losses through fluid pooling in the abdomen and retroperitoneal area, as well as from NG suction, vomiting, and diaphoresis, must be considered and replaced. The intravascular volume deficit may be 30% or greater; therefore, volume restoration should be rapid and efficient.[44] As a rule, crystalloid solutions (such as lactated Ringer's solution) will suffice because the fluid lost into the retroperitoneum has the composition of the extracellular fluid. However, in severe cases of hemorrhagic pancreatitis, blood products and colloid solutions may be needed. With colloid solutions, there may be increased risk of developing ARDS.[45] Because rapid fluid replacement may be needed in some patients to prevent shock, close monitoring of vital signs is mandatory. A urinary catheter is needed to monitor hourly urine output; an hourly output greater than 40 mL is advocated by some authors.[46] Also, it is advisable to monitor the central venous pressure and blood gases at regular intervals.[47] In seriously ill patients, a Swan-Ganz catheter may be needed to monitor central filling pressures and an indwelling arterial line to monitor arterial oxygen tension.

ELECTROLYTE REPLACEMENT

Because hypocalcemia and hypomagnesemia are frequently present in acute pancreatitis, it may be necessary to administer these electrolytes by the parenteral route. Ionized fractions of calcium and magnesium should be measured when possible because they are significant in physiological functioning. When evaluating total calcium or magnesium levels, the effect of hypoalbuminemia should be considered. Hypocalcemia occurs in up to 30% of patients because of calcium precipitation in areas of fat necrosis and hypoalbuminemia.[48] However, the ionized calcium concentration usually remains normal and symptoms of tetany are rare.[49] Hypokalemia is frequently a problem that must be dealt with by potassium replacement.

PAIN MANAGEMENT

The pain of pancreatitis is caused by edema and distention of the pancreatic capsule, obstruction of the biliary tree, and peritoneal irritation caused by pancreatic products. Pain is usually sudden in onset and precedes the development of nausea and vomiting. The pain of acute pancreatitis is usually located in the epigastric and umbilical region and may radiate to the mid or low thoracic region of the back. The pain associated with acute pancreatitis can be quite severe; a constant, knifelike, boring pain is commonly reported. The pain is sometimes partially relieved by sitting and leaning forward or by lying on the side with the knees drawn upward.

Large doses of narcotic medications may be required to control the severe pain often associated with acute pancreatitis. For example, to achieve pain relief from pancreatitis, Soergel[50] recommends the use of meperidine (75–125 mg) every 3 to 4 hours as needed; Friedman[51] recommends meperidine in a dosage up to 100 to 150 mg every 3 to 4 hours as necessary. If severe hepatic or renal dysfunction is present, the dose may need to be reduced.[52] Meperidine is most commonly used because it is believed to have no significant effect on the sphincter of Oddi.[53] (Morphine causes narrowing of the sphincter and increases pressure within the bile duct.) However, others point out that meperidine, like all opioids, can also increase smooth muscle tone in the biliary tract, causing increased pressure in the bile duct.[54,55] The latter authors believe that morphine may be a better choice than meperidine because the analgesic effect of morphine lasts longer; also, repeated doses of meperidine can lead to the accumulation of the meperidine metabolite (normeperidine), which can lead to neuromuscular irritation.[56,57] Because pain associated with acute pancreatitis may be resistant to opioid analgesics, other therapies are being investigated. It has been suggested that octreotide (a long-acting somatostatic analog) may help reduce pancreatitis pain that is unrelieved by opioids.[58] Apparently octreotide is believed to reduce pain by reducing pancreatic secretions. Epidural blocks may also be considered when other techniques fail.[59]

No oral feedings should be given until the patient is pain free; premature introduction of food can exacerbate a severe recurrence.

NASOGASTRIC SUCTION

Nasogastric suction is used for most patients with acute pancreatitis, unless the disease is mild and not associated with significant vomiting or pain.[60] It is definitely needed in patients with protracted nausea and vomiting. A benefit of NG suction is relief from the intestinal ileus so frequently present in acute pancreatitis. Also, theoretically, this therapy helps to "put the pancreas at rest" by stopping the secretin-pancreozymin stimulus to pancreatic secretion. Although this therapy is advocated by

many, its ability to shorten or reduce the severity of an acute attack of pancreatitis has not been demonstrated. Several clinical studies have failed to prove the beneficial effects from NG suction in patients with pancreatitis, unless vomiting is a problem.[61,62]

RESPIRATORY CARE

Supportive respiratory care should be given during the course of acute pancreatitis. A number of respiratory complications have been described in patients with acute pancreatitis (including diaphragmatic elevation, fleeting infiltrates, pleural effusions, atelectasis, and arterial hypoxemia).[63] For this reason, blood gases should be monitored in acutely ill patients and respiratory support provided when indicated (such as humidified oxygen, intratracheal intubation, and assisted ventilation). Nursing management is discussed in the section on Nursing Interventions.

NUTRITIONAL SUPPORT

The patient is not allowed anything by mouth until the ileus and pain have resolved.[64] Small feedings of a high-carbohydrate diet are started once the pain has subsided and bowel sounds have returned.[65] The most reliable indication for beginning oral feedings is hunger.[66] Clear liquids are usually given first and gradually advanced to a low-fat diet, as determined by the patient's tolerance and absence of pain.[67]

Some patients cannot tolerate oral feedings because of persistent pain or nausea and vomiting; but, because they are often hypercatabolic due to the severity of their illness, they require substantial nutrient intake.[68] The problem then becomes one of deciding how to supply nutrients in adequate amounts. The decision as to whether to initiate total parenteral nutrition (TPN) or enteral feedings should be made on an individual basis.

Enteral nutrition is cited by some investigators as the preferred method for initial nutritional support of patients with pancreatitis.[69] Feeding into the jejunum causes less pancreatic stimulation than does feeding into the duodenum or stomach. Also, elemental (amino acid, low-fat) diets cause less stimulation of pancreatic exocrine secretion than do complex diets.[70] Several reports have indicated that small bowel feedings are tolerated by patients with acute pancreatitis.[71–73] Use of enteral feedings may help contain the hypermetabolic stress response to severe pancreatitis and reduce atrophy of the gut.[74] However, it may be difficult to achieve adequate levels of calories and protein because the feeding must be introduced slowly and the rate reduced if intolerance develops. For some patients, it may be necessary to start with TPN and then gradually convert to enteral feeding as tolerance allows.

PERITONEAL LAVAGE

Peritoneal lavage is sometimes used to remove toxins and various metabolites from the peritoneal cavity during attacks of acute pancreatitis; theoretically, this minimizes their systemic absorption.[75] Although in theory this treatment should improve the acutely ill patient's chance for recovery, two controlled studies of peritoneal lavage indicated that it did not affect the morbidity or mortality associated with severe pancreatitis.[76,77] Another study indicated that selected patients (those with more than five risk factors according to Ranson's criteria) who received long-term lavage (7 days), as compared to those who received short-term lavage (2 days), had a decreased mortality rate due to pancreatic abscess formation.[78]

Peritoneal lavage requires the insertion of a peritoneal lavage catheter and the infusion and withdrawal of lactated Ringer's solution (1–2 L/hr) for several days or longer.[79] A response, if it occurs, is most likely in the first 6 to 8 hours.[80]

INSULIN ADMINISTRATION

Small doses of regular insulin may be needed to treat the transient hyperglycemia that may occur in patients with acute pancreatitis. Apparently this is caused by damage to the beta cells (thus decreasing insulin secretion) and increased glucagon release from the alpha cells (elevating the blood sugar level). In some patients, permanent diabetes may follow.

● NURSING ASSESSMENT

Nursing care of the patient with acute pancreatitis is complex and requires sophisticated monitoring for complications and response to medical therapy. The following steps are necessary to detect changes in the patient's often rapidly fluctuating status:

1. Carefully measure and record fluid intake and output (I&O) from all routes. Fluid replacement is partially based on fluid losses that are directly measurable (eg, vomiting and gastric suction). Because of third-space fluid shifts into the retroperitoneum and abdomen, not all of the fluid loss can be measured directly. Therefore, in the early phase of the third-space fluid shift, it is often necessary to give more fluid than would be indicated by measured losses. Fluid replacement is primarily guided by hourly urine outputs, vital signs, and invasive hemodynamic monitoring (such as central venous pressure [CVP] and pulmonary capillary wedge pressures [PCWP]).

2. Monitor for the following signs of hypovolemia due to excessive fluid loss:
   - Decreased skin turgor
   - Dry mucous membranes
   - Initially, postural hypotension; later, decreased systolic pressure in all positions
   - Tachycardia (pulse rate 100/min)
   - Urinary output less than 30 mL/hr in adults. Low urine volume may be a function of insufficient fluid replacement or may indicate renal failure (acute tubular necrosis).
   - BUN elevated out of proportion to serum creatinine level
   - Low CVP
   - Low pulmonary artery capillary pressure
   - Low cardiac output
   - Hematocrit may be elevated (red blood cells are suspended in less plasma as intravascular fluid is shifted into third space)

   Because of sequestering of fluid into the abdominal and retroperitoneal areas plus vomiting and NG suction, fluid loss may be severe enough to induce serious hypovolemia. This situation must be detected before perfusion to vital organs is compromised, leading to permanent renal or cerebral damage. Monitoring I&O alone is not sufficient to guide fluid replacement therapy. With adequate fluid replacement, the above parameters will remain within or return to normal limits.

3. Monitor for the following signs of hemorrhagic shock if the patient has necrotizing hemorrhagic pancreatitis:
   - Hypotension
   - Tachycardia
   - Anxiety
   - Oliguria

- Cool, clammy skin
- Falling hematocrit
- Low CVP
- Low PCWP

Blood loss can be significant in necrotizing hemorrhagic pancreatitis and must be detected before serious perfusion problems develop. Although this condition resembles simple fluid volume deficit, it tends to occur more rapidly and is associated with a decreased rather than an elevated hematocrit.

4. Monitor response to fluid replacement therapy. Fluid replacement therapy should be aggressive enough to keep the vital signs and hourly urine volume within normal limits. If the patient has underlying cardiovascular problems, it may be necessary to monitor the CVP and PCWP. A close working relationship between the nurse and physician is necessary if the correct volume of fluid replacement is to be achieved.

5. Monitor for respiratory distress or infection:
   - Hypoxemia (as evidenced by a low PaO_2)
   - Breath sounds indicating the presence of infiltrates
   - Tachypnea and labored respirations
   - Cyanosis
   - Temperature elevation

   Patients with pancreatitis are predisposed to pulmonary complications, such as ARDS, fleeting infiltrates, pleural effusions, and atelectasis.

6. Monitor for hypocalcemia:
   - Monitor serum calcium levels (consider albumin level and pH if total calcium is measured).
   - Note complaints of numbness or tingling in the extremities or circumoral region.
   - Look for latent tetany as indicated by Trousseau's and Chvostek's signs (see Chap. 2).
   - Expect dysrhythmias to be more frequent if hypocalcemia is present.

   See Chapter 6 for further discussion on hypocalcemia.

7. Monitor for hypomagnesemia:
   - Check laboratory reports for lowered serum magnesium levels. Magnesium deficiency is most likely to be present in patients who were previously malnourished or alcoholic. Note that this imbalance looks much like hypocalcemia. Unfortunately, magnesium is not an ingredient in commonly used IV fluids; for

that matter, neither is calcium (except for the small amount in lactated Ringer's solution). Magnesium is available for parenteral use and is discussed in Chapter 7.
   - Look for tremors, confusion, hallucinations, tachycardia, and positive Chvostek's and Trousseau's signs. See Chapter 7 for a more thorough discussion of assessment for hypomagnesemia.

8. Monitor for hypokalemia:
   - Check laboratory reports for decreased serum potassium levels.
   - Look for arrhythmias, weakness, gastrointestinal hypomotility, and paresthesias. See Chapter 5 for a more thorough discussion of assessment for hypokalemia.

9. Assess for infection by monitoring for pain and elevated body temperature. Consider the location, severity, and duration of pain. Be aware that subtle changes in the nature and frequency of pain may be indicative of pancreatic abscess. Also, be aware that a temperature above the usual low-grade fever associated with acute pancreatitis may signal a complicating infection. Septic complications of acute pancreatitis include pancreatic abscess, infected pancreatic necrosis, and infected pseudocyst.[81]

10. Monitor serum glucose levels to detect hyperglycemia. Serum glucose levels (determined by capillary "sticks") are more valid than urinary glucose levels. Once the renal threshold for glucose has been determined to be normal, one can rely on urine glucose measurements.

11. Assess bowel sounds and abdominal girth at regular intervals to monitor degree of adynamic ileus.

● NURSING DIAGNOSES

Alterations associated with acute pancreatitis involve rapidly changing derangements in fluid, electrolyte, and perhaps acid–base balance. Because of these changes, a number of physiological nursing diagnoses may be appropriate. Clinical Tip: Examples of Nursing Diagnoses Related to Acute Pancreatitis lists examples of several physiological nursing diagnoses related to the care of patients with acute pancreatitis.

CLINICAL TIP

Examples of Nursing Diagnoses Related to Acute Pancreatitis

NURSING DIAGNOSIS	ETIOLOGICAL FACTORS	DEFINING CHARACTERISTICS
FVD related to third-spacing of fluid and gastric loss by vomiting and suction	Escape of secretions into abdomen and retroperitoneum, vomiting, and nasogastric suction (aggravated by fever and diaphoresis)	Tachycardia, hypotension, urine output < 30 mL/hr, concentrated urine, BUN elevated out of proportion to creatinine, poor skin turgor (see Chap. 3)
Ineffective breathing pattern related to immobility, pain, and pleural effusions	Immobility, retained secretions, and pleural effusions (result of inflammation from pancreatic enzymes and extravasation of fluid), aggravated by overzealous fluid administration	Dyspnea, shortness of breath, tachypnea, cyanosis, cough, nasal flaring, decreased arterial oxygenation

BUN, blood urea nitrogen; FVD, fluid volume deficit.

● NURSING INTERVENTIONS

Much of what the nurse does in caring for the critically ill patient with acute pancreatitis revolves around monitoring the current clinical status and working collaboratively with the physician to provide supportive care. The following interventions are often needed:

1. Collaborate with the physician to safely administer fluids and electrolytes based on physiological indices. If desired responses are not achieved, consult with the physician to revise fluid orders (see section on Nursing Assessment).
2. Maintain correct position and patency of the NG tube to alleviate nausea and vomiting and relieve distention.
   - The tip of the tube should be well into the stomach (near the pylorus); if the tip rests high in the stomach, hydrochloric acid may escape through the duodenum and theoretically stimulate secretions.
   - Once the tube has been correctly positioned, mark the exterior portion and make every effort to maintain the position.
   - Maintain patency of the tube by irrigating with about 20 mL isotonic saline every 2 hours. Vis-

cous gastric secretions may necessitate more frequent irrigations.
   - Check suction apparatus periodically to be sure it is working correctly.
3. Implement measures to relieve pain.
   - Administer prescribed analgesics as frequently as indicated. Pain can be quite severe and should be treated with regular analgesic injections. If pain persists despite analgesics, discuss problem with physician. In addition to promoting comfort, pain relief from analgesics decreases restlessness and anxiety, which probably also decreases pancreatic secretions.
   - Assist the patient to achieve a position of comfort. Pain relief may sometimes be partially attained by sitting up or lying curled on the right or left side. Patients with peritoneal irritation are likely to remain very still. (This may present a problem in terms of retained respiratory secretions.)
4. Attempt to prevent or minimize respiratory complications.
   - Turn patient at regular intervals to foster drainage of secretions.
   - Encourage deep breathing at regular intervals.
   - If necessary, suction retained secretions to keep airway open.

- Monitor rate of fluid replacement to avoid overloading the circulatory system and predisposing to pulmonary edema.

The physician may prescribe humidified oxygen to help support the patient. In severe situations, intubation and mechanical ventilation will be indicated. It should be noted that im-paired pulmonary function may occur in all patients with pancreatitis (regardless of severity of illness).

5. Administer insulin per medical directives as indicated, based on capillary blood sugars, to control hyperglycemia.
6. Provide patient with periods of rest between nursing activities and attempt to minimize anxiety-producing situations.
7. Consider the patient's need for nutrients.
   - Administer TPN or jejunal feedings if prescribed. (See section on nutritional support.)
   - Be aware that after NG suction is discontinued, the patient is usually maintained without oral feedings for at least 24 to 48 hours before a low-fat diet is gradually introduced. Great care must be taken to avoid feeding too quickly because this can exacerbate another episode of acute pancreatitis.
   - When the acute phase subsides and clear liquids are allowed by mouth, monitor bowel sounds and watch for recurring pain and nausea.
   - Keep a record of the patient's nutrient intake so that deficiencies can be brought to the attention of the physician and dietitian.

CASE STUDY

● **20-1.** A 50-year-old intoxicated man with a long history of alcoholism was admitted to the hospital for evaluation of epigastric pain that radiated through to the midback. The only way the patient could find relief was to sit in bed with his knees drawn to his chest. He stated he was nauseated and had been vomiting intermittently since the abdominal pain started 2 days earlier.

His vital signs were:
Blood pressure = 108/64 mm Hg
Pulse rate = 120/min
Respiratory rate = 26/min
Temperature = 38.5°C

On examination, his abdomen was diffusely tender to palpation. A chest x-ray revealed a large effusion at the right lung base.

Laboratory results from a venous blood sample were:
Sodium = 143 mEq/L
Potassium = 3.3 mEq/L
Chloride = 92 mEq/L
CO_2 content = 22 mEq/L
Total calcium = 8.2 mg/dL
Magnesium = 1.2 mg/dL
BUN = 48 mg/dL
Creatinine = 1.2 mg/dL
Amylase = 900 IU
Glucose = 200 mg/dL
White blood cell count = 13,400 mm^3

Laboratory results from an arterial sample for blood gases were:
pH = 7.28
$PaCO_2$ = 41 mm Hg
PaO_2 = 56 mm Hg
HCO_3 = 19 mEq/L

Laboratory results from a urinalysis were:
3+ ketones

On the basis of the above findings, a diagnosis of acute pancreatitis was made. The patient was treated with NG suction, IV fluid replacement, and parenteral analgesia. Within the next few days, the abdominal pain, fever, and nausea subsided.

COMMENTARY: Hypotension and tachycardia indicate a low blood volume, as does an elevated BUN (reflective of decreased renal perfusion). A number of potential problems could be present in this patient. For example:

- Hypoxemia (PaO_2, 56 mm Hg) could cause lactic acidosis, a form of high AG metabolic acidosis.
- Absence of food intake (common in alcoholics during heavy drinking spells) and ethanol intoxication could cause alcoholic ketoacidosis, a form of high AG metabolic acidosis (note that the patient had 3+ ketones in the urine).
- Loss of gastric acid by vomiting and NG suction could cause metabolic alkalosis and a lower than normal serum potassium (note

that the patient's potassium is slightly lower than normal).

- The below normal pH indicates acidosis. The lower than normal bicarbonate level indicates *metabolic acidosis*; calculation of the AG indicates that this is a high AG metabolic acidosis due to excessive lactic acid production for hypoxemia (see Chap. 9). The bicarbonate level would have been even lower if vomiting had not been present to cause a predisposition to metabolic alkalosis (and thus an increase in bicarbonate concentration).

- *Respiratory acidosis* is also present. This imbalance can be determined by calculating the expected $PaCO_2$ and comparing that value to the actual reading. Using Winter's formula:

$$\text{Expected } PaCO_2 = 1.5\,(HCO_3) + 8 \pm 2$$
$$= 1.5\,(19) + 8 \pm 2$$
$$= 34.5 \text{ to } 38.5 \text{ mm Hg}$$

Thus, the expected PaCO2 should range between 34.5 to 38.5 mm Hg. Instead, it is 41 mm Hg (indicating a slight degree of carbon dioxide retention in addition to the expected compensatory change).

Note that the patient has a pleural effusion that could be interfering with ventilation, as can abdominal distention and splinting of the diaphragm. It is also thought that release of pancreatic enzymes into the systemic circulation may cause damage to pulmonary tissues.

As noted in Table 20-1, a serum calcium level of less than 8 mg/dL is one indicator of poor outcome after the onset of pancreatitis. Although this patient's serum calcium level is not less than 8 mg/dL, it is below normal. Calcium supplementation may be indicated to prevent cardiac dysrhythmias. Because the patient is acidotic, a greater proportion of calcium exists in the ionized form (making adverse effects of hypocalcemia less prominent).

Like hypocalcemia, hypomagnesemia has at least in part been attributed to precipitation of magnesium ions in the inflamed tissues in and around the pancreas as insoluble magnesium soaps. Losses from vomiting, gastric suction, and diarrhea intensify hypomagnesemia. Because this patient has a history of alcoholism, hypomagnesemia may also be related to the multiple magnesium-lowering effects of alcohol.

REFERENCES

1. Schwartz S, Shires T, Spencer F. *Principles of Surgery*, 7th ed. Baltimore, MD: Williams & Wilkins; 1999:1472.
2. Ibid.
3. Ibid.
4. Ayres S, Grenvik A, Holbrook P, Shoemaker W, eds. *Textbook of Critical Care*, 3rd ed. Philadelphia: WB Saunders; 1995:986.
5. Miskovitz P. Acute pancreatitis: Further insight into mechanisms. *Crit Care Med* 1998;26:816.
6. Soergel K. Pancreatitis. In: Bennett J, Plum F, eds. *Cecil Textbook of Medicine*, 20th ed. Philadelphia: WB Saunders; 1996:730.
7. Mergener K, Baillie J. Acute pancreatitis. *BMJ* 1998;316:44.
8. Muchnick J, Mehta J. Antiotensin-converting enzyme inhibitor-induced pancreatitis. *Clin Cardiol* 1999;22:50.
9. Narins R, ed. *Clinical Disorders of Fluid and Electrolyte Metabolism*, 5th ed. New York: McGraw-Hill; 1994:1026.
10. Kokko J, Tannen R. *Fluids and Electrolytes*, 3rd ed. Philadelphia: WB Saunders; 1996:688.
11. Ibid.
12. Pemberton L, Pemberton D. *Treatment of Water, Electrolyte and Acid–Base Disorders in the Surgical Patient*. New York: McGraw-Hill; 1994:208.
13. Narins, p 1484.
14. Pemberton, Pemberton, p 208.
15. Narins, p 1026.
16. Robertson G et al. Inadequate parathyroid response in acute pancreatitis. *N Engl J Med* 1976;294:512.
17. Narins, p 2202.
18. Ryzen E, Rude R. Low intracellular magnesium in patients with acute pancreatitis and hypocalcemia. *West J Med* 1990;152:145.
19. Narins, p 1053.
20. Lachter J et al. Hypophosphatemia and idiopathic pancreatitis. *American Journal of Gastroenterology* 1986;81:1221.
21. Soergel, p 731.
22. Ibid.
23. Ranson J, Rifkind K, Roses D, et al. Prognostic signs and the role of operative management in acute pancreatitis. *Surg Gynecol Obstet* 1974;139:69.
24. Ranson J. Etiological and prognostic factors in human acute pancreatitis: A review. *Am J Gastroenterol* 1982;77:633.
25. Blamey S et al. Prognostic factors in acute pancreatitis. *Gut* 1984;25:1340.
26. Ranson, p 637.
27. Gorelick F. Acute pancreatitis. In: Yamada T, Alpers D, Owyang C, Powell D, Silverstein F, eds. *Textbook of Gastroenterology*, 2nd ed. Philadelphia: JB Lippincott; 1995:2079.
28. Wilson C et al: Prediction of outcome in acute pancreatitis: a comparative study of APACHE II, clinical assessment and multiple factor scoring systems. *Br J Surg* 1990;77:1260.

29. Steinberg W, Tenner S. Acute pancreatitis. *N Engl J Med* 1994;330:1198.
30. Tran D et al. Prevalence and prediction of multiple organ system failure and mortality in acute pancreatitis. *J Crit Care* 1993;8:145.
31. Tran D et al. Acute renal failure in patients with acute pancreatitis: Prevalence, risk factors, and outcome. *Nephrol Dialysis Transplant* 1993;8:1079.
32. Agarwal N, Pitchumoni C. Acute pancreatitis: A multisystem disease. *Gastroenterology* 1993;1:115.
33. Schwartz, p 1478.
34. Gorelick, p 2075.
35. Schwartz, p 1478.
36. Ibid.
37. Peek G, White S, Scott A et al. Severe acute respiratory distress syndrome secondary to acute pancreatitis successfully treated with extracorporeal membrane oxygenation in three patients. *Ann Surg* 1998;227:572.
38. Willemer S et al. Lung injury in acute experimental pancreatitis in rats. *Int J Pancreatol* 1994;8:305.
39. Agarwal, Pitchumoni, p 121.
40. Gorelick, p 2085.
41. Friedman L. Liver, biliary tract, and pancreas. In: Tierney L, McPhee S, Papadakis M. *Medical Diagnosis & Treatment*, 38th ed. Stamford, CT: Appleton & Lange; 1999:Chap. 15.
42. Gorelick, p 2080.
43. Schwartz, p 1478.
44. Soergel, p 733.
45. Friedman, p 673.
46. Soergel, p 733.
47. Friedman, p 673.
48. Soergel, p 732.
49. Ibid.
50. Ibid, p 733.
51. Friedman, p 673.
52. Ibid.
53. Carey C, Lee H, Woeltje K. *The Washington Manual of Medical Therapeutics*, 29th ed. Philadelphia: Lippincott-Raven; 1998.
54. Lee F, Cundiff D. Meperidine vs morphine in pancreatitis and cholecystitis. (Letter) *Arch Intern Med* 1998;158:2399.
55. Coyne P. Assessing and treating the pain of pancreatitis. *Am J Nurs* 1998;98:14-6.
56. Lee, Cundiff, p 2399.
57. Coyne, p 16.
58. Ibid.
59. Ibid.
60. Schwartz, p 1477.
61. Fuller R, Loveland J, Frankel M. An evaluation of the efficacy of nasogastric suction treatment in alcoholic pancreatitis. *Am J Gastroenterol* 1981;75:349.
62. Switz D. Acute alcoholic pancreatitis: Effect of clinical presentation and therapies on outcome at a VA hospital. *Ann Intern Med* 1973;78:816.
63. Toledo-Pereyra L. *The Pancreas: Principles of Medical and Surgical Practice*. New York: John Wiley & Sons; 1985:184.
64. Schwartz, p 1477.
65. Soergel, p 733.
66. Gorelick, p 2080.
67. Friedman, p 673.
68. Kalfarentzos F, Kehagias J, Mead K et al. Enteral nutrition is superior to parenteral nutrition in severe acute pancreatitis: Results of a randomized prospective trial. *Br J Surg* 1997;84:1665.
69. Ibid.
70. McClave S, Snider H, Sexton L, Owens N. Nutrition in pancreatitis. *The ASPEN Nutrition Support Practice Manual*. Silver Spring, MD: American Society for Parenteral and Enteral Nutrition; 1998:13-5.
71. Kudsk K et al. Postoperative jejunal feedings following complicated pancreatitis. *Nutr Clin Pract* 1990;5:14.
72. McArdle A, Echave W, Brown R et al. Effect of elemental diet on pancreatic secretion. *Am J Surg* 1974;128:690.
73. Nakad A, Piessevaux H, Marot J et al. Is early enteral nutrition in acute pancreatitis dangerous? About 20 patients fed by an endoscopically placed nasogastrojejunal tube. *Pancreas* 1998;17:187.
74. McClave S, Spain D, Snider H. Nutritional management in acute and chronic pancreatitis. *Gastroenterol Clin North Am* 1998;27:421.
75. Schwartz, p 1478.
76. Ihse I et al. Influence of peritoneal lavage on objective prognostic signs in acute pancreatitis. *Ann Surg* 1986;204:122.
77. Mayer A et al. Controlled clinical trials of peritoneal lavage for the treatment of severe pancreatitis. *N Engl J Med* 1985;312:399.
78. Ranson J, Berman R. Long peritoneal lavage decreases pancreatic sepsis in acute pancreatitis. *Ann Surg* 1990;211:708.
79. Schwartz, p 1478.
80. Ibid.
81. Andreoli T, Carpenter C, Bennett J, Plum F. *Cecil Essentials of Medicine*, 4th ed. Philadelphia: WB Saunders; 1997.

Cirrhosis With Ascites

⬤ PATHOPHYSIOLOGY

The incidence of cirrhosis in the United States is about 360/100,000 population, or about 900,000 total patients.[1] Cirrhosis is usually due to alcohol abuse and hepatitis C in the Western world; in contrast, hepatitis B is a major cause in the underdeveloped countries.[2] Other less common causes include drugs and toxins, autoimmune chronic active hepatitis, biliary cirrhosis, chronic hepatic congestion, and certain genetically determined metabolic diseases.[3]

Cirrhosis is characterized by an extensive increase of fibrous tissue within the liver structure. As blood, lymph, and biliary channels become compressed by fibrotic changes, intrahepatic pressure increases, reducing the liver's capacity to fulfill its functions. At first the liver is enlarged with fatty tissue; later, it becomes small, hard, and nodular.

ASCITES FORMATION

Ascites is not a disease but rather a symptom of a disease, such as cirrhosis, in which a collection of serum-like fluid forms within the peritoneal cavity. In cirrhosis, ascitic fluid accumulates as venous outflow is impeded through the fibrotic liver, and then seeps from the surface of the liver into the peritoneal cavity to produce ascites. Because of the fluid's high protein content, it pulls additional fluid from the surfaces of the gut and mesentery by osmosis. A decompensated cirrhotic patient can accumulate more than 15 liters of ascitic fluid; accumulations of up to 28 liters have been reported.[4] Obviously, much discomfort (such as dyspnea, insomnia, and difficulty ambulating) is associated with a large quantity of fluid in the abdominal cavity. Multiple factors contribute to ascites formation. Among these are weeping of fluid from the diseased liver into the peritoneal cavity, which exceeds the capacity of the peritoneum to reabsorb the fluid; hypoalbuminemia (which decreases oncotic pressure); and increased sodium reabsorption by the kidneys.

Exact mechanisms in the pathogenesis of renal sodium retention and ascites formation in cirrhosis is controversial.[5] However, several theories have been proposed, including "overfilling" and "underfilling." Recently, an "integrated" theory has been developed. Early on, intrahepatic hypertension activates a hepatic baroreceptor reflex that enhances renal sodium retention and increases plasma volume. As the cirrhotic dis-ease progresses, this overflow spills into the peritoneal cavity as ascites. The fluid shift from the vascular system into the peritoneal space causes underfilling, which eventually dominates the clinical picture. Stimulation of the renin-angiotensin system increases renal sodium retention and therefore plasma volume.[6]

Decreased Effective Arterial Volume

Decreased effective arterial volume refers to a state in which the total extracellular fluid volume is normal or even expanded, although the kidneys respond as if they were underperfused.[7] They do so by retaining sodium and producing a concentrated urine. Presumably, this is what occurs in the patient with cirrhosis and ascites formation.

Hypoalbuminemia

Severe *hypoalbuminemia* may also contribute to ascites formation. Causes of low serum albumin levels in cirrhotic patients include decreased synthesis of protein by the diseased liver, dilutional effect (due to salt and water retention), and a shift of protein from the vascular space to the peritoneal cavity. The protein content of ascitic fluid may be as high as half that of serum.[8] Because the serum albumin level is below normal, plasma oncotic pressure is reduced, an effect that favors shifting of fluid from the vascular space into the peritoneal cavity.

However, hypoalbuminemia is not nearly as important in ascites formation as is the increased pressure generated by the hepatic postsinusoidal obstruction.[9] Relief from ascites has been reported when portal hypertension is corrected by shunting procedures.

EDEMA

Edema formation in cirrhotic patients has several causes. Increased pressure in the vena cava (secondary to ascitic fluid and enlarged liver size) interferes with venous drainage of the lower extremities. Contributing to edema formation is the hypoalbuminemia that is frequently present in patients with advanced liver disease. By lowering the plasma oncotic pressure, hypoalbuminemia promotes shifting of fluid from the intravascular to the interstitial space. At first, edema appears in dependent areas; later on, it spreads to nondependent areas, varying in severity with the degree of sodium intake.[10] The edema associated with liver disease is of the "pitting" variety (see Fig. 2-3).

FLUID AND ELECTROLYTE DISTURBANCES

The common disorders of fluid, electrolyte, and acid–base metabolism observed in patients with hepatic cirrhosis are fluid volume excess with edema and ascites, hyponatremia, hypokalemia, respiratory alkalosis, and metabolic acidosis.[11]

Fluid Volume Excess

The patient with advanced cirrhotic disease has a complex fluid balance problem. Although there is an excess of total body fluid with an accumulation in the peritoneal cavity (ascites) and in the interstitial space (edema), there is also a problem of decreased effective arterial blood volume. Because of this, the kidneys strive to build up the intravascular volume by retaining sodium and water (although the blood volume may actually be normal or even above normal). Plasma aldosterone levels are often above normal due to increased adrenal secretion and inability of the liver to deactivate this hormone (of course, aldosterone causes sodium and water retention). Nonsteroidal anti-inflammatory drugs should be avoided because they may cause deterioration in renal function (with further fluid retention) if given in sufficient doses to patients with ascites due to liver disease.[12]

Hyponatremia

Hyponatremia is common in patients with advanced hepatic cirrhosis with edema and ascites and is usually caused by intrarenal disturbances in water handling and excessive release of antidiuretic hormone (ADH).[13] This hyponatremia occurs in addition to fluid volume excess. That is, although there is abnormal retention of both sodium and water, a relatively greater degree of water retention occurs. As such, the serum sodium level is diluted below normal although the total body sodium is excessive (see Fig. 4-2A). Other factors that can contribute to hyponatremia are sodium loss through frequent paracentesis or excessive diuretic use or too stringent sodium restriction. When the serum sodium concentration is less than 125 mEq/L, restriction of fluid intake to 800 to 1000 mL/day may be needed.[14] Hyponatremia is associated with increased mortality in patients with liver failure; it is not known if it actually increases mortality or if it is merely a marker of poor hepatic function.[15]

Hypokalemia

Hypokalemia is common in patients with chronic liver disease. Among the causes of hypokalemia are low dietary intake and renal loss of potassium caused by hyperaldosteronism and diuretics, as well as losses from the gastrointestinal (GI) tract.[16] One of the most common causes is diuretic use. In one study, almost two-thirds of the patients with cirrhosis developed a serum potassium level less than 3.1 mEq/L.[17] It has been suggested that potassium depletion can induce hepatic encephalopathy.[18] Additional adverse effects of hypokalemia include ileus, muscle weakness, myocardial irritability, and decreased renal concentrating ability.

Although less common than hypokalemia, *hyperkalemia* is occasionally seen in patients with chronic liver disease. Most often, it is associated with the use of potassium-sparing diuretics (such as spironolactone, amiloride, and triamterene). Use of potassium supplements and potassium-sparing diuretics should be stopped when serum potassium levels exceed 5.5 mEq/L.[19]

Acid–Base Imbalances

All four acid–base imbalances may be encountered in patients with liver disease. The most frequent is respiratory alkalosis.[20] In a study of 91 patients with portal cirrhosis, 64% had respiratory alkalosis.[21] As a rule, the degree of respiratory alkalosis increases as the severity of the hepatic disease increases.[22] It has been postulated that elevated blood ammonia levels stimulate hyperventilation and resultant respiratory alkalosis; however, it is unlikely that increased blood ammonia concentration is the sole factor.[23] Another possible cause is an elevated progesterone level; this hormone (normally degraded by the liver) is a respiratory stimulant.[24] Metabolic alkalosis occurs in many patients with hepatic disease and is usually associated with use of potassium-losing diuretics. It can also be caused by vomiting or nasogastric (NG) suction, or alkali loading from sources such as antacids or citrate from blood transfusions.[25]

High anion gap metabolic acidosis has been observed in 10% to 20% of patients with chronic liver disease.[26] The percentage increases as the severity of disease increases. It has been suggested that patients with liver disease are more susceptible to lactic acidosis because of the decreased ability of their diseased livers to remove lactic acid from the circulation. Also, they are susceptible to increased lactic acid production (as may occur with hypotension secondary to GI hemorrhage).[27]

Other Imbalances

Additional possible fluid and electrolyte disturbances related to cirrhosis of the liver are listed in Table 21-1, along with probable etiological associations.

EFFECTS ON BODY SYSTEMS

Cirrhosis of the liver has an insidious onset and affects most body systems. Brief discussions of the effects on various body systems follow.

Gastrointestinal System

Development of esophageal varices is the most serious complication associated with hepatic failure and portal hypertension. Severity of bleeding from varices is intensified by coagulopathies associated with liver failure. Enlarged abdominal veins and internal hemorrhoids may also be caused by portal hypertension. Malnutrition is common in patients with hepatic failure because the frequently associated anorexia, nausea, and vomiting preclude the recommended dietary intake. Many GI symptoms are related to venous engorgement of the GI organs. Muscle wasting and weight loss may be masked by fluid retention. Fetor hepaticus is often noted.

Cardiovascular System

Right ventricular heart failure often occurs in patients with hepatic failure secondary to high pressure in the portal system. Contributing to cardiac problems is the hypokalemia commonly found in cirrhotic patients as a result of the use of potassium-losing diuretics. Potassium deficiency predisposes to ventricular arrhythmias. Of course, arrhythmias may also result from hyperkalemia, which can occur in patients treated with potassium-sparing diuretics, particularly if renal disease is present.

Renal System

Hepatorenal syndrome (HRS) encompasses a type of renal failure that occurs in patients with hepatic failure. Typically, the kidneys are histologically normal and regain their function in the event of the recovery of hepatic function.[28] That is, when liver transplants are performed on patients with HRS, renal function may become normal.[29] Also, the kidney from a patient with HRS may be transplanted into a patient with normal liver function.[30] Even though there is no major histologic change in the kidneys, HRS is an ominous occurrence because it is usually progressive and fatal. The decline in renal function often follows overzealous diuresis, large-volume paracentesis, or sepsis.[31] HRS is manifested by oliguria, increased serum creatinine (usually > 10 mg/dL), increased blood urea nitrogen (BUN), and a low urinary sodium output (< 10 mEq/L). Before a diagnosis of HRS is made, the physician must consider the possibility of other causes of renal deterioration, such as prerenal azotemia due to fluid volume depletion. To exclude the possibility of prerenal azotemia, it may be necessary to administer a fluid challenge (such as 1,000 mL 0.9% NaCl) or to measure the pulmonary wedge pressure.[32]

Although the cause of HRS is not known, the pathogenesis apparently involves intensive renal vasoconstriction, perhaps because of impaired synthesis of renal vasodilators, such as prostaglandin E_2.[33] Improvement may follow placement of a transjugular intrahepatic portosystemic shunt (TIPS).[34] Because the cause of death in HRS is usually liver failure instead of renal failure, dialysis is generally not helpful; however, if the liver disease is potentially reversible or the patient is a candidate for a liver transplant, dialysis may be considered.[35] Liver transplantation is an accepted treatment for HRS.

Neurological System

Portal systemic encephalopathy (PSE) refers to the syndrome of disordered consciousness and altered neuromuscular activity seen in patients with hepatic failure. It can be classified as acute hepatic encephalopathy (usually occurring with fulminant hepatic failure) or chronic hepatic encephalopathy (as seen in chronic liver disease).[36] With acute hepatic encephalopathy, cerebral edema plays a role and mortality is high; with chronic hepatic encephalopathy, the condition is often reversible and is accompanied by subtle changes in neurological functioning.[37]

Normally, the liver removes nitrogenous by-products and ingested toxic agents and thus protects the systemic circulation from these products. However, in the presence of hepatic failure, these toxins bypass the

TABLE 21-1. Possible Water and Electrolyte Disturbances in Patients With Advanced Cirrhosis and Ascites

Disturbance	Etiology
Increased total ECF volume but decreased effective arterial volume	Enhanced renal tubular reabsorption of sodium
	Increased plasma aldosterone level due to increased adrenal secretion (in response to decreased effective arterial volume) and decreased degradation of this hormone by the diseased liver
Increased water retention, causing dilutional hyponatremia	Impaired renal water excretion related to excess ADH secretion (in response to decreased effective arterial volume)
Hypokalemia	Direct loss in vomiting or diarrhea
	Decreased intake due to anorexia
	Excessive use of potassium-losing diuretics (Note that hypokalemia is especially harmful to patients with hepatic failure because it increases ammonia formation and can induce hepatic coma.)
Hyperkalemia	Excessive use of potassium-sparing diuretics, especially when renal insufficiency is present or potassium-containing salt substitutes are used to make the low-sodium diet more palatable
Elevated serum ammonia level	Under normal circumstances, the large amounts of ammonia formed in the intestines by bacterial action are absorbed into the bloodstream and carried to the liver to be converted to urea for renal excretion. However, in cirrhosis, the liver cannot convert the ammonia to urea; thus, the blood ammonia level increases.
Hypomagnesemia	Loss of magnesium in vomiting and diarrhea, poor dietary intake, and renal wasting of magnesium in patients with cirrhosis due to alcoholism
Hypocalcemia	Possibly a result of inadequate storage of vitamin D by diseased liver; also associated with hypoalbuminemia
Hyperventilation with respiratory alkalosis	May be related to hyperammonemia (high ammonia level may act as a respiratory stimulant)
Respiratory acidosis	May occur if ascites is severe enough to compromise diaphragmatic movement
Metabolic alkalosis	Common in patients treated with potassium-losing diuretics such as furosemide, thiazides, and ethacrynic acid
Mild metabolic acidosis	May occur in patients treated with spironolactone (Aldactone) alone (due to interference by spironolactone with sodium/hydrogen ion exchange in the distal tubules)

ADH, antidiuretic hormone; ECF, extracellular fluid.

liver and enter the systemic circulation in abnormal concentrations. Although the exact toxins are not defined, ammonia is one of the implicated substances. Recall that the normal liver converts ammonia into urea for renal excretion. When this process is altered by a diseased liver, the serum ammonia level may rise sharply. However, the degree of serum ammonia elevation is not always predictive of the severity of PSE. Whatever the precise biochemical trigger of PSE, interference with cerebral metabolism and neurotransmission appears to be the basic underlying mechanism. Symptoms may range from mild (sleep–wake disturbances and ataxia) to severe (coma and seizures). Besides ammonia, other substances that have been implicated as toxins associated with PSE include gamma-aminobutyric acid, other amino acids, mercaptans, and short-chain fatty acids.[38]

Precipitating causes of PSE episodes include fluid volume depletion from overzealous use of diuretics, high-protein diet, digestion of blood from GI bleeding, constipation, infection, progressive liver dysfunction, and hypokalemia with alkalosis. Inability of the liver to convert the end-products of protein metabolism to urea results in an elevated serum ammonia level. Constipation increases the systemic absorption of toxins from the colon. Hypokalemia increases ammonia production and alkalosis promotes movement of ammonia and other toxins into the brain.

Treatment of PSE is aimed at identifying and treating precipitating factors (such as constipation, high dietary protein intake, GI bleeding, central nervous system-depressant drugs, hypokalemia, and overzealous use of diuretics), reducing dietary protein intake, preventing constipation, and administering lactulose to prevent ammonia absorption from the bowel. (See discussion of these modalities later in this chapter.) Prompt control of active bleeding is very important for a number of reasons; one is that blood within the intestinal tract is converted into ammonia by bacteria.[39] Patients with symptoms of PSE should have all narcotics, tranquilizers, and sedatives metabolized or excreted by the liver withheld. Oxazepam may be administered *cautiously* if agitation is severe; this agent is not metabolized by the liver.[40]

In patients with hepatic failure, not all neurological symptoms are due to PSE. They may be related to sodium derangements, especially hyponatremia. For this reason, even mild hyponatremia may be treated aggressively. Another cause of neurological symptoms may be severe malnutrition, which often accompanies hepatic failure. For example, deficiencies of B vitamins can lead to paresthesias, sensory disturbances, peripheral nerve degeneration, palsy of the sixth cranial nerve, and ptosis.

Respiratory System

The primary respiratory complication associated with hepatic failure is decreased lung expansion secondary to upward pressure on the diaphragm from ascites. Lung capacity may also be reduced due to hydrothorax when ascitic fluid leaks through the diaphragm into the pleural cavity. Also, pulmonary hypertension is sometimes associated with uncontrolled portal hypertension. Hypoxemia and hypercarbia may result in all of the above circumstances. However, if a high serum ammonia level is present, hyperventilation with respiratory alkalosis may occur due to stimulation of the respiratory center.

Immune System

The patient with chronic hepatic failure has an increased risk for infection because the liver is no longer able to filter bacteria effectively from the blood. In addition, associated hypersplenism causes a decreased white blood cell count. Infection, particularly full-blown sepsis, places the patient at increased risk for fluid and electrolyte disturbances.

Dermatological System

Dermatological signs of liver failure include varying degrees of jaundice, palmar erythema, hair changes, and spider angiomas. Spider angiomas are small dilated superficial vessels resembling bluish red spiders that may appear in the skin of the face, forearms, and hands. They may represent a large shunting of blood and can bleed profusely.

Hematological System

Anemia may occur in hepatic failure because the hypersplenism caused by portal hypertension increases the rate of red blood cell destruction. Also, the malnutrition that commonly accompanies hepatic failure decreases the rate of red blood cell formation.

Increased bleeding tendencies due to vitamin K deficiency and decreased prothrombin formation leave the patient at risk for excessive bleeding from menses, nosebleeds, gingivitis, GI mucosal changes, and even bruising. Recall that as bleeding in the GI tract is increased, buildup of ammonia secondary to digestion of blood (a protein-containing substance) is increased. Blood transfusions increase the chance of the patient with hepatic failure to develop hyperammonemia if aged whole blood is used (see Chap. 10).

TREATMENT

Treatment of patients with advanced cirrhosis is in part directed at controlling the excess fluid in the peritoneal cavity (ascites) and interstitial space (edema). Among the therapies for these problems are sodium restriction, bedrest, diuretics, water restriction (when hyponatremia is a problem), paracentesis, and various types of shunting procedures. Other interventions for patients with advanced hepatic disease are directed at preventing hepatic coma. Among these are dietary protein restriction and administration of lactulose, bowel-sterilizing antibiotics, and laxatives or enemas.

SODIUM RESTRICTION

Patients with ascites are first treated with sodium-restricted diets. Dietary sodium restriction varies according to need; however, usually no more than 1,000 mg sodium per day is allowed.[41] A more liberal sodium intake (1,500–2,000 mg/day) may be allowed when a diuresis is effected. In hospitalized patients, it may be necessary to restrict sodium intake to 250 to 500 mg; however, in nonhospitalized patients efforts are made to avoid salt restriction because it significantly decreases the palatability of the diet and causes the patient to eat less.[42] Low-sodium diets are discussed in Chapter 3.

BEDREST

Patients with new-onset ascites are managed with bedrest and moderate sodium restriction. Unless life-threatening complications of ascites are present, patients are given a trial of 3 to 4 days of bedrest and sodium restriction.[43] Even patients with massive ascites may undergo spontaneous diuresis in response to bedrest, coupled with sodium restriction.[44] After

diuresis has been initiated, a gradual increase in activity can be allowed.

DIURETICS

Diuretics are considered for patients who do not respond to salt restriction and bedrest. The amount of ascites that can be mobilized through the peritoneal capillaries is limited to about 700 to 900 mL/day in most patients; therefore, diuretic dosage should be determined cautiously.[45] Overvigorous use of diuretics may result in severe contraction of the intravascular fluid volume causing azotemia and worsening of hepatic encephalopathy. Of course, in edematous patients, diuretics promote fluid loss from the tissue space as well as from the pool of ascites. There is not consensus as to what constitutes safe weight loss in patients undergoing diuretic therapy. Some authors believe that the goal of diuretic therapy is a daily weight loss of 0.5 to 1.0 kg in edematous patients with ascites and about 0.25 kg in those having ascites but no edema.[46] These figures are consistent with findings from the classic study reported by Shear and associates in 1970.[47] A more recent study reported that cirrhotic patients without peripheral edema could safely undergo diuresis of 0.75 kg/day as compared to more than 2 kg/day for those with peripheral edema.[48]

Spironolactone (an aldosterone-blocking agent) is usually the first diuretic prescribed when conservative measures (sodium restriction and bedrest) fail to induce an adequate diuresis. Loop diuretics (furosemide, bumetanide, or ethacrynic acid) may be added to spironolactone in patients who fail to respond to spironolactone alone. Because loop diuretics are potassium-losing agents, hypokalemia must be avoided because this imbalance can contribute to the development of hepatic encephalopathy. A frequently advocated method to avoid hypokalemia is the concomitant administration of a potassium-sparing agent, such as spironolactone, with a potassium-losing agent. This not only helps avoid hypokalemia but provides two agents to eliminate excess body sodium.

WATER RESTRICTION

Water restriction is not indicated for all patients. However, if dilutional hyponatremia occurs, a fluid restriction to 1,000 to 1,500 mL/day will usually suffice.[49] For severe hyponatremia, fluid restriction to the amount necessary to replace insensible loss plus urine output may be needed.

PARACENTESIS

Eventually, patients with ascites may become refractory to diuretics and require paracentesis to relieve respiratory distress and symptoms of marked intra-abdominal pressure. Several studies suggested that paracentesis in patients with massive ascites results in a shorter hospital stay and a decreased incidence of fluid and electrolyte disturbances when compared with treatment with diuretics alone.[50–52] In a related study, it was reported that the IV administration of 40 g albumin after each large-volume paracentesis appeared to minimize the risk of intravascular volume depletion due to rapid reaccumulation of ascites.[53] The main complication associated with paracentesis in cirrhotic patients is effective hypovolemia, apparently due to an accentuation of the arteriolar vasodilation already present in these patients.[54]

The desired rate for removing ascites is somewhat unclear. Removing more than 1.5 to 2.0 L/day from patients with ascites but no peripheral edema may lead to a reduction in cardiac output, particularly if albumin infusions are withheld.[55] It is thought that up to 5 liters of ascites can be removed safely if the patient has peripheral edema and the fluid is removed slowly, over 30 to 90 minutes.[56] When large-volume paracentesis is performed, it is often the practice to give IV albumin concomitantly at a dosage of 10 g/L ascites fluid removed; this is done to protect the patient from hypovolemia.[57] However, some authors point out that the cost of albumin is a factor to consider.[58] Rarely, as little as 1,000 mL of fluid removed by paracentesis can lead to circulatory collapse, encephalopathy, and renal failure.[59] When paracenteses are performed regularly, the state of tissue perfusion must be monitored. This can be simply estimated by monitoring the BUN and plasma creatinine concentration; stable levels indicate that renal perfusion and, presumably, that of other organs is well maintained and paracentesis can be safely continued.[60]

ALBUMIN ADMINISTRATION

Recent studies have indicated that albumin infusion is helpful in preventing fluid volume complications when repeated large-volume paracenteses are performed on patients with massive ascites.[61] However, the use of 25% albumin to correct existing intravascular volume depletion is expensive and appears to offer little advantage over crystalloid solutions.[62] Further, albumin administered IV is no substitute for dietary protein. A study conducted in 1949 reported that albumin administered IV passed into the ascites pool in significant quantities, causing the researchers to conclude that albumin was not markedly beneficial in the management of the underlying liver disorder.[63]

SHUNTS

Peritoneovenous shunts (such as the LeVeen shunt) alleviate ascites more rapidly than medical management does; however, overall experience with this technique has not been particularly favorable.[64] Besides high operative morbidity, patients are vulnerable to mechanical and other complications (such as coagulopathies, peritonitis, and septicemia). As an alternative, TIPS provides portal decompression while obviating the need for invasive surgery. TIPS is a percutaneously performed radiologic procedure in which an expandable metal stent is positioned in the liver to connect hepatic veins to portal veins.[65] It can be placed under a local anesthetic and minimizes risk for wound infection and ascites leaks; also, it does not alter the extrahepatic vascular anatomy (an important consideration for patients who are candidates for liver transplantation).[66] Drawbacks to TIPS include a high degree of technical difficulty, risk of encephalopathy, and shunt stenosis.[67]

DIETARY PROTEIN RESTRICTION

Impending hepatic coma is an indication to temporarily restrict the intake of dietary protein to decrease ammonia formation. When this is necessary, adequate nonprotein calories (25–30 cal/kg) must be supplied by the enteral or parenteral route.[68] As the patient improves, more protein can be added in small increments every few days as tolerated. Specialized enteral and parenteral formulas containing branched-chain amino acids are commercially available for malnourished patients with hepatic failure and concomitant hepatic encephalopathy. However, there is no clinical consensus as to the efficacy of these products and their ability to manage hepatic encephalopathy.[69] Although specialized formulas are indicated in some situations, standard formulas are used for most liver patients.[70]

BOWEL-STERILIZING ANTIBIOTICS

Bowel-sterilizing antibiotics, such as neomycin, can reduce ammonia formation caused by excessive bacterial growth in the bowel. Recall that neomycin (given orally, by nasogastric tube, or by enema) kills urease-producing bacteria, causing less urease to be produced, and hence, less urea to be broken down into ammonia. There is a risk of nephrotoxicity and ototoxicity when neomycin is used, particularly in patients with renal impairment. Metronidazole is an agent that is useful for short-term therapy when neomycin is unavailable or poorly tolerated.[71] Long-term use of metronidazole is not recommended because of its neurotoxicity.[72]

LACTULOSE

Constipation should be prevented because the systemic absorption of toxic nitrogenous substances from the intestinal lumen is more likely when constipation is allowed to occur. Lactulose is a poorly absorbed substance used to promote more frequent stools and prevent or treat PSE. About 97% of the lactulose taken orally reaches the colon unabsorbed. The mechanisms by which it reduces PSE are unclear, but several actions have been suggested. First, lactulose is digested by bacteria in the colon to short-chain fatty acids, resulting in acidification of the colon contents. Because the pH of the bowel vasculature is relatively higher than the contents of the colon under treatment with lactulose, ammonia (NH_3) is converted into ammonium (NH_4), preventing the absorption of ammonia. Due to this same pH gradient, absorption of amines (also implicated in PSE) from the colon to the bloodstream is also reduced. Lactulose causes a change in the bowel flora so that fewer ammonia-forming organisms are present. Also, lactulose has a cathartic effect caused by its osmotic effect.

By monitoring the pH of stool (with pH paper) and adjusting lactulose accordingly, it is possible to reach more precisely a desired pH level of 5.[73] Oral dosage begins at 20 to 30 g three or four times a day for 1 or 2 days; the dosage is then adjusted so that two or three soft stools are produced daily.[74]

Lactulose can be administered rectally when it is not tolerated orally or when pulmonary aspiration is a great risk; 300 mL lactulose and 700 mL tap water may be administered two to four times daily.[75] The solution is given through a rectal balloon catheter and retained for 30 to 60 minutes. If not retained, it can be repeated immediately. The process should be repeated every 4 to 6 hours until symptoms of PSE begin to reverse and oral administration can be started. Soapsuds or other enemas with alkalinizing agents are to be avoided because their use can reverse the effects of lactulose.

Concomitant administration of lactulose and neomycin is helpful in selected patients.[76]

● NURSING ASSESSMENT

Nursing assessment of cirrhotic patients with ascites focuses largely on fluid balance parameters, such as fluid gains and losses (as measured by input and output [I&O] records, body weights, and abdominal girth). More specifically, the nurse is responsible for monitoring responses to therapy and for changes indicating metabolic abnormalities. Listed below are some of the more important nursing assessments with a brief discussion of rationales.

1. Monitor response to diuretics and sodium restriction by the following assessments:
   - Determine abdominal girth on a serial basis, measuring the abdomen at the same place each time. To ensure accurate placement of the measuring tape, it is helpful to draw lines above and below the tape on each side of the abdomen. Be sure the tape is not kinked under the patient's body. Measurements should be made with the patient in the same position each time.
   - Measure I&O; expect to see output exceed intake during effective diuresis. Be aware of the danger of excessive diuresis (see rationale).
   - Monitor vital signs at least twice daily. Be alert for hypotension and tachycardia, indications of excessive diuresis and decreased circulating blood volume.
   - Monitor for dependent pitting edema. This is helpful in assessing the degree of sodium and water retention.
   - Measure body weight daily. Weights are most accurate when measured in the early morning before breakfast and after voiding, using the same scale each time. Compare the expected therapeutic weight loss with the actual weight loss (see rationale).
   Rationale: With adequate sodium restriction and diuretic use, a decrease in abdominal girth, a uri-

nary output relatively greater than the intake during period of diuresis, a decrease in peripheral edema, and a decrease in body weight should be anticipated. The desired weight loss with treatment varies with the patient's clinical status. However, an ascitic patient without peripheral edema might be expected to lose 0.25 kg (1/2 lb) per day, whereas an ascitic patient with peripheral edema might be expected to lose 0.5 to 1.0 kg (about 1–2 lb) per day. Also, one study suggested that weight loss might safely occur more rapidly (eg, 0.75 kg/day in ascitic patients without peripheral edema and over 2 kg/day in those with peripheral edema).[77] Because of differences among patients and treatment plans to induce fluid diuresis, the need for careful clinical observations (such as vital sign variations) is evident. The treatment of ascites and edema must be undertaken cautiously. Although the fluid retained as ascites and edema is uncomfortable and cosmetically unpleasing, it is seldom life-threatening. However, overly aggressive therapy can lead to hepatic encephalopathy and compromised renal function.

2. Monitor patients undergoing paracentesis carefully for the following adverse effects:
   - Circulatory collapse (eg, pallor; weak, rapid pulse; hypotension; fall in central venous pressure)
   - Decline in renal function (oliguria, rise in BUN, serum creatinine)
   - Worsening of neurological function (lethargy, confusion, slurred speech)

   Rationale: Hypovolemia is most likely to result when too much fluid is removed at one time. The mechanism involves a rapid reaccumulation of ascitic fluid resulting from flow of sodium and plasma volume. The removal of as little as 1,000 mL may precipitate hypotension in some patients, particularly in those without peripheral edema. However, some sources state that as much as 5 liters may be safely removed in edematous patients, provided the fluid is removed slowly (over 30–90 minutes) and fluid restriction is initiated to avoid hyponatremia.[78] Excessive fluid removal with paracentesis or diuresis can precipitate the hepatorenal syndrome (manifested by oliguria or rise in serum creatinine and BUN) or PSE (manifested by lethargy, confusion, and slurred speech). The administration of albumin helps prevent fluid balance problems after massive paracentesis.[79]

3. Monitor patients receiving diuretics for disturbances in potassium balance.

   Rationale: Patients receiving potassium-losing diuretics (such as furosemide and thiazides) are at risk for hypokalemia. Symptoms include fatigue, muscle weakness, leg cramps, decreased bowel motility, paresthesias, electrocardiographic (ECG) changes (flat T waves and depressed ST segments), arrhythmias, and increased sensitivity to digitalis. On the other hand, patients taking potassium-conserving diuretics (such as spironolactone, triamterene, and amiloride) are at risk for hyperkalemia. Symptoms include weakness, paresthesias, ECG changes (tented T waves), and arrhythmias. See Chapter 5 for a review or nursing responsibilities related to potassium imbalances.

4. Monitor patients receiving neomycin for hearing difficulty.

   Rationale: Large doses of neomycin can damage both the kidneys and the ears; deafness may occur, particularly when neomycin is administered with furosemide (Lasix) or ethacrynic acid (Edecrin).

5. Monitor patients for symptoms of PSE.

   Rationale: This disturbance is particularly likely to occur in individuals who are bleeding into the GI tract. Symptoms include lethargy, loss of memory, slurred speech, personality change, and disorientation. Convulsive seizures and coma may follow untreated or refractory PSE.

6. Monitor patients for hyponatremia.

   Rationale: This imbalance must be detected early so that fluid restriction can be initiated before the imbalance becomes severe. Symptoms are primarily those of cerebral swelling (lethargy and somnolence), making this imbalance difficult to distinguish from other disturbances affecting the neurological status.

● NURSING DIAGNOSES

Examples of nursing diagnoses related to fluid and electrolyte balance in patients with cirrhosis are listed in Clinical Tip: Examples of Nursing Diagnoses Related to Fluid and Electrolyte Problems in Patients With Cirrhosis, along with etiologies and defining characteristics. Nursing interventions and rationales are discussed below.

CLINICAL TIP

Examples of Nursing Diagnoses Related to Fluid and Electrolyte Problems in Patients With Cirrhosis

NURSING DIAGNOSIS	ETIOLOGICAL FACTORS	DEFINING CHARACTERISTICS
ECF volume excess (total body sodium and water increased), but decreased effective arterial volume, related to pathophysiological changes of cirrhosis	Despite increased total ECF volume due to renal retention of sodium and water, body responds as if arterial volume is diminished (decreased effective arterial volume)	Ascites Peripheral edema first noted in lower extremities and later becoming generalized (dependent on sodium intake)
Risk for hypovolemia related to rapid reaccumulation of ascitic fluid after large volume paracentesis	Ascites may reaccumulate rapidly (particularly when albumin is not administered after paracentesis) following the removal of large volumes of ascites	Reduced cardiac output Decreased blood pressure Increased pulse rate
Alterations in thought processes related to increased toxins (such as ammonia)	Elevated serum ammonia level (results when liver is unable to convert ammonia formed in intestines to urea) Bleeding into GI tract increases ammonia formation Excessive diuresis contracts plasma volume and increases concentration of toxins	Slowed response, memory loss, sleep disturbances, confusion, disorientation, personality change, stupor, coma, seizures
Alteration in thought processes related to dilutional hyponatremia	Increased ADH secretion due to decrease in effective arterial volume	Lethargy, somnolence, personality change, serum sodium < 135 mEq/L (see Chap. 4)
Alteration in potassium balance (hypokalemia) related to use of potassium-losing diuretics	Potassium-losing diuretics (such as furosemide or bumetanide)	Fatigue, muscle weakness, leg cramps, decreased bowel motility, arrhythmias, ECG chances (see Chap. 5)
Risk for impaired gas exchange related to decreased lung expansion	Large accumulation of ascites causes diaphragm to press upward on lungs, causing decreased respirations. Condition is aggravated by generalized weakness, lethargy, and immobility	Decreased respiratory depth Increased $PaCO_2$

ADH, antidiuretic hormone; ECF, extracellular fluid; ECG, electrocardiographic; GI, gastrointestinal.

NURSING INTERVENTIONS

Nursing interventions are directed at promoting adaptation and minimizing ill effects of the disease process.

1. Continue ongoing assessment of fluid balance status as the basis for collaborative interaction with the physician in regulation of therapy (see section on Nursing Assessment).
2. Prevent constipation by administering lactulose as prescribed and indicated (goal is to produce two or three soft stools per day).
   • Attempt to minimize the unpleasant sweet taste of lactulose by diluting it with fruit juice, water, or

milk or administering it in foods (such as desserts).

- If lactulose is given through a GI tube, it should be well diluted to prevent vomiting and the risk of pulmonary aspiration.
- If aspiration is likely, it may be necessary to administer the lactulose by retention enema.
- Monitor for excessive loose stools because severe fluid and electrolyte depletion could occur.

Rationale: Constipation should be prevented because it contributes to the accumulation of ammonia. Bleeding in the GI tract increases ammonia formation (due to digestion of blood proteins) and may precipitate hepatic coma. Bowel evacuation removes blood from the intestine and therefore decreases a source of urea and other false neurotransmitters. Use of lactulose (orally and by enema) is described further in the section on treatment.

3. Encourage rest periods in which the patient lies down.

Rationale: Assumption of the supine position is often associated with a spontaneous diuresis, resulting in significant weight loss with mobilization of peripheral edema fluid and ascitic fluid. The diuresis induced by bedrest results from improvement in cardiac output and effective circulating blood volume. The patient with severe ascites is usually better able to tolerate the lateral recumbent position.

4. Maintain a safe environment for the patient with the potential for, or actual presence of, PSE.

- When deemed necessary, remove potential sources of harm (such as matches or sharp objects) from the immediate environment.
- Caution significant others that the patient's ability to drive or perform usual activities (such as cooking) should be closely monitored. Driver's licenses are often restricted or revoked for this group of patients making it necessary for significant others to assume many additional responsibilities for home-bound patients (eg, cooking and transportation to treatment facilities).

Rationale: Because episodes of encephalopathy may interfere with thought and reasoning processes, physical safety of the patient and others must be considered.

5. Initiate patient instruction in self-care.
- Teach home-bound patients how to monitor their fluid I&O and body weights and when to seek intervention from the health care provider.
- Instruct patient or significant other in how to manage a sodium-restricted diet at home; written information that can be taken home is advantageous, as is accessibility of a dietary consultant when questions arise.
- Promote the patient's understanding of the diuretic therapy. For example, the patient should be able to name the diuretic as well as its purpose and common side effects. The desirability of taking the diuretic in the morning to avoid disturbing sleep at night should be emphasized.
- Promote the patient's (or significant other's) understanding of potassium supplements when they are required. The patient or caregiver should be able to name the agent, its dosage, the reason for taking it, and possible side effects. Because some potassium supplements can be unpleasant, the reason for taking the substance should be emphasized (recall that hypokalemia associated with metabolic alkalosis can lead to the development of PSE).
- Promote the patient's understanding of salt substitutes, if used. For example, the patient should be able to name acceptable agents. Instruct patients receiving a combination potassium-conserving, potassium-losing diuretic (such as spironolactone [Aldactazide] or triamterene [Dyazide]) that salt substitutes should be used sparingly, if at all. When only a potassium-conserving diuretic is used, the danger of hyperkalemia is present; for such patients, salt substitutes are generally not recommended. Recall that most salt substitutes contain sizable amounts of potassium (see Table 5-3).

Rationale: Understanding dietary and pharmacological regimens will promote adherence to these treatment modalities and promote optimal wellness.

CASE STUDIES

● **21-1.** A 50-year-old woman with a long history of alcoholism and cirrhosis with ascites was admitted with complaints of difficulty breathing and a weight gain of 13 lb over the past 2 weeks.

On questioning, she stated she had omitted her diuretic (spironolactone) and failed to adhere to her sodium-restricted dietary regimen over this same period.

On physical examination, her abdomen was largely distended with ascites. Her lower extremities were edematous and she had jugular venous distention. Vital signs were: temperature, 98.6°F; pulse rate, 100/min; respiratory rate, 20/min; and blood pressure, 170/98 mm Hg. Laboratory results indicated that all serum electrolytes were within normal limits (serum sodium, 137 mEq/L).

COMMENTARY: The signs of excessive sodium and water retention included acute weight gain, lower extremity edema, ascites, hypertension, and jugular venous distention. Increasing ascitic fluid accumulation placed pressure on the diaphragm and made it difficult for her to breath normally. Because she gained 13 lb over this relatively short period, it can be concluded that she retained about 6 liters of fluid. (One liter of fluid is 2.2 lb.) The increased ascitic fluid accumulation that occurred over the 2-week period did not produce a deficit in the vascular space because it developed relatively slowly, allowing time for sodium and water to be retained by the kidneys to replace fluid shifted from the vascular space to the ascitic pool. Treatment includes diuretics and a sodium-restricted diet. The peritoneum limits the transfer of ascitic fluid into the vascular space to about 750 mL/day. Because she also had peripheral edema, she could be expected to diurese edema fluid in addition to the ascitic fluid (perhaps allowing her to excrete up to 1 liter of fluid per day initially without compromising her intravascular volume). Patients with ascites often are treated with spironolactone (a potassium-sparing diuretic) because it is an aldosterone antagonist that reduces sodium reabsorption by the kidney. It does not cause potassium depletion; this is an important consideration in a cirrhotic patient because hypokalemia increases ammonia production and predisposes to hepatic encephalopathy.

● **21-2.**[80] A confused middle-aged man with cirrhosis of the liver was admitted for evaluation. The following blood work results were obtained:

Serum Na = 133 mEq/L
Serum K = 3.3 mEq/L
Serum Cl = 115 mEq/L

Arterial blood gas values:

pH = 7.44
$PaCO_2$ = 20 mm Hg
HCO_3 = 13 mEq/L

COMMENTARY: Note that the serum sodium and potassium levels were slightly below normal. Probably the slight hyponatremia was related to impaired renal excretion and excessive release of ADH. The mild hypokalemia was likely due to use of potassium-losing diuretics. Most striking in these laboratory results was the low $PaCO_2$ level. This represents primary respiratory alkalosis; the HCO_3 was also low and due to a compensatory change. (Recall that in chronic respiratory alkalosis, the HCO_3 level is expected to decrease by 5 mEq/L for every 10 mm Hg drop in the $PaCO_2$ level. Because the $PaCO_2$ has dropped by 20 (from a normal of 40), the HCO_3 is expected to decrease by 10 (from 24 to 14 mEq/L). Therefore, this patient had chronic compensated respiratory alkalosis. It has been postulated that elevated blood ammonia levels stimulate hyperventilation and result in respiratory alkalosis. Although all four acid–base imbalances may occur in patients with liver disease, respiratory alkalosis is the most frequent.

REFERENCES

1. Friedman S. Cirrhosis of the liver and its major sequelae. In: Bennett J, Plum F, eds. *Cecil Textbook of Medicine*, 20th ed. Philadelphia: WB Saunders; 1996:788.
2. Andreoli T, Bennett C, Carpenter C, Plum F. *Cecil Essentials of Medicine*, 4th ed. Philadelphia: WB Saunders; 1997:339.
3. Ibid, 340.
4. Epstein M. Renal sodium retention in liver disease. *Hosp Pract* September 15, 1995:33.
5. Wong F, Girgrah N, Blendis L. Fluid retention in cirrhosis. *J Gastroenterol Hepatol* 1997;12:437.

6. Schrier RW et al. Peripheral arterial vasodilation hypothesis: A proposal for the initiation of renal sodium and water retention in cirrhosis. *Hepatology* 1988;8:1151.

7. Herrera JL. Current medical management of cirrhotic ascites. *Am J Med Sci* 1991;302:31.

8. Runyon BA. Ascites. In: Schiff L, Schiff E, eds. *Diseases of the Liver*, 7th ed. Philadelphia: JB Lippincott; 1993:992.

9. Ibid.

10. Ibid.

11. Kinouchi T. Fluid, electrolyte, and acid-base disorders in liver cirrhosis. *Nippon Rinsho-Japanese J Clin Med* 1994;52:124.

12. Porayko MK, Wiesner RH. Management of ascites in patients with cirrhosis. *Postgrad Med* 1993;92:194.

13. Akriviadis E et al. Hyponatremia of cirrhosis: Role of vasopressin and decreased "effective" plasma volume. *Scand J Gastroenterol* 1997;32:829.

14. Tierney L, McPhee S, Papadakis M. *Current Medical Diagnosis & Treatment*, 38th ed. Stamford, CT: Appleton & Lange; 1999:654.

15. Arieff A, DeFronzo R. *Fluid, Electrolyte & Acid-Base Disorders*, 2nd ed. New York: Churchill Livingstone; 1995:288.

16. Narins R, ed. *Clinical Disorders of Fluid and Electrolyte Metabolism*, 5th ed. New York: McGraw-Hill; 1994:1159.

17. Sherlock S. Ascites formation and its management. *Scand J Gastroenterol* 1970;7(suppl):9.

18. Narins, p 1160.

19. Ibid, p 1161.

20. Ibid, p 1163.

21. Ibid.

22. Ibid.

23. Ibid, p 1164.

24. Ibid.

25. Ibid, p 1165.

26. Ibid.

27. Ibid.

28. Andreoli et al, p 342.

29. Badalament S et al. Hepatorenal syndrome: new perspectives in pathogenesis and treatment. *Arch Intern Med* 1993;153:1960.

30. Ibid.

31. Andreol et al, p 342.

32. Friedman, p 796.

33. Tierney et al, p 655.

34. Ibid.

35. Kokko J, Tannen R. *Fluids and Electrolytes*, 3rd ed. Philadelphia: WB Saunders; 1996:479.

36. Andreoli, p 343.

37. Ibid.

38. Carey C, Lee H, Woeltje K. *The Washington Manual of Medical Therapeutics*, 29th ed. Philadelphia: Lippincott-Raven; 1998:339.

39. Schwartz S, Shires T, Spencer F et al, eds. *Principles of Surgery*, 7th ed. New York: McGraw-Hill; 1999:1421.

40. Tierney et al, p 655.

41. Carey et al, p 340.

42. McCullough A, Teran C, Bugianesi E. Guidelines for nutritional therapy in liver disease. In: *The ASPEN Nutrition Support Manual*. Silver Spring, MD: American Society for Parenteral and Enteral Nutrition; 1998:12-6.

43. Chiou SS, Changchien CS. Management of end-stage liver disease. *Transplant Proceed* 1993;25:2948.

44. Epstein, p 33.

45. Carey et al, p 340.

46. Porayko, Weisner, p 162.

47. Shear L et al. Compartmentalization of ascites and edema in patients with hepatic cirrhosis. *N Engl J Med* 1970;282:1391.

48. Porayko, Weisner, p 158.

49. Carey et al, p 341.

50. Porayko, Weisner, p 162.

51. Kellerman PS, Linas SL. Large-volume paracentesis in the treatment of ascites. *Ann Intern Med* 1990;11:889.

52. Reynolds TB. Renaissance of paracentesis in the treatment of ascites. *Adv Intern Med* 1990;35:365.

53. Gines P et al. Randomized comparative study of therapeutic paracentesis with and without intravenous albumin in cirrhosis. *Gastroenterology* 1988;94:1493.

54. Vila M, Sola R, Molina L et al. Hemodynamic changes in patients developing effective hypovolemia after total paracentesis. *J Hepatol* 1998;28:639.

55. Reynolds, p 370.

56. Doherty G, Baumann D, Creswell L et al. *The Washington Manual of Surgery*. Boston: Little, Brown; 1997:224.

57. Tierney et al, 654.

58. Ibid.

59. Carey et al, 341.

60. Reynolds, p 368.

61. Gines, p 1493.

62. Arroyo et al. Treatment of ascites in cirrhosis. *Gastroenterol Clin North Am* 1992;21:251.

63. Faloon W et al. An evaluation of human serum albumin in the treatment of cirrhosis of the liver. *J Clin Invest* 1949;28:583.

64. Epstein, p 41.

65. Doherty, p 275.

66. Epstein, p 41.

67. Ibid.

68. Wagner S et al. Pathophysiology and clinical basis of prevention and treatment of complications of chronic liver disease. *Gastroenterol Hepatol* 1991;69:113.

69. Rombeau J, Caldwell M. *Clinical Nutrition: Enteral and Tube Feeding*, 3rd ed. Philadelphia: WB Saunders; 1997:8.

70. Ibid.

71. Carey et al, p 340.

72. Ibid.

73. Bircher J, Sommer W. Portal systemic encephalopathy. In: Prieto C et al, eds. *Hepatobiliary Diseases*. New York: Springer-Verlag; 1992:424.

74. Bircher, Sommer, p 423.

75. Doherty, p 278.

76. Friedman, p 798.

77. Herrera, p 34.

78. Reynolds, p 369.

79. Gines, p 1493.

80. Halperin M, Goldstein M. *Fluid, Electrolyte, and Acid-Base Physiology*, 3rd ed. Philadelphia: WB Saunders, 1999.

CHAPTER 22

Fluid and Electrolyte Disturbances Associated With Oncologic Conditions

Maintaining fluid and electrolyte balance is often difficult in patients with cancer. In some situations, fluid and electrolyte problems are the initial symptoms that cause the individual to seek medical attention. At other times, these problems are related to the development of metastatic disease. Unfortunately, they may also be the consequence of aggressive therapy. A majority of oncology patients will experience a problem with fluid and electrolyte regulation during the course of their illness. Often various fluid and electrolyte disturbances exist simultaneously. The treatment of electrolyte disorders needs to be monitored closely since the correction of one imbalance can lead to the appearance of one or more others (eg, the treatment of hypercalcemia can lead to hypokalemia and hypomagnesemia). Patients with cancer may also suffer from other unrelated health conditions that can cause fluid and electrolyte imbalances; among these are congestive heart failure, hypertension, renal diseases, and gastrointestinal (GI) disorders. The complete picture of the cancer patient needs to be considered when evaluating fluid and electrolyte imbalances. These problems can be acute or chronic and vary significantly in the degree of severity.

Mechanisms responsible for fluid and electrolyte imbalances in cancer patients, as well as the tumors (or associated problems) causing the imbalances are described in this section. Treatment to correct common electrolyte imbalances is also described here. Note that treatment of tumor-related fluid and electrolyte problems initially is directed at relieving immediate life-threatening problems and later at controlling the underlying tumor causing the imbalance. It is essential that the treatment for the malignancy be successful for a permanent resolution of the imbalance.

⬤ HYPERCALCEMIA

One of the more common problems of malignant disease is hypercalcemia. About 10% to 15% of all persons with cancer will develop an elevated serum calcium level during the course of their illness.[1] The incidence increases to 40% in patients with breast cancer and myeloma.[2] Most laboratories report the normal total serum calcium level as ranging between 8.5 to 10.5 mg/dL. Mild to moderate hypercalcemia is often defined as ranging from 12 to 13 mg/dL, whereas severe hypercalcemia is said to exist when the serum calcium level is greater than 14 mg/dL.

LABORATORY MEASUREMENT

If the laboratory measures the total calcium level instead of ionized calcium, it is important to consider the effect that the serum albumin level has on its concentration. This is especially true since cancer patients are often hypoalbuminemic due to malnutrition. A below normal serum albumin concentration causes the total calcium value to appear lower than it actually is. That is, the reported total serum calcium concentration is decreased by 0.8 mg/dL for every 1 g/dL the serum albumin concentration is below normal. For example, a patient with a total serum calcium level of 10 mg/dL and a normal serum albumin level actually has a calcium concentration of 10 mg/dL. In contrast, a patient with a total serum calcium level of 10 mg/dL and a serum albumin that is below normal (such as 2 g/dL) actually has mild hypercalcemia In this case, assuming the albumin concentration is 2 g/dL below normal, one would multiple 2 times 0.8 and add the 1.6 mg/dL to the reported value of 10 mg/dL (making the real total calcium level equal to 11.6 mg/dL). Although most laboratories have the capability of measuring ionized calcium levels, they usually measure the total serum calcium concentration (making it necessary to apply the formula to calculate the actual calcium level). (See Clinical Tip: Correction of Total Serum Calcium When Hypoalbuminemia Is Present).

CAUSES

Malignancy acts to cause hypercalcemia by two major mechanisms. In local osteolytic hypercalcemia, products from tumor cells (such as cytokines) stimulate osteoclastic bone resorption.[3] This form of malignant hypercalcemia is seen in tumors with extensive bone involvement (usually breast cancer, myeloma, and lymphoma). In humoral hypercalcemia of malignancy, systemically active tumor products stimulate bone resorption and, in some cases, decrease calcium excretion.[4] Thus, hypercalcemia is associated with virtually any type of malignancy, from solid tumors with or without bony metastases to hematological malignancies, and may include the following:

1. Solid tumors with bony metastases:
   - Breast
   - Lung
   - Renal
   - Colon
   - Ovary
   - Epidermoid cancers of the head and neck

CLINICAL TIP

Correction of Total Serum Calcium Level When Hypoalbuminemia is Present

A handy formula to use for this purpose is:

Corrected serum calcium = (normal serum albumin − patient's serum albumin) × 0.8 + total calcium level

For example, assume a patient has a laboratory reported total serum calcium level of 7.0 mg/dL and a serum albumin level of 2.0 g/dL.

Although the normal serum albumin level varies according to the laboratory performing the test, it is usually in the range of 3.5 to 5.0 g/dL. Assume for purposes of this formula that a value of 4.0 g/dL is normal.

Corrected serum calcium = (4.0 − 2.0) × 0.8 + 7.0
Corrected serum calcium = (2 × 0.8) + 7.0
Corrected serum calcium = 1.6 + 7.0 (8.6 mg/dL)

Thus, according to the laboratory report, the patient's total serum calcium level indicates hypocalcemia. However, when the value was corrected for the patient's hypoalbuminemia, the value is within the lower range of normal.

---

2. Solid tumors without bony metastases:
   - Lung
   - Head and neck
   - Renal
   - Ovary
3. Hematological malignancies:
   - Lymphoma
   - Leukemia
   - Multiple myeloma

As indicated above, patients with certain malignancies are more likely to develop hypercalcemia than others; among these are breast cancer, renal-cell carcinoma, squamous-cell carcinomas from any site, multiple myeloma, and certain non-Hodgkin's lymphomas.[5]

The only treatment-related cause of hypercalcemia is associated with the use of hormonal therapy (androgens, estrogens, anti-estrogens, and progestins). Metabolic alterations associated with use of these agents cause calcium release from bone into the serum. Obviously, patients receiving these agents should have their serum calcium levels monitored closely. Any marked increase in the calcium level warrants discontinuation of therapy. For example, patients with breast cancer may experience hypercalcemia soon after the institution of tamoxifen therapy; withdrawal of the hormonal agent usually reverses the hypercalcemia.[6] Usually no additional treatment is required once hormonal therapy is stopped.

CLINICAL PRESENTATION

Hypercalcemia can have a wide range of clinical presentations. The symptoms may be so unspecific as to be confused with manifestations of the underlying cancer or its treatment. When the serum calcium concentration rises slowly, the patient may remain relatively asymptomatic for some time, despite a relatively high elevation.[7] The patient with severe hypercalcemia is almost always symptomatic.

The presence of generalized weakness, altered mental status, polyuria, polydipsia, nausea, vomiting, constipation and dehydration should prompt caregivers to suspect hypercalcemia. If the condition is allowed to progress untreated, it can lead to the development of psychotic behavior, bradycardia, ventricular arrhythmias, seizures, coma, renal failure, and death. Although it is true that hypercalcemia is usually associated with a poor prognosis, the aggressive management of this problem can bring about significant improvement in the patient's quality of life.[8] For example, polyuria and nocturia caused by the kidneys' inability to concentrate urine interfere with the patient's rest and sleep. This excessive fluid loss is often accompanied by thirst. Yet, anorexia and vomiting may interfere with drinking and eating. Constipation may lead to the development of fecal impactions.

The muscle weakness and fatigue associated with hypercalcemia cause the patient to be less active; this only serves to worsen hypercalcemia since immobilization favors a shift of calcium from the bones to the extracellular fluid. As hypercalcemia progresses, the patient becomes greatly dehydrated and eventually becomes confused and stuporous. Worsening renal function is manifested by elevated blood urea nitrogen (BUN) and creatinine levels. As indicated above, hypercalcemia is life-threatening when it is severe, perhaps terminating in cardiac arrest or renal failure.

MANAGEMENT

Treatment for tumor-related hypercalcemia is similar to that of other causes of elevated serum calcium levels. (See Chap. 6.) Therapies discussed in this section are those most commonly used in the oncology patient population. The treatment of choice often depends on the severity of the hypercalcemic state, the significance of the side effects for the particular patient, and the clinician's preference. The most effective long-term means of treating cancer-related hypercalcemia is to treat the underlying malignancy.

Hydration and Diuresis

When hypercalcemia is mild to moderate (such as ≤ 13 mg/dL), it may be sufficient to administer isotonic saline (0.9% NaCl) to rehydrate the patient and facilitate renal excretion of calcium (by increasing the glomerular filtration rate) and then to follow with measures directed against the tumor (such as chemotherapy, radiation, or surgery).

When hypercalcemia is severe, large volumes of isotonic saline may be required (such as 4 to 6 liters over the first 24 hours).[9] Before the initiation of any large fluid infusion, renal function needs to be evaluated. It is also advisable to monitor the central venous pressure when fluids are administered rapidly (such as 250 to 500 ml/hr). It is possible to overwhelm the patient's cardiovascular system and cause fluid overload. Among the signs of this condition are shortness of breath, rales (noted on auscultation of the lungs), peripheral edema, and distended neck veins. After the patient is sufficiently rehydrated, intravenous furosemide (such as 20-80 mg every 2 to 4 hours) may be introduced to further facilitate the elimination of calcium by selectively inhibiting its resorption.[10] Diuretics are used only after adequate volume expansion has been achieved (in order to avoid further dehydration). While primarily used to promote calcium excretion, diuretics also serve to prevent volume overload and congestive heart failure in patients with underlying cardiac disease.[11] (Thiazides should be avoided because they inhibit the urinary excretion of calcium.) For patients who cannot tolerate large volumes of isotonic saline, lower volumes (such as 125 ml/hr) may be used (in conjunction with intravenous furosemide once or twice daily).

While rehydration with isotonic saline and the use of furosemide decreases the serum calcium level, they alone are not sufficient to manage severe hypercalcemia. In this situation, additional medications (such as pamidronate, calcitonin, gallium nitrate, plicamycin, and corticosteroids) are needed to produce a sustained decrease in the serum calcium concentration. It should be noted that all antihypercalcemic agents have the potential to cause hypocalcemia; therefore, a careful watch on the serum calcium level is needed during treatment. The drugs are discontinued when the serum calcium concentration returns to normal of near normal.[12]

Bisphosphonates

The bisphosphonates (formerly called diphosphonates) are potent antihypercalcemic agents. Pamidronate (Aredia), inhibits osteoclastic-induced resorption of bone and is the treatment of choice for hypercalcemia in cancer patients. Treatment regimens with pamidronate include a one-time intravenous dose administered over 24 hrs. Onset of action begins 24 to 72 hrs after administration with peak effect in 4 to 9 days. Duration of response rate for pamidronate ranges from 1 to 10 weeks, with an average of 2 to 3 weeks. Another bisphosphonate is disodium etidronate (Didronel); however this agent is less commonly used.

Calcitonin

Synthetic calcitonin may be used to treat hypercalcemia as it promotes calcium excretion by the kidneys (even in patients with compromised renal function). Calcitonin's major advantages include its rapid onset of action (2 to 4 hours) and its comparatively low serious toxicity.[13] A disadvantage is its relatively weak hypocalcemic effect (such as only a 1-3 mg/dL decrease in the serum calcium concentration).[14] Owing to its rapid onset of action, calcitonin is sometimes used in conjunction with pamidronate to treat acute hypercalcemia.[15]

Gallium Nitrate

Gallium nitrate, an agent that inhibits osteoclastic function, has also been used in the treatment of hypercalcemia. One of the major adverse effects of gallium nitrate is its nephrotoxicity.[16] Another drawback is that it requires intravenous therapy for 5 to 7 days. Asymptomatic hypophosphatemia may occur with the use of gallium nitrate and require the administration of oral phosphate supplements.[17]

Plicamycin

Plicamycin (Mithramycin), an antineoplastic antibiotic, lowers the serum calcium level by inhibiting osteoclastic activity; however, its action does not begin until 12 to 24 hours after administration, with maximal results seen usually in 36 to 72 hours. Unfortunately, plicamycin has a high toxic profile. It may cause a precipitous drop in the platelet count. This is particularly problematic for the patient who has received previous chemotherapy and is already thrombocytopenic. Plicamycin is usually reserved for use in patients who are unresponsive to any other therapy.[18]

Glucocorticoids

Glucocorticoids can be helpful in the treatment of hypercalcemia associated with multiple myeloma and in breast cancer patients with metastases to the bone.[19] Unfortunately, it may take several days to lower the serum calcium level. Large doses of hydrocortisone may be required initially, followed by oral maintenace prednisone therapy. Glucocorticoids lower the serum calcium level by increasing urinary calcium excretion and decreasing intestinal calcium absorption.[20] They also inhibit cytokine release and have a direct cytolytic effect on some tumor cells.[21] Side effects can include hyperglycemia, gastrointestinal bleeding, osteoporosis, hypertension, and the development of opportunistic infections.[22]

Oral Phosphates

Oral phosphate therapy (such as Neutra-Phos or Fleet Phospho-Soda) has largely been abandoned now that more effective agents are available.[23] Nonetheless, it is sometimes used to reduce the serum calcium level in patients with chronic hypercalcemia, especially if they are also hypophosphatemic. Oral phosphate therapy works by inhibiting calcium absorption and promoting calcium deposition in bone and soft tissue. Phosphates should be used only if the serum phosphorus level is less than 3 mg/dL and renal function is normal to avoid the complication of soft tissue calcification.[24]

Their use is limited by poor acceptance related to nausea and diarrhea.

Diet

It is generally agreed that restricting the intake of dietary calcium is of little or no benefit in reducing the elevated serum calcium level in oncology patients. This is because the mechanisms involved in hypercalcemia in this population are due to calcium resorption from the bones rather than to the gastrointestinal absorption of calcium.[25] Besides, the dietary restriction of calcium-rich foods is unpleasant and contributes to the chronic malnutrition so often present in the cancer patient.

Maintaining adequate hydration is very important in preventing the development of severe hypercalcemia. When possible, oral fluid intake should be at least 2 to 3 liters per day to promote the excretion of calcium by the kidneys. Medications to treat nausea may be needed to facilitate fluid intake. Also, vomiting and diarrhea should be treated early to avoid the development of dehydration.

Activity

Weight-bearing activities should be encouraged as much as possible since prolonged immobilization enhances bone resorption and is a contributing factor to the development of hypercalcemia. Because ambulation is often associated with pain in cancer patients, it may be necessary to administer pain medications prior to planned exercise and to allow adequate periods of rest between activities.[26]

Antineoplastic Therapy

Although hypercalcemic cancer patients may respond to the above therapies, efforts are obviously necessary to control the source of the hypercalcemia (the malignancy) by antineoplastic therapies, such as chemotherapy, radiation, or surgery.

● HYPONATREMIA

CAUSES

Hyponatremia is a common complication in cancer patients. Among possible causes for decreased serum sodium levels in this population are the following:

1. Ectopic release of an antidiuretic hormone-like substance from certain tumors, especially small-cell lung cancer, leading to the syndrome of inappropriate antidiuretic hormone secretion (SIADH).
2. SIADH secondary to chemotherapeutic agents (such cyclophosphamide, vincristine, vinblastine, and cisplatin)
3. Loss of sodium through vomiting and diarrhea
4. Excessive use of hypotonic intravenous fluids, especially in the presence of SIADH
5. Possible secretion of atrial natriuretic peptide (ANP) by certain tumors

Secretion of inappropriate antidiuretic hormone (SIADH) is associated with certain malignancies. For example, patients with small cell lung carcinoma frequently have hyponatremia at the time of diagnosis.[27] Patients with hyponatremia and SIADH have been shown to have ectopically produced ADH (also called arginine vasopressin [AVP]); when this is the case, the ADH is thought to be the origin of the hyponatremia.[28] Recall that, in normal persons, ADH release by the hypothalamus is controlled by a feedback mechanism that senses the serum osmolality; when the serum osmolality drops, the production of ADH is cut back. However, ectopically produced ADH is not controlled by any feedback mechanism. Therefore, the serum sodium level continues to decrease because of sustained ADH production by the tumor site.

Some patients with small cell lung carcinoma have low serum sodium levels but do not have ectopically produced antidiuretic hormone. It is possible that atrial natriuretic peptide (ANP) production by tumor cells has some relationship to the hyponatremia in these individuals.[29] Among the actions of atrial natriuretic peptide are increased renal excretion of sodium, and decreased biosynthesis and release of aldosterone.[30]

Antitumor agents most frequently associated with hyponatremia include cyclophosphamide (Cytoxan), vincristine sulfate (Oncovin), vinblastine sulfate (Velban), and cisplatin.[31] The mechanism by which all these drugs affect sodium balance is not fully understood. Patients receiving high-dose cyclophosphamie should be monitored closely for hyponatremia. Cisplatin is thought to increase the release of ADH from the posterior pituitary and thus can cause SIADH. Because vigorous hydration is an important component of this nephrotoxic treatment, the problem of water retention is accentuated. If diuretics are also administered, sodium loss in the urine adds to the problem.

Hyponatremia associated with vincristine and vinblastine administration is usually accompanied by other signs of toxicity associated with the drug. The most common of these are ileus and peripheral neuropathy. Because cisplatin, cyclophosphamide, vincristine, and vinblastine are agents commonly used to treat lung cancer (a tumor often associated with hyponatremia), the patient is at even greater risk for developing hyponatremia and should be assessed carefully.

Some cancer patients are treated with narcotics for pain control. Narcotics have also been associated with SIADH. All drugs prescribed to cancer patients should be evaluated for their potential to contribute to hyponatremia as problems may arise from a cumulative hyponatremic effect.

In patients with multiple myeloma, or any state of hyperproteinemia, more non-sodium solids and less water will be present, leading to pseudohyponatremia. Patients with extensive liver metastasis who present with hyponatremia also sometimes have elevated plasma concentrations of ADH and aldosterone and low plasma albumin levels.[32]

CLINICAL PRESENTATION

Table 4-4 details the characteristics of hyponatremia. In some cases, these clinical symptoms may alert the clinician to investigate the possibility of a cancer diagnosis (eg, in a patient with a history of smoking who has no obvious respiratory disorder). The hyponatremia associated with malignancy usually develops gradually; therefore, patients may be relatively free of symptoms until the serum sodium level becomes quite low. (Recall that slowly developing imbalances do not produce symptoms nearly as often as imbalances that develop quickly.)

MANAGEMENT

Successful treatment of the tumor is the most direct treatment of hyponatremia associated with malignancy. Chemotherapy, radiation therapy, or surgery may be used, depending on the malignancy involved. In the majority of patients, chemotherapy for small-cell bronchogenic cancer successfully resolves the hyponatremia. Clinicians who administer any antineoplastic drugs known to induce hyponatremia should closely monitor serum sodium levels and serum osmolality. In the case of drug-induced hyponatremia, discontinuation of the drug usually causes a resolution of the disorder.

Other standard measures to control water excess and restore normal serum sodium concentrations are described in Chapter 4. On a short-term basis, fluid intake is restricted to the extent that negative water balance is induced; this may require restriction to as little as 400 to 700 ml/day. If neurologic symptoms are present, hypertonic saline (3% or 5% NaCl) may need to be cautiously administered. Use of demeclocycline (Declomycin) for long-term control of hyponatremia may be indicated, particularly in patients with uncontrolled malignancies; this agent inhibits the action of ADH on the kidneys, allowing increased urinary output and an increase in serum sodium.[33] Long-term restriction of water is not commonly used as a treatment modality because many patients find this extremely unpleasant.

● HYPOKALEMIA

CAUSES

Hypokalemia has been estimated to occur in up to 75% of cancer patients at some point in their illness.[34] As with any patient, it may be associated with inadequate intake or excessive loss of potassium ions. A decrease in serum potassium related to decreased intake is commonly associated with anorexia or nausea related to cancer pain, depression, tumor obstruction, chemotherapy, or radiation therapy. Administration of potassium-free IV fluids for treatment of dehydration only exaggerates the potassium reduction.

Extrarenal loss of potassium can be associated with excessive vomiting, fistula drainage, diarrhea, and prolonged mechanical GI suction. Vomiting may be associated with chemotherapy and radiation therapy or GI obstruction secondary to the malignancy. Besides the direct loss of potassium in vomitus, the main cause of hypokalemia associated with vomiting is related to the presence of metabolic alkalosis. Recall that prolonged vomiting often causes metabolic alkalosis; as the kidney attempts to conserve hydrogen ions, it increases urinary potassium excretion. In cancer patients, diarrhea may be caused by a variety of factors. A number of malignancies (including villous adenoma of the colon, pancreatic carcinoma, carcinoid syndrome, medullary carcinoma of the thyroid, and small or large intestinal cancers) have been associated with diarrhea. Diarrhea may also be present as a result of antibiotic therapy,

infectious agents in the GI tract (such as Clostridium difficile and candidiasis), radiation therapy to the bowel, and certain antineoplastic drugs. Vomiting and diarrhea can also lead to a state of volume depletion. When this occurs, aldosterone production is increased, causing renal potassium loss.

Hypokalemia is frequently observed in patients with acute myeloid leukemia.[35] Apparently the hypokalemia is related to inappropriate renal potassium loss. Often patients are hypokalemic at the time they first present for treatment. (See Case Study 22-3.) Excessive loss of potassium (due to renal tubular damage) occurs in many patients during induction therapy for acute nonlymphocytic leukemia. Renal tubular damage in this patient population is usually attributed to acute tubular necrosis caused by antineoplastic drugs, anti-infective therapy, or antifungal therapy with amphotericin B.

Certain malignancies release an ACTH-like substance that can cause increased renal loss of potassium, leading to hypokalemia. These malignancies include the following:

- Small-cell carcinoma of the lung
- Thymoma
- Tumors of the adrenal cortex
- Medullary carcinoma of the thyroid
- Carcinoid tumors of the bronchus[36,37]

ACTH stimulates the adrenal cortex to produce glucocorticoids and aldosterone (a mineralocorticoid). Aldosterone has a significant effect on the excretion of potassium and the retention of sodium, whereas glucocorticoids have a lesser effect on these electrolytes. The administration of large doses of prednisone and prednisolone, two drugs that have a mineralocorticoid effect, can result in hypokalemia. These steroids are often used in the treatment of hematological malignancies, spinal cord compression, and sepsis.

Nonabsorbable anions present in certain antibiotics bind to the potassium ion and increase potassium excretion. These antibiotics include penicillin, ampicillin, carbenicillin, and ticarcillin, drugs commonly used in the treatment of infections in cancer patients.[38]

CLINICAL PRESENTATION

Clinical signs of hypokalemia are described in Chapter 5. The most significant problem associated with hypokalemia is the increased risk for cardiac arrhythmias.

MANAGEMENT

The aim of potassium replacement is to eliminate symptoms and avoid life-threatening complications (primarily cardiac arrhythmias). Potassium losses can be replaced with oral supplements, sometimes requiring titration of potassium doses up to 120 mEq/day. Most often the emergent nature of hypokalemia necessitates intravenous potassium supplementation initially. Although the mechanism is not clearly understood, magnesium depletion affects potassium absorption. When hypokalemia is present, the magnesium level needs to be assessed; if decreased, it needs to be corrected before or concurrently with the correction of hypokalemia. The reader is referred to Chapter 5 for a more detailed discussion of the treatment of hypokalemia.

⬤ TUMOR LYSIS SYNDROME

The tumor lysis syndrome can be a life-threatening oncologic emergency situation that follows the massive necrosis of rapidly dividing tumor cells (as in patients with acute leukemia or bulky high-grade lymphomas)[39], usually following the administration of chemotherapy. It usually consists of a combination of hyperuricemia, hyperkalemia, hyperphosphatemia, and hypocalcemia. Treatment is thus directed toward correcting all of these imbalances. Hyperuricemia and each of the electrolyte imbalances is discussed separately below, along with other possible causes of each one.

The most important step in managing this condition is to prevent it from occurring. Measures commonly initiated to prevent the tumor lysis syndrome are presented in Table 22-1.

Hyperuricemia

Hyperuricemia is found most often in conjunction with the tumor lysis syndrome rather than as an isolated imbalance. It occurs with the rapid release of nucleic acids due to tumor cell lysis as a result of chemotherapy or radiation therapy (most commonly noted in patients with lymphoma or leukemia). Rapid elevation of the serum uric acid level presents the danger of acute urate nephropathy caused by crystallization of uric acid in the kidney. A serum urate level greater than 15 mg/dL is associated with a high risk of urate nephropathy.[43]

While hyperuricemia usually follows chemotherapy or radiation, it may also occur spontaneously in the following situations:

• Certain rapidly proliferating neoplasms with a high nucleic acid turnover (even in the absence of previous chemotherapy)
• Overproduction of uric acid precursors by the tumor (most commonly noted in patients with polycythemia vera and chronic granulocytic leukemia)

Diagnosis of hyperuricemia is established by measurement of uric acid in serum and urine. The normal excretory rate for uric acid is 300 to 500 mg/day. Untreated serum uric acid levels may reach 20 mg/dL (normal, 3.0-9.0 mg/dL). The patient may exhibit ureteral colic, oliguria, and azotemia. Hemodialysis should be considered in patients with urate nephropathy.

Prevention of hyperuricemia is the cornerstone of management; prophylactic treatment consists of the following:

• Vigorous hydration
• Administration of allopurinol
• Alkalinization of the urine (See Table 22-1.)

Hyperuricemia must be viewed as a preventable complication rather than as an emergent condition.

Hyperkalemia

Most often hyperkalemia is seen as a component of the tumor lysis syndrome, which may present during or after the successful treatment of leukemias and lymphomas. The rapid cell destruction from the treatment may cause a precipitous release of cellular potassium and an increase in the serum potassium level. This large amount of potassium in the extracellular fluid surpasses the kidney's potassium excretion ability. Lethal cardiac arrhythmias are the most serious consequence of hyperkalemia.[44]

When the hyperkalemia associated with tumor lysis syndrome is mild, increased intravenous administration of 0.9% NaCl with a single dose of furosemide may be sufficient treatment. However, for patients whose serum potassium level is between 5.5 to 6.0 mEq/L, it may be necessary to add an exchange ion resin (such as Kayexalate) to the regimen. If the serum potassium level is > 6.0 mEq/L, or there are cardiac arrhythmias,

TABLE 22-1.   Prevention of the Tumor Lysis Syndrome

Recognize high-risk patients:

Syndrome occurs most often in patients with high-grade lymphomas, leukemias with high leukocyte counts, small cell lung cancer and less commonly solid tumors[40]

When possible, pretreatment IV hydration over 24 hours for 1–2 days before chemotherapy treatment:

Hydration increases urine output; an increased urine volume decreases the concentration of urates in the urine (thus minimizing the danger of renal damage)

Carefully monitor kidney function and for potential fluid overload. Check vital signs and lung sounds, look for edema, and monitor fluid intake and output. Foley catheters may be recommended for accurate monitoring of urine output in certain situations.

Urinary alkalinization by means of sodium bicarbonate added to IV fluid (such as 50–100 mmol/L) to maintain urinary pH ≥ 7:

When monitoring urinary output, observe for any signs of solute precipitation in the urine.

Administration of allopurinol:

Allopurinol is the mainstay of prevention of uric acid nephropathy.[41]

A possible regimen is 600 mg/day by mouth for 1 or 2 days, at least 24 hours before initiating chemotherapy; thereafter, 300 mg/day may be given.[42]

Initial dose often divided into bid schedule; observe for potential side effects (such as fever, rash, eosinophilia, and hypersensitivity reactions).

Monitor laboratory values for potassium, calcium, phosphorus, uric acid, and creatinine levels at frequent intervals (such as every few hours for the first 3–4 days):

Compare these to baseline levels and inform physician immediately of any significant variations.

Assess for symptoms of hyperkalemia, hypocalcemia, hyperuricemia, and hyperphosphatemia.

it may be necessary to administer intravenous calcium gluconate first, and then follow up with intravenous fluids, furosemide, and hypertonic dextrose and regular insulin).[45]

Although hyperkalemia is most commonly associated with the tumor lysis syndrome, there are other possible causes. An increased serum potassium level can result from acute renal failure (as may occur in untreated hyperuricemia, use of nephrotoxic or antineoplastic drugs, or renal malignancy). Also, a falsely high serum potassium level may be reported in the presence of a high white blood cell count. (Increased leukocyte fragility and lysis releases cellular potassium into the clotted serum sample.) Validation of a supposed hyperkalemic state with the expected electrocardiographic changes and other clinical signs of hyperkalemia is needed to determine whether the serum potassium level is truly elevated in a patient with a high white blood cell count due to a leukemic process.

The reader is referred to Chapter 5 for a more thorough discussion of the clinical manifestations and treatment of hyperkalemia.

Hyperphosphatemia

As indicated earlier, massive tumor breakdown due to treatment releases large amounts of uric acid, potassium, and phosphate, creating the tumor lysis syndrome. The elevated serum phosphate level may not occur until 1 or 2 days after treatment is initiated; levels as high as 20 mg/dL may persist for several days afterward. Hyperphosphatemia usually occurs along with hyperuricemia, hyperkalemia, and hypocalcemia. Renal damage (perhaps even acute renal failure) may be a serious problem resulting from the precipitation of calcium phosphate in the kidneys. High phosphate levels must be reduced rapidly to prevent or to correct renal damage. Treatment of tumor lysis syndrome most often corrects hyperphosphatemia. Management of hyperphosphatemia associated with renal failure is described in Chapter 17.

Hypocalcemia

Hypocalcemia is usually related to the tumor lysis syndrome. As the sudden release of cellular phosphates occurs following tumor lysis, there is a reciprocal drop in the serum calcium concentration. Other possible causes of hypocalcemia include:

- Production of calcitonin by medullary carcinomas
- Malabsorption due to extensive bowel resection or loss of small bowel absorptive surface secondary to tumor size
- Magnesium depletion

As indicated earlier, malnutrition with a resultant decrease in the serum albumin level is a major cause of a below-normal total serum calcium value reported by the laboratory. However, this is not a true deficit in the active component of calcium (ionized calcium). If the patient's ionized calcium concentration is markedly reduced, tetany may develop, as may muscle cramps and cardiac arrhythmias. Hypocalcemia can usually be corrected by the intravenous administration of calcium gluconate.[46]

● HYPOPHOSPHATEMIA

Hypophosphatemia may be associated with some untreated rapidly proliferating malignancies (eg, acute leukemia), presumably due to the consumption of phosphate by the tumor cells. However, hypophosphatemia associated with malignant disease usually occurs subsequent to nutritional deprivation and cachexia. Prolonged hyperalimentation, without appropriate phosphate additives, and respiratory alkalosis, which is associated with the septicemic episodes of neutropenic patients, may also result in hypophosphatemia. A recent study found that the incidence of hypophosphatemia in 106 cancer patients undergoing parenteral or enteral nutrition was quite high (24.5%); risk factors include moderate or severe malnutrition and age greater than 60 years.[47] This phenomenon is referred to as the refeeding syndrome and is related to a shift of phosphate from the extracellular fluid into newly formed cells. See case study 8-1 for an example of hypophosphatemia associated with total parenteral nutrition in a cancer patient. Chapters 11 and 12 provide a more thorough discussion of the refeeding syndrome.

Treatment of hypophosphatemia consists of phosphate replacement by either the oral or the IV route. This treatment is described in greater depth in Chapter 8.

● HYPOMAGNESEMIA

Although hypomagnesemia is a common clinical problem for cancer patients in general, it is most prevalent in patients treated with pharmacological agents that cause hypomagnesemia. It may present as a single electrolyte imbalance or in combination with other disorders seen in the cancer patient, such as hypokalemia, hypophosphatemia, and hypocalcemia.

Cisplatin, a potentially nephrotoxic agent used to treat tumors occurring in a variety of sites, causes renal magnesium wasting in a dose-related manner. The cause of the renal magnesium wasting is not clear; among the possible causes are a direct effect of cisplatin on the renal absorption of magnesium and interstitial nephritis due to the drug (causing damage to Henle's loop and reduction in magnesium absorption).[48] Cyclosporine is commonly used for the prevention of transplant rejection in the bone marrow transplant population. Several clinical studies have found a correlation between hypomagnesemia and the use of cyclosporine, although the exact cause is unclear. In addition, amphotericin B (a common agent used in the treatment of fungal infections in the immunocompromised patient) has been associated with hypomagnesemia.[49] Many cancer patients with various diagnoses develop gram-negative sepsis during the course of their treatment. Drugs used to treat this infection have been associated with hypomagnesemia, especially the aminoglycosides. The renal wasting process caused by these drugs is thought to involve an inhibition of magnesium transport by the proximal tubule, leading to increased magnesium delivery to the loop of Henle. The absorptive power of the loop of Henle is exceeded by the magnesium load, causing increased magnesium excretion in the urine.

Malignant cells apparently have a higher magnesium content than do normal tissues.[50] Studies have suggested that hypomagnesemia in cancer patients results from the increased intracellular content of rapidly proliferating cancer cells.[51]

Hypomagnesemia can occur in the cancer patient for the same reasons as in any other (eg, magnesium loss in chronic diarrhea or prolonged diuretic use, and inadequate magnesium supplementation during hyperalimentation). The reader is referred to Chapter 7 for a discussion of other causes of hypomagnesemia as well as its treatment.

● THIRD-SPACE FLUID ACCUMULATION

Cancer patients frequently develop third-space fluid accumulations; these may be due to the following:

- Malignant effusions into the peritoneal, pericardial, or pleural compartments. Direct tumor involvement of the cavity's serous surface appears to be the most frequent cause of effusions in cancer patients. However, peritoneal effusions also known as ascites commonly occur with liver disease secondary to malignancy.
- Edema. This is trapping of excess fluid in the interstitial fluid space due to obstruction of lymphatic drainage or venous return secondary to tumor pressure. Protein seepage through the capillary bed in the edematous site pulls fluid with it, making the edema more severe. Low serum oncotic pressure (due to hypoalbuminemia) along with extremity dependence contributes to ankle and leg swelling in oncology patients who sit for long periods.

Major shifts of water and electrolytes into potential fluid spaces result in extracellular fluid volume deficit (FVD). This condition is manifested by decreased urinary output, increased urinary specific gravity, and postural hypotension. Body weight does not decrease (as it does with actual fluid loss) because fluid is trapped inside the body; in fact, weight may increase with parenteral fluid replacement (given to correct intravascular fluid volume depletion). Unfortunately, administration of intravenous (IV) fluids to correct the FVD also allows an increase in the fluid volume trapped in the third space, which only adds to the patient's discomfort.

In the case of peritoneal effusions, a paracentesis can be performed to drain the fluid for comfort measures; however, replacement of the fluid, electrolytes, and albumin lost during this procedure must be considered. (Refer to Chap. 21 for a discussion of paracentesis for ascites.)

For a long-term resolution of third-space fluid accumulation, the cause of the fluid shift must be corrected. This can only be accomplished if the malignant process producing the third-space fluid accumulation responds to treatment.

As indicated in this chapter, many fluid and electrolyte problems experienced by oncology patients are managed with replacement or restrictive treatment. However, the underlying cause of the electrolyte problem must be considered or a chronic problem will develop. Tumor elimination or control is a primary consideration. Careful, continued observation of the patient is indicated to effectively control the malignancy and its associated fluid and electrolyte problems.

When patients are diagnosed with a malignancy, the nurse's teaching session should include information regarding the fluid and electrolyte imbalances that pose the greatest risk to the particular patient. Patients and family members or caregivers should then be instructed regarding the signs and symptoms of fluid and electrolyte imbalances and the importance of seeking immediate attention from the health care team if symptoms appear. Patients and family members also need to be instructed regarding the importance of continuing mineral supplementation and follow-up laboratory appointments when a disorder has been diagnosed. In some cases, the recurrence of a fluid and electrolyte disorder is the first sign of recurrence of the malignancy; therefore, it is essential that patients and family members understand the critical nature of reporting this information to the health care team. In situations where patients have received significant doses of nephrotoxic chemotherapeutic agents, mineral supplementation may be necessary for the rest of their lives. The chronic nature of this situation must be made clear to both the patient and family. The reader is referred to Chapter 2 for a review of assessment for fluid and electrolyte problems, and Chapters 3 through 9 for information dealing with specific imbalances.

CASE STUDIES

Normal serum laboratory values for reference:
   Sodium = 135–145 mEq/L
   Potassium = 3.5–5.0 mEq/L
   Chloride = 97–110 mEq/L
   Carbon dioxide (CO_2) = 22–31 mEq/L combining power
   Blood urea nitrogen (BUN) = 8–25 mg/dL
   Creatinine = 0.6–1.5 mg/dL
   Uric acid = 3.0–9.0 mg/dL
   Phosphorus = 2.5–4.5 mg/dL
   Albumin = 3.5–4.5 mg/dL
   Calcium = 8.9–10.3 mg/dL
   Magnesium = 1.3–2.1 mEq/L

● **22-1.** Mrs. J is a 61-year-old woman who was initially diagnosed with lymphoma several years ago, and was diagnosed with recurrent lymphoma last month. She presented with anxiety, decreased appetite, dehydration, and feelings of fatigue. Laboratory results included:

Sodium = 133 mEq/L
Potassium = 3.0 mEq/L
Chloride = 95 mEq/L
CO_2 combining = 21 mEq/L
BUN = 14 mg/dL
Creatinine = 0.9 mg/dL
Uric acid = 3.0 mg/dL
Albumin = 3.8 g/dL
Total calcium = 8.8 mg/dL
Magnesium = 0.5 mEq/L

Although she had decreased intake for several days, she had no symptoms of vomiting, diarrhea, or fistula drainage. She also had no obvious signs and symptoms of hypokalemia or hypomagnesemia. To correct the imbalances, she had received cisplatin (Platinol), etoposide (VePesid) and cytarabine (cytosine arabinoside) 3 days previously. She was treated with 100 mEq of potassium and 1 g of magnesium via the IV route. She then received 100 to 120 mEq of potassium orally for 3 days. The day of discharge, her serum potassium and magnesium levels had returned to normal. Discharge medications included: 40 mEq of oral potassium (TID), and 400 mg of magnesium oxide (TID). She was given an appointment to return to the clinic for laboratory evaluation of serum electrolytes in 3 days. A detailed instruction sheet was given to her regarding the administration of her medications. She also received a written list of signs of hyper/ hypokalemia and of hyper/hypomagnesemia and was instructed to report any signs described in the list to the clinic staff. In addition to being told of the importance of continuing the medications as prescribed, she was instructed to call the clinic staff if she had any difficulty taking the medications.

COMMENTARY: This case involves a lymphoma patient 3 days after chemotherapy treatment but does not include the expected picture of tumor lysis syndrome. Instead, the electrolyte disorders of hypokalemia and hypomagnesemia are seen and are probably related to the side effects of cisplatin. Again, the relationship between hypomagnesemia

and hypokalemia is not clearly understood, but magnesium levels must be adequate for the potassium replacement to be effective. Therefore, magnesium supplementation was given in conjunction with potassium.

Because the discharge medications involve significant doses of replacement potassium and magnesium, the patient needs to observe for signs of hyperkalemia and hypermagnesemia. This is because the effect of cisplatin on renal excretion of potassium and magnesium usually reverses a short time after treatment. Thus, although chronic replacement may be necessary, the doses for long-term maintenance may need to be lower than those used at discharge. Repeated laboratory tests are critical in monitoring electrolyte imbalances. Instructing the patient about the signs and symptoms of hypokalemia and hypomagnesemia is important in the event that this situation occurs again after the next chemotherapy treatment. Also, the patient needs to have detailed instructions about taking these medications and about not discontinuing them without direction from the clinic staff.

● **22-2.** A 68-year-old newly diagnosed patient with acute myelogenous leukemia was admitted to the hospital for induction therapy scheduled to begin the next day. Intravenous hydration was begun with 0.9% sodium chloride and added sodium bicarbonate at the rate of 150 mL/hr. Allopurinol (300 mL orally) was ordered to begin the day of admission and to continue daily. All admission blood work was within normal ranges (serum albumin, 4.0 g/dL). The next day, chemotherapy was begun with cytarabine (cytosine arabinoside) by continuous infusion over 7 days and idamycin (idarubicin hydrochloride) once daily for 3 days. On the third day of treatment, the laboratory results from venous blood were as follows:

Potassium = 6.0 mEq/L
Phosphorus = 14.9 mg/dL
Uric acid = 10.3 mg/dL
Calcium = 7.5 mg/dL

Although all of these values were outside the normal range, the patient displayed no symptoms of electrolyte abnormalities. At this time, hydration with 0.9% sodium chloride (with added sodium bicarbonate) was increased to 300 mL/hr.

On the fourth day, the following serum values were reported by the laboratory:

    Potassium = 4.1 mEq/L
    Phosphorus = 10.0 mg/dL
    Uric acid = 8.5 mg/dL
    Calcium = 8.0 mg/dL

All laboratory results returned to within normal ranges on the final day of treatment (5 days after chemotherapy was begun).

COMMENTARY: This patient experienced tumor lysis syndrome secondary to the large amounts of potassium and phosphate ions that shifted from the intracellular space into the serum. This is a common occurrence in a patient with the diagnosis of leukemia undergoing induction therapy. To prevent renal complications of hyperuricemia, large-volume IV hydration (along with sodium bicarbonate to keep the urine alkaline) was given. Allopurinol was given to reduce the production of uric acid (accomplished by inhibiting the chemical reactions that occur immediately preceding its formation). When the patient's laboratory results were abnormal (hyperkalemia, hyperphosphatemia, hyperuricemia, and hypocalcemia), treatment was initiated to correct these imbalances. The basic treatment consisted of increased hydration (preceded by assessment of renal function). The patient had no existing cardiac abnormality and had no symptoms from the hyperkalemia; therefore, no specific treatment of hyperkalemia was initiated. If the laboratory findings on the fourth day did not demonstrate an improvement in the tumor lysis syndrome, additional therapy to correct the hyperkalemia and the hypocalcemia might have been initiated. Although this syndrome can continue for several days after therapy has been completed, this patient had no further problems during this hospitalization.

● **22-3.** A case was reported in which a previously healthy 38-year-old woman complained of a 2-month history of fatigue, muscle weakness, anorexia, increasing polyuria and polydipsia, and 1 week of a low-grade fever.[52]

Physical examination was unremarkable, except for tachycardia (120 beats per minute). Laboratory results indicated the patient had acute myelogoid leukemia (AML). Her serum sodium potassium level was 2.7 mEq/L and her serum sodium level was 177 mEq/L. Induction chemotherapy was instituted and on day 10 after the first course of therapy, the bone marrow was free of blasts and the serum aldosterone level was low. Intravenous potassium replacement was instituted and ultimately corrected the hypokalemia. About one week after completion of chemotherapy, the leukopenic patient developed septic shock and died. Postmortem examination showed bilateral hyperplasia of the zona glomerulosa of the adrenal glands.

COMMENTARY: Often the hypokalemia seen in AML patients is attributed to renal tubular damage following the administration of nephrotoxic agents. However, this patient displayed significant hypokalemia before any such medications were administered. In this patient, the clinical picture, laboratory values, and bilateral hyperplasia of the adrenal cortex point to a case of marked hyperaldosteronism. That is, excessive aldosterone production caused the patient to lose potassium in the urine.[53]

● **22-4.** A case was reported by Elisaf et al. in which a 64-year-old man with multiple myeloma was admitted with complaints of malaise, diffuse bone pain and constipation.[54] Laboratory results confirmed the presence of anemia. Other than severe hypercalcemia, all other electrolyte levels were within normal range:

    Total calcium = 15.4 mg/dL
    Phosphorus = 2.6 mg/dL
    Magnesium = 1.4 mEq/L
    Potassium = 3.6 mEq/L
    Sodium = 136 mEq/L
    Bicarbonate = 25 mEq/L

Following treatment with 6 liters of isotonic saline over a 48 hour period, the serum calcium decreased to 14.4 mg/dL. Pamidronate (90 mg in a liter of 0.9% NaCl) was given over 4 hours and the patient was then monitored for 2 weeks to assess renal function and electrolyte balance. Six days after treatment with pamidronate the serum calcium level had dropped to 7.9 mg/dL (normal range of reporting laboratory, 8.4 - 10.6 mg/dL); at the same time, the serum phosphorus level was decreased to 1.3 mg/dL (normal range 2.5 - 4.5 mg/dL), and the serum magnesium to 0.7 mEq/L (normal range 1.3 - 2.2 mEq/L).

COMMENTARY: The elevated serum calcium level responded to rehydration with isotonic saline and a single dose of pamidronate. However, a number of transient electrolyte imbalances occurred after the pamidronate was administered. The hypocalcemia was asymptomatic and did not require supplementation; this imbalance has been reported in other patients after high-dose (90 mg) pamidronate, especially when in the presence of renal failure.[55] Apparently serum phosphorus levels tend to decrease after the administration of pamidronate, especially when the baseline phosphorus level is low (as it was in this patient). The most likely reason for the hypomagnesemia was magnesium wasting related to the hypophosphatemia. (It is known that phosphate depletion leads to an increase in the renal excretion of magnesium.)[56]

REFERENCES

1. Harvey H. The management of hypercalcemia of malignancy. Support Care Cancer 1995;3:123.
2. Warrell R. Metabolic emergencies. In: DeVita V, Hellman S, Rosenberg S, eds. Cancer: Principles & Practice of Oncology, 5th ed. Philadelphia: Lippincott-Raven; 1997:2486.
3. Dagogo-Jack, S. Mineral and metabolic bone disease. In: Carey C, Lee H, Woeltje K, eds. The Washington Manual of Medical Therapeutics, 29th ed. Philadelphia: Lippincott-Raven; 1998:441.
4. Ibid.
5. Harvey, p 123.
6. Ibid.
7. Jones L. Electrolyte imbalances. In: Groenwald S, Frogge M, Goodman M, Yarbro C, eds. Cancer Symptom Management. Boston: Jones & Bartlett; 1996:Chap. 23.
8. Harvey, p 123.
9. Jones, p 416.
10. Skeel R. Handbook of Cancer Chemotherapy, 5th ed. Philadelphia: Lippincott Williams & Wilkins; 1999:634.
11. Barri Y, Knochel J. Hypercalcemia and electrolyte disturbances in malignancy. Hematol Oncol Clin North Am 1996;10:775.
12. Chisholm M, Mulloy A, Taylor A. Acute management of cancer-related hypercalcemia. Ann Pharmacother 1996;30:507.
13. Warrell, p 2492.
14. Skeel, p 634.
15. Sekine M, Takami H. Combination of calcitonin and pamidronate for emergency treatment of malignant hypercalcemia. Oncology Reports 1998;5:197.
16. Chisholm et al, p 510.
17. Jones, p 419.
18. Chisholm et al, p 510.
19. Skeel, p 637.
20. Chisholm et al, p 510.
21. Dagogo-Jack, p 444.
22. Barri, Knochel, p 778.
23. Harvey, p 125.
24. Dagogo-Jack, p 444.
25. Coward D. Cancer-induced hypercalcemia. Cancer Nurs 1986;9:125.
26. Jones, p 420.
27. Johnson B, Chute J, Rushin J et al. A prospective study of patients with lung cancer and hyponatremia of malignancy. Am J Respir Crit Care Med 1997;156:1669.
28. Johnson B, Damodaran A, Rushin J et al. Ectopic production and processing of atrial natriuretic peptide in a small cell lung carcinoma cell line and tumor from a patient with hyponatremia. Cancer 1997;79:35.
29. Ibid, p 36.
30. Shapiro J, Richardson G. Hyponatremia of malignancy. Crit Rev Oncol Hematol 1995;18:129.
31. Berghmans T. Hyponatremia related to medical anticancer treatment. Support Care Cancer 1996;4:341.
32. Narins R, ed. Clinical Disorders of Fluid and Electrolyte Metabolism, 5th ed. New York: McGraw-Hill; 1994:595.
33. John W, Foon K, Patchell R. Paraneoplastic syndromes. In: DeVita V, Hellman S, Rosenberg S. Cancer: Principles & Practice of Oncology, 5th ed. Philadelphia: Lippincott-Raven; 1997:Chap. 46.
34. Barri, Knochel, p 783.
35. Wulf G, Jahns-Streubel G, Strutz F et al. Paraneoplastic hypokalemia in acute myeloid leukemia: A case of renin activity in AML blast cells. Ann Hematol 1996;73:139.
36. Lind J. Ectopic hormonal production: Nursing implications. Semin Oncol Nurs 1985;1:251.
37. Odell W. Endocrine complications of cancer. In: Calabresi P, Schein P, eds. Medical Oncology, 2nd ed. New York: McGraw-Hill; 1993:177.
38. Gill M et al. Hypokalemic, metabolic alkalosis induced by high-dose ampicillin sodium. Am J Hosp Pharm 1977;34:528.
39. Woodard W, Hogan D. Oncologic emergencies: Implications for nurses. Journal of Intravenous Nursing 1996;19:256.
40. Warrell, p 2494.
41. Skeel, p 407.
42. Ibid, p 630.
43. Rugo H. Cancer. In: Tierney L, McPhee S, Papadakis M. Current Medical Diagnosis & Treatment, 38th ed. Stamford, CT: Appleton & Lange, 1999:Chap. 4.
44. Warrell, p 2494.
45. Skeel, p 361.
46. Warrell, p 2492.
47. Gonzalez A, Rodriguez A, Figueroa G. The incidence of the refeeding syndrome in cancer patients who receive artificial nutritional treatment. Nutr Hosp 1996;11:98.
48. Lam M, Adelstein D. Hypomagnesemia and renal magnesium wasting in patients treated with cisplatin. Am J Kidney Dis 1986;8:164.
49. Narins, p 1103.
50. Barri & Knochel, p 785.
51. Kohli G, Bhagava A, Goel H et al. Serum magnesium levels in patients with head and neck cancer. Magnesium 1989;8:77.
52. Wulf et al, p 141.
53. Ibid.
54. Elisaf M, Kalaitizidis R, Siamopoulos K. Multiple electrolyte abnormalities after pamidronate administration. Nephron 1998;79:337.
55. Ibid.
56. Ibid.

Pregnancy

Although physiologically normal in pregnancy, changes in fluid retention and blood volume expansion and alterations in acid–base and electrolyte balance would be considered abnormal in the nonpregnant woman or in men. These changes are temporary and necessary adaptations to provide for the growing fetus and for maternal health needs during pregnancy. Despite alterations in water and electrolyte balance, pregnancy is considered a wellness state because the changes serve a useful function.

Changes in body water and electrolyte balance in normal pregnancy will be explored in this chapter, as will some abnormal disease or treatment states that directly affect fluid and electrolyte balances.

● NORMAL PHYSIOLOGICAL WATER AND ELECTROLYTE CHANGES

INCREASED BLOOD VOLUME

In a woman pregnant with one fetus, a 30% to 50% blood volume increase may be expected; an even greater increase occurs in a woman pregnant with twins.[1-3] Although both plasma and red blood cell volumes are increased, plasma volume increases disproportionally to red blood cell mass, resulting in the so-called physiological anemia of pregnancy or pseudoanemia. A hematocrit of 33% to 38% and a hemoglobin of 11 to 12 g/dL may be observed. During late pregnancy, a hemoglobin concentration below 11.0 g/dL is usually caused by iron deficiency anemia.[4] When iron stores are adequate, the decline in blood values is usually minimal. The increase in maternal plasma volume may be beneficial to fetal outcome because significant correlations have been found between maternal plasma volume expansion and birth weight.[5]

SODIUM AND WATER RETENTION

To meet her own needs and those of her growing fetus, the pregnant woman must retain additional fluid and electrolytes. To accomplish this, renal excretory responses are modified, resulting in new balances of fluid and electrolytes. The regulation of sodium and water homeostasis involves the hormones arginine vasopressin or antidiuretic hormone (ADH) and the renin-angiotensin-aldosterone system. These systems must also be altered to respond appropriately to this new equilibrium occurring during pregnancy.

In normal pregnancy, retention of about 950 mEq (3–6 mEq/day) sodium and 6 to 8 liters water is expected.[6,7] About 60% of the sodium is used by the fetus and placenta, and the rest is distributed in the maternal blood and extracellular fluid. Most of the sodium retention occurs during the last 8 weeks of pregnancy.[8] Increased amounts of body water in the extracellular spaces accounts for 70% to 75% of the maternal weight gain. Interstitial fluid volume increases 1.5 to 5 liters with the greatest accumulation during the second half of pregnancy.[9] Accumulation of more than 1.5 liters interstitial fluid is associated with edema.

In the past, diuretics and salt restriction were used at the first sign of edema in pregnant women.[10] However, at present diuretics are not routinely used because it is understood that diuretics can cause a number of problems during pregnancy (eg, electrolyte imbalance, hyperglycemia, and hyperuricemia). The body's demand for sodium actually increases during pregnancy due to the normal increased fluid retention.[11] It is now generally agreed that dietary sodium intake should not be restricted during normal pregnancy, although excessive use should be avoided because of the relationship of sodium to the development of hypertension in those at risk for this problem. During pregnancy, it is wise to limit salt intake to a moderate level (such as 5 g/day), but no less than 2 to 3 g sodium should be consumed on a daily basis.[12] Because sodium represents about 40% of the weight of salt (sodium chloride; NaCl), 1 g NaCl is equivalent to 0.4 g sodium. Thus, 5 g salt is equivalent to 2 g sodium. See Chapter 3 for a discussion of low-salt diets.

Edema

By definition, *edema* refers to an expansion of the interstitial fluid volume. Redistribution of fluid between the intracellular and extracellular compartments secondary to sodium retention is associated with the "physiological" edema of many normal pregnancies.[13,14] In fact, 35% to 80% of healthy normotensive women develop edema at some time during pregnancy.[15,16]

Edema can be dependent or generalized. *Dependent edema* of the ankles frequently occurs when the pregnant woman assumes an upright position and is of little physiological significance. Several factors predispose to dependent edema; most significant is venous pressure. Impingement of blood flow through the inferior vena cava by the pregnant uterus causes stagnation of blood in the lower extremities. Increased permeability of the capillary walls may also influence the rate of filtration. *Generalized edema* is manifested by rapid weight gain and edema of the hands and upper half of the body. This type of edema can also occur in normal pregnancy. However, when generalized edema is accompanied by a rise in blood pressure and proteinuria, it is considered a disease process.[17]

In summary, sodium and water retention of normal pregnancy commonly causes mild peripheral edema, particularly in the third trimester when pressure on the inferior vena cava by the enlarged uterus has a contributory effect.[18] When the pregnant woman elevates her legs or lies on her side, the hydrostatic pressure is partially overcome and interstitial fluid is returned to the circulation.[19,20]

The dependent edema associated with normal pregnancy can be quite annoying. Clinical Tip: Example of Nursing Diagnosis and Nursing Process in Care of Patient With Pedal Edema gives an example of the application of the nursing process to deal with this problem.

Plasma Sodium Concentration

Plasma sodium concentration decreases about 5 mEq/L in almost all pregnant women during late pregnancy, and plasma osmolality decreases about 10 mOsm/kg despite the normal ability of the pregnant woman to dilute the urine.[21] These responses are partly due to increased release of ADH (which in turn causes water retention) and the increased thirst common in pregnant women.[22] The lowered plasma sodium level quickly returns to normal after delivery.

CALCIUM BALANCE

Calcium is a particularly important element during pregnancy. Total serum calcium concentration begins to decrease during the second or third month of preg-

---

CLINICAL TIP

Example of Nursing Diagnosis and Nursing Process in Care of Patient With Pedal Edema Problem: Discomfort Related to Pedal Edema

ASSESSMENT

28-year-old sales clerk in last trimester of pregnancy complains of ankle swelling after standing for a few hours at work

Pedal edema present; no edema in face or hands

Blood pressure, 120/82

No proteinuria

INTERVENTIONS

1. Advise client to avoid constrictive garments around the legs.

2. Recommend use of support hose.

3. Advise against prolonged standing; suggest that she obtain a stool to sit on periodically during time at work.

4. Instruct client regarding passive exercises to improve circulation.

5. Advise frequent rest periods when feasible in which lateral position can be assumed (with legs slightly elevated to reduce venous pressure).

6. Advise ample fluid intake (8–10 glasses of water/day).

7. Encourage client to report increase in pedal edema or appearance of edema in face, hands, or other parts of body.

EXPECTED OUTCOME

Client will use self-care measures to increase comfort and decrease edema.

Client will verbalize decrease in discomfort.

Dependent edema will diminish or become no worse.

Client will be knowedgeable about possible abnormal developments.

nancy and reaches its lowest point during the third trimester. In large part, this is caused by the fetal demands for calcium.[23] Large amounts of calcium are transferred against a concentration gradient from the mother to the fetus, the net accumulation of calcium being 25 to 30 g by term.[24]

Women are often advised to consume additional calcium during pregnancy and lactation with a recommendation to increase calcium intake to 1,200 mg/day during both pregnancy and lactation, 33% higher than for nonpregnant women.[25] Recently, however, more has been learned about the changes in calcium homeostasis that occur during pregnancy and lactation. Research indicates that the calcium required for fetal bone mineralization can be obtained by an increased efficiency of maternal calcium absorption in pregnancy, with no detectable mobilization of maternal bone for this purpose.[26,27] These findings indicate that calcium mobilization to the fetus and to breast milk is a result of changes in maternal metabolism. Although it is still unclear what causes these changes in maternal calcium metabolism, they apparently are not influenced by the amount of dietary calcium consumed. After examining all of the available evidence regarding the safety issues and justification for vitamin and mineral supplementation during pregnancy, the Institute of Medicine concluded that routine supplementation of any nutrient, except iron, is unnecessary.[28] Under normal circumstances, therefore, calcium balance in pregnancy is easily maintained by dietary intake, and the nutrient needs of pregnant women, including calcium needs, can be met through dietary sources. Supplements of certain nutrients are, however, recommended whenever a woman's diet is very poor or when significant nutritional risk factors are present. It has been suggested that calcium deficiency during pregnancy may be associated with threatened preterm delivery.[29] As well, hypertension in pregnancy has been associated with an excess in free calcium levels in peripheral blood.[30]

MAGNESIUM BALANCE

The serum magnesium levels decrease by about 6% to 9% in pregnancy.[31] However, rather than reflecting actual hypomagnesemia, this small decrease probably represents the effects of plasma volume expansion and decreased protein binding associated with mild hypoalbuminemia.[32] Of course, actual magnesium deficiency may develop if dietary intake is inadequate. In preg-

nancy, adequate magnesium intake is essential for the formation of new tissues.[33]

POTASSIUM BALANCE

A cumulative retention of about 350 mEq potassium occurs during pregnancy.[34] The retained potassium is stored in the fetus, uterus, breasts, and red blood cells.[35] This retention occurs despite increased circulating levels of mineralocorticoids and increased delivery of sodium to the distal nephron resulting from the increased glomerular filtration rate.[36] Concentration of potassium in the maternal plasma either remains at a prepregnancy level or is slightly decreased. Prolonged nausea and vomiting or the use of diuretics may lead to hypokalemia and metabolic alkalosis.

ACID–BASE CHANGES

Pregnancy is associated with a compensated respiratory alkalosis, which begins early and continues until delivery. The cause is hyperventilation, secondary to the potent stimulating effect of progesterone on the medullary respiratory center.[37] As a result of hyperventilation, the partial pressure of carbon dioxide (PCO_2) decreases from the normal 40 mm Hg to about 30 mm Hg during gestation, causing an arterial pH of 7.44 ± 0.003 compared with the normal measurement of 7.40.[38]

As with any form of chronic respiratory alkalosis, the one associated with pregnancy is compensated for by changes in the serum bicarbonate concentration. This metabolic compensation causes the bicarbonate level to drop to about 20 mEq/L by the third trimester (compared with the normal bicarbonate level of 24 mEq/L).[39] Because the total buffering capacity is reduced by renal compensation, pregnant women are more likely to develop severe acidosis when conditions causing either ketoacidosis or lactic acidosis are present. If the serum bicarbonate level is normal or elevated in late pregnancy, the possibility of a second imbalance (metabolic alkalosis) should be investigated. Possible causes of the latter could be persistent vomiting or excessive use of potassium-losing diuretics.

RESEARCH FINDINGS

There is an increased requirement for nutrients in normal pregnancy, not only due to increased demand, but also to increased loss. Specific nutrient deficiencies or excesses may potentiate the tendency toward complications during pregnancy. A research study was recently conducted in which serum levels of magnesium were compared with those of calcium, sodium, and potassium over the course of pregnancy in normal women and in women who developed preeclampsia.[40] Venous serum samples were collected from 31 pregnant women during their first, second, and third trimesters. Samples were analyzed for ionized and total magnesium, calcium, sodium, and potassium using a biomedical chemistry analyzer. In 22 normal pregnant women, both serum ionized and total magnesium levels decreased significantly with increasing gestational age. No changes in sodium, potassium, or ionized or total calcium were observed. Nine of the 31 women developed preeclampsia by term; serum total magnesium levels decreased significantly by the second trimester in these 9 women when compared to magnesium levels in the 22 normal pregnant women. The researchers concluded that results of this study provide further evidence of decreases in ionized and total magnesium levels with increasing gestational age during normal pregnancy. This study also provides evidence of a magnesium disturbance in women who later developed preeclampsia. The researchers suggest that further studies of magnesium balance in women at risk for developing complications of pregnancy are indicated.

● ABNORMAL CONDITIONS AFFECTING OR AFFECTED BY FLUIDS AND ELECTROLYTES

PREGNANCY-INDUCED HYPERTENSION

Pregnancy-induced hypertension (PIH) is a disease unique to pregnancy and is characterized by progressive hypertension, pathological edema, and proteinuria. According to the Committee on Terminology of the American College of Obstetricians and Gynecologists and the National Institutes of Health Working Group on High Blood Pressure in Pregnancy, there are three clinical types within the classification of PIH. The first is hypertension without proteinuria or edema; second, hypertension with proteinuria, edema, or both; and finally, eclampsia or hypertension with seizures or coma or both.[41,42] The terms *preeclampsia* and *eclampsia* are used to refer to the nature and degree of the symptoms involved in PIH. Preeclampsia is characterized by hypertension with proteinuria, edema, or both, and usually occurs after 20 weeks of gestation. If the pregnant woman develops convulsions, the term eclampsia is used. The terms preeclampsia and PIH are used synonymously.[43]

Pregnancy-induced hypertension occurs in 5% to 7% of all pregnancies and is the third leading cause of maternal death in the United States. It is primarily a disease of the nullipara, usually involving women younger than 20 years or older than 35 years. It develops after the 20th week of gestation and has its highest incidence among women who have a strong predisposition to hypertension. There is a strong familial predisposition to the development of preeclampsia. Preeclampsia occurs more frequently in nulliparous African American women and daughters and sisters of women with a history of preeclampsia. It is associated with multiple pregnancy, polyhydramnios, vascular disease, trophoblastic disease, and abruptio placentae.[44]

The pathogenesis of PIH is unknown; in fact, this condition has long been known as the "disease of theories." Evidently it is somehow related to the physiological changes of pregnancy as the condition improves and the disease apparently disappears after the termination of pregnancy. It has been conjectured that immunological changes, among other factors, have a pathogenetic role. The pathological changes associated with preeclampsia indicate that poor perfusion secondary to vasospasm is a major factor leading to the derangement of maternal physiological functions and increased perinatal morbidity.[45–47]

Sodium Retention and Fluid Distribution Changes

Sodium retention is expected with normal pregnancy; however, the retention that occurs with preeclampsia may be pathological. Although rapid weight gain and sodium retention are characteristic of preeclampsia, they are not universally present or unique to preeclampsia. At most, these signs are a reason for closer observation of blood pressure and monitoring of urinary protein. The primary indicators of preeclampsia are hypertension and proteinuria.

Paradoxically, the plasma volume is often diminished in women with preeclampsia, despite the increase in total body sodium. The intense vasoconstriction characteristic of preeclampsia may result in a shift of the retained sodium and water from the vascular space into the interstitial space, causing a reduced plasma volume (reflected by a rising hematocrit) and increased interstitial fluid volume.[48,49]

Clinical Indicators

Hypertension in the pregnant woman is defined as a blood pressure reading of more than 140/90 mm Hg or a reading that represents an increase over baseline readings of 30 mm Hg systolic or 15 mm Hg diastolic.[50] Two abnormal blood pressure readings taken at least 6 hours apart are required. Note that the typically accepted level of 140/90 mm Hg may be inaccurate in a patient who normally has a low blood pressure. For example, in a woman with a normal baseline blood pressure of 90/50 mm Hg, a reading of 130/80 mm Hg may well represent hypertension. Proteinuria is often the most valid clinical indicator of preeclampsia. Because proteinuria tends to be a late change, PIH *may* be diagnosed without the presence of proteinuria.[51] Significant proteinuria approximates a 2+ urinary protein. The definitive evaluation of the degree of proteinuria is a quantitative analysis of a 24-hour urine collection. (A level of 300 mg is accepted as the upper limit of normal in pregnancy.[52]) Table 23-1 summarizes the suggested nursing assessment parameters for abnormal fluid balance changes associated with preeclampsia and eclampsia.

 TABLE 23-1.   Summary of Nursing Assessment Parameters for Abnormal Fluid Balance Changes Associated with Preeclampsia

Associated Parameter	Comments
Weight changes	Weigh on same scale each time, after voiding, and with same amount of clothing (normal weight curve is a 10-lb weight gain at 20 weeks with a 0.5-lb/wk until 40 weeks. In patients with PIH, weight gain is usually > 30 lb by the third trimester).
BP changes	Establish baseline BP in early pregnancy.
	Assess BP with client in same position and in same arm each visit; use cuff of appropriate size.
	Although 140/90 serves as a rough baseline for hypertension, it is better to look for a degree of elevation over baseline.
	As a rough rule of thumb, consider BP abnormal if systolic elevates > 30 mm Hg or diastolic elevates > 15 mm Hg over first trimester or prepregnancy values.
	Two abnormal readings after 20th week of gestation taken at least 6 hours apart are required for a diagnosis of hypertension.
Edema*	+1 edema: minimal edema of lower extremities
	+2 edema: marked edema of lower extremities (as evidenced by inability to wear usual shoes)
	+3 edema: edema of lower extremities, face, and hands (as in inability to wear rings)
	+4 edema: generalized massive edema including the abdomen and face (puffy eyelids and blunted facial features)
Proteinuria	Obtain clean-catch voided specimen, avoid contamination with vaginal secretions (causes false positive)
	Significant if 1+ or 2+ on two or more occasions or if > 300 mg/L in a 24-hour urine collection

*Edema without other clinical indicators of preeclampsia can occur in normal pregnancy (see text).
BP, blood pressure; PIH, pregnancy-induced hypertension.

Therapeutic Measures

Diuretics are not generally used except in the presence of heart failure. The decreased blood volume resulting from the use of diuretics further decreases the blood flow to the placenta, disrupts the normal electrolyte balance resulting in impairment of some placental functions, and increases the stress on the already compromised kidneys.[53] This is because plasma volume is already decreased in preeclamptic women and the natriuresis associated with diuretic use may be counterproductive.[54,55] Also, some preeclamptic women have insidious sodium losses or are in negative sodium balance because of dietary manipulations. In these women, administration of diuretics may cause severe hyponatremia.[56] Similarly, strict sodium restriction has no role in the prevention or therapy of preeclampsia and may actually be counterproductive (again because of the decreased plasma volume in preeclamptic women).[57] However, moderate sodium restriction may minimize the discomfort of women with significant edema.[58]

Antihypertensive therapy (usually hydralazine) is generally reserved for women with severe hypertension that could lead to intracranial bleeding or left ventricular failure.[59,60] When antihypertensive therapy of preeclampsia is directed at reduction of peripheral vascular resistance, a shift of excess sodium and water from the interstitial into the intravascular space may occur. As a result, excessive expansion of the intravascular space may cause an inadequate response to antihypertensive therapy. To monitor the volume status of seriously ill preeclamptic or eclamptic patients, use of a Swan-Ganz catheter may be necessary to identify patients with elevated wedge pressures who might benefit from the judicious use of diuretics.[61]

Women with preeclampsia may develop oliguria, either because of a diminished intravascular volume or renal problems.[62] Fluid administration in the presence of oliguria must be undertaken cautiously because if the oliguria is renal in origin, fluid overloading is likely to result. Although oliguria due to hypovolemia may be corrected by fluid infusion, excessive fluid administration can lead to congestive heart failure. Also, excessive fluid administration can lead to cerebral edema if the serum sodium level is very low. To avoid lowering the plasma osmolality, hypotonic fluids should not be used (particularly if oxytocin is being administered). Either isotonic electrolyte or colloid-containing fluids may be considered. For the woman with seriously decreased colloid oncotic pressure secondary to hypoalbuminemia, colloid-containing fluids may be indicated. The rate of fluid administration must be closely titrated to urine output and other clinical indicators such as central venous or, preferably, pulmonary wedge pressure.[63]

Magnesium Sulfate as an Anticonvulsant

The therapeutic use of magnesium sulfate ($MgSO_4$) in preeclampsia-eclampsia is due to its pharmacological effects on the central nervous system (CNS) through depression and vasodilation. More specifically, magnesium ions block nerve transmission by presynaptic inhibition, decreasing smooth muscle contractility and depressing CNS irritability.[64] Magnesium also tends to block catecholamine release from the adrenal medulla and may cause peripheral vasodilation.

Magnesium sulfate can be given intramuscularly (IM) or intravenously (IV); however, because the IM administration of large volumes of $MgSO_4$ is painful and the rate of absorption cannot be controlled, this route of administration is seldom used. Magnesium sulfate is commonly given IV with an initial bolus followed by a continuous slow infusion, titrating the rate of administration against maternal deep-tendon reflexes.[65] The desired dosage of $MgSO_4$ varies depending on renal status and the patient's response to the drug. IV administration of magnesium at doses of 2 to 3 g/hr appears to be safe for the patient with normal renal function.[66] However, doses exceeding this level require that serum magnesium concentrations be monitored at least every 2 hours until a steady state has been achieved.

Most authorities agree that $MgSO_4$ is a safe and efficient agent to prevent convulsions. Eclamptic convulsions are usually prevented if plasma magnesium levels are maintained at 4 to 7 mEq/L.[67] (Recall that the normal plasma magnesium concentration is 1.3–2.1 mEq/L.)

The loss of deep-tendon reflexes is the first sign of toxicity; therefore, the presence of deep-tendon reflexes indicates that the serum magnesium concentration is not dangerously high[68] (see Summary of Hypermagnesemia in Chap. 7). However, in addition to monitoring patellar reflexes, rate and depth of respirations should be observed regularly because respiratory paralysis and cardiac arrest can result if serum magnesium levels increase too high. Because magnesium is primarily eliminated by the kidneys, the adequacy of renal function must be monitored during its administration. It is generally agreed that urine output should total at least 100 mL every 4 hours. If toxic symptoms occur from magnesium overdosage, calcium gluconate may be prescribed as an antidote. The normal dose is 10 mL of a 10% solution given slowly over 3 minutes.[69,70] Mechanical respiratory support may also be needed if respirations are severely depressed.

A major advantage of $MgSO_4$ therapy is that at effective anticonvulsant doses it is very safe for the fetus and neonate. Neonatal serum magnesium concentrations are nearly identical to those of the mother. Although amniotic fluid magnesium concentrations increase with prolonged infusion due to fetal renal excretion of magnesium, fetal serum magnesium levels do not increase and there is no evidence of cumulative effects of prolonged magnesium administration on the neonate.[71]

Magnesium sulfate is not a perfect anticonvulsant; some women have convulsions even with high serum magnesium levels. Other anticonvulsants are being studied in clinical trials to assess their efficacy in the care of pregnant women. Specifically, phenytoin has been described as equally effective for the treatment and prophylaxis of eclamptic seizures and could be a reasonable alternative in settings in which magnesium would be best avoided (eg, markedly compromised renal function, myasthenia gravis).[72]

Nursing Interventions

Home care for high-risk obstetric patients by qualified perinatal nurses is increasing.[73] If the preeclampsia is mild and fetal growth retardation is not a problem, management can be accomplished in the home. Home therapy includes two to three weekly medical and nursing assessments, encouraging the patient to participate in the care, dietary modifications, and bedrest.[74]

Of importance is teaching the patient self-assessment of weight, edema, fluid intake and urine output, and assessment of proteinuria as well as recognition of CNS symptomatology (eg, blurred vision, headaches, nausea, and vomiting). An essential part of home management for preeclampsia, home blood pressure monitoring is now less complicated and more reliable as a result of technological advances.[75,76]

Although research indicates that antepartum hospitalization is a significant stressor for high-risk pregnant women, appropriate management for severe preeclampsia and eclampsia can only be accomplished when the woman is hospitalized.[77] The following interventions are often indicated for patients with severe preeclampsia and eclampsia:

1. Maintain bedrest with patient in the lateral recumbent position. (Bedrest in this position increases renal perfusion and, thus, urinary output. Placental perfusion is also increased.)
2. Monitor changes in blood pressure, degree of edema, and degree of proteinuria (see Table 23-1). Frequency of these observations depends on the severity of the patient's condition; for example, they may be needed hourly if the condition is advanced.
3. Provide a quiet, nonstimulating environment (preferably a private room.)
4. Monitor closely for development of labor; monitor fetal status (use fetal monitor).
5. Keep artificial oral airway device at bedside and maintain seizure precautions. Have emergency tray immediately accessible.
6. Monitor for hyperreflexia.
7. Inquire about subjective symptoms such as headaches, epigastric pain, visual disturbances. Record results of daily funduscopic examinations; edema of the retina reflects retinal isch-emia and is a serious development.
8. If prescribed, administer magnesium sulfate according to facility protocol. The goal is to prevent convulsions without creating generalized CNS depression. To prevent overdose of magnesium, it is necessary to:
   - Check patellar reflexes at regular intervals (if depressed, notify physician).
   - Check respirations (12 or less per minute is cause to notify physician).
   - Monitor urine output (notify physician if < 30 mL/hr).
   - Monitor serum magnesium levels, reporting elevations above the therapeutic range designated by physician. The reader is referred to Chapter 7 for the Clinical Tip: Nursing Considerations in Administering IV Magnesium and the Summary of Hypermagnesemia for a list of indicators of hypermagnesemia.
9. Administer oxygen if needed after convulsion. Monitor breath sounds for signs of pulmonary edema.

Research Findings

Since the association between eclampsia and hypertension was first recognized, the measurement of blood pressure during pregnancy has been an essential part of good antenatal care. A study was recently conducted to investigate the clinical and psychological outcome of blood pressure monitoring using a telemetry system at home.[78] Fifty-three previously normotensive women found to have significant hypertension during a routine antenatal visit participated in the study. These women would normally have been hospitalized; however, for purposes of the study, they were allowed to return home and use a telemetry system, which provided regular and accurate monitoring of their blood pressure. Results indicated that home telemetry is a highly acceptable method of managing moderate hypertension in pregnancy. Most frequently the women commented that use of the telemetry system avoided hospital admission and enabled them to remain at home where they were more comfortable and relaxed. Women with young children were particularly positive about the system. Negative responses were mainly associated with the few technical problems that arose with the transmission of blood pressure readings.

HYPONATREMIA AS A COMPLICATION OF OXYTOCIN ADMINISTRATION

Labor induction with oxytocin delivered in an appreciable amount of an aqueous solutions (such as 5% dextrose in water [D_5W]) can lead to water retention, severe hyponatremia, and seizures in both the mother and fetus.[79] Recall that the pharmacological action of oxytocin includes a potent antidiuretic effect causing increased water retention. Although the plasma sodium concentration may return to normal after the water diuresis that follows discontinuance of the infusion, permanent neurological sequelae or even death may occur.[80]

Symptoms of water intoxication (dilutional hyponatremia) include lethargy, headache, blurred vision, twitching, convulsions, and coma. See Chapter 4 for a more complete discussion of this topic. This complication can be prevented by using an electrolyte solution instead of dextrose and water as a vehicle for oxytocin administration, limiting the amount of fluid intake, and monitoring serum electrolytes.[81] Oxytocin should not be infused by gravity because the rate of flow by this method is too erratic to ensure a steady delivery of the drug. Instead, it should be administered by a continuous infusion pump (such as a Harvard pump or a peristaltic-type pump). For induction of labor, the standard dilution is 1 mL (10 units) of oxytocin in 1 liter lactated Ringer's solution or 0.9% NaCl.[82] The initial dose is usually 1–2 mU/min with 1 mU/min increases if the dosing increase interval is 15 minutes (or 0.5 to 1.0 mU/min with increases of 1 to 2 mU/min if the dosing increase interval is 40 to 60 minutes). The maximum dose rarely exceeds 20 mU/min.[83,84]

HYPEREMESIS GRAVIDARUM

Hyperemesis gravidarum is defined as severe vomiting occurring before the 20th week of gestation.[85] Although nausea and vomiting are symptoms encountered in 50% to 90% of pregnant women, the incidence of hyperemesis gravidarum varies from 0.3% to 1%.[87] Excessive vomiting causes fluid volume deficit (FVD), starvational ketoacidosis, and, at times, metabolic alkalosis with hypokalemia. (These imbalances are commonly seen with excessive vomiting; see Chap. 13 for a discussion of fluid and electrolyte disturbances associated with gastric fluid loss.) Significant weight loss may occur and reflects fluid as well as lean tissue loss. Also indicative of FVD is decreased urinary output with a high specific gravity and a high blood urea nitrogen (BUN) level. Ketonuria can occur and is reflective of starvation; excessive ketones in the bloodstream cause metabolic acidosis. Metabolic alkalosis is also a possibility with the loss of gastric acid.

The cause of hyperemesis gravidarum is unknown. It has been postulated that it is related to several factors, including vitamin B_6 deficiency, impaired function of the adrenal cortex, hyperthyroidism and excess human chorionic gonadotropin secretion, change in gastrointestinal physiology, poor nutrition, and emotional state.[87]

Prognosis is good if proper management is instituted. Treatment usually includes hospitalization; however, IV therapy may be initiated in an outpatient setting to correct mild to moderate dehydration. In severe cases, parenteral nutrition is provided until vomiting ceases, oral intake can be initiated, and serum electrolytes return to normal. At times, total parenteral nutrition may be indicated to achieve adequate nutrient intake and allow the gastrointestinal tract to rest. Careful use of antiemetics or mild sedatives may also be indicated for some patients. Attention should be given to handling any psychological component of the patient's illness. Monitoring needs of patients with hyperemesis gravidarum include daily weights, fluid intake and output, vital signs, and laboratory measures of electrolytes and general metabolic status (including potassium, sodium, BUN, glucose, and serum creatinine levels).

FLUID AND ELECTROLYTE DISTURBANCES ASSOCIATED WITH TOCOLYTIC THERAPY

The most widely used drugs for tocolysis or treatment of preterm uterine contractions are the β-mimetics (ie, ritodrine hydrochloride and terbutaline sulfate) and magnesium sulfate. Tocolytic agents are usually initially administered IV. For example, ritodrine is initially administered IV at 50 to 100 μg/min increasing by 50 μg/min every 10 minutes until uterine contractions stop. The usual maintenance dose of ritodrine is 150 to 350 μg/min, continued for 12 hours after contractions have stopped. Oral administration of ritodrine is initiated 30 minutes before discontinuing the IV infusion.[88] Treatment with a β-mimetic is associated with sodium and fluid retention.[89] To avoid this risk, the total amount of IV hydration should be limited to 1,500 to 2,500 mL/24 hr; however, excess fluid volume may result despite limiting IV fluid intake. β-adrenergic drugs also induce a fall in plasma potassium levels.[90] Electrolytes should be monitored before and after 24 hours of treatment with β-adrenergic agents.

Home management of preterm labor may include the oral administration of either ritodrine or terbutaline.[91] The subcutaneous administration of small doses of terbutaline through a terbutaline pump may also be included in home management of preterm labor with the frequency of administration determined by uterine activity and maternal pulse. (Tachycardia is a side effect of β-mimetic drugs.)

Magnesium sulfate decreases uterine activity and is currently being evaluated for its use as a tocolytic agent. Magnesium sulfate is usually administered IV, but may be given IM and orally. Therapeutic maternal serum levels of magnesium range between 4 and 8 mg/dL.[92] Nursing interventions are the same as for the woman receiving magnesium sulfate for severe preeclampsia.

CASE STUDIES

● **23-1.** During her prenatal visit, a 19-year-old primigravida is hospitalized for the treatment of severe preeclampsia. Physical examination reveals that her blood pressure is 164/110 mm Hg, her urine is +2 for protein, her deep-tendon reflexes are 3+ without clonus, and she has 3+ edema. She is treated with $MgSO_4$ to decrease blood pressure and prevent convulsions. On the second day of $MgSO_4$ administration, nursing assessment reveals absent patellar reflexes.
COMMENTARY: The absence of deep-tendon reflexes is a clear sign of magnesium toxicity. The $MgSO_4$ should be discontinued immediately. Magnesium toxicity could even result in respiratory or cardiac arrest. Calcium gluconate, the antidote for magnesium sulfate toxicity, should always be kept at the bedside of any patient receiving $MgSO_4$.

● **23-2.** A 26-year-old gravida 2, 30 weeks' gestation, is being treated for preterm labor. The physician orders an IV infusion of ritodrine hydrochloride, increasing the infusion rate every 10 to 30 minutes depending on uterine response; the IV rate is not to exceed 125 mL/hr. Intake and output are to be strictly measured. Vital signs are to be taken every 15 minutes until stable and then follow hospital protocol. In particular, the patient's pulse rate, regularity, and quality are to be noted. A serum potassium level is to be determined before initiation of the ritodrine infusion and again in 24 hours.
COMMENTARY: Because a common side effect of β-mimetic agents is water retention, adherence to strict guidelines for IV fluid administration and recording of intake and output are important nursing functions. Tachycardia may also be an adverse effect of ritodrine administration. Electrolyte levels should be monitored before initiating the medication to obtain a baseline level and after 24 hours to determine the effect on the patient's potassium level because β-mimetic agents also induce a decrease in plasma potassium.

REFERENCES

1. Guyton A, Hall J. *Textbook of Medical Physiology*, 9th ed. Philadelphia: WB Saunders; 1996:1040.
2. Creasy R, Resnik R. *Maternal-Fetal Medicine*, 4th ed. Philadelphia: WB Saunders; 1999:783.
3. Matteucci E, Giampietro O. Activity of erythrocyte sodium-hydrogen exchange in normal pregnancy. *Clin Sci* 1997;93: 431.
4. Mandeville L, Troiano N. *High Risk & Critical Care Intrapartum Nursing*, 2nd ed. Philadelphia: Lippincott Williams & Wilkins; 1999:15.
5. Theunissen I, Parer J. Fluid and electrolytes in pregnancy. *Clin Obstet Gynecol* 1994;37:6.
6. Creasy, Resnik, p 789.
7. Blackburn S, Loper D. *Maternal, Fetal, & Neonatal Physiology: A Clinical Perspective*. Philadelphia: WB Saunders; 1992:342, 344.
8. Ibid, p 342.
9. Ibid, p 344.
10. Creasy, Resnik, p 125.
11. Lowdermilk S, Perry S, Bobak, I. *Maternity & Women's Health Care*, 6th ed. St. Louis: CV Mosby; 1997:169.
12. Gilbert E, Harmon J. *High Risk Pregnancy & Delivery*, 2nd ed. St. Louis: CV Mosby; 1998:25.
13. Theunissen, Parer, p 3.
14. Creasy, Resnik, p 783.
15. Davison J. Edema in pregnancy. *Kidney Int* 1997;59:S90.
16. Blackburn, Loper, p 346.
17. Gilbert, Harmon, p 499.
18. Blackburn, Loper, p 346.
19. Theunissen, Parer, p 4.
20. Lowdermilk et al, p 146.
21. Paller M, Ferris T. Fluid and electrolyte metabolism during pregnancy. In: Narins G, ed. *Maxwell and Kleeman's Clinical Disorders of Fluid and Electrolyte Metabolism*, 5th ed. New York: McGraw-Hill; 1994:1128.
22. Ibid.
23. Lowdermilk et al, p 169.
24. Creasy, Resnik, p 1032.
25. Ibid, p 162.
26. Ritchie L, Fung E, Halloran B. A longitudinal study of calcium homeostasis during human pregnancy and lactation and after the resumption of menses. *Am J Clin Nutr* 1998;67:693.
27. Laskey M, Prentice A, Hanratty L. Bone changes after 3 mo of lactation: Influence of calcium intake, breast-milk output, and vitamin D-receptor genotype. *Am J Clin Nutr* 1998;67:685.
28. Creasy, Resnik, p 126.
29. Smolarczyk R, Wojcicka-Jagodzinska J, Romejko E et al. Calcium-phosphorus-magnesium homeostasis in women with threatened preterm delivery. *Int J Gynecol Obstet* 1997;57:43.
30. Barbagallo M, August P, Resnick L. Altered cellular calcium responsiveness to insulin in normal and hypertensive pregnancy. *J Hypertens* 1996;14:1081.
31. Paller, Ferris, p 1132.
32. Ibid.
33. Lowdermilk et al, p 162.
34. Paller, Ferris, p 1128.
35. Ibid.
36. Ibid.
37. Ibid, p 1132.
38. Ibid.
39. Ibid.
40. Standley C, Whitty J, Mason B, Cotton D. Serum ionized magnesium levels in normal and preeclamptic gestation. *Obstet Gynecol* 1997;89:1051.
41. Creasy, Resnik, p 833.
42. Mandeville, Troiano, p 159.
43. Krening, C. Perinatal hypertensive crisis. *NAACOG's Clinical Issues in Perinatal and Women's Health Nursing* 1992;3:413.
44. Creasy, Resnik, p 836.
45. Ibid, p 845.
46. Arias F. *Practical Guide to High-Risk Pregnancy and Delivery*, 2nd ed. St. Louis: Mosby–Year Book; 1993:186.
47. Guyton, Hall, p 1041.
48. Arias, p 186.
49. Creasy, Resnik, p 839, 850.
50. Arias, p 186.
51. Gilbert, Harmon, p 497.
52. Arias, p 185.
53. Gilbert, Harmon, p 506.
54. Ibid, p 506.
55. Creasy, Resnik, p 854.
56. Arias, p 199.
57. Creasy, Resnik, p 854.
58. Ibid.
59. Ibid, p 860.
60. Arias, p 194.
61. Creasy, Resnik, p 857.
62. Krening, p 415.
63. Creasy, Resnik, p 861.
64. Ibid, p 858.
65. Arias, p 193.
66. Gilbert, Harmon, p 518.
67. Ibid, p 518.
68. Ibid.
69. Creasy, Resnik, p 859.
70. Gilbert, Harmon, p 520.
71. Creasy, Resnik, p 859.
72. Ibid.
73. Lowdermilk et al, p 710.
74. Ibid.
75. Naef R, Perry K, Magann E et al. Home blood pressure monitoring for pregnant patients with hypertension. *J Perinatol* 1998; 18(3):226.
76. Mooney P, Dalton K, Swindells H, et al. Blood pressure measured telemetrically from home throughout pregnancy. *Am J Obstet Gynecol* 1990;163:30.
77. Heaman M. Stressful life events, social support, and mood disturbance in hospitalized and non-hospitalized women with pregnancy-induced hypertension. *Can J Nurs Res* 1992;24:23.
78. Cartwright W et al. Home measurement of pregnancy hypertension. *Professional Care of Mother and Child* 1993;3:8.
79. Rayburn W, Zuspan F. *Drug Therapy in Obstetrics and Gynecology*, 3rd ed. St. Louis: Mosby-Year Book; 1992:237.
80. Mandeville, Troiano, pp 148, 152.
81. Cherry S, Merkatz I. *Complications of Pregnancy: Medical, Surgical, Gynecologic, Psychosocial, and Perinatal*, 4th ed. Baltimore, MD: Williams & Wilkins; 1991:774.
82. Rayburn, Zuspan, p 235.
83. Wilson, B, Shannon, M, Stang, C. *Appleton & Lange's Nurses' Drug Guide*. Stamford, CT: Appleton & Lange; 1998:1033.
84. American Academy of Obstetricians and Gynecologists. *Induction and Augmentation of Labor*. ACOG Technical Bulletin No. 217. Washington, DC: Author; 1995.
85. Long P, Russell L. Hyperemesis gravidarum. *J Perinatal Neonatal Nurs* 1993;6:22.
86. Theunissen, Parer, p 9.
87. Long, Russell, p 23.
88. Wilson et al, p 1219.
89. Theunissen, Parer, p 9.
90. Ibid, p 10.
91. Lowdermilk et al, p 944.
92. Mandeville, Troiano p 113.

Special Considerations in Children and the Elderly

Fluid Balance in Infants and Children

It is imperative that nurses who care for infants and children know that in addition to the obvious difference in size between infants, children, and adults, significant differences also exist in the rate of metabolism and in the body surface area. Fluid and electrolyte requirements vary, not only with the size of a child but also with the child's age and clinical condition. Fluid and electrolyte imbalances occur much more rapidly in infants and children than in adults. Consequently, nurses need to know that the earlier the imbalances are recognized and treated, the more positive the outcome for the child or infant.

● DIFFERENCES IN WATER AND ELECTROLYTE BALANCE IN INFANTS, CHILDREN, AND ADULTS

BODY WATER CONTENT

The premature infant's body is about 90% water; the newborn infant's body, 70% to 80%; and the adult's body about 60%. Infants have proportionately more water in the extracellular compartment than do adults. For example, 40% of the newborn infant's body water is in the extracellular compartment as compared with less than 20% in the adult.

As the infant becomes older, the ratio of extracellular to intracellular fluid volume decreases. Loss of extracellular fluid (ECF) is attributed to the growth of cellular tissue and the decreasing rate of growth of collagen relative to muscle growth during the early months of life.[1] The decrease is particularly rapid during the first few days of life, but continues throughout the first 6 months. After the first year, the total body water is about 64% (34% in the cellular compartment and 30% in the ECF compartment). By the end of the second year, the total body water approaches the adult percentage of about 60% (36% in the cellular compartment and 24% in the ECF compartment). At puberty, the adult body water composition is attained. It is important to remember that infants and children who are obese have less total body water than those who are not.

DAILY BODY WATER TURNOVER IN INFANTS AND ADULTS

The fact that infants have a relatively greater total body water content than adults does not protect them from excessive fluid loss. On the contrary, infants are more vulnerable to fluid volume deficit (FVD) because they ingest and excrete a relatively greater daily water volume than adults. Infants may exchange half of their daily ECF, whereas the adult may exchange only one-sixth during the same period. Therefore, proportionately, the infant has a smaller reserve of body fluid than does the adult.

The daily fluid exchange is relatively greater in infants, in part because their metabolic rate is two times higher per unit of weight than that of adults. Infants expend 100 kcal/kg body weight, whereas adults expend only 40 kcal/kg. Because of the high metabolic rate, the infant has a large amount of metabolic wastes to excrete. Because water is needed by the kidneys to excrete these wastes, a large urinary volume is formed each day. Contributing to this volume is the inability of the infant's immature kidneys to concentrate urine efficiently. In addition, relatively greater fluid loss occurs through the infant's skin because of the proportionately greater body surface area.

HOMEOSTATIC DIFFERENCES BETWEEN CHILDREN AND ADULTS

Young children have immature homeostatic regulating mechanisms that must be considered when planning water and electrolyte replacement.

Renal Function

The newborn's renal function is not yet completely developed. If infant and adult renal functions are compared on the basis of total body water, the infant's kidneys appear to become mature by the end of the first month of life. However, if body surface area is used as the criterion for comparison, the child's kidneys appear immature for the first 2 years of life. Because the infant's kidneys have a limited concentrating ability and require more water to excrete a given amount of solute, the infant has difficulty conserving body water when it is needed. Also, the infant has difficulty excreting an excess fluid volume.[2] Thus, infants are less able to adapt to too little or too much fluid. Although adults may be able to tolerate fluid imbalances for days, infants may tolerate similar disturbances for only hours before the situation becomes acute.

Acid–Base Homeostasis

Newborn and premature infants have less homeostatic buffering capacity than do older children. They have a tendency toward metabolic acidosis, with pH averages slightly lower (7.30–7.35) than normal.[3] The mild metabolic acidosis (base bicarbonate deficit) is believed to be related to high metabolic acid production and to renal immaturity. Because cow's milk has higher phosphate and sulfate concentrations than breast milk, newborns fed cow's milk have a lower pH than do breast-fed babies.

Body Surface Area Differences

The skin represents an important route of fluid loss, especially in illness. This concept is important when considering fluid balance in infants and young children because their body surface area is greater than that of older children and adults. For example, compared with older children and adults, the premature infant has about five times as much body surface area in relation to weight, and the newborn, three times. The premature infant is very susceptible to fluid and electrolyte losses. Premature infants will lose 10% to 20% of their birth weight compared to 5% to 10% in term infants during the first week of life. This loss of weight appears to result largely from physiological contraction of the extracellular space after birth. The younger the gestational age of the infant, the more pronounced the contraction of the extracellular space and the higher the insensible water loss.[4] In addition, there is increased fluid loss associated with the higher than normal work of breathing experienced by most premature infants and with the use of radiant warmers needed to maintain the infant's temperature. Therefore, any condition causing a pronounced decrease in intake or increase in output of water and electrolytes threatens the body fluid economy of the infant.

The young infant has a relatively greater gastrointestinal membrane surface area than does an older child or adult. Hence, relatively greater losses occur from the gastrointestinal tract in the sick infant than in the older child or adult.

Electrolyte Concentrations

Plasma electrolyte concentrations do not vary strikingly among infants, small children, and adults. Causes of electrolyte imbalances are similar among the various age groups. However, there are some important considerations that are specific for infants and young children.

Calcium and Phosphorus

Serum calcium levels are known to correlate with gestational age, being lower in premature infants. At the time of delivery, the infant's plasma calcium level falls with the abrupt termination of calcium transport across the placenta. This, in turn, causes the release of parathyroid hormone, which mobilizes calcium from the bone. Some infants are not able to achieve this response normally and are thus vulnerable to hypocalcemic tetany because of a transient physiologic hypoparathyroidism (see Case Study 24-2).

The incidence of hypocalcemia in premature infants is extremely high.[5] Other factors that increase the risk of hypocalcemia include low birth weight, intrauterine growth retardation, and feedings with cow's milk. This topic is discussed later in the chapter.

Sodium

Hyponatremia is common in newborns in neonatal intensive care units.[6] Worldwide, up to a third of very low birth weight (VLBW) infants are hyponatremic in the first week after birth, and between 25% and 65% are hyponatremic thereafter.[7] Apparently the hyponatremia is related to renal salt wasting. Sodium is an important nutrient in premature infants because of its association with protein synthesis, bone mineralization, and maintenance of ECF volume.[8] A low serum sodium level in an otherwise healthy premature infant who is greater than 2 weeks old is called "late hyponatremia." Despite standard fortification, human breast milk may not contain an adequate amount of sodium to meet the needs of VLBW infants, especially if the birth weight is less than 1,000 g.[9] Therefore, when the infant's serum sodium level drops below 135 mEq/L, Kloiber et al.[10] state that it may be necessary to alternate human milk with a premature infant formula or to carefully provide sodium chloride supplements.

Hypernatremia may occur in infants for a number of reasons, not unlike older children and adults. However, it is even more likely to occur in infants because of their relatively large obligatory water losses. This topic is discussed later in the chapter.

Magnesium

The serum magnesium concentration is usually low in the first 24 hours after birth. Infants of diabetic mothers are especially inclined to have serum magnesium levels that are lower than normal. Symptoms of hypomagnesemia are difficult to distinguish from those of hypocalcemia[11]; indeed, they often occur together. It is important to note that the infant's serum magnesium concentration may be elevated if the mother received magnesium sulfate for the treatment of eclampsia. The infant with a high serum magnesium level may require artificial respiration or exchange transfusions.[12]

Potassium

The serum potassium concentration rises in the first 24 to 72 hours after birth in premature infants and is apparently related to a shift of potassium from the cells to the extracellular space.[13] The magnitude of the elevation roughly correlates with the degree of immaturity. In very premature infants, the shift can result in serious hyperkalemia.[14]

● NURSING ASSESSMENT

A thorough history and physical examination are required on all infants and children with a suspected or potential fluid and electrolyte imbalance. Establishing a therapeutic relationship as quickly as possible with the child's parents will help the nurse elicit the vital information needed. A review of the child's laboratory data is also important.

HISTORY

Parents usually report that the infant or child has not taken in the usual amount of food and liquids. They may also report numerous episodes of vomiting or diarrhea as well as decreased frequency of voiding. An attempt should be made to estimate the amount of urine, vomitus, and stool eliminated by the child. Parents often report that the child's level of activity has changed as a result of the illness. A change in the child's emotional status is common.

Parents should be asked if the child has any chronic conditions and what, if any, medications the child is currently taking. It is also important to ascertain if the child has been exposed to a communicable illness and to determine if the parents have done anything at home to attempt to help the child (such as administering over-the-counter products to lower body temperature, or if they have used special home remedies). Another important question concerns whether or not there has been an increased intake of any particular type of fluids (such as water, tea, sugar-containing fluids, or electrolyte solutions such as Pedialyte^R or Gatorade^R).[15]

PHYSICAL ASSESSMENT

See Chapter 2 for a review of a systematic approach to assessment of fluid balance status. The following discussion is specific to children and includes the following parameters.

Blood Pressure

Although blood pressure should be measured, it is important to note that it is not considered a reliable sign of fluid volume status in a young child. For example, the elasticity of the blood vessels may keep the blood pressure stable initially even when volume is substantially diminished.[16] Thus, one should not be reassured by a normal blood pressure reading in a dehydrated young child.

Tissue Turgor

Tissue turgor in the child is best palpated in the abdominal areas and on the medial aspects of the thighs (Fig. 24-1). In a normal situation, pinched skin will fall back to its normal configuration when released. In a patient with FVD, the skin may remain slightly raised for a few seconds. Skin turgor begins to decrease after 3% to 5% of the body weight is lost as fluid. Severe malnutrition, particularly in infants, can cause depressed skin turgor even in the absence of fluid depletion.

Obese infants with FVD often have skin turgor that is deceptively normal in appearance. An infant who has lost a relatively greater volume of water than of sodium (FVD with hypernatremia) has a firm, thick-feeling skin. This same phenomenon is observed in the child

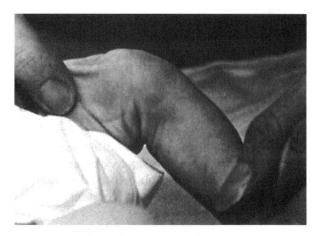

FIGURE 24-1.   Poor skin turgor in infant.

who has sodium excess caused by an excessive sodium intake (such as occurs in salt poisoning). The thickened turgor is believed to be associated with pulling of water from the cells into the hypertonic interstitial fluid.

Mucous Membranes

Dry mouth may be due to FVD or to mouth breathing. When in doubt, the nurse should run a finger along the oral cavity to feel the mucous membrane where the cheek and gums meet. Dryness in this area indicates a true FVD. The tongue of the fluid-depleted child is smaller than normal. Mucous membranes in the child with sodium excess are dry and sticky. Decreased tearing and salivation are signs of FVD that becomes obvious with a fluid loss of more than 5% of the total body weight.

Body Temperature

Fluid volume deficit is often associated with a subnormal temperature because of reduced energy output. However, depending on what caused the FVD, fever may be present; if so, its height should be recorded frequently. The amount of water loss depends on the degree and duration of fever. For example, there is a 12% increase in insensible losses for each 1°C rise in body temperature.[17]

Fever may indicate the presence of an infection, or it may be a sign of FVD with hypernatremia. Despite an elevated body temperature, the extremities of a child with a severe FVD may feel cold to touch due to decreased peripheral blood flow.

Heart Rate and Capillary Refill Time

Tachycardia is considered to be one of the earliest signs of FVD. This is true regardless of the patient's age. A heart rate above 150 beats/min in an infant and above 120 beats/min in a child is indicative of hypovolemia. Decreased peripheral perfusion will cause an increased capillary refill time. In mildly dehydrated children, the capillary refill time is close to normal (2–3 seconds). In moderately dehydrated children, the capillary refill time is increased to 3 to 4 seconds; it is greater than 4 seconds in severely dehydrated children.[18] The skin color in a child with moderate to severe FVD will be ashen or gray due to decreased peripheral blood flow.

Respirations

The child's respiratory rate and work of breathing increase as dehydration develops. Partly this is because dehydration causes metabolic acidosis (secondary to poorly perfused tissues). As the respiratory rate increases, so does the insensible loss of water from the lungs.

Urine Volume and Concentration

A child with FVD has a decreased urinary output and an increased urinary specific gravity (SG). If the FVD is severe, a child may go as long as 18 to 24 hours without voiding and still not have a distended bladder. A child who has a FVD of 5% will have a slight decrease in urine output, whereas a child with greater than a 15% FVD will have marked oliguria and azotemia.[19] If a child with a known FVD excretes large amounts of dilute urine, renal damage probably exists. If the child is receiving a high-solute diet or has a hypercatabolic state (such as fever or infection), the urine volume will be somewhat above normal to help eliminate the increased metabolic wastes.

When possible, all urine should be collected and measured if the child has a real or potential body fluid disturbance. Unfortunately, this is often difficult to do in infants and small children. In this situation, at least the frequency of voiding and the urine's appearance should be noted. In addition, the nurse should estimate the portion of the diaper saturated with urine. One way of measuring the amount of urine in a diaper is to weigh the diaper dry (the same size and brand the child is wearing), and then weigh the diaper after voiding has occurred. For example, a dry diaper may have a weight of 30 g; if, after the child has voided, the same diaper weighs 160 g, one might assume that the additional 130 g represents urine. (A rough estimate is that 1 g of additional weight represents 1 mL urine.) This method has drawbacks. For example, urine may have evaporated from the diaper, especially if the child is under a radiant warmer. Also, it may be difficult to determine how much of the diaper's wetness is due to urine and how much is due to very liquid stool. However, despite possible drawbacks, this method is better than catheterizing the child.

Hourly urinary output reflects the adequacy of hemodynamics and hydration, decreasing as renal perfusion pressure decreases. About normal hourly urine outputs are considered to be the following: premature infant 2 mL/kg/hr, full-term infant 1 mL/kg/hr, and older child 0.5 mL/kg/hr. Because urine flow rates in sick newborns may vary considerably from hour to hour, the average output should be calculated every 6 hours. When an accurate hourly recording of urine is indicated, the nurse must devise a method to collect all the urine passed. A number of devices are available. One could use the diaper weight method described above, or a receptacle to catch the urine can be taped to the child's genitalia. Regardless of the method used, it is important to check frequently for leakage and to provide good skin care to prevent irritation of the genitalia. The urine's concentration can be estimated visually because color of the urine typically becomes a deeper yellow as the urine concentrates. When necessary, the urine's SG can be measured with a refractometer; fortunately, this device requires only a drop of urine for the test. It is common practice to withdraw a small quantity of urine from a disposable diaper by syringe and test its SG with a refractometer or with a urine test strip. Apparently a number of factors affect the accuracy of this practice. Among them are the brand of the disposable diaper, the length of time the urine has been present in the diaper, the volume of urine voided into the diaper, and whether or not the diaper was folded and taped after its removal from the child. A study by Gammage and Yarandi compared the accuracy of urine SG measurements with several brands of disposable diapers, using refractometry and a urine dipstick (N-Multistix SG).[20] They concluded from their study that immediately after a baby voids at least 20 mL urine into any of the diapers, the SG measurement by refractometer and dipstick compare favorably to that made from urine obtained from a urine container. However, because results at 4 hours postvoiding are often inaccurate, the authors recommend that urinary SG measurements (by either refractometer of urine dipstick) be made within 1 hour after voiding.

Weight Changes

If possible, the child's weight before the onset of the illness should be obtained from the parents or from the family physician, who may have a record of the normal weight from a recent office visit. It should be noted that many offices do not obtain naked weights on infants and small children and this can be a problem in determining the child's actual weight.

Weight loss can be caused by loss of fluid or by catabolism of body tissues. The weight loss associated with FVD occurs more rapidly than that caused by starvation. One way of looking at the percentage of FVD is to understand that for every acute loss of 1 kg body weight, there is a deficit of about 1,000 mL. Thus, a child who normally weighs 10 kg and now weighs 9 kg because of FVD is assumed to have a fluid deficit of about 1,000 mL. A mild FVD entails a rapid weight loss of about 3% to 5%, a moderate FVD entails a rapid weight loss of about 5% to 9%, and a severe FVD entails a rapid weight loss of 10% or more. An acute loss of 15% of the body weight will likely cause hypovolemic shock. An accurate method of determining the percentage of the FVD is to use the following equation[21]:

$$\% \text{ Dehydration} = \frac{\text{Preillness weight} - \text{Illness weight}}{\text{Preillness weight}} \times 100$$

Example:

$$\text{Preillness weight} = 10 \text{ kg}$$
$$\text{Illness weight} = 9 \text{ kg}$$
$$(10 - 9)/10 \times 100 = 10\% \text{ deficit}$$

If weighing is not performed accurately, it is useless. Even a minor error is important when the patient is small. The child should be weighed at the same time each day, before eating, and after having voided. The same scales should be used each time. The child should be undressed and covered with a light blanket to protect against chilling while being weighed. (The same blanket should be used each time for consistency.) Intravenous (IV) boards and other equipment attached to the child should be noted on the child's chart next to the recorded body weight.

Other Considerations

The anterior fontanelle will be depressed in infants with moderate to severe FVD. There also will be absence of tearing in infants with severe FVD. The eyes appear increasingly sunken as the severity of dehydration increases. Additional assessment parameters pertaining to evaluation of fluid and electrolyte balance status are presented in Chapters 2 through 9.

Laboratory data are discussed in Chapter 2. A few considerations specific to children are worth noting. For example, a prospective study of 97 children who required IV fluids for acute dehydration found that a low serum bicarbonate concentration (< 17 mEq/L) was a good predictor of the percent of loss of body weight.[22] On the basis of their findings, the investigators suggested that obtaining a serum bicarbonate level might improve the accuracy of predicting the seriousness of dehydration. (Recall that FVD causes reduced tissue perfusion and can lead to metabolic acidosis.) Other investigators used a convenience sample of 40 children requiring IV fluid resuscitation for dehydration to determine the best laboratory predictors of FVD in acutely dehydrated children. They concluded that only the serum blood urea nitrogen (BUN), serum creatinine, and uric acid levels were significantly associated with increasing fluid deficit.[23] Of course, laboratory data should only be used as an adjunct in the context of a careful history and physical examination.

Although electrolytes require frequent monitoring in seriously ill infants and children, it is important to consider the amount of blood withdrawn for this purpose. It has been noted that an important determinant in the need for blood transfusions is the volume of blood sampled. Blood transfusion in a critically ill newborn may be required when 10% or more of the blood volume is withdrawn over a period of less than 2 to 3 days. For example, for a 750-g infant, the withdrawal of as little as 8 mL blood over a short period may necessitate the need for transfusion.[24] Thus, it behooves caregivers to submit the smallest amount of blood possible to the laboratory for testing. Tests can often be grouped in such a way as to minimize the volume of blood needed.

● CONDITIONS IN CHILDREN PREDISPOSING TO FLUID AND ELECTROLYTE DISTURBANCES

See Chapters 10 through 23 for discussion of specific entities; although these chapters are primarily concerned with the care of adults, some information is also applicable to children. The discussion below concerns specific fluid and electrolyte problems occurring in a pediatric population.

CRITICAL ILLNESS OR INJURY

The resuscitation of an infant or child in severe hypovolemic shock or cardiac arrest requires immediate vascular access for the administration of medicines, blood, and fluids. IV access is extremely difficult because of peripheral circulatory collapse, and precious minutes may be wasted in trying to access a peripheral vein.[25] The use of the intraosseous route for parenteral infusions in such emergency situations may be lifesaving.[26] Pediatric advanced life support programs provide training in the technique of intraosseous infusion for the emergency treatment of infants and children. (See the section on the intraosseous route for parenteral infusions later in this chapter.)

A critically ill child will sometimes present with fluid volume excess (FVE). Refer to the chapters on renal and cardiac failure, as well as on the head-injured patient to review causes for FVE. The clinical assessment of a child with FVE may reveal a child with a rapid weight gain as well as systemic, peripheral, and periorbital edema. An infant often demonstrates periorbital edema first, due to the thinness of this tissue. Tachypnea with increased work of breathing, hepatomegaly, and bounding pulses may also be evident.[27]

Daily weights on the same scale at the same time of day are necessary to document any changes in the child's weight. Weight gains that are considered significant and require immediate reporting to the child's physician are: infant, 50 g/24 hr; child 200 g/24 hr; and adolescent 500 g/24 hr.

Auscultation of the child's chest may indicate a gallop rhythm to the heartbeat and rales in the lungs. Children with FVE may have decreasing urine outputs; therefore, accurate measurement of fluid intake and output is very important. Also, the child's abdominal girth should be measured.

BURNS

Children with burns are another challenge to the clinician. Burns are the second leading cause of accidental death in children under the age of 5 years in the United States. Depending on the degree of burn and the amount of body surface area involved, there may be massive fluid losses. Although there is some direct loss of fluid, most of the loss involves a temporary shift of intravascular fluid into the burned tissue (referred to as third-spacing). The goal of fluid therapy is to prevent shock and renal failure due to hypovolemia. There are several accepted formulas for calculating fluid volume replacement; these include the Galveston and Parkland formulas. If the child has sustained burns over greater than 25% body surface area, central venous access should be considered. The nurse needs to be very attentive to the types of resuscitative fluids administered as well as to any ongoing fluid losses. Assessment of the adequacy of tissue perfusion includes monitoring urine output, blood pressure, level of consciousness, and peripheral circulation in unburned tissues. Serum electrolyte levels and blood gases also need to be carefully monitored.

PYLORIC STENOSIS

Pyloric stenosis is a condition in which the circular muscle of the pylorus is elongated and hypertrophic; it produces progressive narrowing of the lumen of the outlet from the stomach to the duodenum and results in vomiting after feedings. The condition becomes evident in the first few weeks of life as vomiting becomes progressive and eventually projectile in nature. In the United States, pyloric stenosis occurs in about 3/1,000 live births; boys are affected four times more often than girls.[28]

Vomiting causes the same imbalances in children as it does in adults. These include metabolic alkalosis, potassium deficit, sodium deficit, and FVD. See Chapter 13 for a discussion of imbalances associated with vomiting. Because of the repeated vomiting, the infants are poorly nourished. Although this condition can be corrected surgically, preoperative correction of the water and electrolyte disturbances caused by the prolonged vomiting is mandatory. Fluid therapy consists of 0.45% to 0.9% NaCl, in 5% to 10% dextrose, with added KCl (30–50 mEq/L).[29] This fluid replacement rehydrates the child and helps correct the metabolic alkalosis. (Potassium is not added to the fluid until the urine output is at an acceptable level.)

The infant with hypertrophic pyloric stenosis has the following symptoms:

- Difficulty in retaining feedings, which becomes progressively worse during the first few weeks of life; eventually, projectile vomiting follows each feeding.
- Signs of malnutrition
- Decreased respiration (compensatory action of lungs to retain carbon dioxide and thus help counteract metabolic alkalosis)
- Tetany accompanying alkalosis (owing to decreased calcium ionization in an alkaline pH)
- Palpable pyloric mass
- Ketoacidosis (may appear if starvation is prolonged)

Once the infant's fluid and electrolyte balance is restored, surgical correction of the pyloric obstruction can be accomplished and oral feedings resumed.

NECROTIZING ENTEROCOLITIS

Necrotizing enterocolitis (NEC) is a serious disease that involves intestinal inflammation, usually of the distal ileum and the proximal colon. The etiology is unknown; however, it is thought to be the result of decreased perfusion, hypoxia, and invasion of bacteria. NEC occurs in about 1% to 5% of all neonatal intensive care admissions. The preterm infant is very susceptible to NEC; conversely, the disease rarely occurs in term infants.[30] The length of intestine that is involved and the degree of necrosis will determine whether surgical resection will be necessary. The amount of intestine resected will determine the degree of electrolyte and nutritional imbalances that will occur.

The clinical manifestations of NEC include:

- Onset is usually within the first 2 weeks of life, often after the initiation of enteral feedings (in VLBW infants, the onset can be as late as 2 months of age).
- Meconium stool is passed normally; however, gastric retention and abdominal distention will be noted (bloody stools are reported in 25% of the infants with NEC).
- Onset can be insidious; the infant's nurse and physician may actually suspect sepsis before NEC.[31]

Treatment of NEC includes the cessation of feedings, nasogastric decompression, IV fluids, and antibiotics. Careful attention to acid–base and electrolyte balance is needed.

If surgery is performed, the length of bowel resected will determine if the infant will be on long-term total parenteral nutrition or on slowly progressing tube feeding (leading to eventual oral feedings). The infant may have an ileostomy postoperatively; therefore, increased fluid losses along with third-spacing from the surgical procedure itself can be a challenge for caregivers. Among the possible complications of NEC following massive intestinal resection are growth failure (due to malabsorption) and sepsis and thrombosis related to the use of central venous catheters for total parenteral nutrition.[32]

DIARRHEA

Diarrhea is a common cause of water and electrolyte disturbances in infants and small children. In the United States, the rotavirus is the pathogen that is responsible for the vast majority of cases. The virus attacks the absorptive cells of the small bowel, which results in watery diarrhea.[33] Rotovirus is estimated to kill one million children worldwide each year. Almost all children are affected by the virus by the time they are 4 years old. In the United States alone, about 55,000 children less than 5 years of age are hospitalized and 550,000 children see their clinicians for treatment.

Fluid Volume and Sodium Balance

A large loss of liquid stools can rapidly deplete the young child's ECF volume, especially when vomiting is also present. Serum electrolytes should be measured in any child with more than a 5% acute weight loss. Usually water and electrolytes are lost in isotonic proportions (FVD or "isotonic dehydration"). In fact, about 70% of the cases of dehydration caused by diarrhea are of the isotonic type. In this form of dehydration, the serum sodium level is between 130 and 150 mEq/L. However, in about 20% of the cases, water is lost in excess of electrolytes (FVD with sodium excess, or "hypertonic dehydration"). This type of dehydration is associated with a serum sodium level greater than 150 mEq/L. Hypernatremic dehydration in the child with diarrhea can be made worse by the ingestion of a high solute-containing formula or an improperly prepared oral electrolyte solution. (Indeed, as discussed later in

the chapter, the latter two can be causes of hypernatremic dehydration in an infant without diarrhea.) In about 10% of the cases of dehydration associated with diarrhea, electrolytes are lost in excess of water (FVD with sodium deficit, or "hypotonic dehydration"); this may occur in children with bacillary dysentery and cholera. In these two diseases, the concentration of sodium in the stool rises with the increasing volume of stool. Hypotonic dehydration is associated with a serum sodium level less than 130 mEq/L.

Other Electrolyte Imbalances

Although sodium is the electrolyte that deservedly receives the most attention, it is important to recognize that the child with diarrhea may also lose substantial quantities of potassium in diarrheal stools. For example, the potassium content in the stool may be as high as 30 to 40 mEq/L.[34] Hypomagnesemia may also occur secondary to magnesium loss. These two conditions are discussed in Chapters 5 and 7.

Metabolic Acidosis

Metabolic acidosis usually accompanies frequent liquid stools. (Recall that the intestinal secretions are alkaline because of their high bicarbonate content; therefore, loss of alkaline secretions in diarrheal stools results in metabolic acidosis.) Decreased dietary intake contributes to metabolic acidosis. In the absence of adequate food intake, the body uses its own fats for energy purposes. The metabolism of these fats causes the accumulation of acidic ketone bodies in the blood, further contributing to the metabolic acidosis caused by bicarbonate loss.

A major symptom of metabolic acidosis is increased depth of respiration. This compensatory mechanism blows off carbon dioxide, thus reducing the carbonic acid content of the blood and influencing the carbonic acid–base bicarbonate balance in the direction of an increased pH. If ketosis of starvation is present, an acetone odor may be noted on the breath.

Treatment

Oral Rehydration
The dehydration that results from diarrhea in infants and children can often be treated by the oral administration of a balanced glucose-electrolyte solution. In many parts of the world, oral rehydration therapy is the only

form of treatment available, and it has been shown to reduce significantly the mortality rate from acute diarrhea.[35] The oral rehydration solution (ORS) recommended by the Diarrhea Disease Control Program of the World Health Organization contains sodium, potassium, chloride, base, glucose, and water. The glucose in the solution facilitates the transport of sodium across the bowel wall.[36] Table 24-1 presents the composition of types of ORS and several other products available in grocery and drug stores throughout the United States. The commercial products are sold with directions for administration. Recommended amounts to use are calculated on the basis of weight and stool frequency.

Oral rehydration consists of three phases: rehydration, replacement of ongoing losses, and maintenance therapy. Oral rehydration should only be attempted in children who are mildly to moderately dehydrated. Parenteral fluids are needed for the child who is severely dehydrated.

Rapid rehydration along with replacement of ongoing losses during the first 4 to 6 hours is advocated, using an appropriate ORS.[37] Rehydration solutions often have a sodium concentration between 75 and 90 mEq/L.[38] Aliquots of 5 to 15 mL can be administered by spoon or syringe every 10 to 20 minutes; the volumes are gradually increased and the interval between feedings decreased as the patient tolerates.[39] After rehydration has been achieved, an orally administered maintenance solution (usually having a sodium concentration of 45–50 mEq/L) is used.[40]

As soon as tolerated, food is reintroduced; the oral electrolyte replacement solution is continued for maintenance and to replace ongoing stool losses. Breast-fed infants can breast feed ad lib; however, they should also receive additional maintenance fluids. Infants who are on formula can either be given lactose-free formula or half-strength lactose-containing formula along with an equal amount of rehydrating solution. Children on regular diets can continue that diet. Caregivers should be cautioned to avoid giving the child foods high in simple carbohydrates.[41] The BRAT (bananas, rice, apples and toast or tea) diet is no longer recommended for children with diarrhea because it has little nutritional value and is low in protein and electrolyte content while being too high in carbohydrates. Also not appropriate are home

TABLE 24-1. Characteristics of Selected Oral Rehydration Solutions

| Solution | Electrolyte content (mEq/L) | | | | Carbohydrate | |
	Na$^+$	K$^+$	Cl$^-$	Citrate	mM	Amount/Liter
Rehydration						
Rehydralyte	75	20	65	30	139	25 g dextrose
World Health Organization	90	20	80	30*	111	4 tbs cane sugar (sucrose)
Maintenance						
Resol solution†	50	20	50	34	111	20 g glucose
Pedialyte solution	45	20	35	30	139	25 g dextrose
Ricelyte	50	25	45	30	167	30 g rice syrup solids‡
Gatorade	20	3	27	3	278	50 g dextrose‡
Gatorade light	15	3	20	3	139	25 g dextrose‡
Lytren	50	25	45	30	111	20 g dextrose‡
Infalyte	50	20	40	30	111	20 g dextrose

*Present as bicarbonate.
†Also contains 4 mEq/L of Mg^{++} and Ca^{++} and 5 mEq/L of PO$_4{}^-$.
‡Value includes nondextrose carbohydrates.
From Alpers D, Stenson W, Bier D. *Manual of Nutritional Therapeutics,* 3rd ed. Boston: Little, Brown, 1995;201 (Table 7-9).

remedies such as decarbonated soda beverages, fruit juices, tea, Kool-Aid[R], and Jell-O[R] because they have inappropriately high osmolalities, which may make diarrhea worse; also, they are low in sodium and thus may cause hyponatremia.[42]

Vomiting is not a contraindication to oral rehydration in most children[43]; however, if vomiting is persistent and oral fluid intake cannot keep up with ongoing losses, IV hydration is needed. Clinicians should caution parents or caregivers that the child should be seen if the diarrhea worsens or the child is incapable of taking oral fluids.

The ORS can be offered by bottle, spoon, or cup. Spoon-feeding appears to minimize vomiting. Throughout the rehydration phase, the solution should be offered in small amounts at frequent intervals. Skin turgor, body weight, and behavioral responses should be assessed frequently to evaluate the child's progress. Nursing strategies for administering oral fluids to infants and young children are discussed later in this chapter.

Parenteral Fluid Therapy

Inability to consume sufficient fluids to keep up with ongoing fluid loss is an indication for parenteral fluid therapy. Other contraindications for oral rehydration include severe FVD with hemodynamic instability, a serum sodium concentration less than 120 mEq/L or greater than 160 mEq/L, altered mental status, severe respiratory distress, and the possibility of an acute surgical abdomen.[44] Children with any of these conditions require parenteral fluid replacement. See the discussion of principles of parenteral fluid replacement in children later in this chapter.

HYPERNATREMIC DEHYDRATION IN EXCLUSIVELY BREAST-FED INFANTS

In the United States, there has been a recognized increase in the incidence of significant morbidity due to breast-feeding failure leading to hypernatremic dehydration.[45] The cause is usually inadequate breast-feeding resulting in the child not consuming sufficient fluid to match the obligatory large fluid losses of infancy. It is difficult to determine the volume of breast milk consumed by an infant; mothers who are not educated to observe for the number and volume of voidings as well as other indications of hydration may not be able to detect the inadequate fluid intake.

In most instances of hypernatremia in breast-fed infants, the problem is not that the breast milk is too high in sodium content (although there have been reports of this occurring).[46] Instead, the problem is inadequate volume intake in relation to fluid output. Some health professionals suggest that the early discharge of infants and mothers due to financial constraints may play a role in the infant's increased chance of developing hypernatremic dehydration (see Case Study 24-2).

USE OF ENEMAS FOR CONSTIPATION

Undesirable effects of enemas for the treatment of constipation in infants and young children are discussed in Chapter 13 (also, see Case Study 24-4). Serious electrolyte complications (primarily hyperphosphatemia, hypocalcemia, and hypernatremia) have been reported with the use of hypertonic sodium phosphate (Fleet[R]) enemas in young children. Excessive absorption of water from tap water enemas can lead to hyponatremia. Parents and caregivers should be instructed to consult the child's clinician before administering an enema to an infant or small child. If an enema is necessary, an appropriate solution is isotonic saline (0.9% NaCl); the solution can be made in the home by dissolving 1 level teaspoon of table salt in 1 pint of tap water.[47] Not only is it important that parents know how to make the isotonic enema solution, they should know how much to administer. Table 24-2 presents guidelines for administering enemas.[48] Nurses should be sure to use terms that parents and caregivers understand.

EXCESSIVE WATER INTAKE

Acute dilutional hyponatremia can develop in infants who are fed excessively diluted formula.[49] Parents need to be instructed on the proper method of preparation for the infant's formula. The parents also need to be instructed on the danger of diluting the infant's formula to make the supply last longer. Some parents have inadvertently given their child too much water during a febrile illness and have caused water intoxication. A somewhat rare cause for water intoxication is the child who swallows large amounts of water during swimming lessons.[50] The condition also can occur in infants who are given tap water enemas because excessive water may be absorbed from the large intestine.[51] Although exceptions apply on rare occasions, Arant

> **TABLE 24-2.**   Guidelines for Administration of Enemas to Children

Age	Amount	Tip Insertion Distance
Infant	120–140 mL (4–8 oz)	2.5 cm (1 in.)
2–4 yr	240–360 mL (8–12 oz)	5.0 cm (2 in.)
4–10 yr	360–480 mL (12–16 oz)	7.5 cm (3 in.)
11 yr	480–720 mL (16–24 oz)	10 cm (4 in.)

From Wong D, ed. *Whaley and Wong's Nursing Care of Infants and Children*, 6th ed. St. Louis: Mosby–Year Book; 1999:1275.

states that a cardinal rule in pediatric fluid therapy is that water without electrolytes is never administered parenterally to an infant or child.[52] For example, the inappropriate use of glucose solutions in water, either as oral or parenteral therapy, to treat infants with dehydration can result in acute dilutional hyponatremia.[53]

As the extracellular sodium dilutes, water shifts to the intracellular space, pulmonary and cerebral edema develop, and intracranial pressure increases. Signs of acute dilutional hyponatremia include:

- Lethargy and irritability
- Subnormal temperature
- Focal or generalized seizures
- Respiratory distress

Treatment is directed toward restricting free water intake and carefully increasing the serum sodium level.[54] With skilled medical and nursing care, the prognosis is good. In a report of 29 infants with acute dilutional hyponatremia, all of whom experienced seizures and 6 of whom required endotracheal intubation, all recovered without apparent sequelae.[55]

EXCESSIVE SODIUM INTAKE

Improperly prepared infant formulas and oral electrolyte solutions can cause serious hypernatremia when too much salt is used. Cases have been reported in which caregivers accidentally substituted table salt for sugar when preparing infant formulas; in other instances caregivers substituted tablespoons for teaspoons of table salt or baking soda (sodium bicarbonate) when preparing electrolyte solutions at home.

A case was recently reported in which a 6-week-old infant developed life-threatening complications following the administration of sodium bicarbonate

(given to help the child "burp").[56] The child's serum sodium level increased to 180 mEq/L and the bicarbonate concentration to 47 mEq/L (about twice normal). The authors recommended that parents be educated to guard against the use of harmful home remedies such as this one. It is disturbing to learn that an informal survey at Johns Hopkins Hospital revealed that 11% of their clinic population had heard of using baking soda as a home remedy, and 4% had actually added baking soda to their infants' formula.[57] Another cause of hypernatremia, mentioned earlier, is the administration of hypertonic sodium phosphate (Fleet[R]) enemas to infants and young children (see Case Study 24-4).

HYPOCALCEMIA

Hypocalcemia of infancy is classified as early or late. Infants at greatest risk for early hypocalcemia are VLBW infants, those born to diabetic mothers, and infants who were subjected to difficult deliveries (see Case Study 24-2). Often the condition is asymptomatic and resolves spontaneously. When clinical manifestations require treatment, it usually consists of the slow IV injection of a 10% solution of calcium gluconate in a dose of about 2 mL/kg.[58] It is important to give the solution slowly while monitoring the cardiac rate for bradycardia. Tissue necrosis may occur if the solution extravasates into the tissue space. Late hypocalcemia can occur in either full-term or premature infants. It is usually caused by the feeding of high-phosphate milk; in this situation, the serum phosphate level increases and causes a reciprocal drop in the serum calcium level. If the normal parathyroid hormone response is not made, the level of serum calcium progressively falls and symptomatic hypocalcemia results. Carpopedal spasm is not usually seen, and Chvostek's sign cannot be interpreted as a sign of hypocalcemia because it is commonly present in newborns.[59] Laryngospasm and apneic episodes may occur.[60]

PRINCIPLES OF PARENTERAL FLUID REPLACEMENT IN CHILDREN

DAILY REQUIREMENTS

Daily requirements for water are related to both caloric consumption and expenditure; these requirements are best met orally. Infants and children who cannot tolerate oral feedings, particularly when abnormal losses are occurring, must receive parenteral fluid therapy to meet maintenance and replacement needs. Maintenance requirements can be computed in several ways. For example, one method to determine 24-hour maintenance fluid requirements based on weight is as follows:[61]

100 mL/kg for first 10 kg
50 mL/kg for next 10 kg
20 mL/kg for each kg above 20 kg

Example: 25 kg child

$(100 \times 10) + (50 \times 10) + (20 \times 5) = 1,600$ mL in 24 hours

Electrolyte needs vary with the child's clinical condition.

Formulas offer only approximations of a child's needs and have to be modified on the basis of assessment data. Factors such as an extremely humid environment or the ability to consume and retain some oral fluids will reduce the amount of IV maintenance fluids to be delivered. Factors such as hyperventilation, an extremely dry environment, or a high body temperature will require an increase in the amount of maintenance fluids.

In addition to the rough guidelines described above, fluid volume replacement must be based on the history of the child's illness, on clinical assessment of circulatory impairment or changes in skin elasticity (discussed earlier), and on laboratory values such as serum electrolytes and osmolality. See Chapter 2 for a discussion of laboratory tests and Chapter 10 for a discussion of water and electrolyte solutions and nursing considerations in their administration.

The amount and type of fluid to be administered to a dehydrated child depends on the degree and type of dehydration (isotonic, hypertonic, or hypotonic), serum electrolyte levels, and any existing acid–base imbalances.

CORRECTION OF ISOTONIC DEHYDRATION (FLUID VOLUME DEFICIT)

Isotonic contraction of body fluids is observable by dry skin and mucous membranes as well as by tachycardia when about 5% of the body weight has been lost during a 24-hour period. Marked circulatory impairment—evidenced by mottled, cool, inelastic skin and sunken eyes—occurs when the child has lost 10% of the body weight over a 1- to 2-day period. Losses of 15% of the body weight over this period can produce a moribund or near-moribund state.[62] When the degree of fluid and electrolyte imbalance has been determined, therapy is administered in three phases (rehydration, replacement of ongoing losses, and maintenance). The objective of the rehydration phase is to expand the ECF volume. In isotonic dehydration, an isotonic fluid (such as 0.9% NaCl or lactated Ringer's solution) is given at a volume of 20 mL/kg.[63] For example, a child with an isotonic volume deficit might be given 20 mL/kg of lactated Ringer's over 30 minutes (this dose may need to be repeated to make the child hemodynamically stable). Following adequate rehydration, a maintenance solution might consist of 5% dextrose in 0.45% NaCl with added KCl (such as 20 mEq/L). Potassium should not be added to IV fluids until renal function has been established and documented.

CORRECTION OF HYPERTONIC DEHYDRATION (FLUID VOLUME DEFICIT WITH HYPERNATREMIA)

Recall that in this type of fluid loss, water loss has exceeded sodium loss. The child will likely have central nervous system involvement, evidenced by irritability, lethargy, nuchal rigidity, and seizures. The principle of therapy is very gradual replacement of water over time so that the brain does not swell. Possible replacement fluids might be 0.45% or 0.3% NaCl. The goal is to lower the serum sodium concentration slowly, such as 0.5 mEq/L/hr; obviously, the serum sodium level must be checked frequently (eg, every 2 hours).[64] Too rapid correction may cause cerebral edema and refractory seizures. (See Chap. 4 for a discussion of safe correction of hypernatremia.)

CORRECTION OF HYPOTONIC DEHYDRATION (FLUID VOLUME DEFICIT WITH HYPONATREMIA)

This condition tends to occur in patients with water and electrolyte loss that is replaced primarily with water; in such instances, the serum sodium level decreases below normal. Management of this condition depends on how low the serum sodium level becomes. If it is extremely low (eg, < 120 mEq/L) and neurological symptoms are present, a 3% solution of NaCl may be needed. It is important that the serum sodium concentration be corrected slowly; too rapid elevation of the sodium concentration can cause central pontine myelinolysis. (See Chap. 4 for a discussion of the treatment of hyponatremia, including principles for administering hypertonic sodium solutions.) The serum sodium level should be monitored very closely during therapy.

THE INTRAOSSEOUS ROUTE FOR PARENTERAL INFUSIONS

The emergency care of infants and children who experience hypovolemic shock or cardiac arrest requires immediate access to the vascular system. In children less than 6 years of age who are critically ill, the intraosseous route is an excellent alternative. The intraosseous route provides an avenue to the rich vascular network within the medullary cavity of the long bones. The intraosseous route is accessed through the anteromedial tibia, 1 to 2 cm below the tibial tuberosity (Fig. 24-2). The technique requires the use of a rigid needle with an inner stylet (14–20 gauge) or a bone marrow needle or one specifically designed for pediatric intraosseous infusions. The insertion site should be cleansed thoroughly, and a local anesthetic agent should be used if the child is responsive to painful stimuli. The needle is inserted at a 90-degree angle through the bone cortex into the medullary space, and placement is confirmed by feeling the "pop" as the needle passes into the marrow and by aspiration of bone marrow. After the needle is flushed with heparinized saline, medicines and volume expanders can be infused. The transfer of medicines and fluids from the medullary cavity to the general circulation is

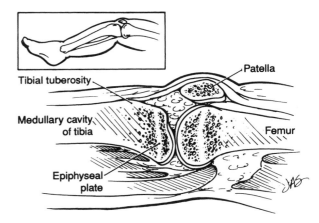

FIGURE 24-2. Structure of the proximal tibia and medullary cavity for intraosseous infusions.

rapid. Dosages of medicines are the same as for IV administration; likewise, the rate of flow for infusing volume expanders is the same.[65]

The infusion site should be observed frequently for signs of infiltration, as with an IV line. Infiltration becomes evident by the swelling of the medial or lateral area of the proximal tibia; it indicates that the needle is not placed properly. Either the needle is too superficial or it has pierced through the bone.

Complications from intraosseous infusion are uncommon. Osteomyelitis is the greatest concern and appears to be related to the length of time that an infusion line is left in place.[66] Once adequate circulation has been restored and an IV line has been established, the intraosseous line should be discontinued.

NURSING CONSIDERATIONS IN INTRAVENOUS FLUID REPLACEMENT

Emotional Preparation

Because children regard IV fluid replacement procedures as intrusive and threatening, they should be given adequate time to develop coping mechanisms. This will be facilitated if the procedure is explained at the child's cognitive level, if the child is given an opportunity to handle the equipment, and if opportunities are provided for play to reduce stress. The IV should be initiated in the treatment room. The child's crib or bed should remain a "safe" place and no intrusive procedures should be done in the child's room. The child should be encouraged to "hold still" during insertion. An adequate number of people (usually two at the most) must be available to help restrain the child if necessary. If at all possible, nurses should avoid using the papoose board to restrain the child. The parents should be offered the opportunity to remain with the child to provide emotional support, if they so choose. Usually parents are most effective if they are near the child's head so the child can see and hear them. Children feel more in control when they can sit up during the insertion procedure. Safety is an important aspect of IV insertions. The nurse needs to be adequately trained to start the IV. In addition to safety, it is important that the person attempting to start the IV knows his or her limitations. Many facilities have an unwritten "three stick" rule. This rule encourages the seeking of a more skilled individual to start the IV to avoid undue pain and injury to the child. If time allows, buffered lidocaine or EMLA® cream (requires 45 minutes to be effective) is sometimes used to anesthetize the insertion site.

The most common sites for infusing fluids are the superficial veins in the arm, wrist, and scalp. The ability to immobilize the area is an important consideration in children. The older child should be allowed site selection, when possible, to promote feelings of control and to lessen interference with activities such as writing or coloring with the preferred hand. For the infant, scalp veins are convenient and accessible (Fig. 24-3). Because there are no valves in these veins, the IV can be infused in either direction. However, the head must be partially shaved for access to the site and the parents must be prepared for this alteration in the infant's appearance. The nurse also should make certain the parents understand that the fluid to be administered will not damage the infant's brain. Some parents might not have any knowledge of the circulatory system in

the region of the scalp. The infant's thumbsucking hand should be avoided if at all possible.

Equipment to Deliver Fluids Safely

Special equipment is used for infusing fluids into children because it is necessary to avoid overloading the smaller system with too large a volume at too rapid a rate. The danger of administering an excessive fluid volume must be a real consideration in all age groups. Infants and small children face special dangers simply because of their size and the fact that fluids tend to be supplied in adult-sized containers. Children are more susceptible to pulmonary edema from excessive fluid overload than are adults because they have greater difficulty excreting excessive fluid volume.

One method to promote safety with gravity flow is to use a microdrip delivery set with a calibrated volume-control chamber (eg, Solu-Set^R or Buretrol^R) that limits the amount of fluid that can be infused. The microdrip delivers a reduced-size drop (60 microdrops/mL) that is one-fourth the size of a macrodrop (usually 15 macrodrops/mL). The calculation for infusion is simplified because the number of prescribed milliliters per hour equals the number of microdrops per minute; for example, 15 mL/hr equals a rate of 15 microdrops/min. In the event of an accident, volume-controlled sets are favored to limit the amount of fluid available for administration. Infusion pumps that can be set at a prescribed rate per hour are an additional safety feature for infants and young children. Overreliance on the accuracy of an infusion pump can cause too little or too much fluid to be infused.[67]

Monitoring Flow Rate and Infusion Site

Although drop-size adapters, small containers, and infusion pumps are used to reduce the possibility of error, the nurse must still keep a close vigil on the flow rate as well as on the child's response to the fluids. The flow rate should be counted at frequent intervals and adjusted as necessary. A pediatric parenteral fluid sheet should be kept at the bedside of infants and small children to record the observed flow rate, the amount of fluid absorbed each hour, the amount of fluid left in the bottle, and the appearance of the infusion site. Such frequent observations and notations greatly reduce the risks of excessive fluid administration and undetected infiltration.[68] Obviously, fluid monitoring is a major aspect of pediatric nursing.

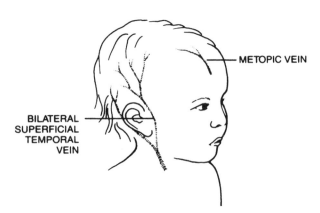

FIGURE 24-3.   Scalp veins in infant.

🔴 APPROACHES FOR ORAL FLUID REPLACEMENT

When infants and children are able to take fluids by mouth and retain them, fluid replacement by the oral route is preferred over the parenteral route. Parenterally administered fluids pass directly into the circulation, whereas fluids taken into the gastrointestinal tract are absorbed slowly. Thus, there is less risk of fluid overload with oral fluid replacement. Also, the child's freedom of movement is not impaired with oral replacement as it is with parenteral replacement.

Oral electrolyte solutions that are available as commercial products are listed in Table 24-1. These solutions are indicated for children who have mild or moderate fluid and electrolyte imbalances and for children who are recovering from acute imbalances that have been treated by parenteral therapy.

Infants and children who are able to take and retain oral fluids may not be willing to do so. Illness often makes them irritable and anorectic, and they cannot understand why they are sick, why their distress cannot be alleviated promptly, and why they need to drink. Children who have gastroenteritis and those who have acute respiratory infections are usually restricted to clear liquids. They may react with frustration when an oral electrolyte solution is offered because they expect and want milk. The phrase "force fluids" is often used in hospital settings, but fluids should never be forced on a child. Attempts to force a child to drink will only increase the child's distress and decrease the likelihood that the child will take and retain the fluid.

Efforts to encourage infants and children to take oral fluids should be gentle and persistent; the process requires patience, perseverance, and creativity. Some recommended approaches for meeting the oral fluid needs of infants and young children are listed below.

- Talk with the child's parents and learn about the child's usual experience in taking fluids at home. What type of fluids does the child usually drink? What amount? What temperature? How often? What method (bottle, cup, or special glass)? What are favorite fluids?
- Plan with the parents to meet the child's fluid needs and involve them in encouraging fluids, measuring amounts, and recording the intake accurately.
- Offer small amounts of fluids in small containers at frequent intervals (at least every hour).

- Use measured containers for precise determination of intake and record the intake accurately.
- Promote the child's comfort before offering fluids. Make certain the child is clean and dry and the upper airway is clear of mucus. (A rubber syringe can be used to remove mucus from the nares.)
- Continue to offer fluids on a regular schedule even though the infant or child may refuse to drink.
- Hold infants before and after offering fluids. Toddlers and preschool children may prefer to sit on the nurse's lap and hold the cup or glass.
- Toddlers may respond positively to a routine, such as offering a drink to a stuffed animal before offering the child a drink. Toddlers might also respond to the opportunity to feed themselves bite-sized pieces of frozen Popsicle or fruit juice.
- Young children like stories and may respond to the power of suggestion in stories about thirsty boys or girls who are looking for a drink.
- Some young children will drink if they have some solid food to hold or mouth, such as a saltine cracker or a vanilla wafer.
- Infants and children who are required to fast before surgery or diagnostic tests should have extra fluids just before the period of fasting to prevent dehydration. A pacifier helps relieve the distress that infants experience while oral feedings are withheld.

Nurses who are patient, perseverent, and creative will be successful in meeting the oral fluid needs of infants and children who are able to take and retain oral fluids.

CASE STUDIES

🔴 **24-1.** Ms. H brought her 10-month-old son to the emergency department of a children's hospital. She stated that she was worried about her baby, Casey, because he looked so sick and had diarrhea that was getting worse. In response to the nurse's questions, Ms. H. explained that Casey had not been "acting right" for nearly a week. He had been cranky and then began vomiting after his feedings. His irritability increased and it was difficult to soothe him. When his diarrhea started 3 days ago, he acted as if he had "stomach cramps." Ms. H stopped giving Casey milk and, for the past 12 hours, had been offering him sugar water in a bottle. His vomiting stopped, but his diarrhea "got worse." In the initial assessment, the nurse noted the following: Casey's color was pale, his anterior fontanelle was slightly sunken, his skin felt very dry and tented when pinched, his mucous membranes were pale and dry, and his extremities felt cool. His apical heart rate was 170 beats/min, his peripheral pulses were weak, and his blood pressure was normal. He became irritable when his blood pressure was measured and made efforts to resist the nurse. Ms. H stated that she thought Casey was urinating normally because his soiled diapers were "so watery." Casey's weight in the emergency department was 9 kg.

COMMENTARY: This baby's deficit is in the high range of moderate dehydration. He requires immediate fluid replacement to prevent the development of shock. This estimate is based on the assessment findings of dry skin and mucous membranes, poor skin turgor, pallor, a sunken fontanelle, tachycardia, and weak peripheral pulses. The assessment findings indicate that Casey has an FVD of at least 8%.

After an IV line was established, Casey received a bolus infusion of 180 mL Ringer's lactate solution. A urine collection bag was placed, and a blood sample was sent to the laboratory for serum electrolytes. A second infusion of 180 mL Ringer's lactate solution was administered over the next 30 minutes. Casey's vital signs, appearance, and behavior were monitored closely. After the second infusion, Casey voided, his heart rate was 160 beats/min, and his peripheral pulses were strong. He became more active and wanted his mother to hold him. He passed a large amount of liquid, watery stool. In addition to fluid replacement requirements in the first 8 hours of treatment, maintenance requirements needed to be met.

After Casey's status improved, an oral electrolyte solution was offered to him in a bottle. The amount that he takes and retains needs to be deducted from the IV fluid maintenance total. Accuracy in calculating, monitoring, and documenting parenteral and oral fluids is a major responsibility in pediatric nursing practice.

Because oral liquids that are high in sugar content and low in sodium exert an osmotic pull in the intestine that increases fluid volume loss through diarrhea, this baby's condition worsened when he was given sugar water. Nurses who care for children have many opportunities to talk with parents about the prevention of diarrhea and the prevention of dehydration when diarrhea does occur. The early administration of an oral electrolyte solution can prevent the potentially devastating consequences of FVD.

● **24-2.** Sheth[69] reported a case in which a 2-week-old infant was brought to an emergency department with a 2-day history of episodes of rapid eye blinking, trembling, and jerking of all four extremities. The episodes occurred several times each day and lasted about 1 minute, followed by a brief period of sleep. No history of trauma, fever, or other illness was present. The infant had not received a formula with high-phosphorus content. No respiratory difficulty was evident. A review of the infant's history revealed that the mother's pregnancy was complicated by gestational diabetes and hypertension and that the father had a family history of seizure disorder. During examination, the infant cried incessantly and had several episodes of seizure activity. Otherwise, the physical examination was normal. Blood work revealed a serum calcium level of 5.2 mg/dL (1.25 mmol/L). (The normal range in most hospital laboratories is 8.5–10.5 mg/dL.) The infant was admitted to the hospital for treatment of hypocalcemia and received oral calcium replacement over the next 3 days. On correction of the low serum calcium level, her symptoms resolved. At the time of discharge from the hospital, she was much less irritable and seizure free and had a serum calcium level of 9.9 mg/dL (2.5 mmol/L). Calcium supplementation was continued for 1 week after discharge and then discontinued. There were no further difficulties.

COMMENTARY: Neonatal seizures are common, with an overall incidence of 1/200 live births.[70] A specific cause can be determined in only about 70% of the cases. One such cause of early onset seizures is hypocalcemia, which is commonly seen in association with infants of diabetic mothers. The seizures are usually brief because the infant's immature neurons are unable to sustain repetitive activity for a prolonged time period. Fortunately, the seizures in this infant did not compromise the airway; also, the cardiovascular status was normal. It was concluded that the infant probably had transient idiopathic hypocalcemia.

● **24-3.** Kaplan et al.[71] reported a case in which an infant was born to a 35-year-old primigravida at term by vaginal delivery. Normal Apgar scores were noted and the baby and mother were discharged 24 hours after delivery. The mother chose to breast-feed the baby exclusively. At 4 days of age, the infant was brought in for an unscheduled visit because the mother was concerned that the baby was not breast-feeding effectively. A greater than 10% weight loss was attributed by the pediatrician to be within acceptable limits for a breast-fed baby. The baby was released to home with advice to supplement breast-feeding as needed. When the infant was 9 days old, the mother returned with the child to the pediatrician's office. At this time, the baby was lethargic, had poor skin turgor, dry mucous membranes, and apparently had not urinated in the past 24 hours. A serum sodium concentration of 191 mmol/L along with a BUN of 177 mg/dL was found, confirming hypernatremic dehydration. The infant developed uncontrollable seizures and subsequently died from a massive intraventricular hemorrhage. (Recall that hypernatremia causes the brain to contract as water is pulled from the cells by the hypertonic ECF; this contraction can produce tearing of cerebral blood vessels.)

COMMENTARY: Maternal breast-feeding failure leading to dehydration of newborn infants has been recognized for many years. A clinical profile identified by some studies includes a well motivated, intelligent primipara of older maternal age who is determined to breast-feed.[72] It is extremely unfortunate that the mother was released from the hospital without the benefit of specific instructions regarding breast-feeding.

● **24-4.** Helikson et al.[73] reported a case in which a 3-year-old girl developed severe hyperphosphatemia and hypocalcemia after the administration of three adult-sized hypertonic phosphate (Fleet) enemas. The child's serum phosphate level rose to 74.7 mg/dL (normal 2.5–4.0 mg/dL) and her ionized calcium level fell to 0.22 mEq/L (normal 1.1–1.6 mEq/L). She also developed metabolic acidosis (pH 7.15). With early intervention and treatment, the child survived without sequelae.

COMMENTARY: The authors pointed out that physicians should be aware of the possible adverse effects that can be caused by hypertonic sodium phosphate enemas; the commonly held notion that these enemas are not absorbed is incorrect. Use of adult-sized sodium phosphate enemas for constipation or bowel cleansing before surgery or diagnostic procedures in children can produce disastrous results. However, not all cases of serious electrolyte disturbances in children after sodium phosphate enemas involve the use of adult-sized enemas. Pediatric-sized sodium phosphate enemas can also cause difficulty.[74] For this reason, the manufacturer of sodium phosphate (Fleet[R]) enemas cautions that adult-sized enemas should not be administered to children under 12 years of age and that the pediatric size should not be administered to children under 2 years of age.[75] They further caution that if after the enema solution is administered there is no return of liquid, the child's physician should be contacted.[76]

REFERENCES

1. Adelman R, Solhaug M. Pathophysiology of body fluids. In: Behrman R, Kliegman R, Arvin A, eds. *Nelson Textbook of Pediatrics*, 15th ed. Philadelphia: WB Saunders; 1996:185.
2. Yared A, Foose J, Ickikawa I. Disorders of osmoregulation. In: Ickikawa I, ed. *Pediatric Textbook of Fluids and Electrolytes*. Baltimore, MD: Williams & Wilkins; 1990:185.
3. Ickikawa I, Narins R, Harris J. Regulation of acid-base homeostasis. In: Ickikawa I, ed. *Pediatric Textbook of Fluids and Electrolytes*. Baltimore, MD: Williams & Wilkins; 1990:84.
4. Lorenz J. Assessing fluid and electrolyte status in the newborn. *Clin Chem* 1997;43:205.
5. Adelman, Solhaug, p 197.
6. Modi N. Hyponatremia in the newborn. *Arch Dis Child Fetal Neonatal Ed* 1998;78:81.
7. Ibid.
8. Kloiber L, Winn N, Shaffer S, Hassanein R. Late hyponatremia in very-low-birth-weight infants: Incidence and associated risk factors. *J Am Diet Assoc* 1996;96:880.
9. Ibid.
10. Ibid.
11. Behrman R, Kliegman R, Arvin A, eds. *Nelson Textbook of Pediatrics*, 15th ed. Philadelphia: WB Saunders; 1996:508.

12. Ibid.

13. Lorenz, p 205.

14. Ibid.

15. Hockenberry-Eaton M. Fluid and electrolytes. In: Wong D, ed. *Whaley & Wong's Nursing Care of Infants and Children*, 6th ed. St. Louis: Mosby–Year Book; 1999:1297.

16. Ibid, p 1299.

17. Adelman, Solhaug, p 207.

18. Merenstein G, Kaplan D, Rosenberg A. *Handbook of Pediatrics*, 18th ed. Stamford, CT: Appleton & Lange; 1997:87.

19. Portal A, Mathias R, Tanney D, Potter D. Kidney and electrolytes. In: Rudolph A, Kamei R, ed. *Rudolph's Fundamentals of Pediatrics*, 2nd ed. Stamford, CT: Appleton-Lange, 1998:551.

20. Gammage D, Yarandi H. The effects of diaper brands, urine volume and time on specific gravity measurements. *J Pediatr Nurs* 1993;9:10.

21. Samson L, Ouzts K. Fluid and electrolyte regulation. In: Curley M et al., eds. *Critical Care Nursing of Infants and Children*. Philadelphia: WB Saunders: 1996:396.

22. Vega R, Avner J. A prospective study of the usefulness of clinical and laboratory parameters for predicting percentage of dehydration in children. *Pediatr Emerg Care* 1997;13:179.

23. Teach S, Yates E, Feld L. Laboratory predictors of fluid deficit in acutely dehydrated children. *Clin Pediatr* 1997;July:395.

24. Lorenz, p. 208.

25. Guy J, Haley R, Zuspan S. Use of intraosseous infusion in the pediatric trauma patient. *J Pediatr Surg* 1993;28:158.

26. Fallon-Smith M. Emergency access in pediatrics. *Journal of Intravenous Nursing* 1998;21:150.

27. Samson, Oustz, p 396.

28. Wyllie R. Pyloric stenosis and other congenital anomalies of the stomach. In: Behrman R, Kliegman R, Arvin A, eds. *Nelson Textbook of Pediatrics*, 15th ed. Philadelphia: WB Saunders; 1996:1060.

29. Ibid.

30. Behrman et al, p 492.

31. Ibid.

32. Ibid, p 493.

33. Jakobowski D, Harmon T, Peck S, Stellar J. Gastrointestinal critical care problems. In: Curley M et al., eds. *Critical Care Nursing of Infants and Children*, Philadelphia: WB Saunders; 1996:738.

34. Merenstein et al, p 552.

35. Samson, Ouzts, p 395.

36. Adelman, Solhaug, p 212.

37. Behrman et al, p 723.

38. Merenstein et al, p 96.

39. Ibid.

40. Ibid.

41. Adelman, Solhaug, p 212.

42. Behrman et al, p 723.

43. Merenstein et al, p 91.

44. Ibid, p 96.

45. Kaplan J, Siegler R, Schmunk G. Fatal hypernatremic dehydration in exclusively breast-fed newborn infants due to maternal lactation failure. *Am J Forensic Med Pathol* 1998;19:19.

46. Behrman et al, p 192.

47. Wong D, ed. *Whaley and Wong's Nursing Care of Infants and Children*, 6th ed. St. Louis: Mosby–Year Book; 1999:1275.

48. Ibid.

49. Keating J, Schears G, Dodge P. Oral water intoxication in infants. *Am J Dis Chid* 1991;145:985.

50. Hockenberry-Eaton, p 1292.

51. Chesney R, Batisky D. Fluid and electrolyte therapy in infants and children. In: Arieff A, DeFronzo R. *Fluid, Electrolyte, and Acid-Base Disorders*, 2nd ed. Mew York: Churchill Livingstone; 1995:Chap 24.

52. Arant B. Fluid and electrolyte abnormalities in children. In: Kokko J, Tannen R, eds. *Fluid and Electrolytes*, 3rd ed. Philadelphia: WB Saunders; 1996:280.

53. Adelman, Solhaug, p 213.

54. Ibid, p 212.

55. Medani C. Seizures and hypothermia due to dietary water intoxication in infants. *South Med J* 1987;80:421.

56. Nichols M, Wason S, Del Rey J, Benfield M. Baking soda, a potentially fatal home remedy. *Pediatr Emerg Care* 1995; 11:109.

57. Ibid.

58. Adelman, Solhaug, p 220.

59. Ibid.

60. Ibid.

61. Merenstein et al, p 86.

62. Feld L, Kaskel F, Schoenman M. The approach to fluid and electrolyte therapy in pediatrics. In: Barness L et al., eds. *Advances in Pediatrics*. Chicago: Year Book Medical Publishers, 1988:508.

63. Merenstein et al, p 88.

64. Ibid, p 91.

65. Fallon-Smith, p 150.

66. Ibid.

67. Ibid.

68. Handler E. Superficial compartment syndrome of the foot after infiltration of intravenous fluid. *Arch Phys Med Rehabil* 1990; 71:58.

69. Sheth D. Hypocalcemic seizures in neonates. *Am J Emerg Med* 1997;15:638.

70. Ibid.

71. Kaplan et al, p 19.

72. Ibid.

73. Helikson M, Parham W, Tobias J. Hypocalcemia and hyperphosphatemia after phosphate enema use in a child. *J Pediatr Surg* 1997;31:1244.

74. Sotos J et al. Hypocalcemic coma following two pediatric phosphate enemas. *Pediatrics* 1977;60:305.

75. *Physician's Desk Reference*, 53rd ed. p 1012. Montvale, NJ:Medical Economics; 1999:1012.

76. Ibid.

CHAPTER 25

Fluid Balance in the Elderly Patient

CHANGES IN WATER AND ELECTROLYTE HOMEOSTASIS ASSOCIATED WITH AGING

Because the percentage of elderly in the population is increasing, nurses in all settings must be aware of the risk of fluid and electrolyte imbalances in the elderly. Fluid balance in the elderly is marginal at best because of physiological changes associated with aging. Under normal conditions, older adults can usually maintain homeostasis; however, they may require more time to return to normal when deficits or excesses are imposed by disease or environmental stress.[1] Older adults do not possess the fluid reserves or ability to adapt readily to rapid changes. Alterations in fluid and electrolyte balance frequently accompany acute illness, particularly in aged persons. Medicare expenditures for hospital treatment of dehydration are substantial, with about 4.6% of those over age 85 admitted with a diagnosis of hypovolemic dehydration.[2,3]

Normal aging changes that affect fluid and electrolyte balance are summarized in Table 25-1. Included also are nursing implications related to these changes.

Renal structural changes associated with aging result in a decreased glomerular filtration rate and a decrease in the older person's ability to concentrate urine when fluid intake is restricted. The nurse must remain alert to this when aged patients are subjected to fluid restriction for any reason. It becomes even more important when older patients are unable to provide for their own fluid needs due to disorientation or functional loss.

Aged kidneys have a slower response to sodium and potassium imbalances. For example, half-time for reduction in urinary sodium after salt restriction is 17 hours in young people but increases to 31 hours in elderly people. Hyponatremia may occur in an older patient who is placed on a strict sodium-restricted diet. Hyperkalemia can develop quickly in the aged when intravenous (IV) potassium is administered.[4]

Cardiovascular and respiratory changes combine to contribute to a slower response to stress in the aged. As a result, the aged person cannot respond as quickly to blood loss, fluid depletion, shock, and acid–base imbalances.

Current research indicates that thirst sensation diminishes with aging.[5,6] In a comparison of 24-hour water deprivation in two age groups, the elderly group reported a lack of thirst sensation after the 24-hour period.[7] Decreased thirst has been demonstrated in elderly subjects with normal mental status, ability to communicate needs, and ability to physically obtain water. Ratings of perceived thirst did not correspond to the rise in serum osmolality after a period of dehydration.[8–10] Rather than being regulated by thirst, fluid intake may be closely associated with food intake. In a study of well elders, living in their own homes, normal amounts of fluid were consumed by drinking fluids with food. Subjects were asked to maintain a diary for 7 consecutive days of everything they ate and drank and their subjective state of thirst. The strongest predictor of the amount of fluid ingested was not thirst but the amount of solids ingested. Thus, a person who is eating poorly is probably drinking poorly as well.[11]

Adding to the problem of decreased thirst is the conscious restriction of fluid by incontinent elderly patients in an effort to limit involuntary urination. Unfortunately, the restriction of fluid only increases the incontinence by concentrating the urine, which irritates the bladder wall. This increases voiding contractions and further increases incontinence.[12]

Elderly patients experience a decreased acuity for the taste of salt; thus, they may salt food heavily in an attempt to satisfy this taste sensation.[13] The caregiver carefully must weigh the issue of limiting salt against the potential medical benefits. The end result of salt restriction may be poor appetite, which may create additional problems.

For all of these reasons, the aged are at risk for dehydration (hypernatremia) and hyperosmolarity. One should be aware that the elderly are often slow in adapting to change and may lack the physiological reserves to respond adequately to stress.

ASSESSMENT OF THE ELDERLY PATIENT

Fluid imbalances, particularly dehydration (hypernatremia), are seen quite frequently in aged patients in all settings. To make accurate nursing diagnoses, a thorough physical and functional assessment must be done.

TABLE 25-1.   Normal Aging Changes Affecting Fluid Balance: Related Nursing Implications

Physiological Component	Normal Aging Changes	Nursing Implications
Total body water	About 6% reduction in total body water Decrease in ratio of intracellular fluid	Increased risk for fluid volume deficit
Renal function	Reduction in renal weight by 50 g between ages 40 and 80 Loss of 30–50% of glomeruli by age 70 Thickening of glomerular and tubular basement membranes 46% decrease in glomerular filtration rate from age 20–90 Decrease in ability to concentrate urine (maximum ability to concentrate urine is 1.022–1.026)	Greater difficulty in eliminating heavy solute loads (drugs, glucose, protein, electrolytes) Slower conservation of fluids in response to fluid restriction
Regulatory functions sium	Decrease in secretion of aldosterone from adrenal cortex Decreased response to zona glomerulosa Decreased response of distal tubule to vasopressin Decreased ability to form and excrete ammonia Decreased glucose tolerance Decreased sensation of thirst	Diminished ability to conserve sodium and excrete potas- Reduced ability to correct an acid–base imbalance Increased risk for hyperglycemia and osmotic diuresis Decreased ability to recognize a fluid deficit
Skin changes	Decreased skin elasticity Atrophy of sweat glands Diminished capillary bed	Skin turgor is a poor indicator of state of hydration Skin is less effective in cooling body temperature
Cardiovascular function	Decreased baroreceptor sensitivity Decreased cardiac output (1%/yr from age 20–80) Decreased stroke volume (0.7%/yr from age 20–80) Decrease in renal plasma flow from 600 mL/min in 2nd decade to 300 mL/min by 8th decade Decreased elasticity of arteries Increased vascular rigidity causing increased peripheral resistance	Diminished ability to manage hypotension associated with shock Increased frequency of peripheral edema Increased risk for orthostatic hypotension, dizziness, falls
Respiratory function	Decreased compliance of chest wall Decreased elasticity of lung tissue Decreased number of alveoli Decreased strength of expiratory muscles Decreased normal partial pressure of oxygen	Increased difficulty in regulation of pH if experiencing major illness, surgery, burns, or trauma
Gastrointestinal function	Decreased volume of saliva Decreased volume of gastric juice Decreased calcium absorption	Mouth may be dryer Increased risk for hyponatremia and hypokalemia during vomiting and gastric suction Increased need for dietary calcium and vitamin D

Adopted from Ebersole P, Hess P. *Toward Healthy Aging.* St. Louis: CV Mosby, 1998:85–95; Kenney R. *Physiology of Aging.* Chicago, Year Book Medical Publishers, 1989:13–21; Garner B. Guide to changing lab values in elders. *Geriatr Nurs* 1989;10:144.

CORRELATION OF PHYSICAL FINDINGS WITH LABORATORY DATA

Only sparse amount of research has tried to correlate laboratory values indicative of dehydration with physical signs. One study correlated laboratory values with tongue dryness, longitudinal tongue furrows, dryness of mucous membranes of the mouth, upper body weakness, confusion, speech difficulty, and sunken eyes.[14] If using these measures, one must be aware of the older adult's usual upper body strength, mental status, and speech patterns and check for any medications that may be contributing to the oral dryness. A study where moisture under the axilla was correlated with blood urea nitrogen (BUN) and serum osmolality revealed that moisture under the axilla was not a reliable sign.[15]

SKIN TURGOR

Usual measures for assessing fluid balance may need to be altered for the elderly; for example, testing skin turgor on the forearm is not a valid measure for the elderly because skin loses elasticity with age. Skin turgor can best be observed in the older patient by tenting the tissue on the forehead or over the sternum because alterations in skin elasticity are less marked in these areas.

RATE OF VEIN FILLING

Rate and degree of filling of small veins in the foot has been used to assess hydration status. A dorsal foot vein can be occluded by finger pressure at a distal point and emptied of its blood by stroking proximally with another finger. In a well hydrated patient, the vein will fill instantly when the pressure is released. In a volume-depleted patient, the vein will fill slowly, over a period longer than 3 seconds. Researchers using this measure found that changes in the rapidity and degree of foot vein filling provided the best means for evaluating changes in hydration of elderly subjects.[16]

INTAKE AND OUTPUT

Although intake and output (I&O) records are often crucial in managing patients with fluid imbalances, research has indicated that frequent inaccuracies make these records less than reliable. According to Pflaum,[17] daily weights may be a more accurate measure of a patient's fluid status. However, one must be aware that inaccuracies also occur in measuring body weights. Therefore, *both* I&O and weight records should be maintained to monitor fluid status. In general, a gain or loss of 1 kg body weight in a short period is equivalent to a gain or loss of 1 liter fluid.

Decline in food intake has been correlated with a decline in fluid intake. Staff documentation of a decreased percent food intake was highly associated with increased BUN/creatinine ratio and serum sodium.[18]

BLOOD PRESSURE

Monitoring for positional changes in blood pressure is another measure that is helpful in assessing hydration. Research has indicated that a drop of at least 15 mm Hg in the systolic pressure and 10 mm Hg in the diastolic pressure occurs when volume-depleted patients are quickly shifted from a lying to a standing position.[19]

BODY TEMPERATURE

In younger individuals, a temperature elevation above normal (37.8°C [98.6°F]) may be an indicator of dehydration (hypernatremia). However, when assessing aged patients, it is important to remember that their normal body temperature is often lower than 37.8°C (98.6°F), possibly closer to 36.1°C (97.8°F). Thus, a temperature of 37.8°C (98.6°F) may represent a significant elevation in an aged patient.

ABILITY TO OBTAIN FLUIDS

Functional assessment of an aged patient's ability to obtain fluids is essential before determining nursing diagnoses and appropriate interventions. For example, problems with vision may make it difficult to locate the glass or pitcher of water. Tremors or stiffness of hands and fingers may impair the older adult's ability to grasp the pitcher or glass. Alterations in mental status may significantly interfere with the patient's ability to participate in the plan of care to meet the intake goals. Additionally, fluid preferences must be determined.[20]

DELIRIUM

Acute confusion is often the first sign of dehydration. Often, dehydration is the primary precipitating factor in the development of acute confusion in frail elders.

Research has focused on identification of risk factors for development of delirium in hospitalized elders.[21] Of 107 elderly medical patients 70 years or older, 27 (25%) developed delirium during their hospital stay. A predictive model was developed and validated. Results identified four independent baseline risk factors for delirium:

1. Vision impairment
2. Severe illness
3. Cognitive impairment
4. Dehydration (BUN/creatinine 18:1)

Signs of delirium include decreased ability to focus, perceptual disturbances, and drowsiness. Delirium can be detected by simple tests that require attention, such as saying the days of the week backward or saying as many examples of fruits, animals, colors, or towns within 1 minute (should be able to say 15).[22]

The physical signs of dehydration are difficult to interpret in the older adult. Because poor fluid intake is associated with poor food intake, reports by staff that dietary intake has declined may offer the first clue that dehydration is developing.

● SPECIAL PROBLEMS IN THE ELDERLY PATIENT

Elderly patients with specific problems can be identified as having a potential for fluid imbalances. The care plans for these patients should include a nursing diagnosis reflecting this potential. Interventions should be used to monitor for these imbalances and prevent them from occurring when possible.

HYPERNATREMIA RELATED TO POOR INTAKE OR INCREASED WATER LOSS

Hypernatremia associated with a decreased extracellular fluid (ECF) volume is a common problem in the elderly. It may be induced by free-water losses from diuresis, diarrhea, vomiting, and hyperglycemia. Usually it will not occur unless oral intake is restricted.[23]

Hypernatremia related to poor intake has been recognized as a major problem within long-term care. According to Campbell,[24] the prevalence of dehydration may be as high as 25% in residents in long-term care facilities. Left untreated, mortality may be as high

as 50%. Consequently, the government regulators of long-term care have mandated completion of an assessment of dehydration as part of the Minimum Data Set that must be completed on all nursing home admissions receiving Medicare reimbursement.[25]

The problem of dehydration in long-term care is complex. Some have referred to dehydration as an indicator of neglect. Residents are often unable to ambulate, pour their own fluids, or express feelings of thirst. A study comparing fluid intake practices of institutionalized and noninstitutionalized elderly found that the average daily intake for institutionalized persons was 1,507 mL, as compared with 2,115 mL for those not confined to institutions.[26] In addition, those not confined to institutions tended to consume water in greater amounts than the institutionalized subjects. Another interesting finding was that subjects outside institutions had greater access to very cold and very hot liquids; the extent to which this influenced fluid intake is not known.

A number of research studies have attempted to identify risk factors for dehydration in elders in long-term care. Results of these studies indicate that those elderly at risk for dehydration are over 80 years old, are women, and suffer from multiple chronic diseases. The role of mental status and functional status as predictors of dehydration in long-term care remains inconclusive.[27-32]

Researchers suggest that the minimal amount of fluid intake for the typical older adult is 1,500 mL. The recommended formula for determining fluid needs is 100 mL fluid/kg for the first 10 kg actual body weight, 50 mL fluid for the next 10 kg, and 15 mL/kg for the remaining.[33] A recent study in which nursing home residents were observed around the clock by investigators revealed that a majority of nursing home residents barely reached an intake of 1,000 mL. This is at least 500 mL below the recommended intake. A significant correlation was found between the number of times a resident received medications and the amount of fluids given. The concern is that if the resident is not receiving medications, additional fluids may not be provided other than at mealtimes. In this study, 79% of fluid intake was consumed during meals.[34]

The role of the caregiver in preventing hypernatremia by early recognition of inadequate fluid intake and provision of needed fluids cannot be overemphasized. Functional elders can be made aware of their fluid needs and can actively participate in attaining those goals. Hoffman[35] suggests that prescriptions be given to these elders to consume a certain number of glasses of fluid. The older adult can keep a record by marking on the picture of the glass, the level of the fluid consumed (Fig. 25-1). Other suggestions include use of attractive colorful pitchers and glasses, frozen liquids such as lemon ice and Popsicles, and blenderized juice combinations such as kiwi and strawberry, ginger ale and cranberry, orange and pineapple, and ginger ale and sorbet.[36]

For residents whose muscle rigidity prevents the normal tilting of the head with drinking, a semicircle can be cut from the rim of a paper cup. This allows space for the nose as the cup is tipped. Offering fluids with a syringe should be considered a last resort. The ability to eat and drink may be the only remaining functional ability. Replacing this with syringe feeding may destroy the last element of dignity. Before being syringe fed, the elder should be exam-

ined by a speech pathologist to determine that there is an intact pharyngeal state. The elder should be seated at a 90-degree position with the chin tipped downward. The caregiver must get the elder's attention, tell what liquid is being offered, and deposit 5 mL fluid on the side of the tongue in the front one-third of the mouth.[37,38]

Older adults suffering from Alzheimer's disease or other forms of dementia present special challenges. These elders may fail to recognize a glass of water and frequently will not remember how to get the glass of water from the table to the mouth. To get the resident to drink, the nurse may have to prompt each step. For example, "Put your hand around this cup. Lift the cup to your mouth. Tip the cup so that you can get a drink." In addition, elders who have Alzheimer's disease frequently wander around the facility much of the day. Nurses must be alert that this older adult is losing

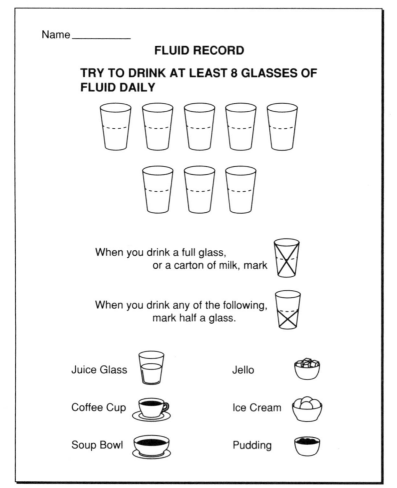

FIGURE 25-1. Fluid record. (Decatur Memorial Hospital Patient Fluid Record. Developed by Sherry Robinson, RNCS, MSN(R), PhD. 1994.)

additional fluids through increased metabolism and insensible loss. Medicine cups and adaptive devices such as spouted cups may be helpful.[39]

Obviously, fluid intake is a special concern in the long-term care setting. Hydration programs using a multidisciplinary approach must be instituted.[40] Nurses should encourage elders to consume a full glass of water with medications. The dietitian should ensure that residents are receiving foods with high fluid content such as fresh oranges. The activity director should incorporate fluids into all recreational and diversional activities. A fluid cart, stocked with a variety of fluids, should make regular and frequent rounds. One facility created a volunteer program where each volunteer was teamed with a resident. The volunteer was taught the specific feeding techniques to maximize intake for that particular resident.[41]

Development of hypernatremia as a result of high-protein (hypertonic) tube feedings is not as common today because of the widespread use of isotonic tube feedings. However, fluid balance of tube-fed aged patients should be closely monitored because extra fluid may be needed even when isotonic feedings are used. Recall that elderly individuals are not as able to concentrate urine as their younger counterparts because of changes in renal structure. (See Chap. 12 for further discussion of this topic.)

Delirium, related to hypernatremia, is a frequent problem in acute care settings as well as in long-term care settings. When an elderly client experiences a change in mental status, the nurse should immediately assess fluid status. When fluid is limited for any reason, there is an increase in serum sodium concentration, and mental functioning can be impaired. Using the case study method, Jana and Jana[42] studied four confused elderly dehydrated (hypernatremic) patients. With restoration of fluid volume, all subjects became oriented and cooperative. Seymour et al.[43] examined 71 patients older than age 70 admitted to a hospital in acute confusional states. Assessment of mental status and fluid status was done on admission and 1 week later after measures to restore hydration. Results indicated a significant relationship between mental scores on admission and degree of dehydration. Because of the large number of subjects, the study provides strong evidence for the relationship between confusion and dehydration (hypernatremia). Another study found a significant change in mental status in elderly patients depleted of fluids in preparation for diagnostic procedures.[44] Clinical Tip: Mini-

Mental State Examination (MMSE) is an example of a mental status questionnaire.

A care plan for an elderly client with a nursing diagnosis of altered mental status related to inadequate fluid intake is shown in Clinical Tip: Nursing Care Plan for an 80-Year-Old Woman With a Nursing Diagnosis of Alteration in Thought Process Related to Inadequate Fluid Intake.

IMBALANCES ASSOCIATED WITH USE OF DIURETICS

Diuretics are the most frequently prescribed drugs for treatment of hypertension and congestive heart failure in the elderly. Both thiazides and furosemide (Lasix) are potassium-losing diuretics, and they have a greater tendency to induce hypokalemia in the aged than in the younger adult. Hypokalemia potentiates the action of digitalis and can precipitate toxic symptoms. Use of a potassium-sparing diuretic, such as spironolactone (Aldactone) or triamterene (Dyrenium), has been shown to produce a higher incidence of hyperkalemia in the aged.[45]

Hyponatremia has also been attributed to thiazide diuretic use. Persons of small body mass, low fluid intake, or excessive intake of low-sodium nutritional supplements are at greater risk for effects of fluid and electrolyte imbalance caused by diuretics.[46]

Because of the orthostatic hypotension associated with diuretic-induced fluid volume deficit (FVD), an older patient may become dizzy on position change and experience a fall. Indeed, use of diuretics has been identified as a characteristic of patients at risk for falls.[47]

Patients on diuretic therapy should be weighed daily. Serum electrolyte levels should be determined at regular intervals. In addition, older patients should be monitored closely for signs of weakness, lethargy, and postural hypotension. One should also monitor for confusion, thirst, and muscle cramps.[48]

IMBALANCES RELATED TO CONSTIPATION, LAXATIVE ABUSE, AND DIARRHEA

Reduced motility of the intestinal tract and a lessened sense of the need to eliminate can lead to chronic constipation with laxative and enema dependency. In addition to decreased gastrointestinal motility with aging, certain drugs, such as anticholinergics and antacids containing calcium carbonate or aluminum hydroxide,

---

CLINICAL TIP

Mini-Mental State Examination (MMSE)

QUESTIONS	POINTS
1. What is the Year? Season? Date? Day? Month?	5
2. Where are we? State? County? Town or City? Hospital? Floor?	5
3. Name three objects (Apple, Penny, Table), taking 1 second to say each. Then, ask the patient to tell you the three objects. Repeat the answers until the patient learns all three.	3
4. Serial 7s. Subtract 7 from 100. Then, subtract 7 from that number, etc. Stop after five answers.	5
5. Ask for the names of the three objects learned in #3.	3
6. Point to a pencil and a watch. Have the patient name them as you point.	2
7. Have the patient repeat "No ifs, ands, or buts."	1
8. Have the patient follow a three-stage command: "Take the paper in your right hand. Fold the paper in half. Put the paper on the floor."	3
9. Have the patient read and obey the following: "CLOSE YOUR EYES." (Write in large letters.)	1
10. Have the patient write a sentence of his or her own choice.	1
11. Have the patient copy the following design (overlapping pentagons).	1

Total points = 30

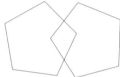

Scoring

24–30 = No cognitive impairment
18–23 = Mild cognitive impairment
0–17 = Severe cognitive impairment

Folstein M, Folstein S, McHugh P. Mini-Mental Mental State. A practical method for grading the cognitive state of patients for the clinician. Psychiatry 1975;12:189–198. With permission.

---

predispose to constipation. It has been reported that persons over age 70 take laxatives twice as often as those in the 40- to 50-year-old age group. Prolonged use of strong laxatives predisposes to hypokalemia and FVD. Metabolism of drugs by the aged person is generally slower than in a younger person. Abnormal prolongation of the effect of some over-the-counter laxatives containing phenolphthalein has been seen. There is an increase in the half-life of the drug and, therefore, diarrhea may result as the drug's action continues.

Unfortunately, use of laxatives in the aged often becomes a habit, requiring larger and more frequent doses to achieve results.[49]

Increased fluid and bulk intake, in addition to regular exercise, should be encouraged to correct constipation. Stool softeners are useful physiological tools, and a glass of warm water or hot coffee first thing in the morning can stimulate the evacuation reflex. Natural laxative mixtures composed of raisins, currants, prunes, figs, and dates have also been found to be useful.[50]

CLINICAL TIP

Nursing Care Plan for an 80-Year-Old Woman With a Nursing Diagnosis of Alteration in Thought Process Related to Inadequate Fluid Intake

ASSESSMENT	GOAL	INTERVENTIONS	EVALUATION CRITERIA
Disoriented	Restore normal mental status	Increase oral intake to 2,000 mL/day	Score on Mental Status Questionnaire will improve.
Score on MMSE is 18 (normal is 24)		**Follow this schedule:**	
Behavior changes		8:00 breakfast 300 mL	Behavior will improve.
Skin turgor poor on forehead		9:00 water 120 mL 10:00 lemonade 120 mL 11:00 water 120 mL	Oral intake will reach 2,000 mL in 24 hours.
Tongue dry and furry		12:00 lunch 300 mL 1:00 water 120 mL	Physical assessment will reveal improved
No pool of saliva under tongue		2:00 water 120 mL 3:00 orange juice 120 mL	skin turgor, pool of saliva under tongue,
BP 160/80 (supine), 128/62 (standing)		4:00 water 120 mL 5:00 water 120 mL	normal vein filling, and absence of marked
Foot vein fills in 6 seconds		6:00 supper 300 mL 7:00 water 120 mL	postural hypotension on position change.
Oral intake 900 mL/day		8:00 water 120 mL	
Able to swallow		Continue assessment of fluid and mental status every shift	
Unable to pour fluids due to arthritis in hands			
Favorite fluids • Water • Lemonade • Orange juice			
MMSE, Mini-Mental State Examination			

These nursing interventions are preferable to drugs in reducing the problem of constipation and thereby preventing fluid and electrolyte problems associated with laxatives and enemas.

Aging changes can also predispose the older adult to development of diarrhea from infectious agents. With aging, there is a decreased immune response. Constipation can predispose the older adult to colonization by enteropathogens. In addition, the decrease in gastric acid from atrophy of the gastric mucosa or secondary to histamine antagonists results in a reduced barrier to infection. If stressed by an infectious agent, diarrhea and resulting fluid imbalances may occur quickly.[51]

IMBALANCES ASSOCIATED WITH PREPARATION FOR DIAGNOSTIC TESTS

Standard colon-cleansing techniques for diagnostic studies usually include dietary restrictions (liquid diet the day before, NPO after midnight the day before the test), purgatives (such as magnesium citrate, Dulcolax), and numerous cleansing enemas. These techniques constitute a threat to elderly persons who are only marginally hydrated. Studies have indicated that the rigorous catharsis associated with this kind of preparation leads to significant shifts of fluid among body compartments. If the shifts occur rapidly in an elderly person with cardiovascular disease, the results can be dangerous. Computed tomography has been recommended rather than a barium enema for the initial investigation of the large bowel in frail elderly.[52]

In a study of elderly persons undergoing preparation for a barium enema, a significant number of indicators of FVD was detected on nursing assessment. In addition, there was a slow response to restore fluid balance to baseline, indicating the need to encourage fluid intake after the test.[53]

Much of the gastrointestinal testing is now done as an outpatient service. It is often impossible to observe the elderly person undergoing rigorous bowel preparation for adverse reactions. Consequently, it is critical for the person who provides the patient teaching before the testing to stress the importance of increasing fluid intake before and after the test. It is most appropriate to include a nursing diagnosis in the care plan that reflects the potential for FVD related to bowel preparation. The need for close observation is reflected in the care plan in Clinical Tip: Nursing Care Plan for an 84-Year-Old Man With a Nursing Diagnosis of at Risk for Hypernatremia With Fluid Volume Depletion Related to X-Ray Preparation. Care should be taken to perform the procedure correctly the first time to avoid the need for repeated radiographs, requiring more

cathartics, more enemas, and more fluid restrictions. The elderly can ill afford to undergo one test after another without a rest period; it is frequently up to the nurse to intervene in this area on the patient's behalf.

OSTEOPOROSIS

Calcium deficiency has been associated with osteoporosis development in the elderly. Annually, 1.5 million fractures (mainly of the spine, wrist, and hip) are attributed to osteoporosis. In 1995, functional loss associated with osteoporosis resulted in 180,000 admissions to nursing homes. About 14% of patients who suffer hip fractures must be cared for in nursing homes. Risk factors for fracture include low bone mineral density; history of a fracture of the hip, wrist, or vertebrae in a first-degree relative; lowest quartile in weight, and current cigarette smoking. Obesity appears to offer some protection against osteoporosis because the added weight increases skeletal mass by creating stress on the skeleton.[54]

Back pain is the most frequent symptom of osteoporosis, and spinal deformity is the most common sign. "Dowager's hump" (a hunchback posture due to severe loss of anterior vertebral height) is a frequent finding.

CLINICAL TIP

Nursing Care Plan for an 84-Year-Old Man With a Nursing Diagnosis of at Risk for Hypernatremia With Fluid Volume Depletion Related to X-Ray Preparation

ASSESSMENT	GOAL	INTERVENTIONS	EVALUATION CRITERIA
To receive rigorous colon preparation on Tuesday	To prevent hypernatremia with fluid volume depletion	Physical assessment of fluid balance every shift	Intake exceeds 2,000 mL/day on day before x-ray
Fluid restriction (NPO) after midnight Tuesday		2,000–3,000 mL fluid orally the day before x-ray; give 150 mL/hr from 8:00 AM to 10:00 PM	Intake exceeds 2,000 mL/day after x-ray
Decreased renal function, related to advanced age		Obtain order for IV fluids if unable to drink above amount	No change in baseline physical assessment parameters
Alert and functionally able to obtain own fluids		Force fluids (150 mL/hr) after x-ray until HS	
Baseline physical assessment of fluid balance within normal limits		Explain need for fluids to patient; give schedule to him; assist as needed	

HS, hour of sleep (bedtime)

The patient's height may be 1 to 6 inches shorter than the arm span if multiple wedge-compression fractures have occurred. Loss of 2 inches in height has been found to be an accurate screening mechanism to detect osteoporosis. Early detection of osteoporosis, before the development of symptoms, is best accomplished through bone mineral density studies, which are recommended for women with risk factors. Laboratory blood tests provide little information because serum concentrations of calcium, phosphate, and alkaline phosphatase are normal, although deficits of total body calcium, phosphate, and nitrogen exist. Currently, there is promising research identifying biochemical markers that measure bone turnover.

Current public health recommendations for the prevention of osteoporosis based on research emphasize that no single treatment can protect people forever from suffering osteoporotic fractures. Daily intake of calcium should be between 1,000 and 1,500 mg along with a daily intake of 400 IU to 800 IU of vitamin D. Walking is the most beneficial exercise, and smoking should be discouraged.[55]

Numerous studies have drawn similar conclusions: estrogen intervention reduces the rate of loss of skeletal tissue by reducing bone remodeling. All routes of administration (oral, transdermal, or subcutaneous) are equally effective. To protect the endometrium, women who have not had a hysterectomy may be given progestin. It should be remembered, however, that large daily doses of estrogen have been associated with sodium retention, hypertension, myocardial infarction, and increased risk of endometrial carcinoma. Many physicians believe that the anticatabolic effect of estrogen, which reduces bone resorption, outweighs the risk of these untoward effects.[56]

Other treatment options are now available for women who choose not to take estrogen. Alendronate has been shown to be effective in reducing spine, hip, and wrist fractures. Calcitonin has been useful in the treatment of vertebral fractures by rebuilding vertebral bone, thus reducing back pain.[57]

Because of the lack of longitudinal studies, the exact relationship of exercise and the skeleton remains incompletely defined. The particular type of exercise that has the greatest impact on skeletal mass has not been determined. One hour of walking three or four times per week is the current recommendation to satisfy weight-bearing requirements. There are numerous benefits to any kind of exercise, including increased strength, coordination, and flexibility that may in themselves prevent falls and the resultant fractures.[58,59]

Education in the areas of nutrition, proper exercise, and safety must be included in the care plans of patients with osteoporosis.

Nutrition

1. Encourage the intake of adequate calcium in the diet. At least 1 quart of skim milk daily is recommended; whole milk or cheese products may be used if the patient's physical condition allows. Most women will require calcium and vitamin D supplements.
2. Encourage adequate protein intake.
3. Encourage intake of sufficient calories to maintain normal body weight.

Exercise

After assessing for abilities and disabilities, consider the following interventions:

1. Encourage patients who swim, golf, or bicycle to continue to do so. Jogging should be avoided because of the possibility of joint damage. Some form of weight-bearing exercise should be included in the exercise program.
2. For sedentary individuals who cannot perform weight-bearing exercise, encourage any exercise that affects strength, balance, and range of motion. These will indirectly prevent fractures through the reduction of falls.
3. Suggest the following exercises for sedentary individuals:
   A. Arm circles
      i. Sit erect, arms extended.
      ii. Form circles by moving arms backward and then forward.
   B. Angle stretch
      i. Lie on bed (not floor), legs straight, feet together, and arms at side.
      ii. Slide arms and legs to a spread-eagle position and return.
   C. Stationary rocking
      i. Sit erect on chair, feet flat on floor, arms at side.
      ii. Lean forward and press floor with toes.
      iii. Lean back to upright position and press floor with heels.

Recommend extension and isometric abdominal exercises for those diagnosed with spinal osteoporosis. Teach them to avoid any flexion exercises of the spine because this action may cause compression or frac-tures.[60]

Safety

1. Teach the patient to avoid sudden bending, twist-ing, lifting, or carrying of heavy objects.
2. Teach the patient to use assistive devices, such as canes or walkers, if needed, to prevent falls.
3. Teach the patient to wear properly fitted, low-heeled shoes (athletic shoes should be suggested).
4. Teach the patient to use long-handled utensils and cleaning tools if needed.
5. Assess the patient's environment. Make sure the home is well lighted and has nonskid rugs. Look for objects that might cause falls.

HYPERTHERMIA

The greatest number of cases of heatstroke occurs in the elderly. Sweating, the major mechanism for heat dissipation, is altered in the aged. Not only is the num-ber of operative sweat glands decreased in aged per-sons, it takes longer for them to begin sweating, and they produce less sweat than in their younger years. Loss of subcutaneous adipose tissue reduces the effec-tiveness of the skin as an insulator and enhances water loss from the deeper tissues.

Elderly persons seem to have an impaired sense of warmth perception. Also, the elderly exhibit little change in cardiac output in response to heat stress. The circulatory system cannot dissipate efficiently the heat through peripheral vasodilation and evaporation of perspiration.[61] In addition, a number of medications frequently prescribed for aged patients can interfere in some way with thermoregulation (eg, diuretics, antiparkinsonian drugs, propranolol, antihistamines, phenothiazines, tricyclic antidepressants). Other risk factors for hyperthermia in the elderly include recent diarrhea or febrile illness, obesity, sleep deprivation, and dehydration.[62]

Mortality related to heat stress increases progres-sively in those older than 70 years. Because of their greater susceptibility to heat stress, it is important to teach these individuals to take the following precau-tions during a heat wave:

- Avoid excessive physical activity.
- Wear light-colored cotton fabrics to facilitate sweat-ing.
- Increase dietary consumption of carbohydrates and fluids.
- Use air conditioners or fans when available.
- Contact health provider if cessation of sweating occurs.[63]

The nurse must be cautious when assessing the older person for heat stress. Normal body temperature decreases with age; as such, the older adult may be experiencing heat stress with a temperature of 37.2°C (99.8°F).

⬤ SPECIAL CONSIDERATIONS RELATED TO THE PERIOPERATIVE PERIOD

Elderly persons tolerate major surgery and its compli-cations less well than younger adults; therefore, preop-eratively, every effort should be made to treat condi-tions likely to cause postoperative problems. Cardiac complications are a common cause of postoperative mortality; pneumonia and atelectasis also occur fre-quently.[64] Conscientious preoperative preparation often means the difference between success or failure of surgery in the aged because the decreased body homeostatic adaptability of these patients predisposes to difficulty when they are exposed to stress.

The following facts apply to the aged surgical patient:

- Moderate FVD and decreased circulating blood vol-ume are not uncommon in the elderly *before* surgery. Because many patients are admitted the day of surgery, the nurse who provides preoperative instruc-tion must be alert to assess for existing problems. The patient may be on diuretic therapy or may have had a problem with nausea and vomiting. FVD pre-disposes to renal insufficiency, particularly in elderly individuals. Administration of oral fluid replacement must be encouraged before the NPO period. Ade-quate IV fluids before surgery will improve renal blood flow and renal function; in contrast, adminis-tration of the same fluids after induction of anesthe-sia will have only minimal effect in increasing renal blood flow. It is important that parenteral fluids be started before surgery and an adequate urine volume established before induction of anesthesia. Urine flow should be at least 50 mL/hr (preferably 75–100 mL/hr).[65,66]

- In the operating room, the older patient is at risk for hypothermia. In addition to the cool environment, the patient is rapidly infused with cool IV fluids and possibly blood. Rinsing the skin with cool solutions also increases the risk of hypothermia. Use of a cap, warm gown, stockinette on unaffected limbs, and warmed flannelette blankets is recommended.[67,68]

- Because diminished respiratory function interferes with carbon dioxide elimination, many aged patients are in a state of impending respiratory acidosis. Because of this decline in pulmonary function, the nurse must help the aged patient achieve maximal ventilation. This can be accomplished by keeping the respiratory tract free of excessive secretions, providing maximal allowed activity, turning the bed-fast patient from side to side at regular intervals, and avoiding restrictive clothing and chest restraints.

- Because renal response to pH disturbances is not as efficient in the aged, imbalances occur more quickly. There is a tendency toward metabolic acidosis as a result of decreased renal function. It behooves the health care team to detect imbalances early and to intervene early.

- Changes in pH are less well tolerated in the aged. In addition to decreased renal and pulmonary reserves, presence of anemia, with its decreased hemoglobin, depletes one of the major buffer systems. Blood should be administered as needed to correct anemia, preferably several days before the operation. Emphysema is not uncommon in the aged and also disrupts pH control. Measures to improve pulmonary function should also be used preoperatively.

- Hypotension is poorly tolerated by the aged and, unless corrected quickly, is frequently complicated by renal damage, stroke, or myocardial infarction. Shock becomes irreversible earlier than in young patients.

- The aged patient will develop sodium deficit faster than younger adults; thus, the nurse should be particularly alert for this imbalance when the patient is losing body fluids containing sodium. Hyponatremia is particularly apt to occur when there is a free intake of water orally or when excessive volumes of 5% dextrose in water are administered IV.

- Hyponatremia may also result from excessive water retention associated with the stress of hospitalization and anticipation of surgery. Stress mediates the release of antidiuretic hormone (ADH). Research has shown that relocation and separation from loved ones, as occur with hospitalization, cause greater stress in the aged. This stress has been shown to contribute to the development of water intoxication (dilutional hyponatremia).[69]

- Malnutrition is more common in aged than in younger adults and contributes to the increased incidence of postoperative complications. Preoperative dietary management is particularly important. Optimal nutrition helps the aged patient withstand the electrolyte deficits and pH changes occurring with surgery. If the patient is unable to eat, tube feedings or parenteral nutrients are indicated to meet nutritional needs and build up operative reserves. (Tube feedings are discussed in Chap. 12 and parenteral nutrition is discussed in Chap. 11.)

- Ambulation and activity improve appetite and sleep and prevent the complications of bedrest. Bedrest in the preoperative period can be damaging to the aged patient because it predisposes to negative nitrogen balance, osteoporosis, muscle weakness, pneumonia, phlebitis, pressure ulcers, bladder and bowel dysfunction, decrease in myocardial reserve, and diminished pulmonary ventilation and tidal volume.

Intravenous therapy for treatment of fluid imbalances is common in long-term care, community, and clinic settings.[70] Coulter[71] recommends the use of a small 22- to 24-gauge catheter and a rehydration rate of 80 to 100 mL/hr. In maintaining patency of the IV site in a restless elderly person, restraints should be avoided. Use of restraints creates anxiety and agitation, as well as respiratory and cardiovascular problems. IV tubing can be hidden under long-sleeved shirts or covered with flexible elastic netting. Turtleneck shirts can be used to protect central lines from manipulation by confused elders. Because of the older person's increased skin fragility, a skin protectant should be applied before tape is applied; excessive tape should be avoided in securing the IV site, and extreme care should be taken when removing the tape to prevent skin tears.

Treatment of dehydration by hypodermoclysis is on the rise in long-term care settings in Canada and Europe. Hypodermoclysis is the use of subcutaneous fluid as a method of rehydration. Recent research comparing this method with IV infusions has found both to be comparable in restoration of hydration. Hypodermoclysis is advantageous because many elderly have difficult veins to cannulate and because functional status is not limited by immobilizing limbs.[72–74] A concentration of kCl greater than 10 mEq/L should not be infused subcutaneously, to avoid tissue trauma.

HYPEROSMOLAR HYPERGLYCEMIC NONKETOTIC SYNDROME

Most patients who develop hyperosmolar hyperglycemic nonketotic syndrome (HHNS) are elderly with relatively mild (perhaps undetected) diabetes mellitus. Unconscious patients may present in the emergency room with a history of 3 to 7 days of decreased fluid intake. Precipitating factors in the diabetic elderly may include medications such as osmotic diuretics, phenytoin sodium (Dilantin), steroids, and immunosuppressive agents, infections such as pneumonia, hyperosmolar tube feedings, and high-carbohydrate infusion loads (as in total parenteral nutrition).[75] Normal aging changes affecting kidney function create a greater potential for fluid imbalance in the older diabetic patient. Monitoring fluid intake adequacy in the elderly diabetic patient is an important nursing assessment that can lead to earlier detection of HHNS. A thorough discussion of HHNS is presented in Chapter 18.

CASE STUDY

● **25-1.** Mr. D is an 89-year-old gentleman who has been admitted to the hospital with a diagnosis of hypernatremic dehydration (sodium, 150 mEq/L; BUN, 54 mg/dL; creatinine, 1.5 mg/dL; BUN/creatinine ratio, 36:1). Mr. D also has Alzheimer's disease and has been residing in a long-term care facility for about 1 year. He is disoriented and does not recognize his wife who accompanies him to your unit. He is restless, combative, and very anxious. The emergency room personnel inserted an IV into his right arm and secured his hands with wrist restraints.
COMMENTARY: There are several alternatives to wrist restraints that could be used to maintain IV fluids. Due to Mr. D's usual state of dementia, the restraints will only make nursing management more difficult. Ask his wife to stay with him if possible. Ask her to hold his left hand, gently stroke his arm, and reminisce with him about their earlier life together (he may have retained some long-term memory and thinking about something familiar is usually comforting and quieting). If she cannot stay, there still are some other alternatives. Disguise the IV by running the IV tubing along his arm and by placing a long-sleeved shirt on him. If this option is not effective, Posey mitts or Nerf balls placed in each hand and secured with burn net may be beneficial. By using these options, his arms can remain free and he will probably be less restless.

The patient's mental status should improve, although he will always have some cognitive deficits. In this situation, dementia (a chronic confusional state) is compounded by delirium (acute confusional state). The dehydration, the elevated sodium, the elevated BUN, the restraints, and relocation to a strange environment are all contributing to the acute confusional state aggravating the chronic confusional state.

Because of his age, the IV fluids should not be infused too rapidly (no more than 120 mL/hr). During any calm periods, approach Mr. D. Gently, place a glass of water in his hand and gently help him to raise it to his lips. Remember that a person with Alzheimer's disease may no longer be able to recognize a glass of water and may have forgotten how to bring the glass to his lips and drink it. Also, provide him with fresh fruit slices like oranges to improve hydration. When Mr. D is rehydrated, approach the doctor about discontinuing the IV fluids and returning him to long-term care. It is important to return the patient with Alzheimer's disease to his normal routine and environment as soon as possible. The staff in the long-term care facility must be extremely attentive to his fluid needs. Because most people with Alzheimer's will wander within the facility, the long-term care nurse must recognize the increased fluid needs required by the increased metabolism and constant movement of the wanderer. Every staff member should be alerted to offer him frequent drinks and finger foods high in fluids.

REFERENCES

1. Hoffman A. Dehydration in the elderly: Insidious and manageable. *Geriatrics* 1991;46:35.
2. Weinberg A, Minaker K. Dehydration: Evaluation and management in older adults. *JAMA* 1995;279:1552.
3. Ciccone A, Allegra J, Cochrane D, Cody R, Roche L. Age-related differences in diagnoses within the elderly population. *Am J Emerg Med* 1998;16:43.
4. Cape R, Coe R, Rossman I. *Fundaments of Geriatric Medicine.* New York: Raven; 1983:71B74.
5. Porth C, Erickson M. Physiology of thirst and drinking: Implications for nursing practice. *Heart Lung* 1992;21:273.
6. Rolls B, Phillip P. Aging and disturbances in thirst and fluid balance. *Nutr Rev* 1990;48:137.
7. Phillips P et al. Reduced thirst after water deprivation in elderly healthy men. *N Engl J Med* 1984;311:753.
8. Menully G. Thirst threshold changes pose dehydration risk. *Geriatrics* 1985;40:91.
9. Mack G, Weseman C, Langhans G. Body fluid balance in dehydrated healthy older men: thirst and renal osmoregulation. *J Appl Physiol* 1994;76:1615.
10. Forsling M, Rolls B, Phillips P, Ledingham J, Smith R. Altered water excretion in healthy elderly. *Age Aging* 1987;16:285.
11. Decastro J. Age-related changes in natural spontaneous fluid ingestion and thirst in humans. *J Gerontol* 1992;47:321.
12. Stone J, Syman J, Salisbury S. *Clinical Gerontological Nursing: A Guide to Advanced Practice.* Philadelphia: WB Saunders; 1999:203.
13. Ebersole P, Hess P. *Toward Healthy Aging.* St. Louis: CV Mosby; 1998:443.
14. Gross C, Lindquist R, Wooley A et al. Clinical indicators of dehydration severity in elderly patients. *J Emerg Med* 1992;10:267.
15. Eaton D, Bannister P, Mulley G, Connolly M. Axillary sweating in clinical assessment of dehydration in ill elderly patients. *BJM* 1994;308:1271.
16. Robinson S, Demuth P. Diagnostic studies for the aged: What are the dangers? *J Gerontol Nurs* 1985;11:6.
17. Pflaum S. Investigation of intake-output as a means of assessing body fluid balance. *Heart Lung* 1979;8:495.
18. Pals J, Weinberg A, Beal L, et al. Clinical triggers for detection of fever and dehydration: Implications for long-term care nursing. *J Gerontol Nurs* 1995;21:13.
19. Robinson, Demuth, p 6.
20. Sansevero A. Dehydration in the elderly: Strategies for prevention and management. *Nurse Pract* 1997;22:41.
21. Inouye S, Viscoli C, Horwitz R, Hurst L, Tinetti M. A predictive model for delirium in hospitalized elderly medical patients based on admission characteristics. *Ann Intern Med* 1993;119:474.
22. Mentes J, Buckwalter K. Getting back to basics: Maintaining hydration to prevent acute confusion in frail elderly. *J Gerontol Nurs* 1997;2348.
23. Sadat A, Paulman P, Mathews M. Hypernatremia in the elderly. *Fam Pract* 1989;40:125.
24. Campbell S. Maintaining hydration status in elderly persons: Problems and solutions. *Support Line* 1992;247.
25. Weinberg, Minaker, p 1552.
26. Adams F. How much do elders drink? *Geriatr Nurs* 1988;9:218.
27. Himmelstein D, Jones A, Wollhander S. Hypernatremic dehydration in nursing home patients: An indicator of neglect. *J Am Geriatr Soc* 1983;31:466.
28. Gaspar P. What determines how much patients drink? *Geriatr Nurs* 1988;9:221.
29. Lavizzo-Maurey R, Johnson J, Stotley P. Risk factors for dehydration among elderly nursing home residents. *J Am Geriatr Soc* 1988;36:213.
30. Snyder N, Feigal D, Arieff A. Hypernatremia in elderly patients: A heterogenous, morbid, and iatrogenic entity. *Ann Intern Med* 1987;107:309.
31. Aaronson L, Seaman L. Managing hypernatremia in fluid deficient elderly. *J Gerontol Nurs* 1989;15:29.
32. Foreman M. Confusion in the hospitalized elderly: Incidence, onset, and associated factors. *Res Nurs Health* 1989;12:21.
33. Chidester J, Spangler A. Fluid intake in the institutionalized elderly. *J Am Diet Assoc* 1997;97:23.
34. Armstrong-Brown K, Armstrong-Esther D, Sander L. The institutionalized elderly: Dry to the bone! *Int J Nurs Stud* 1996;33:619.
35. Hoffman, p 35.
36. Zembrzuski C. A three-dimensional approach to hydration of elders: administration, clinical staff, and in-service education. *Geriatr Nurs* 1997;18:20.
37. Soriano R. Syringe feeding: Current clinical practice and recommendations. *Geriatr Nurs* 1994;15:85.
38. Yen P. When swallowing is a problem. *Geriatr Nurs* 1991;12:313.
39. Alford D. Tips on promoting food and fluid intake in the elderly. *J Gerontol Nurs* 1991;17:44.
40. Zembrzuski, p 20.
41. Musson D, Frye G, Nash M. Silver spoons: Supervised volunteers provide feeding of patients. *Geriatr Nurs* 1997;18:18.
42. Jana D, Jana L. Hypernatremic psychoses in the elderly: Case reports. *J Am Geriatr Soc* 1983;31:473.
43. Seymour D et al. Acute confusional states and dementia in the elderly: The role of dehydration/volume depletion, physical illness, and age. *Age Ageing* 1980;9:137.
44. Robinson, Demuth, p 6.
45. Todd B. Diuretics' danger. *Geriatr Nurs* 1989;10:212.
46. Sonnenblick J, Friedlander Y, Rosin A. Diuretic-induced severe hyponatremia. *Chest* 1993;103:601.
47. Watson M, Mayhew P. Identifying fall risk factors in preparation for reducing the use of restraints. *Medsurg Nurs* 1994;3:25.
48. Todd, p 212.
49. Yakaborwich M. Prescribe with care: The role of laxatives in the treatment of constipation. *J Gerontol Nurs* 1990;16:7.
50. Beverly L, Travis I. Constipation: Proposed natural laxative mixtures. *J Gerontol Nurs* 1992;18:5.
51. Bennett R, Greenough W. Approach to acute diarrhea in the elderly. *Gastroenterol Clin North Am* 1993;22:517.
52. Day J, Freeman A, Coni N, Dixon A. Barium enema or computed tomography for the frail elderly patient? *Clin Radiol* 1993;48:48.
53. Robinson, Demuth, p 8.
54. National Osteoporosis Foundation. *Osteoporosis: Review of the Evidence for Prevention, Diagnosis, and Treatment and Cost-Effectiveness Analysis.* Springer: National Osteoporosis Foundation; 1998:2.
55. National Osteoporosis Foundation, p 5.
56. Heaney R. Bone mass, nutrition, and other lifestyle factors. *Am J Med* 1993;95(suppl 5a):29s.
57. National Osteoporosis Foundation, p 5.
58. Chesnut C. Bone mass and exercise. *Am J Med* 1993;95(suppl 5a):34s.
59. National Osteoporosis Foundation. p 47.
60. Aisenbrey J. Exercise in the prevention and management of osteoporosis. *Phys Ther* 1987;67:1100.

61. Vassallo M, Gera K, Allen S. Factors associated with high risk of marginal hyperthermia in elderly patients living in an institution. *Postgrad Med J* 1995;71:313.

62. Dematte J, O'Mara K, Buescher J et al. Near-fatal heat stroke during the 1995 heat wave in Chicago. *Ann Intern Med* 1998;129:173.

63. Delaney K. Heatstroke: Underlying processes and lifesaving management. *Postgrad Med* 1992;91:379.

64. Latz P, Wyble R. Elderly patients perioperative nursing implications. *AORN J* 1987;46:238.

65. Saleh K. The elderly patient in the post-anesthesia care unit. *Nurs Clin North Am* 1993;28:507.

66. Martin J, Larsen P. Dehydration in the elderly surgical patient. *AORN J* 1994;60:666.

67. White H, Thurston N, Blackmore K, Green S, Hannah K. Body temperature in elderly surgical patient. *Res Nurs Health* 1987;10:317.

68. Moddeman G. The elderly surgical patient—a high risk for hypothermia. *AORN J* 1991;53:1270.

69. Booker J. Severe symptomatic hyponatremia in elderly outpatients. *J Am Geriatr Soc* 1985;33:108.

70. Baldwin D. Provision of intravenous therapy in a skilled nursing facility. *Journal of Intravenous Nursing* 1991;14:366.

71. Coulter K. Intravenous therapy for the elder patient: Implications for the intravenous nurse. *Journal of Intravenous Nursing* 1992;15(suppl 2):s18.

72. Challiner Y, Jarrett D, Hayward M, Al-Jubouri M, Julious S. A comparison of IV and Subq hydration in elderly acute stroke patients. *Postgrad Med J* 1994;70:195.

73. Rochon P, Gill S, Litner J et al. A systematic review of the evidence for hypodermoclysis to treat dehydration in older people. *J Gerontol A Biol Sci Med Sci* 1997;52:M169.

74. Worobec G, Brown M. Hypodermoclysis therapy in a chronic care hospital setting. *J Gerontol Nurs* 1997;23:23.

75. Lorber D. Nonketotic hypertonicity in diabetes mellitus. *Med Clin North Am* 1995;79:39.

INDEX

Page numbers followed by *f* refer to figures; page numbers followed by *t* refer to tables; page numbers followed by *b* refer to text in shaded boxes.